Developmental Dyslexia across Languages and Writing Systems

This volume presents the first truly systematic, multidisciplinary, and cross-linguistic study of the language and writing system factors affecting the emergence of dyslexia. Bringing together a team of scholars from a wide variety of disciplines, it places a dual focus on the language-specific properties of dyslexia and on its core components across languages and orthographies, in order to challenge theories on the nature, identification, and prevalence of dyslexia, and to reveal new insights. Part I highlights the nature, identification, and prevalence of dyslexia across multiple languages including English, French, Dutch, Czech and Slovakian, Finnish, Arabic, Hebrew, Japanese, and Chinese, while Part II takes a cross-linguistic stance on topics such as the nature of dyslexia, the universals that determine relevant precursor measures, competing hypotheses of brain-based deficits, modeling outcomes, etiologies, and intergenerational gene–environment interactions.

LUDO VERHOEVEN is Professor of Communication, Language, and Literacy in the Behaviour Science Institute at Radboud University Nijmegen and at the University of Curaçao.

CHARLES PERFETTI is Distinguished University Professor of Psychology and Director of the Learning Research and Development Center at the University of Pittsburgh.

KENNETH PUGH is Professor of Psychology at the University of Connecticut and Associate Professor of Linguistics and Medicine at Yale University, and he is President and Director of Research, and Senior Scientist at Haskins Laboratories.

Developmental Dyslexia across Languages and Writing Systems

Edited by

Ludo Verhoeven

Radboud University Nijmegen and the University of Curaçao

Charles Perfetti

University of Pittsburgh

Kenneth Pugh

Yale University

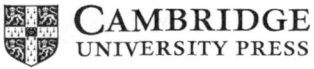

CAMBRIDGE
UNIVERSITY PRESS

University Printing House, Cambridge CB2 8BS, United Kingdom

One Liberty Plaza, 20th Floor, New York, NY 10006, USA

477 Williamstown Road, Port Melbourne, VIC 3207, Australia

314-321, 3rd Floor, Plot 3, Splendor Forum, Jasola District Centre, New Delhi - 110025, India

103 Penang Road, #05-06/07, Visioncrest Commercial, Singapore 238467

Cambridge University Press is part of the University of Cambridge.

It furthers the University's mission by disseminating knowledge in the pursuit of
education, learning and research at the highest international levels of excellence.

www.cambridge.org
Information on this title: www.cambridge.org/9781108451000
DOI: 10.1017/9781108553377

First published 2019
First paperback edition 2022

A catalogue record for this publication is available from the British Library

Library of Congress Cataloging in Publication data
Names: Verhoeven, Ludo Th., editor. | Perfetti, Charles A., editor. | Pugh, Ken
(Kenneth R.), editor.
Title: Developmental dyslexia across languages and writing systems / edited by
Ludo Verhoeven, Charles Perfetti, Kenneth Pugh.
Description: New York, NY: Cambridge University Press, [2019] | Includes
bibliographical references and index.
Identifiers: LCCN 2019010033 | ISBN 9781108428774 (alk. paper)
Subjects: LCSH: Dyslexia – Case studies. | Reading disability – Case studies. |
Language and languages.
Classification: LCC RC394.W6 D484 2019 | DDC 616.85/53–dc23
LC record available at https://lccn.loc.gov/2019010033

ISBN 978-1-108-42877-4 Hardback
ISBN 978-1-108-45100-0 Paperback

Contents

Figures

Tables

Contributors

MIKKO ARO *University of Yyväskylä*

BRIAN BYRNE *University of New England*

MARKETA CARAVOLAS *Bangor University*

S. HÉLÈNE DEACON *Dalhousie University*

ANDREA FACOETTI *University of Padua*

SANDRO FRANCESCHINI *University of Padua*

STEPHEN J. FROST *Haskins Laboratories*

NADINE GAAB *Harvard University*

JOHN D. E. GABRIELI *Massachusetts Institute of Technology*

SIMONE GORI *University of Bergamo*

ELENA GRIGORENKO *University of Connecticut*

LINDSAY HARRIS *Northern Illinois University*

FUMIKO HOEFT *Haskins Laboratories*

JANICE M. KEENAN *University of Denver*

ANNA KUCHASKÁ *Charles University, Prague*

KARIN LANDERL *University of Tübingen*

NICOLE LANDI *Haskins Laboratories*

ORLY LIPKA *University of Haifa*

HEIKKI LYYTINEN *University of Yyväskylä*

W. EINAR MENCL *Haskins Laboratories*

MARÍNA MIKULAJOVÁ *Pan-European University, Bratislava*

CATHERINE MIMEAU *Laval University*

ELIZABETH S. NORTON *Northwestern School of Communication*

RICHARD K. OLSON *University of Denver*

CHARLES PERFETTI *Pittsburgh University*

CONRAD PERRY *Swinburne University of Technology*

KENNETH PUGH *Haskins Laboratories*

ULLA RICHARDSON *University of Yyväskylä*

STEFAN SAMUELSSON *Linköping University*

MICHAL SHANY *University of Haifa*

DAVID L. SHARE *University of Haifa*

LAN SHUAI *Haskins Laboratories*

LILIANE SPRENGER-CHAROLLES *CNRS Paris*

LI HAI TAN *Shenzhen University*

XIULI TONG *University of Hong Kong*

LUDO VERHOEVEN *Radboud University Nijmegen*

CHENG WANG *University of California, San Francisco*

TAEKO N. WYDELL *Brunel University*

MIN XU *Shenzhen University*

JASON D. ZEVIN *University of Southern California*

MARINA ZHUKOVA *Saint Petersburg State University*

JOHANNES C. ZIEGLER *Aix-Marseille University*

MARCO ZORZI *University of Padua*

1 Introduction

Developmental Dyslexia – A Cross-Linguistic Perspective

Ludo Verhoeven, Charles Perfetti, and Kenneth Pugh

Reading involves decoding written language in order to understand it. In learning to read, children implicitly learn how their writing system encodes their spoken language and how they can decode printed words into spoken words to derive meaning (see Verhoeven & Perfetti, 2017). However, many children around the world encounter problems learning to read, fail to develop fluent decoding, and are thus diagnosed as dyslexic.

A large body of research supports the conclusion that a phonological deficit underlies most developmental dyslexia. Much of the existing evidence, however, is based on studies of children learning to read in English. It is important to note that English has an opaque orthography that creates challenges beyond those facing children who read more transparent orthographies. In recent years, the research base for developmental dyslexia has broadened across languages, allowing the question of differences and similarities across languages and writing systems to receive attention. It has been suggested, for example, that developmental dyslexia can involve not only phonological problems but also – particularly for writing systems that are more transparent than that of English – delayed development of decoding fluency. Other processing factors, such as rapid automatized naming and visual attention, have been argued to play a role in the occurrence of developmental dyslexia. And language factors beyond phonology, especially morphological processing, become visible when languages beyond English are considered. Whether the observed cross-linguistic differences in developmental dyslexia reflect more or less superficial variation around a common, underlying phonological disturbance or result from deeper, more fundamental variation in the causes of developmental dyslexia still remains to be seen (see Pugh & Verhoeven, 2018). Indeed, this question is a special case of the more general question of universal reading procedures and the adaptations that these procedures make to specific writing system and language factors (Perfetti, 2003; Perfetti & Harris, 2013).

The time is thus ripe to bring together what we know about reading problems and their underlying etiology across languages and writing systems. The present volume starts with a review of what is known about developmental dyslexia for nine different languages and orthographies (Part I) and then addresses the possible underlying mechanisms (Part II). Our selection of languages is based on the seventeen languages (and five writing systems) that were reviewed in Verhoeven and Perfetti (2017), in a collection of chapters that examined the languages, their writing systems, and research on learning to read in those languages. We chose nine of these languages for follow-up in the present volumes. We chose these nine languages to represent four major writing systems, excluding only alphasyllabaries, for which research on dyslexia is sparse. Our aim was to have some contrast among languages and writing systems (e.g., Finnish and Dutch (alphabetic), Chinese (morphosyllabic), Hebrew (abjad)) for which there has been substantial dyslexia research. We limited our examination to developmental dyslexia, excluding acquired dyslexia, thus allowing examination of risk factors, biological bases, interventions, and other important aspects of dyslexia that accompany children's difficulties in reading.

In this introductory chapter, we set the stage for taking a comparative perspective on developmental dyslexia by briefly reviewing the acknowledged universals for learning to read in general, and the definition, treatment, and neurocognitive foundations of dyslexia.

1.1   Learning to Read across Languages and Writing Systems

Several models have been proposed to account for the processing of visual word forms. The central assumption underlying so-called dual-route theories of reading, which are applied specifically to alphabetic writing, is that two independent routes can be followed to generate the pronunciation of a word: the nonlexical route or the lexical route. The nonlexical, computational route involves the computation of an orthographic code via the application of orthography-to-phonology mapping rules for the reading of letters, words, and text. The lexical retrieval route involves accessing a word's *written* representation from the so-called orthographic input lexicon followed by retrieval of the word's *spoken* form from the so-called phonological output lexicon (e.g., Coltheart et al., 2001). It is important to note that familiarity with a given writing system generally is thought to shift word reading from the computational to the retrieval route on these accounts (Pugh et al., 2013). Indeed, this is one of the conclusions considered to be universal based on comparisons across seventeen writing systems (Perfetti & Verhoeven, 2017). That is, computational routines are called upon for the reading of unknown or infrequent words and thus during the early stages of learning to read as well.

Sublexical mappings of phonology or morphology to orthography are used to determine the pronunciation (and meaning) of the whole word. With increased word familiarity and retrieval from memory on the basis of a few identified features of the whole word, computation becomes less necessary. This assumption also represents a more general observation about the nature of memory-based information processing by humans: Non-computational retrieval processes operate more frequently as experience establishes addressable memory forms. It should be noted here that alternative classes of computational models, such as the Division of Labor connectionist account (Harm & Seidenberg, 2004), challenge some key assumptions in the dual-route theories (such as independent pathways) while accounting for the same observed shifts with reading experience and the contrasts remains an active research domain.

Learning to read entails discovering how a writing system encodes a spoken language. The basic assumption underlying our understanding of the processes of reading and learning to read is that fluent reading draws upon lexical representations contain both orthographic and phonological components (see Perfetti, 1997). As we know, however, writing systems can show minor but *significant* variation in the mapping of spoken linguistic units to written linguistic units (see Dehaene, 2009). In Figure 1.1, it is shown how language units are related to graphic units across writing systems and orthographies. It is assumed that both reading and spelling draw upon lexical representations that contain orthographic and morpho-phonological constituents (see Verhoeven &

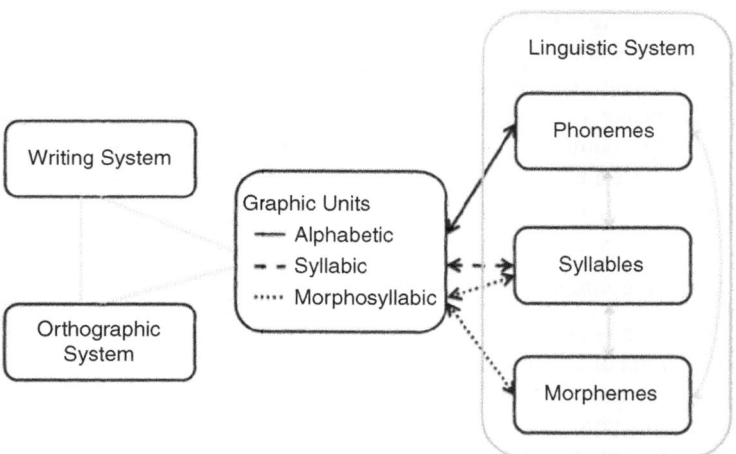

Figure 1.1 How graphic units mediate the relationship between writing systems and orthographies, on the one hand, and linguistic units, on the other hand

Perfetti, 2017). Accordingly, writing systems can reflect a dominance of mapping at the level of *morphemes*, with graphs corresponding to the basic units of meaning or morphemes), *syllables*, with graphs corresponding to spoken syllables, or *phonemes*, with graphs corresponding to the minimal units of speech, or phonemes.

Stated differently, writing systems have been found to show a varying predominance of phonological mapping at the morphemic, syllabic, and phonemic levels. According to the Universal Phonological Principle (Perfetti, Zhang, & Berent, 1992), word reading entails the activation of phonology at the lowest linguistic level encoded by the relevant writing system: the phoneme, the syllable, the morpheme, or the word. For systems using alphabetic writing, phonological activation is typically driven by grapheme-to-phoneme mappings. Even within the family of alphabetic writings, however, variation in orthographic depth or the extent to which the written language deviates from a simple grapheme-to-phoneme correspondence has been found to affect the course of the word-identification process (Frost, Katz, & Bentin, 1987). Grapheme–phoneme consistency (high for shallow orthographies, low for deep orthographies) and morpheme recovery (higher for deep orthographies, and reliance on morphemic as opposed to phonemic information for word decoding/reading) might produce corresponding variations in reading processes and processes of learning to read (Daniels & Share, 2018). Other writing systems, such as those of Japanese Kanji and Chinese, encourage direct activation of not only morphological but also syllabic information on the basis of orthographic form (Perfetti, Liu, & Tan, 2005).

Given that reading development requires learning how a writing system encodes the spoken language, it can be posited that universal operating principles guide children's perception, analysis, and use of a writing system to master a language's orthography. As is displayed in Figure 1.2, learning to read universally requires children to become linguistically aware, build orthographic representations, and develop routines for efficient word-to-text integration (see Verhoeven & Perfetti, 2017).

1.1.1   Becoming Linguistically Aware

Learning to read is known to be facilitated by the development of a sensitivity to the spoken units of a language. To the extent that visual word identification requires the connection of familiar sound units to to-be-learned or familiar orthographic units within a given language, the quality of the child's morphophonological knowledge and phonological processing will be essential. However, the speech signal is continuous and rapid with sharp modulations in both frequency and amplitude, making it difficult to segment the speech stream and identify the relevant units for reading. Moreover, the same speech

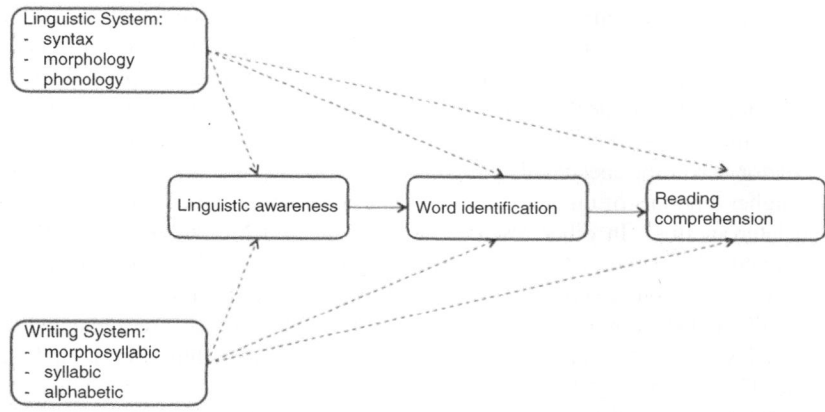

Figure 1.2 How the linguistic system and writing system impact the development of linguistic awareness, word identification, and reading comprehension

sound can manifest itself differently depending on the phonetic environment, the prosody, and the rate of speech. To solve this so-called variability problem, the speech signal can be normalized. Acoustic variants can then be mapped onto canonical phonemes and, in turn, onto spoken word representations within the mental lexicon (see McQueen & Cutler, 1997). It is already known that, with exposure to speech, infants begin to segment the incoming acoustic signal into consistent, replicable chunks that come to represent phonemes (cf. Kuhl et al., 1997). Stress, intonation, and the rhythm of the incoming speech signal can further alert children to significant units of speech and help them build high-quality, speech-based lexical representations. The quality of the representation is important, as precise and stable representations at the level of the phoneme are needed for the efficient retrieval of word forms. And word representations that are only partially specified may set the stage for impoverished reading development (see Goswami, 2000).

Learning to read in an alphabetic orthography builds upon a child's emerging phonological awareness (Snowling, 2000); that is, its ability to attend to the sounds of language independent of meaning. Stated generally, this awareness entails the ability to isolate words within sentences. More specifically, phonological awareness entails the ability to identify sublexical units, syllables, rhymes, the beginnings of words, the ends of words, and phonemes. Attention to salient syllabic, onset–rime, or phoneme boundaries within words is therefore highly important for children's reading development. Phonological awareness is usually assessed using tasks that measure segmentation, blending, or the manipulation of speech sounds. It has been found to progress from the syllable and onset–rime levels to the phoneme level (cf. I. Y. Liberman & Shankweiler, 1985; Shankweiler & I. Y. Liberman, 1989; Treiman & Zukowski, 1996). In recent research, when Moll et al. (2014) compared the roles of differential phonological processing (phonological awareness and memory vs. rapid naming) in reading development across various orthographies, rapid naming was found to be the best predictor of reading speed while phonological awareness and memory accounted for higher amounts of unique variance in the accuracy of the children's reading and later spelling. In other research, Shu, Peng, and McBride-Chang (2008) examined the nature of phonological awareness in 4–6-year-old Chinese children. They found syllable and rime awareness, but also tone awareness, to gradually and steadily increase, while awareness of phoneme onset remained at chance levels until the start of instruction on phonological coding (Pinyin) in first grade. The variance in Chinese character recognition was then best explained by phonological processing tasks measuring syllable awareness, tone awareness, and naming speed.

Children must not only attend to spoken language but also obviously have opportunities to link spoken to written linguistic forms in order to learn to read. With attention to salient script signs, they can acquire the inventory of graphic forms for a given writing system and gain insight into the orthographic units (graphemes) connected to the spoken units within the language (phonemes and morphemes). As a result of further analysis of the constituent sounds (phonemes, syllables) and graphemes of familiar words, they may then discover the more general mapping principle. And such self-learning is likely to be applicable across writing systems and orthographies. However, at least for alphabetic orthographies, the outcomes of research suggest that spontaneous self-discovery is not sufficient for most children to learn to read. More systematic instruction on the so-called alphabetic principle and the specific grapheme–phoneme correspondences within a language is required (de Graaff et al. 2009; Torgerson, Brooks, & Hall, 2006). Given such instruction, considerable research has shown phonological precursors as measured in preschool to predict later literacy development (cf. Blachman, 2000; Goswami, 2001).

Across a variety of orthographies (English, Finnish, Swedish), early phonological awareness and rapid naming (measured in kindergarten) have been found to correlate with later word-reading and spelling skill (measured in first and second grade; Furnes & Samuelsson, 2011). In a meta-analysis on correlates of later reading outcomes, Swanson et al. (2003) showed phonological awareness and rapid naming to moderately correlate with the reading of real words, but weaker associations were found within groups of poor as opposed to skilled readers. Strong support has consistently been found for associations between poor phonological abilities and problems learning to read (Elbro & Scarborough, 2004; Torgesen et al., 1997). More specifically, poor readers appear to have less precise phonemic discrimination and also problems with phoneme segmentation and other tests of phonological awareness (Høien & Sundberg, 2000; Wagner, Torgesen, & Rashotte, 1994). In sum: Phonological awareness has been found to play a key role in literacy outcomes, with later literacy problems often stemming from early and persistent deficits in phonological awareness.

1.1.2   Building Orthographic Representations

The building of the underlying orthographic representations needed for fluent reading requires the additional learning of graphic forms that might extend beyond beginning reading experiences, depending on the writing system. Alphabetic writing systems have the advantage of calling upon a relatively small inventory of graphs (letters). This inventory can usually be mastered during the first year of instruction or even prior to this. In contrast, the alpha-syllabaries of the languages in South and Southeast Asia are more demanding than those of – for example – English and Dutch. This is due to more graphs to start with and greater variation among the consonant graphs. Chinese requires the largest inventory of graphs, with over 6,000 graphs commonly in use and even more in dictionaries containing traditional characters. Mastering the Chinese writing system is therefore known to place the greatest demand on learning and requires more continuous learning than mastering the writing systems of other languages.

Across languages, written words can become familiar perceptual objects, which can then be recognized at a glance. According to Jorm and Share (1983) and Share (1995), a first encounter with a written word can lead to *phonological recoding*, which is then fed back to the word's orthographic representation to thereby initiate the word-specific reading identification process. With the aid of this mechanism, only a few exposures to the same word may thus be sufficient to create a high-quality, orthographic representation with sufficient prevision and redundancy for subsequent quick recognition (Perfetti, 1992, 2003, 2007; Share, 2004). Beyond making words familiar, experience with reading can produce gains in word-reading fluency as well. And highly fluent word reading, in other words, entails an effortless perceptual response to visual information, automatization of word decoding, and familiarity-based memory retrieval (see Verhoeven & van Leeuwe, 2009). Across different orthographies, research shows parallel developmental gains in both the speed and accuracy of word decoding immediately following the start of explicit reading instruction and steady improvements in lexical retrieval during the years thereafter. Retrieval of word representations on the basis of familiarity can be assumed to be universal (Verhoeven & Perfetti, 2017; Ziegler & Goswami, 2005). And given that such familiarity-based retrieval has been shown to be important for fluent alphabetic reading, it can similarly be assumed to be important – or possibly even more important – for such morpheme-based orthographies as Chinese. It should then be kept in mind that most reading problems have been shown to stem from limited reading fluency (Torgesen & Hudson, 2006).

Most current models of learning to read have focused on how letter strings are converted into phonological strings (pronunciations) but have essentially ignored the internal structure of words or morpheme units, which constitute the core of such morpheme-based orthographies as Chinese. The reading of more complex words across languages and writing systems nevertheless requires the processing of morphological structure in addition to the identification of grapheme–phoneme connections and the retrieval of whole words from memory. The processing of morphological structure or, in other words, morphological decomposition, can be viewed as an acquired sensitivity to the systematic associations between the surface forms of words and their under-lying meanings (cf. Plaut & Gonnerman, 2000; Seidenberg & Gonnerman, 2000). Morphological decomposition can be graded rather than all-or-none, depending on the degree of phonological and semantic transparency character-izing the language. Transparent associations between the orthographic, phonological, and semantic representations within a language can facilitate recognition of written forms and activation of meaning to thereby promote reading comprehension. And such transparent associations can be seen to constitute an important cornerstone for interventions with poor readers (Bowers, Kirby, & Deacon, 2010).

1.1.3   Word-to-Text Integration

The ultimate goal of reading is, of course, comprehension of a written text. The comprehension of a text starts from the identification of words for integration into the ongoing representation of the text. Word-to-text integra-tion entails each individual word being connected to a larger syntactic phrase, leading to the integration of words and phrases into sentences and larger text frames (Hagoort, 2005; Verhoeven & Perfetti, 2008). It is important to note that identified words are attached to not only syntactic phrases but also their underlying meanings of the semantic representation of a text. The referential integration of the meanings of words thus feeds the situation model being created by a written text. Word-by-word processing leads to word-to-text integration. And readers must then call upon prior knowledge to integrate the meaning of successive sentences and update the linguistic representation of the text being read and its underlying situation model. A situation model can also help the reader identify comprehension problems and find solutions for those problems (see Kintsch, 1988, 1998). When word identification is hampered as in the case of poor reading, however, comprehension will also be hampered (Stanovich, 2000).

In the *simple view of reading* as initially proposed by Hoover and Gough (1990), reading comprehension is presumed to be completely accounted for by word decoding and listening comprehension. That is, the pronunciation of a word is determined and, on the basis of this internal pronunciation, the meaning of the word and text is discerned. Reading comprehension is assumed to be the same as listening comprehension, once the decoding of a word (or word identification; Tunmer & Hoover, 1993) has taken place. And further in the simple view of reading, the reader's spoken language skill is assumed to determine the entire comprehension processes: the parsing of sentences into their constituent parts, the drawing of inferences to make the relations within and between sentences sufficiently apparent, the further facilitation of the integration of information, and the identification of the propositional structure (micro structure) underlying a text along with the global gist (macro structure) of the text (see Balota, Flores d'Arcais, & Rayner, 1990).

Extending from the simple view, the importance of lexical knowledge for reading comprehension cannot be overestimated. Both knowledge of word meanings (vocabulary) and the fluent retrieval of this knowledge on the basis of written words are critical for reading comprehension. The reading comprehension of both children and adults is supported by their knowledge of words and of the relevant orthographic, phonological, and semantic representations that can vary in their precision and interconnectedness. According to the lexical quality hypothesis (Perfetti & Hart, 2001), not only the sheer number of available words but also the quality of the reader's lexical representations can directly affect reading comprehension. There is a well-documented and strong association between vocabulary size and reading comprehension (cf. Torgeson et al., 1997; Verhoeven, 2000; Verhoeven, van Leeuwe, & Vermeer, 2011; Verhoeven & Perfetti, 2011).

1.2   Developmental Dyslexia: Definition and Intervention

1.2.1   Definition

Developmental dyslexia is typically defined as a specific learning disability "characterized by difficulties with accurate and/or fluent word recognition and by poor spelling and decoding abilities" (International Dyslexia Association: https://dyslexiaida.org/definition-of-dyslexia/). The disability occurs despite the receipt of normal classroom instruction and sociocultural stimulation and opportunities. Although there are no uniform criteria for dyslexia and its genetic or neurocognitive underpinnings (see Elliott & Grigorenko, 2014), it is generally accepted that developmental dyslexia can be considered a neurobiological disorder with a genetic origin (e.g., Eden & Moats, 2002; Shaywitz & Shaywitz, 2008). As a case in point, Byrne et al. (2008) report that

40 percent of children with a familial risk for dyslexia do indeed develop reading deficits that manifest themselves within a few months of the start of formal reading instruction in a language with a relatively transparent orthography. The prevalence of developmental dyslexia varies according to the definition adhered to. By means of computational modeling, Perry, Zorzi, and Ziegler (2019) have recently identified subtypes of dyslexia stemming from problems with the nonlexical route for word identification, the lexical route, or both. In many places throughout the world, a cut-off criterion in terms of standard deviations below the population mean for word and pseudoword decoding and spelling tasks is adopted to identify cases of dyslexia. And using such a criterion, 5 to 10 percent of children are then identified as having dyslexia. In the current version of the *Diagnostic and Statistical Manual of Mental Disorders* (i.e., the *DSM-5*), dyslexia is classified in the broad category of specific learning disorders, which entails three main subtypes: reading disorders, mathematics disorders, and written expression disorders. For reading disorders, the components of word-reading accuracy, reading rate, reading fluency, and reading comprehension are distinguished. And according to Snowling and Hulme (2012), two different types of reading disorders can be distinguished on the basis of this information: decoding disorders and comprehension disorders. Children identified as having a decoding disorder generally suffer from developmental dyslexia and show difficulties mastering the relationships between the spelling patterns in words and their pronunciations. These children typically show slow and inaccurate reading, and they also show spelling problems.

Children identified as having a comprehension disorder are able to read words accurately and fluently but show difficulties understanding what they have read. Although dyslexia can be distinguished in a number of ways from other neurobiological disorders, it is often observed along with other impairments. For example, comorbidity with attention-deficit disorders has been found. Children with attention-deficit disorders often suffer from dyslexia as a consequence of an incapacity for sustained attention (Willcutt & Pennington, 2000). Dyslexia has also been found to show comorbidity with specific language disorders. Children with a specific language impairment (SLI), for example, show a significant spoken language deficit that cannot be attributed to neurological damage, hearing impairment, or intellectual disability (Leonard, 2014); SLI is known to affect about 7 percent of the population. Finally, as Bishop and Snowling (2004) have shown, distinguishing specific phonological as opposed to more general linguistic dimensions of impairment can help us identify neurobiologically and etiologically coherent subgroups, which reinforces the potential value of brain-based research models in this domain. Phonological skills form the basis for learning to read, whereas vocabulary and grammar are essential for reading comprehension.

1.2.2   Intervention

An important question that now arises is: To what extent can developmental dyslexia be treated? Luckily the results of research on the effectiveness of early literacy programs can help us answer this question. In a meta-analysis, Ehri et al. (2001) evaluated the effects of instruction for phonemic awareness on learning to read and spell. The effect sizes from fifty-two studies showed a large impact on children's phonemic awareness and a moderate impact on reading and spelling development. The instruction not only helped typically developing readers, but also both at-risk and disabled readers with preschool, kindergarten, and first-grade levels of reading and varying socioeconomic backgrounds. The instruction for phonemic awareness was more effective when taught with letters than without, when provided in small groups, and when the instruction was intensive. In another meta-analysis, Bus and van IJzendoorn (1999) evaluated the results of randomized or matched group intervention aimed at promoting phonological awareness on reading gains. The combined effect size for phonological awareness and reading gain was moderate. Even in the early stages of early development, thus, phonemic awareness can be trained – also among children at risk for dyslexia. In other research, the effectiveness of treatment for children with demonstrated reading failures has been demonstrated. When Snowling and Hulme (2011) reviewed the characteristics of successful interventions for children with dyslexia, phonics-based interventions with a focus on the training of letter sounds, phoneme awareness, and the linking of graphemes and phonemes through writing and reading from texts were found to be most successful and this is a similar conclusion to those drawn by many large-scale assessments (e.g., National Reading Panel, 2000). Intervention programs that were more systematic, structured, multi-sensory, and direct-teaching-based were also found to be more successful than intervention programs without these characteristics (Snowling, 2013).

In still other research, various treatment approaches for children and adolescents with reading disabilities were compared. Galuschka et al. (2014) analyzed the effects of twenty-two randomized controlled trials with a total of forty-nine comparisons for experimental and control groups. The comparisons involved phonics-related interventions (e.g., training of phonemic awareness, decoding, or reading fluency) versus other types of interventions (e.g., auditory perception training, medical treatment, treatments using special lenses, or motor exercises). Explicit phonics instruction was found to be the only approach to significantly improve children's reading achievement. The results further showed that severe reading and spelling difficulties could only be helped with treatment. And individual variation was also found to play a role in the success of treatment efforts. More generally, about half of successfully trained children maintain the gains made in reading ability over the years. Interestingly, the predictors of early reading success (i.e., phonological awareness, rapid naming, and letter knowledge) also hold for predicting the success of training for children with dyslexia (Snowling, Gallagher, & Frith, 2003). Thus, while many alternative treatments have been put forward, focused on various hypothesized core deficits (sensory attentional, etc.), the vast consensus at this point is that the only reliable means of reaching children with reading problems is to focus on those processes key to print and language connections.

1.3   The Underlying Nature of Developmental Dyslexia

1.3.1   The Phonological Deficit Hypothesis

As we have seen in the preceding section, the most prominent models of dyslexia have been concentrated on the presence of phonological processing deficits. This focus is predicated on the finding that the core difficulty in the reading deficiencies of the vast majority of struggling readers occurs at the level of phonological processing. To successfully learn to read in an alphabetic writing system, for example, the child must recognize the segmented nature of speech and appreciate that spoken words can be broken down into smaller segments or phonemes. This phonemic awareness and the understanding that the constituents of the printed word (i.e., written letters) bear a relationship to the phonemes of the spoken language allows beginning readers to connect printed words to word representations in the speech lexicon. There is considerable evidence showing phonological awareness to be characteristically deficient (or even lacking) in young readers suffering from dyslexia. Such readers encounter difficulties with the development of efficient routines for the mapping of alphabetic characters onto the phonetic constituents that they represent (Bradley & Bryant, 1983 A. M. Liberman, 1992). And although the mechanisms underlying the development of phonemic awareness are not fully understood, support exists – at least in part – for the assumption that the difficulties experienced by children with dyslexia reside in the phonological component of a larger human specialization for spoken language. When that component is disturbed, the perception of phonemes and thus important linguistic distinctions in spoken and written language may be impaired. For children with no phonological deficit, in contrast, the orthographic, phonological, and semantic codes required for reading are part of high-quality lexical representations and are well integrated (Perfetti et al., 2007). All of this then means that word decoding normally becomes more fluent and automatic with sufficient reading practice (Pugh et al., 2013).

In an extension of the phonological deficit hypothesis, there is widespread agreement that skilled word decoding in any writing system demands adequate binding of orthographic phonologic and semantic codes (Harm & Seidenberg,

2004; Perfetti & Hart, 2001): as noted above, dual-route models assume a phonological pathway in which the phonological representation of a printed word is computed via specific orthography-to-phonology mapping routines and a lexical-semantic pathway in which orthography-to-semantic mapping routines operate directly (i.e., without the intervention of phonological analysis). Deficits in phonological representations will negatively impact orthography-to-phonology mapping and ultimately limit adequate development of both pathways. The phonological deficit hypothesis framed much of the existing work on the neurobiological bases of both skilled and less-skilled reading development. In the left hemisphere of the brain, the dorsal and ventral networks have been shown to support both orthographic-to-phonologic and orthographic-to-semantic mapping, with dorsal hubs most tuned to the former, and ventral hubs to the latter mappings. Both left-hemisphere circuits are poorly organized in untreated dyslexia, and this specifically manifests as unstable and reduced activation, and diminished functional connectivity in these pathways in dyslexia (Pugh et al., 2013; Richlan, 2012, 2014).

1.3.2   Neurocognitive Foundations

Alternative theoretical explanations for the phonological deficit in dyslexia are available today. In line with the phonological deficit hypothesis, it is often suggested that the observed reading problems arise from insufficiently specified phonological representations. Children with dyslexia will then find it hard to segment words into their phonological constituents, especially at the level of the phoneme (Ramus, 2014; Snowling, 2000). Alternatively, underlying phonological representations may be relatively intact, but the child has problems accessing the representations (Boets et al., 2013). Indeed, recent neuroimaging indicates that the phonological representations of individuals with known dyslexia are more or less intact, but not accessed efficiently (Boets et al., 2013). Support for the hypothesis that a deficit in accessing phonological representations characterizes dyslexia, rather than a deficit in phonological representations, has thus been found (cf. Ramus, 2014; but see Lallier et al., 2017, for contrasting claims).

   In another theoretical account, phonemic representations are presumed to be intact and accessible, but the building of the orthographic representations required to read is somehow impaired. According to Share (2004), phonological recoding gives children a self-teaching device for the incremental building of the orthographic representations associated with specific words. For successful phonological recoding, children must obviously discover the shared units within the orthography and phonology of their language and then integrate these via cross-modal processing (Blomert, 2011). Once the child is able to recode an entire written word, the orthographic representation can be formed and subsequently addressed directly during word reading. Several studies have shown that just a few exposures to a word are often sufficient for the detection and storage of word-specific orthographic information (e.g., Ziegler, Perry, & Zorzi, 2014). And with additional exposure, this information is known to provide an alternative lexical/orthographic foundation for future word reading (Stanovich, 2000).

In still another account, it has been asserted that it is not so much the computation of orthographic word forms that is the problem for children with dyslexia but, rather, the retrieval of already existing orthographic word representations from memory. Recent neurocognitive research has been interpreted to suggest that word recognition across languages may activate orthography-specific neural pathways (cf. Cohen & Dehaene, 2009; Das et al., 2011). The naming-speed impairments characteristic of dyslexia may reflect ventral orthographic retrieval problems, dorsal phonological recognition problems, or possibly both – leading to a so-called double deficit (Wolf & Bowers, 1999). Research on this and on how it might vary across languages is currently very active (cf. Norton et al., 2014).

While it is widely accepted that phonological processing is vulnerable in dyslexia, attempts have also been made to link the problems with phonology to non-language mechanisms including: auditory processing (Marshall, Snowling, & Bailey, 2001; Tallal, 1980), sensorimotor processing (Goswami et al., 2011), visual attention processing (Bosse & Valdois, 2009), statistical learning (Vicari et al., 2005), or procedural learning (Nicolson & Fawcett, 2007). In the domain of auditory processing, problems with categorical perception have indeed been found to impede the determination of phoneme boundaries among children with dyslexia. A high sensitivity for phonetic distinctions that are not represented in the native language has even been demonstrated in cases of dyslexia (Serniclaes et al., 2004). And such allophonic speech perception may then result in unclear phonological representations in the brain (Dufor et al., 2009).

Within the language domain, insufficient morphological awareness has been shown to impede the development of adequate word decoding (Kirby et al., 2012). In the so-called multifactorial framework related to this research, it is further recognized that dyslexia symptomology can be quite heterogeneous, and it is therefore posited that many etiological paths (and combinations of deficits) can thus lead to the same end state (Pennington, 2006). Of particular relevance for the current volume, then, is the possibility that the various models of reading development and dyslexia – from canonical to multifactorial – may be more or less relevant, depending on the transparency of the writing system to be mastered, which we will turn to next.

1.3.3   A Cross-Linguistic Perspective

An important question is how the apparent or possible universals and particulars of developmental dyslexia across languages and writing systems can be explained. Dual-pathway cognitive or brain-based explanations are generally adopted to account for the processing of visual word forms in many languages. The majority of the dual-pathway models have been developed with alphabetic reading in mind. The principles underlying the dual-pathway models should nevertheless apply to all writing systems in which written words are composed of constituents that can be assembled to lead to initial word identification, followed only later by whole-word retrieval from memory (see Daniels & Share, 2018; Ziegler et al., 2008). The research base on children's reading development and literacy problems has broadened recently to include insights from a variety of languages and writing systems, making the time ripe to adopt a cross-linguistic perspective on the observations across languages and writing systems. Therefore, our focus in the present volume is on those aspects of developmental dyslexia that appear to be language-specific (i.e., specific to a particular writing system) and those aspects that appear to be common across languages and orthographies.

As noted earlier, fluent word reading must depend to some extent on *both* the quality of underlying phonological word representations *and* the development of rapid word access with phonological awareness and rapid naming as important precursors. But according to some researchers, the contributions of such factors as phonological awareness and rapid naming to dyslexia can clearly vary across writing systems (see Wimmer, Mayringer, & Landerl, 2000, but also Caravolas et al., 2013, for an alternative viewpoint). The question of whether one or the other cognitive test is actually indicative of fundamental differences in the etiology of dyslexia also remains to be answered and is thus open to debate. Despite phonological awareness showing a bidirectional association with word-decoding skill, and word-decoding skill unfolding relatively quickly for transparent writing systems, it is still possible that the importance and predictive role of phonological awareness may be limited in languages relying on other writing systems. Additional cross-linguistic data on the developmental transition to literacy that also gives attention to the neurocognitive bases is needed to clarify the universal and language-specific aspects of reading development and causes of dyslexia. For insight into the possibly universal and language-specific factors playing a role in typical and atypical reading development, comparison of results for alphabetic languages (with varying degrees of orthographic transparency) and those for languages with consonantal root-based writing systems such as Arabic and Hebrew, but also non-alphabetic morphosyllabic writing systems such as Chinese, promise to be informative. It is possible, for example, that parallels do not exist for the orthography-to-phonology and orthography-to-semantics division of labor that characterizes learning to read in alphabetic systems. This may be due to the larger grain size of the phonological units in Chinese. Neurocognitive evidence nevertheless suggests that cross-linguistic similarities may exist for both typical reading development (Rueckl et al., 2015) and dyslexia (Hu et al., 2010). These similarities are posited despite other research presenting evidence for *significant neurocognitive variation* in underlying aspects of phonology and morphology (Perfetti et al., 2007; Siok et al., 2004), including neuroanatomical differences (Siok et al., 2008. It is thus important at this juncture that more extensive, cross-linguistically diverse, developmental data become available and our analyses of these data be informed by the results of computational modeling and brain imaging. Only then can we identify what is universal and what is not.

1.4   The Present Volume

The aim of this volume is to advance theoretical models of developmental dyslexia through systematic analyses of different languages, writing systems, and orthographies in relation to the conceptualization and etiology of reading disabilities. We assume reading to entail – among other things – an acquired sensitivity to the systematic (statistical) relationships occurring in a writing system between the surface forms of words and their underlying meanings. This is assumed to be a universal aspect of reading, but given that the statistical organization can vary across writing systems there should be some computational differences, despite general universality in neurocognitive organization (Frost, 2012); failures to detect and/or master these relationships located are thought to be at the core of dyslexia as a universal disability. Given that languages substantially differ, on the one hand, in their phonological, morphological, and syntactic structure, and, on the other hand, in their script characteristics, language-specific disturbances can also be expected across orthographies and writing systems.

The present volume is divided into two parts. In Part I, an account of developmental dyslexia for nine different orthographies is presented. To shed light on the role of cross-linguistic differences, reading researchers examine how reading disabilities manifest themselves for typologically different languages and writing systems. The implications of these insights for the conceptualization of developmental dyslexia are then discussed. To examine the universal and particular cognitive principles underlying developmental dyslexia, alphabetic orthographies with varying levels of orthographic depth (English, Dutch, French, Czech-Slovakian, Finnish, and Russian) are contrasted with the unvoweled root-based orthography of Hebrew, the syllable-based (Kana) orthography of Japan, and the morpheme-syllable based orthographies of Chinese and Japanese Kanji. In each of the chapters in Part I of this volume, attention is paid to the processes of learning to read, the problems encountered by children learning to read, the neurocognitive and behavioral underpinnings of dyslexia, and the possibilities for intervention.

In Part II, the behavioral and neural markers of dyslexia are examined from a cross-linguistic perspective. Of particular interest are the possibly universal markers of dyslexia, the behavioral and neural precursors to dyslexia, the neuro-cognitive markers of dyslexia, the modeling of dyslexia across alphabetic languages and other writing systems, and the etiology of dyslexia and its intergenerational transmission. Each of these chapters begins with a theoretical introduction to the marker being considered. The cross-linguistic evidence for various claims, explanatory frameworks, and alternative hypotheses is then considered.

In a final chapter, the implications of the within- and cross-language comparisons presented in this volume are considered for the conceptualization of developmental dyslexia, clinical practice, and future research.

References

Balota, D. A., FloresD'Arcais, G. B., & Rayner, K. (1990). *Comprehension processes in reading*. Mahwah, NJ: Lawrence Erlbaum.

Bishop, D. V. M., & Snowling, M. J. (2004). Developmental dyslexia and specific language impairment: Same or different? *Psychological Bulletin, 130*, 858–888.

Blachman, B. A. (2000). Phonological awareness. In M. L. Kamil, P. B. Mosenthal, P. D. Pearson, & R. Barr (Eds.), *Handbook of reading research* (Vol. III; pp. 483–502). Mahwah, NJ: Erlbaum.

Blomert, L. (2011). The neural signature of orthographic-phonological binding in successful and failing reading development. *Neuroimage, 57*, 695–703.

Boets, B., Op de Beeck, H. P., & Vandermosten, M. et al. (2013). Intact but less accessible phonetic representations in adults with dyslexia. *Science, 342*, 1251–1254.

Bosse, M., & Valdois, S. (2009). Influence of the visual attention span on child reading performance: A cross-sectional study. *Journal of Research in Reading, 32*, 230–253.

Bowers, P. N., Kirby, J. R., & Deacon, S. H. (2010). The effects of morphological instruction on literacy skills: A systematic review of the literature. *Review of Educational Research, 80*, 144–179.

Bradley, L., & Bryant, P. E. (1983). Categorizing sounds and learning to read – a causal connection. *Nature, 301*, 419–421.

Bus, A. G., & van IJzendoorn, M. H. (1999). Phonological awareness and early reading: A meta-analysis of experimental training studies. *Journal of Educational Psychology, 80*, 403–414.

Byrne, B., Coventry, W. L., Olson, R. K. et al. (2008). A behavioral-genetic analysis of orthographic learning, spelling, and decoding. *Journal of Research in Reading, 3*, 8–21.

Caravolas, M., Lervåg, A., Defior, S., Málková, G. S., & Hulme, C. (2013). Different patterns, but equivalent predictors, of growth in reading in consistent and inconsistent orthographies. *Psychological Science, 24*, 1398–1407.

Cohen, L., & Dehaene, S. (2009). Ventral and dorsal contribution to word reading. In M. S. Gazzaniga (Ed.), *Cognitive neuroscience* (pp. 789–804). Cambridge, MA: MIT Press.

Coltheart, M., Rastle, K., Perry, C., Langdon, R., & Ziegler, J. (2001). DRC: A dual route cascaded model of visual word recognition and reading aloud. *Psychological Review, 108,* 204–256.

Daniels, P. T., & Share, D. L. (2018). Writing system variation and its consequences for reading and dyslexia. *Scientific Studies of Reading, 22,* 101–116.

Das, T., Padakannaya, P., Pugh, K. R., & Singh, N. C. (2011). Neuroimaging reveals dual routes to reading in simultaneous proficient readers of two orthographies. *NeuroImage, 54,* 1476–1487.

de Graaff, S., Bosman, A. M. T., Hasselman, F., & Verhoeven, L. (2009). Benefits of systematic phonics instruction. *Scientific Studies of Reading, 13,* 318–333.

Dehaene, S. (2009). *Reading in the brain.* London: Penguin Viking.

Dehaene, S., & Cohen, L. (2011). The unique role of the visual word form area in reading. *Trends in Cognitive Sciences, 15,* 254–262.

Dufor, O., Serniclaes, W., Sprenger-Charolles, L., & Démonet, J.-F. (2009). Left pre-motor cortex and allophonic speech perception in dyslexia: A PET study, *NeuroImage, 46,* 241–248.

Eden, G., & Moats, L. (2002). The role of neuroscience in the remediation of students with dyslexia. *Nature Neuroscience, 5,* 1080–1084.

Ehri, L., Nunes, R. S., Willows, D., Schuster, B. V., Yaghoub-Zadeh, Z., & Shanahan, T. (2001). Phonemic awareness instruction helps children learn to read: Evidence from the National Reading Panel's meta-analysis. *Reading Research Quarterly, 36,* 250–287.

Elbro, C., & Scarborough, H. S. (2004). Early intervention. In P. Bryant & T. Nunes, (Eds.), *Handbook of children's literacy* (pp. 361–381). Dordrecht: Kluwer.

Elliott, J. G., & Grigorenko, E. L. (2014). *The dyslexia debate.* Cambridge, UK: Cambridge University Press.

Frost, R. (2012). Towards a universal model of reading. *The Behavioral and Brain Sciences, 35*(5), 263–279. doi: http://dx.doi.org/10.1017/S0140525X11001841.

Frost, R., Katz, L., & Bentin, S. (1987). Strategies for visual word recognition and orthographic depth: A multilingual comparison. *Journal of Experimental Psychology: Human Perception and Performance, 13,* 104–115.

Furnes, B., & Samuelsson, S. (2011). Phonological awareness and rapid automatized naming predicting early development in reading and spelling results from a cross-linguistic longitudinal study. *Learning and Individual Differences, 21,* 85–95.

Galuschka, K., Ise, E., Krick, K., & Schulte-Körne, G. (2014). Effectiveness of treatment approaches for children and adolescents with reading disabilities: A meta-analysis of randomized controlled trials. *PLoS One, 9*(2), e89900.

Goswami, U. (2000). Phonological and lexical processes. In M. L. Kamil, P. B. Rosenthal, P. D. Pearson, & R. Barr (Eds.), *Handbook of reading research* (Vol. III; pp. 251–268). Mahwah, NJ: Erlbaum.

Goswami, U. (2001). Early phonological development and the acquisition of literacy. In S. Neuman & D. Dickinson (Eds.), *Handbook of research in early literacy for the 21st century* (pp. 111–125). New York: Guilford Press.

Goswami, U., Wang, H. L., & Cruz, A. et al. (2011). Language-universal sensory deficits in developmental dyslexia: English, Spanish, and Chinese. *Journal of Cognitive Neuroscience, 23,* 325–337.

Hagoort, P. (2005). On Broca, brain, and binding: A new framework. *Trends in Cognitive Sciences, 9,* 416–423.

Harm, M. W., & Seidenberg, M. S. (2004). Computing the meanings of words in reading: Cooperative division of labor between visual and phonological processes. *Psychological Review, 111*, 662–720.

Høien, T., & Sundberg, P. (2000). *Dyslexia: From theory to intervention.* Dordrecht: Springer.

Hoover, W. A., & Gough, P. B. (1990). The simple view of reading. *Reading and Writing, 2*, 127–160.

Hu, W., Lee, H. L., & Zhang, Q. et al. (2010). Developmental dyslexia in Chinese and English populations: Dissociating the effect of dyslexia from language differences. *Brain, 133*, 1694–1706.

Jorm, A. F., & Share, D. L. (1983). Phonological recoding and reading acquisition. *Applied Psycholinguistics, 4*, 103–147.

Kintsch, W. (1988). The use of knowledge in discourse processing: A construction-integration model. *Psychological Review, 95*, 163–182.

Kintsch, W. (1998). *Comprehension: A paradigm for cognition.* Cambridge, UK: Cambridge University Press.

Kirby, J. R., Deacon, S. H., & Bowers, P. N. et al. (2012). Children's morphological awareness and reading ability. *Reading and Writing, 25*, 389–410.

Kuhl, P. K., Andruski, J. E., & Chistovich, I. A. et al. (1997). Cross-language analysis of phonetic units in language addressed to infants. *Science, 277*, 684–686.

Lallier, M., Molinaro, N., Lizarazu, M., Bourguignon, M., & Carreiras, M. (2017). Amodal atypical neural oscillatory activity in dyslexia: A cross-linguistic perspective. *Clinical Psychological Science, 5*, 379–401.

Leonard, L. B. (2014). Specific language impairment across languages. *Child Development Perspectives, 8*, 1–5.

Liberman, A. M. (1992). The relation of speech to reading and writing. *Advances in Psychology, 94*, 167–178.

Liberman, I. Y., & Shankweiler, D. (1985). Phonology and the problems of learning to read and write. *Remedial and Special Education, 6*(6), 8–17.

Marshall, C. M., Snowling, M. J., & Bailey, P. J. (2001). Rapid auditory processing and phonological ability in normal readers and readers with dyslexia. *Journal of Speech, Language, and Hearing Research, 44*, 925–940.

McQueen, J. M., & Cutler, A. (1997). Cognitive processes in spoken-word recognition. In W. J. Hardcastle & J. D. M. H. Laver (Eds.), *The handbook of phonetic sciences* (pp. 566–585). Oxford, UK: Blackwell.

Moll, K., Ramus, F., & Bartling, J. et al. (2014). Cognitive mechanisms underlying reading and spelling development in five European orthographies: Is English an outlier orthography? *Learning and Instruction, 29*, 65–77.

National Reading Panel. (2000). *Report of the National Reading Panel: Teaching children to read: An evidence-based assessment of the scientific research literature on reading and its implications for reading instruction: Reports of the subgroups.* Washington, DC: National Institute of Child Health and Human Development, National Institutes of Health.

Nicolson, R. I., & Fawcett, A. J. (2007). Procedural learning difficulties: Reuniting the developmental disorders? *Trends in Neurosciences, 30*, 135–141.

Norton, E. S., Black, J. M., & Stanley, L. M. et al. (2014). Functional neuroanatomical evidence for the double-deficit hypothesis of developmental dyslexia. *Neuropsychologia, 61*, 235–246.

Pennington, B. F. (2006). From single to multiple deficit models of developmental disorders. *Cognition, 101*, 385–413.

Perfetti, C. A. (1992). The representation problem in reading acquisition. In P. B. Gough, L. C. Ehri, & R. Treiman (Eds.), *Reading acquisition* (pp. 145–174). Hillsdale, NJ: Lawrence Erlbaum.

Perfetti, C. A. (1997). The psycholinguistics of spelling and reading. In C. A. Perfetti, L. Rieben, & M. Fayol (Eds.), *Learning to spell: Research, theory, and practice across languages* (pp. 21–38). Mahwah, NJ: Lawrence Erlbaum Associates.

Perfetti, C. A. (2003). The universal grammar of reading. *Scientific Studies of Reading, 7*, 3–24.

Perfetti, C. A. (2007). Reading ability: Lexical quality to comprehension. *Scientific Studies of Reading, 11*, 357–383.

Perfetti, C. A., & Harris, L. N. (2013). Universal reading processes are modulated by language and writing system. *Language Learning and Development, 9*(4), 296-316.

Perfetti, C. A., & Hart, L. (2001). The lexical quality hypothesis. In L. Verhoeven, C. Elbro, & P. Reitsma (Eds.), *Precursors of functional literacy* (pp. 189–214). Amsterdam: John Benjamins.

Perfetti, C. A., Liu, Y., & Fiez, J. et al. (2007). Reading in two writing systems: Accommodation and assimilation of the brain's reading network. *Bilingualism: Language and Cognition, 10*, 131–146.

Perfetti, C. A., Liu, Y., & Tan, L. H. (2005). The Lexical Constituency Model: Some implications of research on Chinese for general theories of reading. *Psychological Review, 12*(11), 43–59.

Perfetti, C. A., Zhang, S., & Berent, I. (1992). Reading in English and Chinese: Evidence for a "universal" phonological principle. In R. Frost & L. Katz (Eds.), *Orthography, phonology, morphology, and meaning* (pp. 227–248). Amsterdam: North-Holland.

Perfetti, C. A. & Verhoeven, L. (2017). Epilogue: Universals and particulars in learning to read across seventeen orthographies. In L. Verhoeven & C. A. Perfetti (Eds.), *Learning to read across languages and writing systems* (pp. 455–480). Cambridge, UK: Cambridge University Press.

Perry, C., Zorzi, M., & Ziegler, J. C. (2019). Understanding dyslexia through personalized large-scale computational models. *Psychological Science, 30*(3), 386–395.

Plaut, D. C., & Gonnerman, L. M. (2000). Are non-semantic morphological effects incompatible with a distributed connectionist approach to lexical processing? *Language and Cognitive Processing, 15*, 445–485.

Pugh, K. R., Landi, N., & Preston, J. L. et al. (2013). The relationship between phonological and auditory processing and brain organization in beginning readers. *Brain and Language, 125*, 173–183.

Pugh, K. R., & Verhoeven, L. (2018). Introduction to this special issue: Dyslexia across languages and writing systems. *Scientific Studies of Reading, 22*, 1–6.

Ramus, F. (2014). Neuroimaging sheds new light on the phonological deficit in dyslexia. *Trends in Cognitive Sciences, 18*, 274–275.

Richlan, F. (2012). Developmental dyslexia: Dysfunction of a left hemisphere reading network. *Frontiers in Human Neuroscience, 6*, 120.

Richlan, F. (2014). Functional neuroanatomy of developmental dyslexia: The role of orthographic depth. *Frontiers in Human Neuroscience, 8*, 347.

Rueckl, J. G., Paz-Alonso, P. M., & Molfese, P. J. et al. (2015). Universal brain signature of proficient reading: Evidence from four contrasting languages. *Proceedings National Academy of Sciences, 112*, 15510–15515.

Seidenberg, M. S., & Gonnerman, L. M. (2000). Explaining derivational morphology as the convergence of codes. *Trends in Cognitive Sciences, 4*, 353–361.

Serniclaes, W., Van Heghe, S., Mousty, P., Carré, R., & Sprenger-Charolles, L. (2004). Allophonic mode of speech perception in dyslexia. *Journal of Experimental Child Psychology, 87*, 336–361.

Shankweiler, D., & Liberman, I. Y. (Eds.). (1989). *Phonology and reading disability: Solving the reading puzzle.* Ann Arbor, MI: The University of Michigan Press.

Share, D. L. (1995). Phonological recoding and self-teaching: Sine qua non of reading acquisition. *Cognition, 55*, 151–218.

Share, D. L. (2004). Orthographic learning at a glance: On the time course and developmental onset of reading. *Journal of Experimental Child Psychology, 87*, 267–298.

Shaywitz, S. E., & Shaywitz, B. A. (2008). Paying attention to reading: The neurobiology of reading and dyslexia. *Development and Psychopathology, 20*, 1329–1349.

Shu, H., Peng, H., & McBride-Chang, C. (2008). Phonological awareness in young Chinese children. *Developmental Science, 11*, 171–181.

Siok, W. T., Niu, Z. Jin, Z., Perfetti, C. A., & Tan, L. H. (2008). A structural-functional basis for dyslexia in the cortex of Chinese readers. *Proceedings of the National Academy of Sciences, 105*, 5561–5566.

Siok, W. T., Perfetti, C. A., Jin, Z., & Tan, L. H. (2004). Biological abnormality of impaired reading constrained by culture: Evidence from Chinese. *Nature, 431*, 71–76.

Snowling, M. J. (2000). Language and literacy skills: Who is at risk and why? In D. V. M. Bishop & L. B. Leonard (Eds.), *Speech and language impairment in children: Causes, characteristics, interventions and outcome* (pp. 245–260). Hove, UK: Psychology Press.

Snowling, M. J. (2013). Early identification and interventions for dyslexia: A contemporary view. *Journal of Research in Special Educational Needs, 13*, 7–14.

Snowling, M. J., Gallagher, A., & Frith, U. (2003). Family risk of dyslexia is continuous: Individual differences in the precursors of reading skill. *Child Development, 74*, 358–373.

Snowling, M. J., & Hulme, C. (2011). Evidence-based interventions for reading and language difficulties: Creating a virtuous circle. *British Journal of Educational Psychology, 81*, 1–23.

Snowling, M. J., & Hulme, C. (2012). Interventions for children's language and literacy difficulties. *International Journal of Language & Communication Disorders, 47*, 27–34.

Stanovich, K. E. (2000). *Progress in understanding reading: Scientific foundations and new frontiers.* New York: Guilford Press.

Swanson, H. L., Trainin, G., Necoechea, D. M., & Hammill, D. D. (2003). Rapid naming, phonological awareness, and reading: A meta-analysis of the correlation evidence. *Review of Educational Research, 73*, 407–440.

Tallal, P. (1980). Auditory-temporal perception, phonics, and reading disabilities in children. *Brain and Language, 9*, 182–198.

Torgerson, C. J., Brooks, G., & Hall, J. (2006). *A systematic review of the research literature on the use of phonics in the teaching of reading and spelling* (Research Report No. 711). London: DfES Publications.

Torgesen, J. K. & Hudson, R. (2006). Reading fluency: Critical issues for struggling readers. In S. J. Samuels & A. Farstrup (Eds.). *Reading fluency: The forgotten dimension of reading success.* Newark, DE: International Reading Association.

Torgeson, J. K., Wagner, R. K., Rashotte, C. A., Burgess, S., & Hecht, S. (1997). Contributions of phonological awareness and rapid automatic naming ability to the growth of word-reading skills in second-to fifth-grade children. *Scientific Studies of Reading, 1,* 161–195.

Treiman, R., & Zukowski, A. (1996). Children's sensitivity to syllables, onsets, rimes, and phonemes. *Journal of Experimental Child Psychology, 61,* 193–215.

Tunmer, W. E., & Hoover, W. A. (1993). Components of variance models of language-related factors in reading disability: A conceptual overview. In R. J. Joshi & C. K. Leong (Eds.), *Reading disabilities: Diagnosis and component processes* (pp. 135–173). Dordrecht: Kluwer.

Verhoeven, L. (2000). Components in early second language reading and spelling. *Scientific Studies of Reading, 4,* 313–330.

Verhoeven, L., & Perfetti, C. (2008). Advances in text comprehension: Model, process, and development. *Applied Cognitive Psychology, 22,* 293–301.

Verhoeven, L., & Perfetti, C. (2011). Introduction to this special issue: Vocabulary growth and reading skill. *Scientific Studies of Reading, 15,* 1–7.

Verhoeven, L., & Perfetti, C. (2017). *Learning to read across languages and writing systems.* Cambridge, UK: Cambridge University Press.

Verhoeven, L., & van Leeuwe, J. (2009). Modeling the growth of word decoding skills: Evidence from Dutch. *Scientific Studies of Reading, 13,* 205–223.

Verhoeven, L., van Leeuwe, J., & Vermeer, A. (2011). Vocabulary growth and reading development across the elementary school years. *Scientific Studies of Reading, 15,* 8–25.

Vicari, S., Finzi, A., & Menghini, L. et al. (2005). Do children with developmental dyslexia have an implicit learning deficit? *Journal of Neurology, Neurosurgery & Psychiatry, 76,* 1392–1397.

Wagner, R. K., Torgesen, J. K., & Rashotte, C. A. (1994). Development of reading-related phonological processing abilities: new evidence of bidirectional causality from a latent variable longitudinal study. *Developmental Psychology, 30,* 73–87.

Willcutt, E. G., & Pennington, B. F. (2000). Comorbidity of reading disability and attention-deficit/hyperactivity disorder: Differences by gender and subtype. *Journal of Learning Disabilities, 33,* 179–191.

Wimmer, H., Mayringer, H., & Landerl, K. (2000). The double-deficit hypothesis and difficulties in learning to read a regular orthography. *Journal of Educational Psychology, 92,* 668–680.

Wolf, M., & Bowers, P. G. (1999). The double-deficit hypothesis for the developmental dyslexias. *Journal of Educational Psychology, 91,* 415–438.

Ziegler, J. C., Castel, C., & Pech-Georgel, C. et al. (2008). Developmental dyslexia and the dual route model of reading: Simulating individual differences and subtypes. *Cognition, 107,* 151–178.

Ziegler, J. C., & Goswami, U. (2005). Reading acquisition, developmental dyslexia, and skilled reading across languages: A psycholinguistic grain size theory. *Psychological Bulletin, 131,* 3–29.

Ziegler, J. C., Perry, C., & Zorzi, M. (2014). Modelling reading development through phonological decoding and self-teaching: Implications for dyslexia. *Philosophical Transactions of the Royal Society, B: Biological Sciences, 369,* 20120397.

Part I

Developmental Dyslexia across Languages and Writing Systems

2   Developmental Dyslexia in English

Charles Perfetti and Lindsay Harris

2.1   Introduction

It is probably a stretch to say that dyslexia was made for the English language. However, there is a special suitability for a discussion of dyslexia to center on English as the paradigm case. For one thing, the history of reading disability, or dyslexia, is populated by English-language papers from medicine, psychology, and education. Of course, the Germans deserve credit too. Adolf Kussmaul, a German physician, is credited with the earliest (1878) observations on an adult patient with impaired reading (acquired dyslexia), and Rudolf Berlin may have been the first to use the word "dyslexia" in an 1887 book *Eine Besondere Art der Wortblindheit (dyslexie)* [A Special Type of Word Blindness (Dyslexia)]. The English-language reports of dyslexia began shortly after with the 1896 publication by W. Pringle Morgan, an English physician in the *British Journal of Medicine* and then the ophthalmologist Hinshelwood (1917), both of whom referred to "word blindness." The 1925 publication by the American Samuel T. Orton on word blindness in children became a highly cited landmark publication for developmental dyslexia; his argument that whole-word reading instruction may contribute to this condition has credibility in the context of contemporary thinking (Orton, 1929).

A second reason for English as a paradigm for dyslexia springs from the specific nature of English orthography. Its lack of mapping consistency between its letters and its phonemes creates challenges to learning to read, and these difficulties naturally leak through the tissue separating reading challenges from reading disability. This leads to high (and unreliable) estimates of dyslexia in the English-speaking world and to explanations of dyslexia that dwell on orthographic vs. phonological sources that correspond to English spelling patterns. One can speculate that only research in English reading could have led to the elaboration of dyslexia into subtypes of surface/orthographic vs. phonological (e.g., Shallice, Warrington, & McCarthy, 1983; Patterson & Marcel, 1977).

From an international perspective, the English language provided a focal point for psycholinguistic descriptions of dyslexia that led to theories of multiple routes to word identification (Coltheart, 1978; Coltheart et al., 1993) and their diagnostic implications: Dyslexia emerges through the impairment of one or the other reading route, e.g., orthography-to-sublexical phonology, or orthography-to-whole-word phonology and meaning. When other languages are considered, especially across writing systems and language groups, departures from the English model might be expected.

2.2 Learning to Read English

2.2.1 English Language and Its Orthography

English is widely spoken as both a first and second language, with the largest population of speakers residing in the United States. British English, American English, Australian English, South African English, and Scottish English are a few of the varieties of English spoken around the world, with numerous dialects within these broad varieties. More than a first language, however, English is the world's most learned second language.

Explaining how children learn, and fail to learn, to read depends on specific language features that are variable across languages. The phonological and grammatical (morphology and syntax) systems of a language are the basic machinery of spoken language. Reading, with the addition of an orthographic system, requires written symbols to be mapped onto spoken language units combined through this machinery. Historical developments of English and descriptions of its contemporary systems are described in a chapter by Perfetti and Harris in *Learning to Read across Writing Systems* (2017). Here we provide a brief summary of the essential facts of English that are the most important for reading and dyslexia.

One historical note is especially relevant, however – the Great Vowel Shift in English. This shift or, better, drift (because it stretched out over three centuries) gradually caused the loss of the pure vowels that continued to be part of European languages. For example, the lower back vowel [a] moved forward and up in distinct phases to become [e:], the long vowel we now hear in the English word "name," which earlier would have been pronounced to rhyme with "Tom." An even more radical shift occurred in dialects that stretched this vowel to a diphthong [ei], with the pure vowel [a] giving way to a vocal glide across two vowels. This great vowel drift played a part – but only a part – of the irregularities of English spelling.

2.2.1.1 English Phonology Across the dialects of English, the phoneme inventory varies between thirty-seven and forty-two, well above the language average of thirty phonemes (Hay & Bauer, 2007). Twenty-four consonants, more or less, serve all varieties of English, with vowels, of course, producing the largest variation in dialects. British Received (upper-class) English has more vowels, including many diphthongs, than Australian English, which in turn has more than standard American English. All varieties of English, however, use diphthongs freely. The large number of phonemes, especially vowels, creates a problem for grapheme-to-phoneme mapping English's twenty-six-letter alphabet.

Important also for reading is the internal structure of syllables, which is commonly identified as onset + rime (vowel + coda). The significance of this structure is that it separates the vowel nucleus (sonorant peak) from the onset of the syllable, producing /s/ + /æt/ rather than /sæ/ +/t/ for "sat" and /sp/ + /at/ over / s/ + /pat/ for "spat." Although the CVC (consonant + vowel + consonant) pattern could show either structure – onset + rime, or nucleus (onset + vowel) + coda – the onset + rime structure applies more generally to English. Kessler and Treiman (1997) found that the statistics of CVC sequences showed more constraint imposed by the vowel within VC (vowel + consonant) than by the consonant within CV (consonant + vowel). This tighter binding of the vowel with the final consonant suggests the reality of the rime unit in English. Other languages, with less influence from initial consonant clusters, can show a different structure (Geudens & Sandra, 2003; Yoon et al., 2002). The significance of internal consonant structure for reading is the reason for the recommendation to provide English-speaking children with onset + rime-based phoneme awareness and reading practice (Goswami & Bryant, 1990).

Finally, English words show phonological richness: they are largely multisyllabic with a full range of both simple consonants and consonant clusters and both open and closed syllables. Being able to read VC or CVC patterns helps a reader of English, but its usefulness is limited given this complexity.

2.2.1.2 English Morphology   English follows the root + affix paradigm of inflectional morphology, but with relatively simple grammatical paradigms: inflections for number on noun roots and verbs, tense on verb roots, and a case and number paradigm for pronouns, which are marked for gender (*he, she, it*). Verb tense is only partly regular, with many verbs showing stem alterations with tense changes instead of affixation. The regular affixation pattern regular adds *–ed* to root spellings, which is phonemically realized as /t/ (*kicked*), /d/ (*jogged*), or /ed/ (*surrounded*). Irregulars such as *run/ran/* and *ride/rode* show the stem alteration pattern. Plural markings have this same dual system: The morphophoneme [s] is added to noun roots as the regular pattern and realized according to its phonemic environment as /s/, /z/, /às/, or /əz/, yielding different pronunciations for the plural affix in *bits, bids*, and *roses*. Irregular plurals are formed by vowel changes (*foot/feet; mouse/mice*) and other devices.

English derivational morphology shows a very rich word-formation process. Noun compounding abounds – *saltwater, seawater*; but in writing, spaces mark resistance to compounding – *spring water* and *river water*. Derivational processes freely create adjectives from verbs – *drink/drinkable, kiss/kissable, watch/watchable, live/livable.* Many human nouns add *-er* to a stem with inanimate semantics (*village/villager, bank/banker, farm/farmer*), and others are created through alterations to a noun stem: *library/librarian.* Nominalization is rampant, with nearly any verb or adjective likely to yield a noun form; sometimes the form does not change, as when the verb *read* becomes the noun *read.* This is but a small sample of the tricks of word formation in English that confront the reader with a large variety of related forms.

2.2.1.3 English Orthography Written English, for all its irregularities, belongs squarely to the alphabetic writing system. Its linear array of twenty-six Roman letters can appear in various scripts, from standard print and computer fonts to handwriting, where ligatures produce scripts called *cursive* (United States) or *joined-up writing* (United Kingdom). Written words are separated by spaces, which makes words, but not morphemes, visually prominent.

English departs substantially from the alphabetic ideal. Its forty-four or so phonemes are coded by twenty-six letters, several of which combine as digraphs to map consonant phonemes (‹sh›, ‹th›, ‹ch›); a larger number combine as digraphs for vowels (e.g., ‹ee› ‹ie› ‹ei› ‹ay› ‹oo›), including diphthongs (e.g., ‹au›, ‹ou›, ‹oy›, ‹ow›, ‹oi›). Three of the five consonant digraphs are the only spelling of the consonant sound and the two that are not (‹ck› and ‹ph›) are limited by positional or vocabulary constraints. However, nearly all the English long vowels and diphthongs have multiple spellings. The challenge this presents for reading is not only that the same letter can map onto more than one phoneme, as is the case with ‹a› in *cat, car, care, Cal*, and *cape.* A letter may be part of a digraph that maps onto a pure phoneme or a diphthong, as is the case with the multiple strings that contain ‹o›, ou›, ‹oy›, ‹ow›, ‹oi›. Because the variable mapping works in the opposite direction, spelling any phoneme has multiple options.

The reasons for the inconsistent mappings in English are many, including shifts in pronunciation that were not accompanied by changes in spelling and the related preservation of spellings from the multiple languages that came to make up English – most notably its Germanic roots and substantial Latin and French influences. Its inconsistencies have earned English a place at the opaque end of the transparency dimension among alphabetic orthographies; Finnish, Welsh, and other alphabetic languages anchor the transparent end of the scale. The word "opaque" nicely captures the difficulty of "seeing through" the letters of an English word to its pronunciation. English has also been labeled as orthographically "deep" (Katz & Frost, 1992), a recognition that its spellings sometimes preserve meaning (morphology) at the cost of pronunciation. Thus, although "health" has a deviant pronunciation of the vowel letters ‹ea›, this spelling exposes its morphemic relation to "heal." It would be nice if this trade-off of morphology and pronunciation explained all the inconsistencies in English writing; however, the countless counterexamples of inconsistencies show that it does not.

Nevertheless, English spelling is less chaotic than often assumed. Measures of inconsistencies tend to count the number of context-free mappings of a grapheme, ignoring both the relative frequencies of mappings and constraints on their positions. Kessler (2003) notes this example: In American English the phoneme /a/ is usually spelled ‹o›, as in *lock, rot, flop*, etc. However, when it precedes /r/ in the same syllable, it is spelled with ‹a›, as in *car, start*, and *harp*. Additional constraints come from lexical stress; e.g., ‹ai› is usually pronounced as the tense vowel /ey/ in a stressed syllable (*daisy, regain*); but ‹ai› is pronounced as a lax vowel in an unstressed syllable (*certain*). For this, a reader does not need a rule – just knowledge of English spoken words and their stress patterns. Thus, taking into account the linguistic environment of a letter reduces the mapping uncertainty substantially. This uncertainty is further reduced by weighing the token frequencies of letter–phoneme mappings. For any grapheme some mappings are much more frequent than others. English orthography becomes considerably more consistent when phonotactic constraints of the spoken language and the statistical patterns spellings are taken into account (Kessler, 2003).

2.2.2   Challenges in Learning to Read English

Its very large vocabulary and opaque orthography combine to make English a challenge for learning to read. The learner must come to recognize many words without reliance on consistent connections between letters and phonemes. Cross-language comparisons show that English-speaking children lag behind their peers in learning to decode, compared with children who speak German (Frith, Wimmer, & Landerl, 1998; Wimmer & Goswami, 1994), Spanish and French (Goswami, Gombert, & de Barrera, 1998), Greek (Goswami, Porpodas, & Wheelwright, 1997), and Dutch (Patel, Snowling, & de Jong, 2004). Seymour, Aro, and Erskine (2003)'s comparison of children after one year of instruction found that English children showed only a 40 percent accuracy rate in reading words and nonwords. Most other European samples were above 90 percent and the worst among the remainder, France and Denmark, were much higher on word reading.

Are these documented disadvantages and strategy variations due to English orthography? Many factors differ across national settings in addition to orthography itself – the language, the culture and its emphasis on literacy, variations among children and families, instructional method, and the familiarity of specific words used to test reading. One study, less influenced by these factors, suggests that English may encourage decoding strategies that rely less on phonological information than those used by children learning to read other European languages. Ellis and Hooper (2001) compared two groups of six- and seven-year-olds in Wales. One group began reading instruction in English and the second began reading instruction in Welsh, following the standard practice in Wales in which children learn both Welsh, a very transparent orthography, and English. Errors in oral reading provided a window on decoding strategies: Unlike the close decoding errors of Welsh-reading children, the English-reading children produced errors that suggested non-decoding, whole-word strategies. The English-reading children were twice as likely as the Welsh-reading children to give a null response during a word-reading task, and were nearly twice as likely to make a whole-word substitution error. This result suggests a specific influence of orthographic transparency on the development of reading strategies. Overall, however, reading differences across languages have multiple possible sources and orthography remains only one possibility.

2.3   Reading Difficulties in English

It is useful to consider reading difficulties broadly – taking into account the fact that many children struggle in learning to read outside the special category of dyslexia that is assigned to some of these struggling children. This section provides a brief historical and cultural context for reading difficulties, followed by a characterization of dyslexia.

2.3.1   *Historical and Cultural Context*

Over 120 years have passed since the first report of "congenital word blindness" by Pringle Morgan (1896). This report, and especially the much later paper by Orton (1925), *Word Blindness in School Children*, established the hypothesis of a specific reading disorder with a biological basis. However, understanding this specific disorder can benefit from a broader perspective about the challenges of learning to read faced by many children.

Although a goal of universal literacy is the norm in English-speaking countries, this is a relatively recent development (Resnick & Resnick, 1977). Only when everyone is expected to learn to read does the difficulty in learning become noticed. In the United States, low rates of reading success have led to the publication of several national reports concerning reading difficulties and what to do about them (e.g., Snow, Burns, & Griffin, 1998). Central to this question has been how reading should be taught; should the method be meaning-based or decoding-based? To argue for a meaning-based instruction when the writing is based on phonemes rather than meaning would be laughable for a pure alphabet. However, for English, the inconsistency of grapheme–phoneme mappings, along with other perhaps more important factors, have allowed non-alphabetic, meaning-based teaching to become dominant at various times. The consistency problem has been somewhat exaggerated, as I noted in the previous section. More so than orthography, differing views on child development and the demeaned role of "skills training" in education fed controversies about how to teach reading. A landmark study by Marilyn Adams (1990) reviewed the cultural history and educational prescriptions that gave rise to the great debates about teaching reading. From twentieth-century emphases on meaning-based "Look and Say" reading to vigorous criticisms of this method (Flesch, 1955), the best-way-to-teach-reading dispute has been a fixture on the American educational landscape. The USA does not have a national curriculum, but policy incentives have led to a stronger emphasis on phonemic awareness and decoding since the 2001 National Reading Report (National Institute of Child Health and Development, 2000).

The situation has been similar in the UK, Australia, and New Zealand, although the countries are at different points on the swinging pendulum. Reversing the UK's whole-language approach, Scotland took the lead in moving instruction to a decoding basis, implemented as synthetic phonics and relying on a research-based report by Johnston and Watson (2007). England followed suit and the UK generally now emphasizes phonemic awareness and systematic phonics. New Zealand followed its own path, with a national literacy strategy based on whole-language ideas, and continues to not include an emphasis on decoding instruction. Australia, which, like New Zealand, has not emphasized decoding, appears gradually to be adding phonemic awareness and phonics to its national curriculum.

International comparisons suggest that the English-speaking world has been variable in its reading achievement relative to other countries. The 2016 PIRLS report (Progress in International Reading Literacy Study) shows that Ireland, Northern Ireland, and England are among the top ten countries in overall fourth grade reading scores, with the U.S.15th. However New Zealand is 33rd, behind Australia (21st) and Canada (23rd). This variation shows that factors beyond English orthography are at issue. Heterogeneous populations within and across these English-speaking countries and the economic inequities, language backgrounds, and cultural factors that affect educational opportunities and outcomes are all part of the story. Instruction, which ranges from whole-language approaches in low-scoring countries to various degrees of phonics and decoding in the higher-scoring ones, is another factor.

The level of achievement relative to some meaningful standard is a different, difficult issue. If we take the lowest literacy standard of the PIRLS – the retrieval of explicitly stated information from texts – as a standard, then the failure rates range from 2 to 7 percent among English-speaking countries. In the United States, the NAEP (National Assessment of Educational Progress) attempts to provide a standards-based assessment of reading comprehension every other year. For 2015, NAEP reports that 31 percent of US fourth-grade students failed to achieve the NAEP standard for "basic" text comprehension (Nation's Report Card, 2015). The lesson is that reading achievement assessments are highly variable because of differences in instruments, definitions of standards, and sampling schemes, and other challenges. Thus, although it is useful to ground an assessment of dyslexia, for example its prevalence, on general assessments of reading difficulty, this is challenging.

What cannot be ignored in the English context are the within-nation disparities in reading achievement and educational outcomes. Failures in learning to read occur disproportionately among African American students in the United States, in Australia to its indigenous people, and in England, to its language-minority immigrants. This deep embedding of achievement inside socioeconomic, cultural, and racial factors is important in reading problems and academic achievement outside the traditional medically grounded discussion of dyslexia.

2.3.2   *Identification and Prevalence of Dyslexia*

Dyslexia has always been about biology. From its origins as a brain-based condition in adults (acquired dyslexia) to its diagnosis in children (developmental dyslexia), dyslexia has been assumed to have a neuronal source, and in the case of developmental dyslexia, a genetic origin. What has changed over a hundred-plus years is the science behind the biological hypotheses.

Identifying dyslexia is not yet a matter of brain scans, although such a diagnostic tool is not science fiction. Instead, a longstanding tradition of diagnosis through behavioral assessments continues. Important to the dyslexia community of special educators, parents, and dyslexic children and adults is the specialness of the diagnosis. Dyslexia has been defined generally as a failure to learn to read despite adequate opportunity and, usually, adequate intelligence. However, the International Dyslexia Association adopted a more causally loaded definition in 2002:

Dyslexia is a specific learning disability that is neurobiological in origin ... characterized by difficulties with accurate and/or fluent word recognition and by poor spelling and decoding abilities. These difficulties typically result from a deficit in the phonological component of language that is often unexpected in relation to other cognitive abilities and the provision of effective classroom instruction ...[1]

---

[1] https://dyslexiaida.org/definition-of-dyslexia/. International Dyslexia Association, 2002.

Striking in this definition is its commitment to a deficit in phonology; although the qualifier "typically" allows hedging room, no secondary causes are suggested. Of further interest is that there is no reference to normal or adequate intelligence, which was a primary exclusionary criterion applied to dyslexia in English for many years, at least since (Critchley, 1970). Other contemporary definitions, including that of the British Dyslexia Association and that of the National Institutes of Health, agree: "Dyslexia is a specific learning disability that is neurobiological in origin. It is characterized by difficulties with accurate and/or fluent word recognition and by poor spelling and decoding abilities" (Lyon, Shaywitz, & Shaywitz, 2003, p. 2).

Definitions matter, because access to dedicated remedial services can be legally restricted to children meeting diagnostic criteria. The contemporary definitions permit more flexibility than older definitions that required IQ standards (which varied) to be met.

The prevalence of dyslexia in English is subject to some guesswork because of criteria that are variable and shifting across regions. For the United States, estimates of 6 to 17 percent have been cited, depending on the severity of the reading problem (Fletcher, 2009). For the UK, Canada, Australia, and New Zealand most sources cite 10 percent rates, e.g., the British Dyslexia Association, although the source of these estimates is not clear.[2] The impression is that a single source estimate is being duplicated across all English-speaking countries.

Dyslexia in English occurs more among boys than girls. While concerns have been raised that some of the sex-linked disparity results from statistical and referral biases, the evidence from several careful large sample studies is that dyslexia in English occurs from 1.5 to 2 times more often among boys than girls (Rutter, Caspi, Fergusson et al., 2004). Finally, dyslexia often occurs with other disabilities, including speech disorders, mathematic disability (dyscalculia), and attention deficit disorders. The high rates of these "co-morbidities" undermine the assumption of a prevalent "pure reading disorder" if that is understood as a failure at learning to read or write to the exclusion of all other problems.

2.4   Behavioral and Neurocognitive Evidence

Unknown hundreds of research papers have been published on dyslexia among English-speaking populations in specialty journals (*Annals of Dyslexia, Dyslexia*), and journals of reading research and learning disabilities. What follows is a selective review that provides the larger recurring conclusions.

---

[2] www.bdadyslexia.org.uk/.

2.4.1   Nature of Reading Problems in English

Research with acquired dyslexia patients provides some of the earliest observations of two basic varieties of impaired reading, corresponding to visual-orthographic and phonological dyslexia (Marcel & Patterson, 1977; Shallice et al., 1983). These two varieties reflect the two routes to identifying (naming) English words, one through direct lookup of the word-level orthographic string (the lexical route) and one through conversion of sublexical strings of graphemes to phoneme strings. Thus, some cases of dyslexia could be attributed to failures of the visual-orthographic pathway to retrieve a familiar (even if irregular) word that should be stored in memory; others would result from a failure of grapheme–phoneme conversion to produce the phonology of a regular word.

The evidence came from errors made by patients in reading words aloud. Shallice et al. (1983) reported that patient H.T.R. made pronunciation errors such as *move* to rhyme with *stove* and *gone* to rhyme with *bone*. These indicate a heavy reliance on grapheme–phoneme consistency for words that should be familiar orthographically. H.T.R. also "sounded out" less familiar words such as *circuit*, producing /kurkut/, *colonel*, producing /kalanul/, and *sword*, producing /swo:rd/. For this patient, these errors reflected a general deterioration of memory functions that forced her to sound out words rather than retrieving their pronunciation from memory based on their visual-orthographic form.

Patterson and Marcel (1977) reported on two patients who showed the opposite pattern: an intact visual-orthographic pathway, but a low functionality of the grapheme–phoneme conversion pathway. Thus, D.E. produced "near-miss" whole words, such as "organ" for *origin* and "patient" for *patent* and generally did better for words of high ("marriage") rather than low imageability, which can be considered a stand-in for semantic support for word identification.

These early reports on adults who had suffered brain lesions provided a way to link dyslexia, a severe difficulty in reading, to ideas about the process of reading words. Normal word reading in English could occur along two pathways that were differentially effective for words with regular spellings and words with irregular spellings, and differentially used according to the strength of orthographic memory. Word reading could be disrupted by weakened connections along either pathway. These pathways are variably described but correspond to a direct retrieval of a word identity based on its visual-orthographic form or its indirect assembly from grapheme–phoneme conversion.

2.4.1.1   From Acquired to Developmental Dyslexia   It was natural to extrapolate results from brain-injured patients to children learning to read. They too could be expected to show one or the other of the two forms of impairments and be subtyped accordingly. Castles and Coltheart (1993), presenting comparisons

of dyslexic and non-dyslexic children, argued that developmental dyslexia includes these complementary subtypes, one an impairment to the lexical route and the other to the sublexical route. These were referred to as surface and phonological dyslexia, respectively, consistent with descriptors from patient studies. The bases for this subtyping were the discrepancies between children's performance in reading words with irregular grapheme–phoneme correspondences (also termed "exception words"), which require the lexical route, and nonwords, which require the sublexical route. Whereas performances on words and nonwords were highly correlated among normal-developing children, this was not the case for the dyslexic sample of Castles and Coltheart: Forty-five of the fifty-three dyslexics showed a significant dis-association between exception word and nonword performance. Of these, twenty-nine showed the phonological dyslexia profile: Their nonword reading did not reach the level predicted by their exception-word reading. Sixteen showed the surface-dyslexia pattern, with their exception-word reading failing to reach the level predicted by their nonword reading. These disassociations were found even when age was taken into account. Important in this study and in many others is the higher prevalence of phonological dyslexia relative to surface dyslexia. Finally, thirty-two of the fifty-two children were low on both nonwords and irregular words, a "mixed" pattern, but twenty-seven were assigned to one or the other disassociation patterns because they were higher on one or the other test.

2.4.1.2 Criteria for Subtyping   Subtyping based on dissociation of exception word and nonword reading seemed compelling, showing a theory-based diagnosis in both acquired dyslexia and developmental dyslexia. However, there is reason to consider this criterion more critically, as did Manis, Seidenberg, Doi, McBride-Chang, and Petersen (1996). Their study followed the approach of Castles and Coltheart (1993) and found the same two profiles. They also found that most of the dyslexic children showed impaired reading of both exception and nonwords. Because this pattern was also found by Castles and Coltheart, it seems clear that, with this diagnostic approach, most dyslexics show problems in both nonwords and exception words. The number of cases in which a child is in the normal range on one type and below normal on the other appears smaller: eighteen of fifty-three in Castles and Coltheart (1993) and ten of fifty-one in Manis et al. (1996).

The interpretation of a dissociation pattern when children are below normal on both exception words and nonwords is not straightforward, as Manis et al. argued. Because (1) normal-developing readers also show discrepancies between nonword and exception-word reading, and (2) any individual test result includes measurement error, classification based on these single-test discrepancy scores can be misleading. One approach to the first problem has been to use reading level rather than age-matched controls (Bryant & Impey, 1983). Thus a dyslexic is compared with a younger child whose score on a test of word reading is the same as that of the dyslexic. This approach has its own problems, however, because it implies the two groups, if they differ, will have to differ on nonword reading because they are matched on word reading, as Coltheart (1987) pointed out. An alternative approach is to test the subtyping diagnosis against independent tests that are theoretically sensitive to the process for which a deficit is hypothesized. Thus, a phonological dyslexic should do poorly on phonemic awareness or some other phonology-dependent task and a surface dyslexic should do poorly on test of orthographic recognition. Manis et al. (1996) designed such independent tasks and confirmed the validity of the two profiles.

2.4.2   Underlying Causes of Reading Problems in English

2.4.2.1   Cause of Disassociated Deficits   The two complementary profiles seem to have validity, but the cause of the disassociated deficits is another question. Whereas the original interpretation is that the two deficits reflect impairments to one or the other route to word reading, there are other possibilities. One is that surface dyslexia does not result from an impaired lexical route, but instead from a developmental delay. Manis et al. (1996) observed that the performance of children classified as surface dyslexics based on better nonword reading than exception-word reading was similar to that of normal-developing, but younger, readers. They argued, accordingly, that the surface dyslexic pattern reflects a general delay in acquiring readings skills. The delay itself could reflect an underlying deficit in making use of reading experience. Put another way, delay reflects experience that is inadequate to compensate for the deficit. On either framing, it implies that some children with the surface-dyslexia profile, but with enough reading experience, should show gains in reading. Not all cases of surface dyslexia can be attributed to a general delay, but many can. Fourteen of the fifteen surface dyslexics in Manis et al. (1996) showed discrepancy profiles that overlapped with those of normal-developing younger readers. A pure deficit specific to orthography appears to be real but very rare. Finally, it is important to emphasize that most surface dyslexics are also worse than normal-developing children on regular words and nonwords. Thus difficulties in learning to recognize words, including exception words, can be imposed by phonological problems that limit the benefit of experience.

The complementary profiles in exception and nonword reading could be explained as a single-cause model that places phonological problems at the center. Such a model might not be plausible for a pure case of surface dyslexia, but the evidence reviewed above showed phonological problems for most children with the surface profile. Manis et al. (1996) argued that the connectionist learning model of Seidenberg and McClelland (1989) can account for the dual impairments on exception words and nonwords. It does so by assuming degraded phonological representations, which negatively affect the pronunciation of all letter strings, but those of nonwords more than words. This is because, like the child, the model is exposed to real words and must learn to generalize pronunciation patterns to apply to nonwords as they are experienced for the first time. Exception words, given some experience with atypical spelling patterns and mild phonological degrading, will be read reasonably well, at an intermediate level between regular words and nonwords. However, and ironically, a severe phonological deficit severely impairs exception-word reading. A model reported in Harm and Seidenberg (1999) carried this demonstration further by simulating the effects of pre-literate phonological processes on the reading system that is acquired.

2.4.2.2 The Ascendance of the Phonological Deficit Hypothesis

An overwhelming consensus across many behavioral studies points to phonological problems as central to dyslexia. These results do not depend solely on carefully defined small sample studies of the kind reviewed above. Rack, Snowling, and Olson (1992) reviewed a number of studies that together involved over 400 children, which led them to conclude that most dyslexic children have phonological decoding skills that are below what is expected according to their overall word-recognition ability. In contrast to subtyping approaches, their evidence suggested a continuum of the phonological decoding skill.

What became known as the phonological deficit hypothesis emerged with growing evidence over at least thirty years, getting boosts from research on the development of syllabic and phonemic awareness and its relation to reading acquisition (Liberman et al., 1974), a critique of visual-deficit hypotheses (Vellutino, 1981), and evidence that training on phonemic awareness improved the reading of low-achieving children (Bradley & Bryant, 1983). The evidence grew to include a broader range of phonological processing and memory deficits (Brady & Shankweiler, 1991; Snowling, Stackhouse, & Rack, 1986) and to connect "garden-variety" low-skill readers with dyslexics, both of whom seem to have a core phonological deficit with varying adaptations (Stanovich, 1988). Later adding force to this hypothesis is a review of sixteen acquired-dyslexic patient studies by Ramus (2003), who concluded that, although some patients had visual, cerebellar, or auditory problems, all sixteen showed a phonological deficit.

Brain-imaging studies provide results that converge with this picture. Reading problems are associated with failure to engage the left-hemisphere language areas during reading (Simos et al., 2007, Shaywitz et al., 2004; Turkeltaub et al., 2003), as predicted by Orton. The primacy of a phonological deficit does not mean that there are no other causes of dyslexia. Hypotheses of visual deficits continued throughout this period (e.g., Livingstone et al., 1991; Stein & Walsh, 1997) and the possibility of rare visual anomalies remains open. However, the phonological deficit hypothesis – that dyslexia specifically and low reading skill generally are caused by problems in phonological processing – has accumulated sufficient evidence and advocates that it is now the standard theory.

2.4.2.3 Beyond Phonology: Automatized Naming

There is one other prominent and heavily researched factor, rapid auto-matized naming (RAN). This is assessed through digits, pictures, or colors that are presented in grouped displays for rapid serial naming of each stimulus; from its development by Denckla and Rudel (1976) onward, RAN has proved to be a strong correlate of reading development and reading difficulties (Wolf, 1991; Norton & Wolf, 2011). When measured concurrently with reading, RAN, as well as phonological awareness, is highly correlated with reading skill. More important is RAN's ability to be predictively diagnostic of reading problems. Two longitudinal studies drew different conclusions about the role of RAN in predicting children's reading development. Scarborough (1998) found that RAN scores in the second grade did not predict reading outcomes at eighth grade for children who had been at normal reading level in second grade; their eighth-grade reading was well predicted by their second-grade reading. However, the reading and spelling outcomes at eighth grade for children who had been delayed in reading at second grade were well predicted by RAN. Torgesen et al. (1997) found a different pattern in a longitudinal study of second-to-fourth and third-to-fifth grades. The RAN indicator was predictive of children's reading two years later only if their early reading levels were ignored. When earlier reading levels were included, RAN was no longer predictive – although phonological awareness remained a unique predictor. Scarborough (1998), in explaining the contrasting results, pointed to the key role played by actual reading achievement, which in turn is related to individual differences among samples, and perhaps instruction; that is, the predictive value of RAN may emerge only when previous reading achieve-ment does not predict future reading achievement.

Since these studies, the evidence for the significance of RAN has accumu-lated (Norton & Wolf, 2011). Studies, including a large-sample longitudinal study of kindergarten through second grade by Schatschneider et al. (2004), show that RAN joins phonological awareness (and phonological processing) and letter naming as the most consistent predictors of future reading difficulty in English. Two questions about the role of RAN have been challenging. One is its relation to phonological processing. On one view, rapid naming is tapping a phonological process because it requires the retrieval of phonological codes (Torgesen et al., 1997). However, this is true of almost any language process, and it is not obvious that the phonological component is the dominant challenge in the RAN task, compared with automatic retrieval in the context of attention control and eye movements. A metanalysis by Swanson et al. (2003) concluded that the correlation between phonological awareness and RAN was moderate, overall $r = 0.38$.

The other question about RAN is its processing significance, as opposed to its correlational significance. The significance of phonological awareness is predicated on the relationship between written units and the spoken units of a language. In the case of RAN, the connection is less clear or at least more complex. It does not seem to be a stand-in for general processing speed, but may reflect connections between visual and speech circuits in the brain, as argued by Norton and Wolf (2011). At a general level, RAN's significance may be characterized as an indicator of fluency, the rapid access, retrieval, and integration of visual and linguistic information that make up the recurring cognitive processes of skilled reading. Still, how to apply this description to the failure to read a single word or nonword, which is diagnostic for dyslexia, is not straightforward. Indeed, Norton and Wolf (2011) argue that RAN should be most related to reading fluency, broadly conceived, beyond speed of word retrieval. Both phonological awareness and rapid automatized naming can be sources of reading difficulty for a child, according to the double-deficit hypothesis (DDH) of Wolf and Bowers (1999). DDH children show the most severe reading problems.

2.4.3   The Search for Deeper Causes

The question becomes, what exactly is the nature of the phonological deficit? Or the RAN deficit? The search for underlying causes – described in cognitive or neural terms – has led to a number of proposals and observations concerning the phonological system (Berent et al., 2012; Goswami, 2011; Ramus, 2008; Serniclaes, 2004; Tallal, 2004). Serniclaes (2004) reported that dyslexics are overly sensitive to nonsystematic variation in the speech signal and thus have problems categorizing speech input into phoneme categories; Berent et al. (2012) found that (Hebrew) adult dyslexics had speech discrimination problems (e.g., pa/ba) but no problems at the level of the phonological grammar, e.g., distinguishing illegal duplication in nonwords (*titug*) from legal duplication (*gitut*). Ramus (2008) concluded that dyslexics do not suffer from impaired phonological *representations*; rather their *access* to these representations is limited in tasks that make demands on cognitive resources.

The search for an explanation of a phonological deficit has led to both of the two basic dimensions of acoustic input. Tallal (2004) pointed to a temporal processing disorder, a failure to detect rapid changes in frequency, which would affect the ability to use the rapid frequency shifts that distinguish among stop consonants. This hypothesis has generated research and led to remediation programs. Also in the acoustic domain, Goswami (2011), based on a time-sampling speech-perception framework, proposed that the ability to perceive amplitude modulation, specifically the rise time to the vocalic peak of a syllable, is deficient in dyslexics. Goswami et al. (2012) found that dyslexic 11-year-olds required twice the voice rise time difference (100 ms) to perceive a difference as did reading-level control children (50 ms). The bigger idea is that the ability to detect amplitude shifts is important in developing phonological representations and can lead to the broader phonological problems that are central to dyslexia.

These ideas differ in their focus but most seem to share the assumption that the cause of a phonological deficit – or for that matter any deficit – can be sought in general perceptual/cognitive levels closer to neural mechanisms. The brief temporal dynamics of acoustic inputs, their rapid amplitude and frequency shifts, are attractive at this level. Although each of these hypotheses has accumulated evidence in its favor, it is unclear whether any one of them captures a substantial share of the etiology of dyslexia. One might summarize the state of affairs as showing clear evidence for two markers of dyslexia, one reflecting problems in the phonological system with clear evidence for causal status; and one reflecting problems with the automatized integration of perceptual, attention, and memory retrieval processes with less clear causal status.

The search for deeper or more general explanations has led to multiple potential causes at the cognitive, perceptual, and neural levels. Much of this effort can be characterized as a reductionist approach to explanation. Terms grounded in behavioral operations (lack of phonemic awareness, poor rapid naming) are abandoned as causal terms: first in favor of terms of cognitive theory (poor phonological representations, slow memory access and retrieval); then in psychophysical terms (poor rise time sensitivity, poor temporal dynamics sensitivity); then in large-grain neuroanatomy terms (lack of hemisphere lateralization of reading, anomalies in visual word form area); and then to genetic, biochemical, and fine-grain neurodevelopmental (neuronal migration) explanations. Viewed this way, the proliferation of causes of dyslexia is less diffuse than it may seem, especially when these different levels of analysis can be connected.

2.5   Intervention

Interventions for struggling readers and for younger children at risk for reading problems have been developed that are consistent with the causes of dyslexia identified through research. Increasingly, there is evidence to support the principles underlying some of these interventions, including both behavioral and neuroimaging studies. (The US Institute for Education Sciences maintains a periodically updated *What Works Clearing House* (ies.ed.gov) to provide research outcomes for literacy interventions. Of seventy listed in 2016, twelve were intended for children with learning disabilities.) Because of evidence that risk for reading failure can be observed prior to schooling, there has been a strong emphasis on early interventions in kindergarten and first grade. However, identification of individual children who will turn out to struggle in reading after instruction is underway is a low-reliability effort, especially given the expense of extensive screening of all children.

2.5.1   Response to Intervention (RTI)

An alternative approach is to use how an individual child responds to classroom instruction to determine whether specific interventions are needed. This RTI framework requires that the classroom instruction follow sound, evidence-based principles that include some focus on direct instruction in decoding. A child who shows signs of not learning from such instruction then receives specifically tailored instruction. With variation, the principle is to offer a child support early, as soon as signs of struggling are present – no dyslexia diagnosis needed. Instead, this framework allows increasingly intense interventions as needed. Vaughn, Denton, and Fletcher (2010), in reviewing some of the ways to make interventions sufficient for such children, emphasized the importance of explicit instruction in decoding, with active student engagement and extended opportunities to practice skills with teacher support and feedback. Interestingly, a good response to intervention may be predictable from the state of the brain's reading network prior to the intervention (Rezaie et al., 2011). For Rezaie et al.'s struggling middle-school readers, activation in left middle, superior temporal, and ventral occipital temporal regions prior to intervention predicted their gains in reading a year after the intervention.

In the UK, where there is a national curriculum that emphasizes phonics, RTI is not common. Data for individual children are routinely available, however, and Snowling (2015) reports that teachers' ratings of students on a national assessment instrument, the Early Years Foundation Stage Profile (EYFSP), at age 5 predicts literacy attainment two years after. In Australia and especially New Zealand, the primary intervention is Reading Recovery, an individualized program that is not focused on phonology and decoding. Applied in second grade, the use of the program awaits failure in learning to read. A study of a scale-up of Reading Recovery in the United States over four years found that the program produced gains in reading relative to untreated controls (May et al., 2016); however, questions were raised about the study, including its elimination of the lowest achieving students (Chapman & Tunmer, 2016). Additionally, comparisons with other interventions are lacking and it is certain that doing nothing, as in an untreated control, is seldom a good intervention. The relative expense associated with the program on a per-child basis further highlights the need for comparisons with other programs.

2.5.2 Phonology-Centered Interventions

The strong evidence for phonological deficits is consistent with efforts to support struggling readers' awareness of phonology, their learning of English grapheme–phoneme correspondences, and their ability to read words using orthography-to-phonology mappings. A large number of interventions have been developed and a fair number have been studied for their effectiveness.

A sound research strategy is to compare programs with control treatments that allow comparable levels of special attention rather than with untreated control groups (e.g., Lovett, Steinbach, & Frijters, 2000). Especially useful are comparisons of interventions developed from relevant theories. For young children beginning reading instruction, interventions based on spoken language and decoding are obvious choices. Children who enter school with poorly developed language skills are at high risk for dyslexia. For such children, Bowyer-Crane et al. (2008) compared an intervention with a focus on phonology and decoding with one designed to improve spoken language skills. After twenty weeks in one or the other program, children in the phonology and decoding program showed and maintained higher gains in phonemic awareness, reading, and spelling than those in the language program, with many being raised to the typical reading levels.

Torgesen (2005) reviewed eight studies using phonology and decoding interventions with severely disabled children (mainly aged 8–10, with one study that included eighth grade). Especially important across interventions is the consistency of gains in phonemic coding and word identification, as modeled in growth rates that take into account the number of hours in the intervention. Torgesen's conclusion makes the important point clearly: "Even children with severe difficulties in the phonological domain can acquire productive and generative phonemic decoding skills if they are taught with intensity and skill" (2005, p. 110). Interventions based on phonology and decoding have also produced changes in the brain's left-hemisphere reading network, including the inferior frontal gyrus, middle temporal gyrus (Shaywitz et al., 2004), and left-temporal parietal regions (Simos et al., 2007). Further, Simos et al. found that only children who showed these left-hemisphere changes benefited from their intervention, which included first a phonological focus and then rapid word recognition practice.

The diagnostic status of children undergoing interventions adds another issue. Is a phonological intervention effective for children who also show a deficit in rapid naming, thus having a double deficit (Wolf & Bowers, 1999)? Lovett et al. (2000) implemented a comparison of interventions: phonological training, which included spoken language and direct instruction in decoding, and a metacognitive strategy program, which draws attention to four different word-identification strategies centered on phonological and orthographic analyses (WIST, Word Identification Strategy Training.) The results showed the effectiveness of these two phonologically based programs. Even the most disabled readers, including those with the double-deficit diagnosis, showed gains on speech and reading assessments of phonological processes. Children who had only a RAN deficit showed gains in word-reading accuracy and phonological processes, but not in naming times, demonstrating that instruction can be designed to improve the skills it teaches, but not necessarily something only related to what it teaches. A program (RAVE-O) that directly addresses the rapid naming deficit was designed by Wolf, Miller, and Donnelly (2000) to be implemented along with phonologically based programs. Morris et al. (2010) report positive results for combining RAVE-O with either of the two interventions of Lovett et al. (2000). Quite aside from its effectiveness, it is encouraging to see the combining of theoretically motivated interventions. Another example of a multi-component program that includes phonology (Fast ForWord) was developed from the temporal processing disorder hypothesis (Tallal, 2004). One of the earliest imaging studies of intervention effects on the brain showed gains for 8–12-year-old dyslexic children (Temple et al., 2003).

2.5.3   Intervention Challenges

A summary of results can mask the interpretative challenges that face intervention research. Variations in instructional delivery factors (teachers, school ecologies), duration of the study, deficit severity under study, and specific reading components targeted by interventions all challenge the generalizations that can be drawn from studies(Lyon & Moats, 1997). One of special importance is the relation between severity and prior instruction. A child with a mild disability who has had weak instruction, when tested, will show a larger reading impairment than a child of comparable disability who has received better instruction. In fact, as observed by Torgesen (2005), really effective instruction might make this child undetectable as reading disabled and would block him or her from the intervention study. Meanwhile, the child who shows a disability even with good instruction is more likely to have a serious disability. Any study of children diagnosed with reading failure following instruction needs to consider how to take this into account. Otherwise, a formula for a confirmatory outcome is to find a classroom with poor instruction.

2.6   Discussion and Conclusion

English offers a special suitability for the study of reading problems in the context of cross-language comparisons. Although English is an outlier among alphabetic orthographies to some extent (Share, 2008), it is not clear what a typical language or writing system is. The world has more Mandarin speakers (as a first language) than any other, so on a token speaker basis, maybe Chinese is more typical. With second-language speakers added, Chinese and English are comparable, both exceeding all other languages. So maybe the typical language and writing system is the average of Chinese and English, something interesting to consider.

English maps alphabetically but has enough multi-grain units to also mimic morphological mapping. Its spelling–phoneme mappings are inconsistent. International comparisons show slower development of decoding skill in English-speaking children, which may or not be caused by the language's inconsistent mappings. It is also clear that its inconsistency is considerably less noticeable when larger units are taken into account. Its real challenge for literacy may be its large vocabulary, which provides a multiplier effect on its inconsistencies, as well as being one cause of them. However, dyslexia is not caused by English orthography. The factors that contribute to problems in reading English contribute to those in alphabetic reading generally.

The development of dual-route theories of reading and, correspondingly, of dual-route theories of reading failure, is closely related to English orthography. Observations of errors implicated complementary weaknesses in reading pathways, a lexical basis and a sublexical (phonological basis) for dyslexia. Problems with irregular words (implicating whole-word retrieval) and non-words (implicating sublexical phonology) tend to co-occur in English dyslexia, although patterns of dissociation between the two problems have been verified. However, problems in the lexical route are often a matter of delayed reading skill or reading experience that has limited the learner's opportunities to experience the full range of English exception words and unusual spelling patterns. Learning models in the connectionist tradition are able to simulate both lexical and sublexical patterns of reading disability through a single learning mechanism that builds on phonological knowledge.

Indeed, phonological problems are at the core of reading disability, and much of recent theory and research has been directed at trying to explain what causes those problems. At least partly independent from phonological problems is the automatization of serial naming. It is possible that the two problems are linked to both shared and distinct components of reading, decoding, and fluency.

Many successful interventions have been developed, influenced by the research that shows phonological deficits as the major source of reading problems. The effectiveness of some of these interventions has been demonstrated in neuroimaging studies as well as behavioral studies. Most promising may be multi-component interventions in which each component has specific evidence linking it to reading problems.

References

Adams, M. J. (1990). *Beginning to read: Thinking and learning about print*. Cambridge, MA: MIT Press.

Berent, I., Vaknin-Nusbaum, V., Balaban, E., & Galaburda, A. M. (2012). Dyslexia impairs speech recognition but can spare phonological competence. *PLoS One, 7*, e44875.

Berlin, R. (1887). *Eine Besondere Art der Wortblindheit (Dyslexie)*. Wiesbaden: J. F. Bergmann.

Bowyer-Crane, C., Snowling, M. J., Duff, F. J. et al. (2008). Improving early language and literacy skills: Differential effects of an oral language versus a phonology with reading intervention. *Journal of Child Psychology & Psychiatry, 49*(4), 422–432.

Bradley, L., & Bryant, P. E. (1983). Categorizing sounds and learning to read: A causal connection. *Nature, 301*, 419–421.

Brady, S., & Shankweiler, D. (Eds.) (1991). *Phonological processes in literacy: A tribute to Isabelle Y. Liberman*. Hillsdale, NJ: Erlbaum.

Bryant, P. E., & Impey, L. (1986). The similarities between normal readers and developmental and acquired dyslexics. *Cognition, 24*, 121–137.

Castles, A., & Coltheart, M. (1993). Varieties of developmental dyslexia. *Cognition, 47*, 149–180.

Chapman, J. W., & Tunmer, W. E. (2016). Is Reading Recovery an effective intervention for students with reading difficulties? A critique of the i3 scale-up study. *Reading Psychology, 37*(7), 1025–1042.

Coltheart, M. (1978). Lexical access in simple reading tasks. In G. Underwood (Ed.), *Strategies of information processing* (pp. 151–216). New York: Academic Press.

Coltheart, M. (1987). Varieties of developmental dyslexia: A comment on Bryant and Impey. *Cognition, 27*, 97–101.

Coltheart, M., Curtis, B., Atkins, P., & Haller, M. (1993). Models of reading aloud: Dual-route and parallel-distributed processing approaches. *Psychological Review, 100*, 589–608.

Critchley, M. (1970). *The dyslexic child*. London: Heinemann Medical Books.

Denckla, M. B., & Rudel, R. G. (1976). Rapid automatized naming (R.A.N.): Dyslexia differentiated from other learning disabilities. *Neuropsychologia, 14*, 471–479.

Ellis, N. C., & Hooper, A. M. (2001). Why learning to read is easier in Welsh than in English: Orthographic transparency effects evinced with frequency-matched tests. *Applied Psycholinguistics, 22*, 571–599.

Flesch, R. (1955). *Why Johnnie can't read: And what you can do about it*. New York: Harper & Brothers.

Fletcher, J. M. (2009). Dyslexia: The evolution of a scientific concept. *Journal of the International Neuropsychological Society, 15*, 501–508.

Frith, U., Wimmer, H., & Landerl, K. (1998). Differences in phonological recoding in German- and English-speaking children. *Scientific Studies of Reading, 2*, 31–54.

Geudens, A., & Sandra, D. (2003). Beyond implicit phonological knowledge: No support for an onset-rime structure in children's explicit phonological awareness. *Journal of Memory and Language, 49*, 157–182.

Goswami, U. (2011). A temporal sampling framework for developmental dyslexia. *Trends in Cognitive Sciences, 15*(1), 3–10.

Goswami, U., & Bryant, P. (1990). *Phonological skills and learning to read.* London: Erlbaum.

Goswami, U., Gombert, J., & de Barrera, F. (1998). Children's orthographic representation and linguistic transparency: Nonsense word reading in English, French and Spanish. *Applied Psycholinguistics, 19*, 19–52.

Goswami, U., Huss, M., Mead, N., Fosker, T., & Verney, J. P. (2012). Perception of patterns of musical beat distribution in phonological developmental dyslexia: Significant longitudinal relations with word reading and reading comprehension. *Cortex, 49*(5), 1363–1376.

Goswami, U., Porpodas, C., & Wheelwright, S. (1997). Children's orthographic representations in English and Greek. *European Journal of Psychology of Education, 12*(3), 273–292.

Harm, M. W., & Seidenberg, M. S. (1999). Phonology, reading acquisition, and dyslexia: Insights from connectionist models. *Psychological Review, 106*(3), 491–528.

Hay, J., & Bauer, L. (2007). Phoneme inventory size and population size. *Language, 83*, 388–400.

Hinshelwood, J. (1917). *Congenital word blindness.* London: H K. Lewis & Co.

Johnston, R., & Watson, J. (2007). *Teaching synthetic phonics.* Exeter, UK: Learning Matters.

Katz, L., & Frost, R. (1992). Reading in different orthographies: The orthographic depth hypothesis. In R. Frost & L. Katz (Eds.), *Orthography, phonology, morphology, and meaning* (pp. 67–84). Amsterdam: Elsevier North Holland Press.

Kessler, B. (2003). Is English spelling chaotic? Misconceptions concerning its irregularity. *Reading Psychology, 24*, 267–289.

Kessler, B., & Treiman, R. (1997). Syllable structure and the distribution of phonemes in English syllables. *Journal of Memory and Language, 37*(3), 295–311.

Kussmaul, A. (1877). Diseases of the nervous system and disturbances of speech. In H. von Ziemssen (Ed.), *Cylopedia of the practice of medicine* (pp. 770–778). New York: William Wood.

Liberman, I. Y., Shankweiler, D., Fischer, F. W., & Carter, B. (1974). Explicit syllable and phoneme segmentation in the young child. *Journal of Experimental Child Psychology, 18*(2) 201–212.

Livingstone, M. S., Rosen, G. D., Drislane, F. W., & Galaburda, A. M. (1991). Physiological and anatomical evidence for a magnocellular defect in developmental dyslexia. *Proceedings of the National Academy of Sciences, 88*(18), 7943–7947.

Lovett, M. W., Steinbach, K. A., & Frijters, J. C. (2000). Remediating the core deficits of developmental reading disability: A double-deficit perspective. *Journal of Learning Disabilities, 33*(4), 334–358.

Lyon, G. R., & Moats, L. C. (1997). Critical conceptual and methodological considerations in reading intervention research. *Journal of Learning Disabilities, 30*, 578–588.

Lyon, G. R., Shaywitz, S. E., & Shaywitz, B. A. (2003). A definition of dyslexia. *Annals of Dyslexia, 53*, 1–14.

Manis, F. R., Seidenberg, M. S., Doi, L. M., McBride-Chang, C., & Petersen, A. (1996). On the bases of two subtypes of developmental dyslexia. *Cognition, 58*(2), 157–195.

May, H., Sirinides, P. M., Gray, A., & Goldsworthy, H. (2016). Reading Recovery: An Evaluation of the Four-Year i3 Scale-Up. Philadelphia: Consortium for Policy Research in Education. http://repository.upenn.edu/cpre_researchreports/81

Morris, R. D., Lovett, M. W., Wolf, M. et al. (2010). Multiple-component remediation for developmental reading disabilities: IQ, socioeconomic status, and race as factors in remedial outcomes. *Journal of Learning Disabilities, 45*(2), 99–127.

Mullis, I. V. S., Martin, M. O., Foy, P., & Drucker, K. T. (2012). *PIRLS 2011 International Results in Reading.* Chestnut Hill, MA: TIMSS & PIRLS International Study Center, Boston College.

National Institute of Child Health and Development. (2000). Report of the National Reading Panel. *Teaching children to read: An evidence-based assessment of the scientific research literature on reading and its implications for reading instruction:* Reports of the subgroups. NIH Publication No. 00–4754. Washington, DC: US Government Printing Office. www.nichd.nih.gov/sites/default/files/publications/pubs/nrp/Documents/report.pdf.

Nation's Report Card (2015). National achievement level results. Online source. *Nation's Report Card.* www.nationsreportcard.gov/reading_math_2015/.

Norton, E. S., & Wolf, M. (2011). Rapid automatized naming (RAN) and reading fluency: Implications for understanding and treatment of reading disabilities. *Annual Review of Psychology, 63,* 427–452.

Orton, S. (1925). Word blindness in school children. *Archives of Neurology and Psychiatry, 14,* 581–615.

Orton, S. T. (1929). The three levels of cortical elaboration to certain psychiatric symptoms. *American Journal of Psychiatry, 8,* 647–659.

Patel, T. K., Snowling, M. J., & de Jong, P. F. (2004). A cross-linguistic comparison of children learning to read in English and Dutch. *Journal of Educational Psychology, 96*(4), 785–797.

Patterson, K. E., & Marcel, A. J. (1977). Aphasia, dyslexia and the phonological coding of written words. *Quarterly Journal of Experimental Psychology, 29*(2), 307–318.

Perfetti, C. A., & Harris, L. (2017). Learning to read English. In L. Verhoeven & C. A. Perfetti (Eds.), *Learning to read across languages and writing systems* (pp. 347–370). Cambridge, UK: Cambridge University Press.

Pringle Morgan, W. (1896). A case of congenital word blindness. *British Medical Journal, 2,* 1378.

Rack, J. P., Snowling, M. J., & Olson, R. K. (1992). The nonword reading deficit in developmental dyslexia: A review. *Reading Research Quarterly, 27*(1), 29–53.

Ramus. F. (2003). Developmental dyslexia: Specific phonological deficit or general sensorimotor dysfunction*? Current Opinion in Neurobiology, 13,* 212–218.

Ramus, F., Rosen, S, Dakin, S. C. et al. (2003). Theories of developmental dyslexia: Insights from a multiple case study of dyslexic adults, *Brain, 126*(1), 841–865.

Ramus, F., & Szenkovits,G. (2008). What phonological deficit? *Quarterly Journal of Experimental Psychology, 61*(1), 129–141.

Resnick, D., & Resnick, L. (1977). The nature of literacy: An historical exploration. *Harvard Educational Review, 47*(3), 370–385.

Rezaie, R., Simos, P. G., Fletcher, J. M. et al. (2011). Temporo-parietal brain activity as a longitudinal predictor of response to educational interventions among middle school struggling readers. *Journal of the International Neuropsychological Society*, *17*, 875–885.

Rutter, M., Caspi, A., Fergusson, D. et al. (2004). Sex differences in developmental reading disability: New findings from 4 epidemiological studies. *The Journal of the American Medical Association*, *291*, 2007–2012.

Scarborough, H. S. (1998). Predicting the future achievement of second graders with reading disabilities: Contributions of phonemic awareness, verbal memory, rapid naming, and IQ. *Annals of Dyslexia*, *48*, 115–136.

Schatschneider, C., Fletcher, J. M., Francis, D. J., Carlson, C. D., & Foorman, B. R. (2004). Kindergarten prediction of reading skills: A longitudinal comparative analysis. *Journal of Educational Psychology*, *96*(2), 265–282.

Seidenberg, M. S., & McClelland, J. L. (1989). A distributed, developmental model of word recognition and naming. *Psychological Review*, *96*, 523–568.

Serniclaes, W., Van Heghe, S., Mousty, P., Carré, R., & Sprenger-Charolles, L. (2004). Allophonic mode of speech perception in dyslexia. *Journal of Experimental Child Psychology*, *87*, 336–361.

Seymour, P. H. K., Aro, M., & Erskine, J. M. (2003). Foundation literacy acquisition in European orthographies. *British Journal of Psychology*, *94*(2), 143–174.

Shallice, T., Warrington, E. K., & McCarthy, R. (1983). Reading without semantics. *The Quarterly Journal of Experimental Psychology Section A*, *35*(1), 111–138.

Share, D. L. (2008). On the anglocentricities of current reading research and the practice: The perils of overreliance on an 'outlier' orthography. *Psychological Bulletin*, *134*, 584–615.

Shaywitz, B. A., Shaywitz, S. E., Blachman, B. A. et al. (2004). Development of left occipito-temporal systems for skilled reading in children after a phonologically-based intervention. *Biological Psychiatry*, *55*(9), 926–933.

Simos, P. G., Fletcher, J. M. Sarkari, S. et al. (2007). Altering the brain circuits for reading through intervention: A magnetic source imaging study. *Neuropsychology*, *21*(4), 485–496.

Snow, C. E., Burns, M. S., & Griffin, P. (Eds.) (1998). *Preventing reading difficulties in young children*. Washington, DC: National Academic Press.

Snowling, M. J. (2015). The dyslexia debate. *Child and Adolescent Mental Health*, *20*, 127–128.

Snowling, M. J., Stackhouse, J., & Rack, J. P. (1986). Phonological dyslexia and dysgraphia: A developmental analysis. *Cognitive Neuropsychology*, *3*, 309–339.

Stanovich, K. E. (1988). Explaining the differences between the dyslexic and the garden-variety poor reader: The phonological-core variable-difference model. *Journal of Learning Disabilities*, *21*(10), 590–604.

Stein, J., & Walsh, V. (1997). To see but not to read: The magnocellular theory of dyslexia. *Trends in Neuroscience*, *20*(4), 147–152.

Swanson, H. L., Trainin, G., Necoechea, D. M., & Hammill, D. D. (2003). Rapid naming, phonological awareness, and reading: A meta-analysis of the correlation evidence. *Review of Educational Research*, *73*, 407–440.

Tallal, P. (2004). Improving language and literacy is a matter of time. *Nature Reviews Neuroscience*, *5*, 721–728.

Temple, E., Deutsch, G. K., Poldrack, R. A. et al. (2003). Neural deficits in children with dyslexia ameliorated by behavioral remediation: Evidence from functional MRI. *Proceedings of the National Academy of Sciences, 100*(5), 2860–2865.

Torgesen J. (2005). Remedial interventions for students with dyslexia: National goals and current accomplishments. In S. O. Richardson & J. Gilger (Eds.), *Research-based education and intervention: What we need to know*. Baltimore, MD: International Dyslexia Association.

Torgesen, J. K., Wagner, R. K., Rashotte, C. A., Burgess, S., & Hecht, S. (1997). Contributions of phonological awareness and rapid automatic naming ability to the growth of word-reading skills in second-to fifth-grade children. *Scientific Studies of Reading, 1*(2), 161–195.

Turkeltaub, P. E., Gareau, L., Flowers, D. L., Zeffiro, T. A., & Eden, G. F. (2003). Development of neural mechanisms for reading. *Nature Neuroscience, 6*, 767–773.

Vaughan, S., Denton, C. A., & Fletcher, J. M. (2010). Why intensive interventions are necessary for students with severe reading difficulties. *Psychology in the Schools, 47* (5), 432–444.

Vellutino, F. R. (1981). *Dyslexia: Theory and research*. Cambridge, MA: MIT Press.

Wimmer, H., & Goswami, U. (1994). The influence of orthographic consistency on reading development: Word recognition in English and German children. *Cognition, 51*, 91–103.

Wolf, M. (1991). Naming speed and reading: The contribution of the cognitive neurosciences. *Reading Research Quarterly, 26*, 123–141.

Wolf, M., & Bowers, P. (1999). The double-deficit hypothesis for the developmental dyslexias. *Journal of Educational Psychology, 91*, 1–24.

Wolf, M., Miller, L., & Donnelly, K. (2000). Retrieval, automaticity, vocabulary elaboration, orthography (RAVE-O): A comprehensive, fluency-based reading intervention program. *Journal of Learning Disabilities, 33*(4), 375–386.

Yoon, H-K., Bolger, D. J., Kwon, O-S., & Perfetti, C. A. (2002). Subsyllabic units in reading: A difference between Korean and English. In L. Verhoeven., C. Elbro, & P. Reitsma (Eds.), *Precursors of functional literacy* (pp. 139–163). Amsterdam/ Philadelphia: John Benjamins.

3   Developmental Dyslexia in French

Liliane Sprenger-Charolles

3.1   Introduction

Reading comprehension requires the ability to both accurately and fluently identify written words and to understand spoken language (Perfetti, 1985, 2007). The main task facing beginning readers, then, is to find a means of understanding written texts as skillfully as they process spoken language. To this end, and to be able to allocate a large part of their processing capacity to reading comprehension, children must develop precise and rapid access to written words. Dyslexics' reading problems, by definition, are about identifying written words (Lyon, Shaywitz, & Shaywitz, 2003). To understand the problems facing dyslexic readers, it is necessary to determine what is involved in reading in their writing system; which, for French-speaking children, is an alphabetic system. In such systems, graphemes (e.g., ‹b›, ‹oo›, and ‹t›, in the written word *boot*) must be mapped onto phonemes (/b/-/u/-/t/ in the spoken word), the smallest units of sounds that differentiate words, such as ‹u› /y/ and ‹ou› /u/ in French (differentiating *pur* [pure] from *pour* [in order to]).

The first problem facing beginning readers is that, at least on its first encounter, reading the word *boot* requires the child to map each grapheme to a phoneme. Therefore, beginning readers must be able to segment spoken words into phonemes. This skill, called *phonemic awareness*, is not easy to acquire because phonemes cannot be isolated within a syllable: *boot* is pronounced in one articulatory gesture. The second problem of literacy acquisition in an alphabetic system relates to the level of grapheme–phoneme consistency, which has an impact on both typical and atypical (dyslexia) reading acquisition. French orthography, for instance, is more consistent than English, but less so than German and Spanish (Sprenger-Charolles, 2003). The third problem relates to the fact that reading calls for visual skills which contrast with those used to perceive objects, and indeed written words are processed by a particular area in the left occipito-temporal cortex, the visual word form area (Dehaene et al., 2011). Two characteristics of this area seem to be responsible for this specialization: its location, which is particularly appropriate for the discrimination of small letter shapes, and its interconnections to the left superior temporal and inferior frontal language areas (Dehaene, 2014).

In the present chapter, after a summary of studies on French orthography and on learning to read in French, three issues related to dyslexia in French are examined: the historical context of reading difficulties, as well as their identification and prevalence; behavioral and neurocognitive evidence on deficits in reading skill and reading-related skills; and the results of intervention studies.

3.2   Learning to Read French

3.2.1   *French Language and Its Orthography*

Standard French has seventeen consonants, ten to sixteen vowels, and three semi-vowels.

With regard to vowels, differences between close-mid vowels (/a/, /e/, /ø/, /o/) and open-mid vowels (/ɑ/, /ɛ/, /œ/, /ɔ/) are related to the syllabic structure: The four first vowels are mostly found in open syllables (*ma* [my], *thé* [tea], *feu* [fire], *do* [do]) whereas the other four are mostly found in closed syllables (*mal* [bad], *mer* [sea], *peur* [fear], *bol* [bowl]). Therefore, most phoneticians (e.g., Delattre, 1965) consider that there are only seven oral vowels (/a(ɑ)/, /e(ɛ)/, /ø(œ)/, /o(ɔ)/, and /i/, /y/, /u/), plus three to four nasal vowels (/ɑ̃/, /ɔ̃/, /ɛ̃/, /œ̃/, e.g.: *danse* [dance], *don* [don], *Tintin* [Tintin], and *un* [one]), with most French speakers confusing /ɛ̃/ and /œ̃/. In addition, the final printed ‹e› is most of the time entirely mute in French, and thus not transcribed by a phonetic symbol (e.g., *balle*: /bal/ [ball]). The three French semi-vowels are /w/ (‹oi›, *loi* [low]), /ɥ/ (‹u›, *huile* [oil]), and /j/, the latter of which can be written with ‹i/y›, ‹il(l)›, or ‹ll› (*yeux* [eyes]). Among the seventeen French consonants, there are six stop consonants (/p/-/t/-/k/, /b/-/d/-/g/), the same number of fricative consonants (/f/-/s/-/ʃ/, /v/-/z/-/ʒ/), two liquids (/l/-/r/), and three nasals (/m/-/n/ and /ɲ/, written ‹gn›).

French orthography developed under the influence of two antagonistic views: one, centered on etymology, in which letters are written to reflect the origins of the word. Thus *seven* is written with a ‹p› (*sept*) even though it is not pronounced in French, honoring its origins in the Latin word *septem*. The other view, centered on phonology (promoted by writers such as Ronsard and Voltaire), called for the strictest possible mapping between graphemes and phonemes. Most inconsistencies in French orthography are a consequence of these antagonisms, along with two additional facts (Catach, 2001). First, whereas there are thirty to thirty-six phonemes in French (Delattre, 1965), there were no more than twenty-four letters as French writing developed. It was therefore necessary to design new symbols to encode the phonemes that the alphabet had no way to differentiate: for instance, oral vowels (e.g., ‹a› /a/ in *chat* [cat]) from nasal vowels (‹an› /ã/ in *chant* [song]). Second, most of the consonants at the end of written words are silent. This is the case for consonants used to support derivations or inflections (‹t› in *petit* [little], from which are derived the words *petitesse* [littleness] and *petite* [little, for a girl]) as well as for those used to indicate inflections, such as ‹s› indicating either the plural form of nouns and adjectives (*petits pantalons* [little pants]) or the second-person singular of verbs (*tu chantes* [you sing]). These units are called morpho-phonograms.

Peereman, Sprenger-Charolles, and Messaoud-Galusi (2013) computed statistics on the consistency of grapheme–phoneme and phoneme–grapheme correspondences (GPC and PGC) for the 10,000 most frequent word-forms (with inflections) from Manulex, a lexical database based on 54 primary textbooks (Lété, Sprenger-Charolles, & Colé, 2004). Morpho-phonograms denoting gender and number inflections for nouns and adjectives, verbal inflections, and final consonants used to support inflections or derivations were coded. As shown by the data presented in Table 3.1, the strong inconsistencies observed for PGC at the end of words decreased when morpho-phonograms were taken into account.

3.2.2 Challenges in Learning to Read French

Two reading routes can be used to pronounce written words (Coltheart et al., 2001; Ziegler, Perry, & Coltheart, 2003; Ziegler, Perry, & Zorzi, 2014): a lexical route, which relies on a large set of meaningful units (mainly words); and a sublexical (or phonological) route, which relies on a small set of meaningless units (mainly GPCs). The reading of high-frequency irregular words is used to assess the lexical route for two reasons: first, because these words' frequency means that they are stored in the reader's internal lexicon; and second, because their irregularity means that using the phonological route to read them leads to the production of phonological errors (e.g., ‹qu› in *quay*

Table 3.1 *French GPC and PGC consistencies computed by token (textual frequency) based on Peereman et al. (2013)*

Position in the word	GPC consistency		PGC consistency	
	Without morphology	With morphology	Without morphology	With morphology
Beginning	96%	96%	87%	87%
Middle	74%	75%	72%	72%
End	78%	80%	66%	75%

read-aloud /kw/ like in *quality*). The phonological route is mainly assessed using the reading of non-existent words (pseudowords), because no lexical strategy is available in these cases unless the item shares most of the spelling pattern of a real word (*mable* vs. *table*).

The processes used by beginning readers must depend on general principles, common to all languages, and on the peculiarities of their own language (Sprenger-Charolles, 2003; Ziegler & Goswami, 2005). In particular, reading acquisition in any alphabetic writing system strongly depends on the level of decoding skills (i.e., the successful development of the phonological reading route: general principle), which in turn depends on the degree to which the writing system represents the spoken language it encodes (language-specific). In support of the former claim, Deacon, Desrochers, and Levesque (2017) note strong resemblances between the early literacy development of French-speaking children and that of native speakers of English. For instance, children in the two groups face similar obstacles linked to the reading of single- versus multiple-letter graphemes, and inconsistent GPCs. In support of the latter claim, they report that young French-speaking readers outperform their English-speaking peers (e.g., Goswami, Gombert, & de Barrera, 1998) and that, by the end of first grade, they reach a high level in reading (e.g., Sprenger-Charolles et al., 2003). Furthermore, studies in morphology indicate that French children master the use of inflectional markers very late (around age 10; Fayol et al., 1999). Deacon and colleagues also note that there is ongoing debate as to whether this learning (like the acquisition of other orthographic features which are not grounded in phonology) is based on statistics or on rules (Pacton, Fayol, & Perruchet, 2005). Evidence that early reliance on decoding skills constitutes a bootstrapping mechanism for reading acquisition (Share, 1995; Ziegler et al., 2014) has been provided by longitudinal studies indicating that decoding skills predict future reading of irregular words (Sprenger-Charolles et al., 2003). Comparisons between good and poor decoders, indicating that decoding skills predict reading comprehension, also support this view (Gentaz, Sprenger-Charolles, & Theurel, 2015).

3.3   Reading Difficulties in French

3.3.1   *Historical and Cultural Context*

In France, a recent set of laws and regulations provides for the recognition of children with a severe reading deficit as "disabled" (Expertise collective INSERM, 2007). To facilitate these children's schooling, a personalized plan is drawn up, which may take different forms: (a) participation in mainstream classrooms; (b) integration in classes for children with special needs; (c) adaptation of the time spent in school to facilitate relevant out-of-school activities (especially, speech therapy); (d) help from a classroom assistant; (e) arrangements for exams.

3.3.2   Identification and Prevalence

Dyslexia is characterized by problems with accurate and/or fluent word recognition. In France, these reading skills are usually assessed using the Alouette reading test (Lefavrais, 1967; for a comparison with other tests, see Bertrand et al., 2010). The test involves reading aloud a 265-word text, which includes low-frequency words and misleading contextual information (e.g., after *lac* [lake], *poison* [poison] rather than *poisson* [fish]). This test therefore assesses word-level reading skills rather than word-in-context reading. Reading scores are computed by combining total reading time and errors. To be recognized as a dyslexic reader, the child's reading level must be at least 18 months behind that of typical readers of the same chronological age (e.g., Casalis, Colé, & Sopo, 2004; Lassus-Sangosse, N'guyen-Morel, & Valdois, 2008; Monzalvo et al., 2012; Serniclaes et al., 2001; Ziegler et al., 2010). For adults, no acknowledged standardized reading test exists, although the Alouette is used in some studies (e.g., Martin et al., 2010; Szenkovits & Ramus, 2005).

Reading difficulties affect 3 to 15 percent of the French population in unselected samples (Expertise collective INSERM, 2007), similar to the proportions observed in studies with English-speaking children (Shaywitz et al., 2009). The differences depend on the threshold levels chosen to identify reading deficits. However, the proportion of poor readers in France, as in other countries, is higher in children from a low socioeconomic status (SES) background. For instance, Gentaz et al. (2013) found that 30 percent of 346 first graders from low-SES families had Alouette reading test scores at least 1 standard deviation (SD) below the mean.

3.4   Behavioral and Neurocognitive Evidence

3.4.1   Nature of Reading Problems in French

Given that phonological reading skills are impaired in dyslexia (Lyon et al., 2003), and that early reliance on the phonological reading route is a bootstrapping mechanism for reading acquisition (Share, 1995; Ziegler et al., 2014), lexical reading skills may be impaired as well, at least in comparison between dyslexics and typical readers of the same chronological age (CA controls). Indeed, the results of a comparison of adult dyslexic and typical readers of French, English, and Italian (Paulesu et al., 2001) indicate that French and English dyslexic readers made significantly more errors than Italian dyslexic readers for both words and pseudowords (see Supplemental Table 1, Paulesu et al., 2001).[1] These results confirm the negative impact of orthographic inconsistency on reading skills observed in studies with beginning readers (see Section 3.2.2, above). However, regardless of orthographic consistency, the deficit of dyslexic readers is greater on pseudowords than on words, as indicated by the magnitude of the differences (in Cohen's *d*) between dyslexic and typical readers in naming time for pseudowords versus words (for French participants, −1.53 vs. −1.18; for English participants, −2.01 vs. −1.78; for Italian participants, −2.93 vs. −2.07). The underlying impairment of French-speaking dyslexic readers thus does not seem to differ from that of English or Italian dyslexic readers: The impairment is greater when they are required to use the phonological reading route without the aid of lexical knowledge.

To assess processing time for word-level reading skills, Paulesu and collea-gues (2001) relied on naming time (the time from the word's appearance on the computer screen to the onset of the vocal response), a commonly used measure with French adults (Martin et al., 2010) and children (Sprenger-Charolles et al., 2000; Ziegler et al., 2008). This measure is more precise than fluency measures being used in other French studies (e.g., Lallier, Thierry, & Tainturier, 2013; Lassus-Sangosse et al., 2008; Lobier, Zoubrinetzky, & Valdois, 2012; Reilhac et al., 2012; Zoubrinetzky, Bielle, & Valdois, 2014), since it includes the time taken to read all words (even those incorrectly read or correctly read after self-corrections) plus the duration of the vocal response. Differences between dyslexic readers and CA controls (Cohen's *d*), computed for the scores on pseudoword and irregular word reading found in the aforementioned studies, are presented in Table 3.2. Deficits in both reading routes were observed in all studies. However, contrary to Paulesu et al. (2001), most studies found the lexical reading route to be at least as impaired as the phonological route. This is probably because Paulesu and colleagues used regular words, while the other studies used only irregular words. Regular words, unlike irregular words, can be correctly read through both the lexical and the phonological reading route.

Comparisons with younger typical readers of the same reading level (RL controls) allow researchers to examine whether the developmental trajec-tory of dyslexic readers is *deviant* or merely *delayed* (Bryant & Impey, 1986). If the trajectory is delayed, the comparison should reveal equal phonological and orthographic reading skills in the two groups; if the trajectory is deviant, only the phonological skills of dyslexic readers should be poorer than those of controls. Differences between dyslexic readers and RL controls (Cohen's *d*) were computed for the scores on pseudoword and irregular word reading found in three of the aforementioned studies (Martin et al., 2010; Reilhac et al., 2012; Sprenger-Charolles et al., 2000), and in another study (Sprenger-Charolles

---

[1] For Supplementary Table 1, see: https://science.sciencemag.org/content/suppl/2001/03/14/291 .5511.2165.DC1.

Table 3.2 *Differences (Cohen's d) in processing speed (fluency or naming time, NT) between dyslexic readers and CA controls for pseudowords vs. irregular words*

	Sprenger-Charolles et al., 2000	Ziegler et al., 2008	Martin et al., 2010	Reilhac et al., 2012	Lallier et al., 2013	Lobier et al., 2012	Zoubrin-etzky et al., 2014	Lassus-Sangosse et al., 2008	
Chronol. age	10	10	22	11	11	11	10;6	11	11
No. of Dyslexic children	N=31[a]	N=24[a]	N=15[a]	N=12[a]	N=16[a]	N=14[b]	N=71[c]	N=13[d]	N=13[e]
Measure	NT	NT	NT	Fluency	Fluency	Fluency	Fluency	Fluency	Fluency
Pseudoword	−1.39	−0.92	−1.18	−1.18	−1.77	−3.45	−2.36	−4.23	−2.41
Irregular word	−1.20	−1.19	−1.11	−1.15	−1.87	−3.28	−2.00	−3.31	−1.97

a: Unselected samples of dyslexic readers; b–e: dyslexic readers with a specific profile (b: with a visual-attention deficit; c: with a mixed profile; d: with a phonemic awareness deficit; e: with no phonemic awareness deficit).

Table 3.3 *Differences (Cohen's d) between dyslexic readers (DR) and RL controls for pseudowords vs. irregular words*

	Sprenger-Charolles et al., 2009	Reilhac et al., 2012		Sprenger-Charolles et al., 2000		Martin et al., 2010
DR Reading level	7	7;6		8		10;5
DR Chronol. age	9	11		10		22
No. of dyslexic children	N= 15	N= 12		N= 31		N= 15
Measure	Accuracy	Accuracy	Fluency	Accuracy	Naming-time	Naming-time
Pseudoword	−1.07	−0.73	−0.53	−0.64	−0.36	−0.65
Irregular word	+0.06	+0.26	−0.06	−0.02	+0.19	−0.33

et al., 2009). The results are presented in Table 3.3. As reported in reviews of accuracy-based English studies (Van IJzendoorn & Bus, 1994; Metsala, Stanovich, & Brown, 1998), only a deficit of the phonological reading route emerged in these studies. This deficit was found only for long pseudowords in the accuracy-based study with younger RL controls (Sprenger-Charolles et al. 2009), and only for response times among older dyslexic readers (Martin et al., 2010).

Other studies have assessed the orthographic skills of dyslexic readers and RL controls using different paradigms (Doignon-Camus et al., 2012; Grainger et al., 2003; Reilhac et al., 2012). In Grainger et al. (2003) dyslexic readers and RL controls had to choose which of two letters was present in three types of briefly presented items: words, pseudowords (pronounceable items with legal letter strings), and nonwords with unpronounceable or illegal letter strings. Only the difference between pseudowords and nonwords was significant (pseudoword superiority effect), regardless of group. The pseudoword superiority effect can be due to the frequency of sublexical orthographic units, such as bigram frequency, which is higher for pseudowords than for nonwords. Reilhac et al. (2012) reported similar findings from a task in which participants had to indicate whether or not two sequentially presented words, pseudowords or nonwords, were identical. The results of a study investigating syllabic processing (Doignon-Camus et al., 2012) also suggest a preserved sensitivity to bigram frequency in dyslexic readers in comparison to RL controls. It must be added that dyslexic readers underperformed RL controls in two of these studies that assessed sublexical phonological skills with a pseudoword reading-aloud task (Grainger et al., 2003; Reilhac et al., 2012).

The reviewed studies indicate that, in comparisons to RL controls, dyslexic readers' sublexical phonological reading skills are less well preserved than either their lexical or sublexical orthographic skills (for lexical compared to sublexical orthographic skills, see Grainger & Ziegler, 2011).

3.4.2   Prevalence of Phonological, Surface, and Mixed Profiles

In order to examine to what extent there is prevalence of phonological, surface, and mixed profiles in French as compared to English, we reviewed a meta-analysis of six multiple-case studies by Sprenger-Charolles et al. (2011): three with French-speaking children (Génard et al., 1998; Sprenger-Charolles et al., 2000; Ziegler et al., 2008) and three with English-speaking children (Castles & Coltheart, 1993; Manis et al., 1996; Stanovich, Siegel, & Gottardo, 1997). In all of these studies, children were said to have phonological dyslexia when only their phonological reading skills (assessed with pseudoword reading) were impaired, and surface dyslexia when only their lexical reading skills (assessed with high-frequency irregular-word reading) were impaired; when both skills were deficient, they were said to have a mixed profile.

In comparison with CA controls, mixed profiles were the most common for both accuracy and speed (data available only for the French group). When, in French studies, both accuracy and speed are considered, 86 percent of dyslexic readers showed a mixed profile. Differences were observed in the proportion of dissociated profiles between French and English studies. In accuracy-based French studies, surface dyslexia was more frequent than phonological dyslexia, but this was not the case in accuracy-based English studies. These findings are probably due to the fact that pseudoword reading in transparent orthographies is easier than in opaque orthographies, and seem to indicate that, in consistent orthographies, reading speed must be used to detect deficits in phonological reading skills.

Two main profiles can be found in comparison with RL controls: a delayed profile, characterized by the absence of a performance difference between dyslexic readers and controls on both irregular words and pseudowords, and a deviant profile, characterized by dyslexic readers underperforming controls on phonological reading skills only. The results reported here are drawn from three accuracy-based French studies (Casalis, 2003; Sprenger-Charolles et al., 2000, 2009). The threshold chosen to define a skill as deficient was 1.65 SDs. In Sprenger-Charolles et al. (2000), 61 percent of the thirty-one dyslexic readers were classified as delayed, 26 percent as having a deviant phonological profile, and 13 percent as having a deviant surface profile. Among the forty-five dyslexic readers of Casalis (2003), the proportion of delayed profiles was also higher than that of deviant phonological profiles: 56 vs. 40 percent, plus 4 percent of deviant surface profiles. A greater proportion of deviant phonological profiles was found in Sprenger-Charolles et al. (2009): 60 percent, compared to 27 percent of dyslexic readers with a delayed profile, and none with a surface profile (see the results on long pseudowords vs. short irregular words). These results suggest that the proportion of deviant phonological profiles increases with the severity of the reading disorder. As a matter of fact, all the fifteen dyslexic readers from Sprenger-Charolles et al. (2009) were enrolled in a special program for children with severe reading difficulties; all the forty-five dyslexic readers from Casalis (2003) had received a long-term speech-therapy; this was not the case for most of the thirty-one dyslexic readers from Sprenger-Charolles et al. (2000). These results also indicate that the surface profiles almost disappear in the RL comparison. Therefore, as suggested by some researchers (e.g., Manis et al., 1996), dyslexic readers with a surface profile can be considered to be delayed in reading progress.

3.4.3   Problems with Processing of Morphological Information

For derived words, readers can rely on the convergence between form and meaning (e.g., *amical* [friendly] from *ami* [friend]), and dyslexic readers can take advantage of their relatively preserved semantic skills to develop a morpho-semantic level of representation. Quémart and Casalis (2015) examined the processing of morphological information using priming effects in a lexical decision task with dyslexic readers and CA controls (around age 13), as well as RL controls (around age 9). In two experiments, significant priming effects were observed in a morphologically transparent condition (*ami* primed by *amical*) for all groups. In the first experiment, significant priming effect also was obtained in a pseudo-morphological condition (*rat* [rat] primed by *rater* [to miss]), but only in the control groups. Dyslexic readers thus were influenced only by the semantic properties of morphemes, whereas CA and RL controls were influenced by both their semantic and formal properties. Since, for all groups, priming effects were not observed in a semantic condition (*fleur* [flower] primed by *tulipe*), these results could not be due solely to the meaning of the items. In the second experiment, the only other significant priming effects were observed with dyslexic readers in two non-transparent morphological conditions (*dent*, with a silent ‹t› [tooth] primed by *dentiste*, or *clair* [clear] primed by *clarté* [clarity]). The authors interpreted these results in the framework of the dual-route account of orthographic processing (Grainger & Ziegler, 2011): Effects observed with slight orthographic modifications between primes and targets indicate that dyslexic readers do not code letter position or identity within morphemes in a strict fashion, but with coarse-grained orthographic units.

Another study examining the processing of silent inflectional markers found that only 10-year-old typical readers were sensitive to inflectional markers written at the end of words, while dyslexic readers of the same chronological age and younger RL controls (age 8) were not (Casalis, Leuwers, & Hilton,

2013). As also suggested by other results (e.g., Fayol et al., 1999), it thus seems that only typical readers master inflectional morphology, and only very late.

3.4.4   Underlying Deficits

3.4.4.1 Deficit in Phonemic Awareness   As observed in most behavioral studies with English participants (Melby-Lervåg, Lyster, & Hulme, 2012), most studies with French-speaking dyslexic participants have found them to have lower levels of phonemic awareness than CA controls (e.g. for children: Altarelli et al., 2013; Bogliotti et al., 2008; Casalis et al., 2004, 2013; Monzalvo et al., 2012; Ziegler et al., 2008; e.g. for adults: Dufor et al., 2007; Martin et al., 2010; Paulesu et al., 2001; Szenkovits & Ramus, 2005). Some of these studies (e.g., Bogliotti et al., 2008; Casalis et al., 2004, 2013) also reported differences with RL controls. Deficient phonemic awareness skills have been found not only in phonological dyslexia, but also in surface dyslexia (Sprenger-Charolles et al., 2000; Ziegler et al., 2008). Such a deficiency has also been observed prior to reading acquisition in future dyslexic readers in comparison to future typical readers (Sprenger-Charolles et al., 2000). Furthermore, a high proportion of dyslexic readers show deficient phonemic awareness skills (e.g., 83 percent in Ziegler et al., 2008). At the brain level, an area involved in native language phonemic processing, the left planum temporale (Chang et al., 2010) is the main structure whose activation correlates with several behavioral measures, especially phonemic awareness (Monzalvo et al., 2012; but see Altarelli et al., 2014).

However, a few studies have failed to find significant differences in phonemic awareness between dyslexic readers and CA controls, including some studies that also reported significant results (e.g., Martin et al., 2010; Talli, Sprenger-Charolles, & Stavrakaki, 2015). In other cases, significant differences were only found in a subgroup of dyslexic readers (e.g., Bosse, Tainturier, & Valdois, 2007). Most of these contradictory findings may be explained by differences in task difficulty (e.g., deletion of the first phoneme of consonant-vowel-consonant pseudowords vs. consonant-consonant-vowel pseudowords, the first task being easier than the second) or in the measure used (accuracy vs. speed). For example, some studies (e.g., Martin et al., 2010; Talli et al., 2015) have found deficits only for accuracy on the more difficult task, or only for speed on the easier task.

3.4.4.2 Deficit in Phoneme Discrimination   Phoneme discrimination skills are assessed with tasks using pairs of syllables which differ by one phonemic feature: for instance, voicing (/do/ vs. /to/) or place of articulation (/ba/ vs. /da/). Scores on such tasks reach a *ceiling level* very early (around age 6: see Piquard-Kipffer & Sprenger-Charolles, 2013), and deficits have been found in French-speaking dyslexic readers only in challenging conditions, such as a noisy environment (Ziegler et al., 2009). In addition, phoneme discrimination skills prior to reading acquisition predict future reading skills (Piquard-Kipffer & Sprenger-Charolles, 2013) and phoneme discrimination training leads to reading improvements (see Section 3.6).

Phoneme discrimination skills are also assessed with different continua in which pairs of stimuli differ acoustically and are perceived either as indistinguishable by native speakers (acoustically distinct stimuli equally perceived as /to/, called *within category*) or as different because they straddle a phonemic boundary (/to/ vs. /do/, called *between category*). Bogliotti et al. (2008) found the prevalence of phoneme discrimination deficits (characterized by small differences between judgments on between-category and within-category pairs) to be high in dyslexic readers and low in CA and RL controls. Another question is that of the specificity of the phoneme discrimination deficit, which was assessed in some studies (e.g., Serniclaes et al., 2001) by the use of the same stimuli presented first as whistles and then as speech sounds: a synthetic / ba-da/ place-of-articulation continuum produced using sine-wave analogs of speech sounds. At the behavioral level, dyslexic children showed reduced discrimination of between-category pairs and increased discrimination of within-category pairs, both of which appear to be specific to speech (Serniclaes et al., 2001). At the brain level, using the same continuum, two other studies reported differences between the speech and non-speech conditions: one with EEG and fMRI data collected from unimpaired adults (Dehaene-Lambertz et al., 2005), and one with PET data collected from dyslexic adults and CA controls (Dufor et al., 2007). In the non-impaired readers of these two studies, significant differences among the processing of between- versus within-pairs were only found in the speech mode and in a specific brain area, the supra-marginal gyrus (SMG). In contrast, Dufor et al. (2007) reported hypo-activation of the same brain area in dyslexic adults compared to CA controls in speech mode. These findings confirm previous results on the role of the SMG in speech processing and its hypo-activation in dyslexia (Ruff et al., 2002).

Some of these studies (Bogliotti et al., 2008; Serniclaes et al., 2001) indicate that dyslexic readers exhibit an enhanced sensibility to within-phoneme category pairs (called allophones), a deficit whose prevalence is high in dyslexic readers compared to both CA and RL controls (Bogliotti et al., 2008). Yet another study did not find an enhanced sensitivity to allophonic contrasts in French-speaking dyslexic adults, at least at the behavioral level (Dufor et al., 2009; for negative results from studies conducted in other languages, see Noordenbos et al., 2013a and 2013b, in Dutch; and Messaoud-Galusi, Hazan, & Rosen, 2011, in English). Importantly, however, two of these studies (Dufor et al., 2009; Noordenbos et al., 2013) found significant differences between dyslexic and typical readers at the brain level. Other studies report associations between brain data and impaired skills at the phonemic level in dyslexic adults (Lehongre et al., 2013; Lehongre et al., 2011) and children (Monzalvo et al., 2012). For instance, Lehongre et al. (2011) observed a reduced left hemisphere bias in phonemic processing in auditory cortex during passive listening to white noise with a range of amplitude modulations broadly covering the syllabic versus phonemic sampling range. Similar results are reported by Lehongre et al. (2013) during passive viewing of audiovisual movies.[2] These results show that dyslexic readers suffer from deficits in skills at the phonemic level that differ from those assessed by the classical phonemic awareness tasks. They indicate the need to assess these skills with fine-grained methods and with both behavioral and brain data.

3.4.4.3 Deficit in Visual Attention   The hypothesis that dyslexic readers have a visual attention (VA) deficit – that is, a limitation in the number of elements they can process in parallel from a brief visual display – has been assessed mostly using five consonant-strings (e.g., RHSDM) presented briefly (200 ms), with the task being either to orally report the whole string (global report), or a single cued letter (partial report). Some studies conducted with French participants have corroborated the hypothesis (e.g., Bosse et al., 2007; Valdois, Bosse, & Tainturier, 2004).

Two caveats must be applied to the VA tasks described above, however: They use verbal stimuli, and they require a verbal response. To assess to what extent the VA deficit might be caused by a more general VA deficit, Ziegler et al. (2010) used strings of symbols (e.g.:}, §, /), in addition to strings of letters or digits. They found deficits in dyslexic readers with letters and digits, but not with symbols. Similar findings were reported in another study that compared adult readers with dyslexia associated to a VA deficit (assessed by the global report) to CA controls on a categorization task involving strings of letters, digits, and non-alphanumeric items (Lobier et al., 2014). This might be because the processing of alphanumeric items requires the mapping of visual codes to phonological codes, an ability that is well known to be deficient in dyslexia. The overall conclusion is that research on French children with dyslexia does not show a substantial visual-attention effect when the task is designed to minimize orthographic and phonological processing, a condition not met in most studies that report visual-attention effects (e.g., Zoubrinetzky et al., 2014).

---

[2] Other French studies suggest that phonological representations are not impaired in dyslexic readers, either in adults (e.g., preserved sensitivity to phonotactic probabilities: Szenkovits & Ramus, 2005; and for a review Ramus & Szenkovits, 2008) or children (e.g., preserved hierarchy of sonority: Maïonchi-Pino et al., 2013). Studies in other languages using tasks like those used in the aforementioned studies have reported contradictory findings (e.g., sensitivity to phonotactic probabilities in dyslexic adults: Noordenbos et al., 2013a). More research is thus needed in this domain.

3.4.5   Neurocognitive Underpinnings   Several studies suggest a link between dyslexia and abnormal specialization of an occipito-temporal area of the left hemisphere, the visual-word-form area (VWFA). This area is unresponsive to written words in nonreaders (Dehaene et al., 2010), and quickly increases its responses during reading acquisition (Maurer et al., 2010). A cross-linguistic PET study (Paulesu et al., 2001) observed dyslexic readers and CA controls while they performed different reading tasks: an explicit reading-aloud task with words and pseudowords, and an implicit task involving the detection of graphic features within written words, pseudowords, and false-font strings. Whatever the task or language, brain activity was reduced in dyslexic readers compared to CA in the VWFA. N170 tuning also provides electrophysiological support for suggested links between dyslexia and abnormal specialization of left occipito-temporal areas: neural activity in the VWFA is linked with this component, which exhibits left lateralization in response to letter strings. In a study with French-speaking adults (Mahé et al., 2012), dyslexic readers and CA controls performed a lexical decision task with non-alphabetic symbols versus words, pseudowords, and nonwords. Only CA controls showed larger left occipito-temporal negativities for word-like stimuli than for symbols, suggesting impaired visual expertise in dyslexic readers. Noteworthy, these dyslexic readers were also found to have impaired phonological reading skills shown by inaccurate and slowed pseudoword reading.

In an fMRI study aimed at probing functional brain architecture with an implicit task (to reduce task difficulty effects), dyslexic children and CA controls from both low- and high-SES families (Monzalvo et al., 2012) detected a target star while viewing written words, faces, buildings, and moving checkerboards. The words minus blank screen fMRI responses identified a cluster in the left fusiform gyrus, the location of the VWFA, which was more activated in controls than in dyslexic readers. Reading scores were correlated with fMRI activity in this area. Dyslexic readers' responses to checkerboards and houses were normal. Deficits in children with dyslexia in both SES groups emphasized the existence of a core set of brain activation anomalies in dyslexia, independent of SES. A subsequent study found reduced thickness in the region of the left hemisphere responsive to words in dyslexic children, even in comparison with RL controls (Altarelli et al., 2013). As the authors explained "although requiring cautious interpretation," the comparison with RL controls "suggests that there might be a primary structural defect in dyslexic children precisely in the left occipito-temporal sub-region that eventually becomes the visual word form area" (p. 11300).

Additionally, correlation of the findings of experiments with written and spoken language can be used to identify spoken-language predictors of VWFA activation. Thereby, Monzalvo et al. (2012) found stronger correlations between written and spoken language responses in typical than in dyslexic readers predominantly in classical left-hemispheric language areas of the superior temporal gyrus. These finding suggests that the processes of written and spoken language are better integrated in typical than in dyslexic readers.

With respect to environmental factors (linguistic environment, SES background), one study (Paulesu et al., 2001) observed a neurobiological deficit in dyslexic readers regardless of orthographic opacity, and another study (Monzalvo et al., 2012) found such a deficit in dyslexic readers regardless of SES. However, Mahé, Bonnefond, and Doignon-Camus (2013) observed a neurobiological impairment only in dyslexic readers, not in poor readers from low-SES backgrounds matched to them on reading level. More research is needed in this domain, as the majority of studies have involved dyslexic readers from middle- to high-SES backgrounds, because of the exclusionary criteria used to define dyslexia.

3.5   Intervention

There have been a few training studies with French-speaking dyslexic readers. Some (e.g., Habib et al., 2002) were conducted to examine Tallal's hypothesis of rapid auditory processing deficits (Tallal, 1980). The results remain inconclusive (see Mody, 2003), as do those of most studies on this issue based on a meta-analysis (Strong et al., 2011). Other studies have focused on the effect of training that incorporates an audiovisual phoneme discrimination task using pairs of phonemes that differ by one phonemic feature, such as voicing (/p/-/b/; /t/-/d/; see Section 3.5.2). In these trainings (Ecalle et al., 2009; Magnan et al., 2004), the participants listen to a consonant-vowel syllable (/pa/) and must decide which of two printed alternatives (⟨pa⟩ or ⟨ba⟩) is the same as the syllable they have just heard. Improvement in reading skills has been observed in both young and older dyslexic readers after brief but intensive training (8 to 10 hours). These results are in agreement with the fact that phonemic-skills training helps dyslexic readers, especially when the training involves the association of phonemes with graphemes (for reviews, see Ehri et al., 2001; Serniclaes, Collet, & Sprenger-Charolles, 2015).

3.6   Discussion and Conclusion

3.6.1   *Evidence of a Phonological Deficit*

At the behavioral level, deficits in phonological reading skills were evidenced in dyslexic readers compared to RL controls (e.g., Reilhac et al., 2012). In young children with dyslexia these deficits were reflected in accuracy and speed, in older dyslexic readers only by speed (e.g., Martin et al., 2010). In the same comparison, relatively preserved lexical and sublexical orthographic skills were observed (e.g., Grainger et al., 2003). In multiple-case studies, again in comparison to RL controls, most dyslexic readers showed either a delayed profile or a deviant phonological profile; the latter is widespread in severely impaired dyslexic readers (Sprenger-Charolles et al., 2009). Comparisons among French-, English-, and Italian-speaking dyslexic readers indicated that the more opaque the orthography, the poorer are the performances (Paulesu et al., 2001). Deficits at the behavioral level were also observed in phonemic awareness in comparison with RL controls (e.g., Casalis et al., 2004), even before reading acquisition in children subsequently classified as dyslexic (Sprenger-Charolles et al., 2000). Furthermore, phonemic discrimination skills predicted future reading levels when assessed prior to reading acquisition (Piquard-Kipffer & Sprenger-Charolles, 2013), and improvements in reading skills were obtained in young and older dyslexic readers after audiovisual phonemic discrimination training (e.g., Magnan et al., 2004). In addition, dyslexic readers perceived phonetic differences that were not relevant to processing their native language (e.g., Bogliotti et al., 2008; Serniclaes et al., 2001). This subtle deficit, found even in comparison with RL controls, is prevalent (Bogliotti et al., 2008). Although some studies reported visual attention deficits (e.g., Bosse et al., 2007), it is not clear that these deficits are purely visual, since the task involved verbal stimuli, requiring a verbal response. The argument that reported visual attention deficits actually have a verbal component receives support from studies in which deficits in visual attention are found for the processing of alphanumeric, and not for non-alphanumeric symbols (e.g., Ziegler et al., 2010).

At the brain level, hypo-activations were observed in dyslexic readers compared to CA controls in regions involved in phonemic computations, mainly left temporo-parietal regions, often in combination with hyper-activations of inferior frontal regions, generally interpreted as the result of compensatory responses (e.g., Dufor et al., 2009). Hypo-activations of a left occipito-temporal region (VWFA) in dyslexic readers compared to CA controls were found in dyslexic adults (Paulesu et al., 2001) and children (Monzalvo et al., 2012). A different kind of impairment (cortical thickness) located in the same brain region was found in dyslexic children even in comparison with RL controls (Altarelli et al., 2013). Other findings suggest that written and spoken language processing are better integrated in typical than in dyslexic readers (Monzalvo et al., 2012). To conclude, there is abundant evidence from behavioral and neurocognitive studies that children with dyslexia generally show a phonological deficit.

3.6.2   Clinical Implications

With respect to clinical implications, it is important to consider that most of the reviewed studies with French-speaking dyslexic readers follow a research design that controls for the effects of reading experience (Goswami, 2015): the use of RL comparisons, longitudinal data with pre-readers, and training studies. In addition, the prevalence of deficits in reading and reading-related skills is examined in most studies. The outcomes of most of these studies are consistent with the phonological explanation of this developmental disorder (e.g., Ramus, 2003; Shaywitz et al., 2009; Sprenger-Charolles, Colé, & Serniclaes, 2006; Ziegler et al., 2014). In an alphabetical writing system like French, reading acquisition requires the establishment of connections between graphemes and phonemes. The establishment of these connections involves changes in the reader's behavior, from a slow and laborious decoding of each word based on grapheme–phoneme correspondences to the proficient reading of a word in a few milliseconds. It also involves changes in the brain. Indeed, certain brain areas progressively become functionally specialized for reading, and new connections develop between these areas and areas functional in language (Dehaene, 2014; Dehaene et al., 2011). The successful implementation of these connections depends on the consistency of the relationship between graphemes and phonemes in the writing system in which children learn to read. Nonetheless, whatever the opacity of the orthography, early reliance on phonology-based procedures is a bootstrapping mechanism in reading acquisition (Share, 1995; Ziegler et al., 2014). The automation of written-word identification also depends on the children's level of phonemic awareness, and more generally on their skills at the phonemic level. A child who has difficulty grasping that the word *pat* contains three distinct speech sounds (phonemes) will also have difficulty in learning to read. Furthermore, sensitivity to phonetic contrasts which are not relevant to the processing of the child's native language (allophonic perception) has obvious implications for reading acquisition, because it impedes the establishment of relationships between phonemes and graphemes, turning even completely transparent writing systems opaque. This may be the case in at least some dyslexic children and adults, and could explain why their word-reading skills are not well automated (Serniclaes & Sprenger-Charolles, 2015; Shaywitz et al., 2009).

Although impaired phonological reading skills characterize the word-reading problems of dyslexic children, they also have an impact on their reading comprehension. Since reading comprehension problems can be due to difficulties in listening comprehension and/or in written-word identification, a modality effect between listening and reading comprehension can be expected. In two studies with 9–10-year-old dyslexic readers along with CA controls (Casalis et al., 2013; Talli et al., 2015), written and spoken comprehension were assessed with a task in which, after either reading or hearing a short utterance, children were asked to choose the picture that corresponded to the utterance they had just read or heard, out of a set of four options. In both studies it was indeed found that dyslexic readers performed worse in reading comprehension than in listening comprehension, a modality effect which did not appear in the CA control groups. The results of these two studies are consistent with the definition of dyslexia (Lyon et al., 2003) in which reading comprehension deficits are said to be a mere consequence of a deficit in written-word identification.

References

Altarelli, I., Leroy, F., & Monzalvo, K. et al. (2014). Planum temporale asymmetry in developmental dyslexia: Revisiting an old question. *Human Brain Mapping*, *37*, 5717–5735.

Altarelli, I., Monzalvo, K., Iannuzzi, S., Fluss, J., Billard, C., Ramus, F., & Dehaene-Lambertz, G. (2013). A functionally guided approach to the morphometry of occipitotemporal regions in developmental dyslexia: Evidence for differential effects in boys and girls. *Journal of Neuroscience*, *33*, 11296–11301.

Bertrand, D., Fluss, J., Billard, C., & Ziegler, J. C. (2010). Efficacité, sensibilité, spécificité: Comparaison de différents tests de lecture. *L'Année Psychologique*, *110*, 299–320.

Bogliotti, C., Serniclaes, W., Messaoud-Galusi, S., & Sprenger-Charolles, L. (2008). Discrimination of speech sounds by dyslexic children: Comparisons with chronological age and reading level controls. *Journal of Experimental Child Psychology*, *101*, 137–175.

Bosse, M. L., Tainturier, M. J., & Valdois, S. (2007). Developmental dyslexia: The visual attention span deficit hypothesis. *Cognition*, *104*, 198–230.

Bryant, P., & Impey, L. (1986). The similarities between normal readers and developmental and acquired dyslexics. *Cognition*, *24*, 124–137.

Casalis, S. (2003). The delay-type in developmental dyslexia: Reading processes. *Current Psychology Letters: Behavior, Brain, & Cognition*, *10*(1). http://journals.openedition.org/cpl/95

Casalis, S., Colé, P., & Sopo, D. (2004). Morphological awareness in developmental dyslexia. *Annals of Dyslexia*, *54*, 114–138.

Casalis, S., Leuwers, C., & Hilton, H. (2013). Syntactic comprehension in reading and listening: A study in French dyslexic children. *Journal of Learning Disabilities*, *46*, 201–219.

Castles, A., & Coltheart, M. (1993). Varieties of developmental dyslexia. *Cognition*, *47*, 149–180.

Catach, N. (2001). *Histoire de l'orthographe française*. Paris, France: Honoré Champion.

Chang, E. F., Rieger, J. W., Johnson, K., Berger, M. S., Barbaro, N. M., & Knight, R. T. (2010). Categorical speech representation in human superior temporal gyrus. *Nature Neuroscience*, *13*, 1428–1432.

Coltheart, M., Rastle, K., Perry, C., Langdon, R., & Ziegler J. C. (2001). DRC: A dual route cascaded model of visual word recognition and reading aloud. *Psychological Review*, *108*, 204–256.

Deacon, S. H., Desrochers, A., & Levesque, K. (2017). Learning to read French. In C. Perfetti & L. Verhoeven (Eds.), *Learning to read across languages and writing systems* (pp. 243–269). Cambridge, UK: Cambridge University Press.

Dehaene, S. (2014). Reading in the brain revised and extended: Response to comments. *Mind & Language, 29,* 320–335.

Dehaene, S., Dehaene-Lambertz, G., Gentaz, E., Huron, C., & Sprenger-Charolles, L. (2011). *Apprendre à lire: Des sciences cognitives à la salle de classe.* Paris, France: Editions Odile Jacob.

Dehaene, S., Pegado, F., & Braga, L. W. et al. (2010). How learning to read changes the cortical networks for vision and language. *Science, 330,* 1359–1364.

Dehaene-Lambertz, G., Pallier, C., Serniclaes, W., Sprenger-Charolles, L., Jobert, A., & Dehaene, S. (2005). Neural correlates of switching from auditory to speech perception. *NeuroImage, 24,* 21–33.

Delattre, P. (1965). *Comparing the phonetic features of English, French, German and Spanish.* Heidelberg, Germany: Jumius Gross Verlag.

Doignon-Camus, N., Seigneuric, A., Perrier, E., Sisti, A., & Zagar, D. (2012). Evidence for a preserved sensitivity to orthographic redundancy and an impaired access to phonological syllables in French developmental dyslexic. *Annals of Dyslexia, 63,* 117–132.

Dufor, O., Serniclaes, W., Sprenger-Charolles, L., & Démonet, J. F. (2007). Top-down processes during auditory phoneme categorization in dyslexia: A PET study. *Neuroimage, 34,* 1692–1707.

Dufor, O., Serniclaes, W., Sprenger-Charolles, L., & Démonet, J. F. (2009). Left pre-motor cortex and allophonic speech perception in dyslexia: A PET study. *Neuroimage, 46,* 241–248.

Ecalle, J., Magnan, A., Bouchafa, H., & Gombert, J. E. (2009). Computer-based training with ortho-phonological units in dyslexic children: New investigations. *Dyslexia, 15,* 218–238.

Ehri, L. C., Nunes, S. R., Willows, D. M., Schuster, B. V., Yaghoub-Zadeh, Z., & Shanahan, T. (2001). Phonemic awareness instruction helps children learn to read: Evidence from the National Reading Panel's meta-analysis. *Reading Research Quarterly, 36,* 250–283.

Expertise collective INSERM. (2007). *Dyslexie, dysorthographie, dyscalculie: Bilan des données scientifiques.* Paris, France: Institut National de la Santé et de la Recherche Médicale (INSERM).

Fayol, M., Thenevin, M. G., Jarousse, J. P., & Totereau, C. (1999). From learning to teaching to learn French written morphology. In T. Nunes (Ed.), *Learning to read: An integrated view from research and practice* (pp. 43–64). Dordrecht, The Netherlands: Kluwer.

Génard, N., Mousty, P., Alegria, J., Leybaert, J., & Morais, J. (1998). Methods to establish subtypes of developmental dyslexia. In P. Reitsma & L. Verhoeven (Eds.), *Problems and interventions in literacy development* (pp. 163–176). Dordrecht, The Netherlands: Kluwer.

Gentaz, E., Sprenger-Charolles, L., & Theurel, A. (2015). Differences in the predictors of reading comprehension in first graders from low socio-economic status families with either good or poor decoding skills. *PLos One, 10*(3), e0119581.

Gentaz, E., Sprenger-Charolles, L., Theurel, A., & Colé, P. (2013). Reading comprehension in a large cohort of French first graders from low socio-economic status families: A 7-month longitudinal study. *PLos One, 8*(11), e78608.

Goswami, U. (2015). Sensory theories of developmental dyslexia: Three challenges for research. *Nature Reviews Neuroscience, 16,* 43–54.

Goswami, U., Gombert, J. E., & Barrera, L. F. (1998). Children's orthographic representations and linguistic transparency: Nonsense word reading in English, French and Spanish. *Applied Psycholinguistics, 19*, 19–52.

Grainger, J., Bouttevin, S., Truc, C., Bastien, M., & Ziegler, J. C. (2003). Word superiority pseudoword superiority and learning to read: A comparison of dyslexic and normal readers. *Brain and Language, 87*, 432–440.

Grainger, J., & Ziegler, J. C. (2011). A dual-route approach to orthographic processing. *Frontiers in Psychology, 2*, 54. doi: http://dx.doi.org/10.3389/fpsyg.2011.00054.

Habib, M., Rey, V., Daffaure, V., Camps, R., Espesser, R., Joly-Pottuz, B., & Démonet, J. F. (2002). Phonological training in children with dyslexia using temporally modified speech: A three-step pilot investigation. *International Journal of Language and Communication Disorders, 37*, 289–308.

Lallier, M., Thierry, G., & Tainturier, M. J. (2013). On the importance of considering individual profiles when investigating the role of auditory sequential deficits in developmental dyslexia. *Cognition, 126*, 121–127.

Lassus-Sangosse, D., N'guyen-Morel, M. A., & Valdois, S. (2008). Sequential or simultaneous visual processing deficit in developmental dyslexia. *Vision Research, 48*, 979–988.

Lefavrais, P. (1967). *Test de l'Alouette*. Paris, France: Les Editions du Centre de Psychologie Appliquée (ECPA).

Lehongre, K., Morillon, B., Giraud, A. L., & Ramus, F. (2013). Impaired auditory sampling in dyslexia: Further evidence from combined fMRI and EEG. *Frontiers in Human Neurosciences, 7*, 454. doi: http://dx.doi.org/10.3389/fnhum.2013.00454.

Lehongre, K., Ramus, F., Villiermet, N., Schwartz, D., & Giraud, A. L. (2011). Altered low-g sampling in auditory cortex accounts for the three main facets of dyslexia. *Neuron, 72*, 1080–1090.

Lété, B., Sprenger-Charolles, L., & Colé, P. (2004). MANULEX: A grade-level lexical database from French elementary school readers. *Behavior Research Methods, Instruments, & Computers, 36*, 156–166.

Lobier, M., Peyrin, C., Pichat, C., Le Bas, J. F. & Valdois, S. (2014). Visual processing of multiple elements in the dyslexic brain: Evidence for a superior parietal dysfunction. *Frontiers in Human Neurosciences, 8*, 479. doi: http://dx.doi.org/10.3389/fnhum.2014.00479.

Lobier, M., Zoubrinetzky, R., & Valdois, S. (2012). The visual attention span deficit in dyslexia is visual and not verbal. *Cortex, 48*, 768–773.

Lyon, G. R., Shaywitz, S. E., & Shaywitz, B. A. (2003). A definition of dyslexia. *Annals of Dyslexia, 53*, 1–14.

Magnan, A., Ecalle, J., Veuillet, E., & Collet, L. (2004). The effects of an audio-visual training program in dyslexic children. *Dyslexia, 10*, 131–140.

Mahé, G., Bonnefond, A., & Doignon-Camus, N. (2013). Is the impaired N170 print tuning specific to developmental dyslexia? A matched reading-level study with poor readers and dyslexics. *Brain and Language, 127*, 539–544.

Mahé, G., Bonnefond, A., Gavens, N., Dufour, A., & Doignon-Camus, N. (2012). Impaired visual expertise for print in french adults with dyslexia as shown by N170 tuning. *Neuropsychologia, 50*, 3200–3206.

Maïonchi-Pino, N., Taki, Y., & Yokoyama, S. et al. (2013). Is the phonological deficit in developmental dyslexia related to impaired phonological representations and to universal phonological grammar? *Journal of Experimental Child Psychology, 115*, 53–73.

Manis, F. R., Seidenberg, M. S., Doi, L. M., McBride-Chang, C., & Peterson, A. (1996). On the basis of two subtypes of developmental dyslexia. *Cognition, 58*, 157–195.

Martin, J., Colé, P., Leuwers, C., Casalis, S., Zorman, M., & Sprenger-Charolles, L. (2010). Reading in French-speaking adults with dyslexia. *Annals of Dyslexia, 60*, 238–264.

Maurer, U., Blau, V. C., Yoncheva, Y. N., & McCandliss, B. (2010). Development of visual expertise for reading: Rapid emergence of visual familiarity for an artificial script. *Developmental Neuropsychology, 35*, 404–422.

Melby-Lervåg, M., Lyster, S. A. H., & Hulme, C. (2012). Phonological skills and their role in learning to read: A meta-analytic review. *Psychological Bulletin, 138*, 322–352.

Messaoud-Galusi, S., Hazan, V., & Rosen, S. (2011). Investigating speech perception in children with dyslexia: Is there evidence of a consistent deficit in individuals? *Journal of Speech, Language, and Hearing Research, 54*, 1682–1701.

Metsala, J. L., Stanovich, K. E., & Brown, G. D. A. (1998). Regularity effects and the phonological deficit model of reading disabilities: A meta-analytic review. *Journal of Educational Psychology, 90*, 279–293.

Mody, M. (2003). Rapid auditory processing deficits in dyslexia: A commentary on two differing views. *Journal of Phonetics, 31*, 529–539.

Monzalvo, K., Fluss, J., Billard, C., Dehaene, S., & Dehaene-Lambertz, G. (2012). Cortical networks for vision and language in dyslexic and normal children of variable socio-economic status. *Neuroimage, 61*, 258–274.

Noordenbos, M. W., Segers, E., Mitterer, H., Serniclaes, W., & Verhoeven, L. (2013a). Neural evidence of the 501 allophonic mode of speech perception in adults with dyslexia. *Clinical Neurophysiology, 124*, 1151–1162.

Noordenbos, M. W., Segers, E., Serniclaes, W., & Verhoeven, L. (2013b). Neural evidence of allophonic perception in children at risk for dyslexia. *Neuropsychologia, 50*, 2010–2017.

Pacton, S., Fayol, M., & Perruchet, P. (2005). Children's implicit learning of grapho-tactic and morphological regularities. *Child Development, 76*, 324–339.

Paulesu, E., Démonet, J. F., & Fazio, F. et al. (2001). Dyslexia, Cultural diversity and Biological unity. *Science, 291*, 2165–2167.

Peereman, R., Sprenger-Charolles, L., & Messaoud-Galusi, S. (2013). The contribution of morphology to the consistency of spelling-to-sound relations: A quantitative analysis based on French elementary school readers. *L'Année Psychologique, 213*, 113–133.

Perfetti, C. A. (1985). *Reading ability*. New York, NY: Oxford University Press.

Perfetti, C. A. (2007). Reading ability: Lexical quality to comprehension. *Scientific Studies of Reading, 11*, 357–383. doi: http://dx.doi.org/10.1080/10888430701530730.

Piquard-Kipffer, A., & Sprenger-Charolles, L. (2013). Early predictors of future reading skills: A follow-up of French-speaking children from the beginning of kindergarten to the end of the second grade (age 5 to 8). *L'Année Psychologique, 113*, 491–521.

Quémart, P., & Casalis, S. (2015). Visual processing of derivational morphology in children with developmental dyslexia: Insights from masked priming. *Applied Psycholinguistics, 36*, 345–376.

Ramus, F. (2003). Developmental dyslexia: Specific phonological deficit or general sensorimotor dysfunction? *Current Opinion in Neurobiology, 13*, 212–218.

Ramus, F., & Szenkovits, G. (2008). What phonological deficit? *Quarterly Journal of Experimental Psychology, 61*, 129–141.

Reilhac, C., Jucla, M., Iannuzzi, S., Valdois, S., & Démonet, J. F. (2012). Effect of orthographic processes on letter identity and letter-position encoding in dyslexic children. *Frontiers in Psychology*, *3*, 154. doi: http://dx.doi.org/10.3389/fpsyg .2012.00154.

Ruff, S., Cardebat, D., Marie, N., & Démonet, J. F. (2002). Enhanced response of the left frontal cortex to slowed down speech in dyslexia: An fRMI study. *Neuroreport*, *13*, 1285–1289.

Serniclaes, W., Collet, G., & Sprenger-Charolles, L. (2015). Review of neural rehabilitation programs for dyslexia: How can an allophonic system be changed into a phonemic one? *Frontiers in Psychology*, *6*, 190. doi: http://dx.doi.org/10.3389/fps yg.2015.00190.

Serniclaes, W., & Sprenger-Charolles, L. (2015). Reading impairment: From behavior to brain. In R. Bahr & E. Silliman (Eds.), *Handbook of communication disorders* (pp. 34–45). London: Routledge.

Serniclaes, W., Sprenger-Charolles, L., Carré, R., & Demonet, J. F. (2001). Perceptual discrimination of speech sounds in developmental dyslexia. *Journal of Speech, Language, and Hearing Research*, *44*, 384–399.

Share, D. L. (1995). Phonological recoding and self-teaching: Sine qua non of reading acquisition. *Cognition*, *55*, 151–218.

Shaywitz, S. A., Gruen, J., Mody, M., & Shaywitz, B. A. (2009). Dyslexia. In R. G. Schwartz (Ed.), *The handbook of child language disorders* (pp. 115–139). Boca Raton, FL: Psychology Press.

Sprenger-Charolles, L. (2003). Reading acquisition: Cross linguistic data. In T. Nunes & P. Bryant (Eds.), *Handbook of children's literacy* (pp. 43–66). Dordrecht: Kluwer.

Sprenger-Charolles, L., Colé, P., Kipffer-Piquard, A., Pinton, F., & Billard, C. (2009). Reliability and prevalence of an atypical development of phonological skills in French-speaking dyslexics. *Reading and Writing*, *22*, 811–842.

Sprenger-Charolles, L., Colé, P., Lacert, P., & Serniclaes, W. (2000). On subtypes of developmental dyslexia: Evidence from processing time and accuracy scores. *Canadian Journal of Experimental Psychology*, *54*, 88–104.

Sprenger-Charolles, L., Colé, P., & Serniclaes, W. (2006). *Reading acquisition and developmental dyslexia (Essays in developmental psychology)*. New-York, NY: Psychology Press.

Sprenger-Charolles, L., Siegel, L. S., Béchennec, D., & Serniclaes, W. (2003). Development of phonological and orthographic processing in reading aloud, in silent reading, and in spelling: A four-year longitudinal study. *Journal of Experimental Child Psychology*, *84*, 194–217.

Sprenger-Charolles, L., Siegel, L. S., Jiménez, J. E., & Ziegler, J. C. (2011). Prevalence and reliability of phonological, surface, and mixed profiles in dyslexia: A review of studies conducted in languages varying in orthographic depth. *Scientific Studies of Reading*, *6*, 498–501.

Stanovich, K. E., Siegel, L. S., & Gottardo, A. (1997). Converging evidence for phonological and surface subtypes of reading disability. *Journal of Educational Psychology*, *89*, 114–127.

Strong, G. K., Torgerson, C. J., Torgerson, D., & Hulme, C. (2011). A systematic meta-analytic review of evidence for the effectiveness of the "Fast ForWord" language intervention program. *Journal of Child Psychology and Psychiatry*, *52*, 224–235.

Szenkovits, G., & Ramus, F. (2005). Exploring dyslexics' phonological deficit I: Lexical versus sub-lexical and input versus output processes. *Dyslexia, 11*, 253–268.

Valdois, S., Bosse, M. L., & Tainturier, M. J. (2004). Cognitive correlates of developmental dyslexia: Review of evidence for a selective visual attentional deficit. *Dyslexia, 10*, 1–25.

Tallal, P. (1980). Auditory temporal perception, phonics, and reading disabilities in children. *Brain and Language, 9*, 182–198.

Talli, I., Sprenger-Charolles, L., & Stavrakaki, S. (2015). Is there an overlap between specific language impairment and developmental dyslexia? New insights from French. In S. Stavrakaki (Ed.), *Language acquisition and language disorders* (pp. 57–88). Amsterdam: John Benjamins.

Van IJzendoorn, M. H., & Bus, A. G. (1994). Meta-analytic confirmation of the non-word reading deficit in developmental dyslexia. *Reading Research Quarterly, 30*, 266–275.

Ziegler, J. C., Castel, C., Pech-Georgel, C., George, F., Alario, F. X., & Perry, C. (2008). Developmental dyslexia and the dual route model of reading: Simulating individual differences and subtypes. *Cognition, 107*, 151–178.

Ziegler, J. C., & Goswami, U. (2005). Reading acquisition, developmental dyslexia and skilled reading across languages: A psycholinguistic grain size theory. *Psychological Bulletin, 131*, 3–29.

Ziegler, J. C., Pech-Georgel, C., Dufau, S., & Grainger, J. (2010). Rapid processing of letters, digits, and symbols: What purely visual-attentional deficit in developmental dyslexia? *Developmental Science, 13*, F8–F14.

Ziegler, J. C., Pech-Georgel, C., George, F., & Lorenzi, C. (2009). Speech-perception-in-noise deficits in dyslexia. *Developmental Science, 12*, 732–745.

Ziegler, J. C., Perry, C., & Coltheart, M. (2003). Speed of lexical and nonlexical processing in French: The case of the regularity effect. *Psychonomic Bulletin & Review, 10*, 947–953.

Ziegler, J. C., Perry, C., & Zorzi, M. (2014). Modelling reading development through phonological decoding and self-teaching: Implications for dyslexia. *Philosophical Transactions of the Royal Society B, 369*, 20120397.

Zoubrinetzky, R., Bielle, F., & Valdois, S. (2014). New insights on developmental dyslexia subtypes: Heterogeneity of mixed reading profiles. *PLoS One, 9*(6), e99337.

4 Developmental Dyslexia in Dutch

Ludo Verhoeven

4.1 Introduction

Although Dutch can be considered a transparent orthography, a substantial number of children in the Netherlands suffer from severe reading and spelling problems. Over the past decades, research has focused on the question of how problems with learning to read and spell in Dutch can best be understood. Importantly, policymakers have recognized the results of ongoing research efforts and protocols are now being followed nationwide for the diagnosis of developmental dyslexia and conduct of interventions.

In this chapter, we start with a short introduction to the Dutch language and its orthography. We then review what is known about the processes of learning to read and spell in Dutch as evidenced by research with typical children (see also Verhoeven, 2017). Next, we sketch the historical and cultural context leading up to the identification of problems with learning to read in Dutch and the diagnosis of developmental dyslexia in the Netherlands. We then review the state of the art with regard to behavioral and neurocognitive research on the underpinnings of reading and spelling problems in Dutch, on the one hand, and the effectiveness of current reading and spelling interventions, on the other. We conclude with a general discussion of what is known about dyslexia in Dutch and the relevance of this information for children who are having problems with learning to read and spell in general – also those learning in other languages.

4.2 Learning to Read Dutch

4.2.1 Dutch Language and Its Orthography

Dutch is a West Germanic language related to both German and English. Dutch did not, however, undergo the High German consonant shift and also does not have the extensive grammatical case system of German. This has resulted in a relatively simple morphology. And while most Dutch words originate from Germanic, there are also many loan words from Roman languages (Latin and

French). Dutch vowels are pronounced according to the phonological features of place of articulation (frontal, central, back) and height (low, middle, high). There is also an opposition between long and short vowels: Long vowels tend to be tense and short vowels lax. Dutch has three diphthongs: frontal ɛı as in *hei* "heath," central ʌü as in *bui* "shower," and back ɑu as in *dauw* "dew." The Dutch system of consonants is relatively simple, with place and manner of articulation, in addition to voicing, as the main distinctive features. The vast majority of Dutch monosyllabic words follow a Consonant-Vowel-Consonant (CVC) pattern, although consonant clusters can occur in both initial and final word positions. In polysyllabic words, the main stress tends to be on the pre-final syllable. And with the exception of only the schwa, all vowels in Dutch can receive stress. In nominal and verbal compounds, primary stress is on the first part and secondary stress on the second. Word formation in Dutch is primarily accomplished via affixation and compounding (cf. Booij, 1977). For affixation, the processes of declination, conjugation, and derivation can be distinguished. There are more or less regular devices available to form the plural, possessive, comparative, and superlative. Sentence intonation is rather flat in Dutch. Unmarked Dutch declarative sentences have a low declining contour at the beginning, a high declining contour in the middle, and a final low declining contour at the end. Interrogative sentences (i.e., questions) have a high declining contour at the end.

Dutch orthography is largely phonemic (Nunn, 1998). That is, a rather straightforward mapping of graphemes onto phonemes occurs in short Dutch words while this is not always the case in longer Dutch words. The mapping between letters and phonemes in monosyllabic words is highly consistent, moreover. In CVC words, the basic grapheme-to-phoneme correspondences are almost strictly one-to-one and invariant. Dutch syllable structure, in contrast, is quite complex because multiple consonants can occur in both the onset and coda positions (i.e., word initial and final positions). Dutch words can thus contain multi-letter graphemes (e.g., *leeuw* "lion") and morphological analogies (e.g., *vriend* "friend," which receives a final –*d* because of its plural *vrienden*). In longer words, further deviations from the one-to-one correspondence between letters and sounds occur. A case in point is the vowel *e*, which can represent three different sounds in polysyllabic words: Occurring in a closed stressed syllable, it is pronounced /ɛ/; occurring in an open stressed syllable, it is pronounced /e/; and occurring in an unstressed syllable, it is pronounced /œ/. The Dutch word *wegnemen* ("take away") is thus pronounced / wɛgnemœn/. In addition, the phonological status of the schwa occurring as the central vowel in unstressed syllables in polysyllabic words can be quite unclear in Dutch and is thus represented by the letters <e>, <ij>, as in *bodem* ("bottom"), *gevaarlijk* ("dangerous"), and *vredig* ("peaceful"), at times. A schwa is also inserted in sonorant consonant clusters in unstressed final syllables, as in *kever* ("beetle"). Yet another deviation in Dutch phonology and orthography concerns the written reduplication of vowels and consonants. Vowels that are normally spelled with reduplication <aa>, <ee>, <oo>, are written with a single letter when occurring in pre-final word position; the plural of *maan* ("moon") is thus spelled *manen*. In contrast, a single-letter consonant is reduplicated when it occurs in an intervocalic position after a stressed short vowel; that is, the plural of *man* ("man") is spelled *mannen*. These examples show that in Dutch the transparency from orthography to phonology is much larger than the other way around (cf. Bosman & Van Orden, 1997).

4.2.2 Challenges in Learning to Read Dutch

In preschool and kindergarten in the Netherlands, storybook reading and emergent literacy activities are part of daily routines aimed at strengthening the oral communication skills and vocabularies of most children, and thus their phonological awareness and emergent literacy. When Vloedgraven and Verhoeven (2007, 2009) examined the development of children's early phonological awareness in relation to their reading skills in kindergarten and first grade, they found performance on four different tasks to reflect a single underlying ability. The tasks ranged in difficulty with rhyming being easiest, phoneme blending and phoneme identification occurring in between, and phoneme segmentation proving most difficult. In addition, strong growth in phonological awareness was observed between kindergarten and first grade. In other research, de Jong and van der Leij (1999) documented changing associations between phonological awareness and the reading abilities of children over time. In particular, children's initial kindergarten phonological awareness did not relate to their later reading skill while their phonological awareness in first grade did relate to their later reading skill. This effect was tentatively explained at the time in terms of the transparent nature of Dutch orthography. However, a later comparison of the capacities of phonological awareness and alphanumeric naming speed to predict the later word decoding of Dutch versus English school-aged children revealed no significant differences for the prediction of word-decoding speed or word-decoding accuracy in a relatively transparent language (i.e., Dutch) versus a relatively opaque language (i.e., English; Patel, Snowling, & de Jong, 2004).

In still other research, Verhoeven et al. (2016) showed differential relations between measures of the precursors to lexical quality and the emergence of letter knowledge and word decoding in kindergarten. The children's early phonological awareness and rapid naming related to the development of their letter knowledge while their phonological awareness and letter knowledge related to the development of their word decoding during the kindergarten year. A lifespan perspective was taken on the development of rapid naming by van den Bos,

Zijlstra, and Iutje Spelberg (2002), and its impact on word-reading fluency was evidenced by van den Bos, Zijlstra, and van den Broeck (2003). The role of visual attention in the development of reading has also been recently examined and has been shown to significantly add to the prediction of reading and spelling skill after control for phonological awareness and rapid-naming speed (van den Boer, van Bergen, & de Jong, 2015). The researchers nevertheless argue that the observed role of visual attention span may simply reflect the quality of the associations already established between the orthographic and phonological units required for reading and spelling in Dutch.

The basic task confronting children learning to read in Dutch is to progress from sequential, grapheme-to-phoneme decoding of words to fast, parallel, and largely phonology-based decoding processing of different word classes. Given what we know about learning to read in Dutch, initial reading instruction across schools in the Netherlands already involves a large amount of phonics instruction with a focus on the decoding of regular CVC word patterns. In a period of about four months, all of the regular grapheme–phoneme correspondences are taught – within the contexts of individual words and small bits of text. In the subsequent months, the instruction is extended to include the reading of monosyllabic words containing consonant clusters and disyllabic words. By the end of first grade, Dutch children are expected to be able to decode simple and regularly written Dutch words. In second grade, the length of the words is increased and irregularities or specific context-sensitive mapping rules for sounds to letters and letters to sounds are introduced. In subsequent years, the automatization of the decoding of words is stimulated via practice with a variety of book-reading routines.

In a longitudinal study, the acquisition of Dutch word decoding throughout the elementary years was examined by Verhoeven and van Leeuwe (2009, 2011). Mastery of words that varied in orthographic transparency was analyzed (cf. Nunn, 1998): regular CVC words, complex monosyllabic words with consonant clusters in initial and final word positions, and polysyllabic words. The word decoding of the beginning readers started out slow and laborious with a fair number of mistakes but reached a level of virtual mastery quickly by the beginning of second grade (i.e., 7 years of age). These results show the growth of Dutch word-decoding skill to be largely a matter of increasing speed. The three measures of word decoding further showed considerable commonalities and strong longitudinal interrelationships over the years. The unique variance accounted for by the individual word-decoding skills also showed that specific orthographic complexities have to be learned over the years. The rapid increases observed in the speed and accuracy of children's word decoding and the finding that the speed and accuracy of their word decoding continually relate to each other over the years in the studies by Verhoeven and van Leeuwe are fully commensurate with the restricted interactive model of lexical presentation as put forth by Perfetti

(1997). According to this model, word-decoding practice increases the number of orthographically addressable words and modifies individual word representations.

The overlap observed in early Dutch word-decoding skills is fully commensurate with a study by Keuning and Verhoeven (2007) showing a single ability to underlie the decoding means for a representative set of Dutch words throughout the elementary years. However, evidence of specific orthographic complexities comes from a range of experimental studies examining the role of morphology in the development of Dutch word decoding. Similarly, when Verhoeven, Schreuder, and Haarman (2006) examined morphological sensitivity by having both children and adults read bisyllabic words with varying morphological constituents in Dutch, they found both beginning and advanced readers to successfully apply the necessary conversion rules. Young children were aware of not only elementary grapheme–phoneme correspondences but also correspondences for larger orthographic (morpheme-based) units. In other research, Verhoeven, Schreuder, and Baayen (2006) examined the learning of autonomous graphotactic rules in relation to morphological awareness. These rules were specifying that the contrast between long and short vowels be expressed by an alternation between single- versus double- consonant letters in open syllables but by single- versus double-vowel letters in closed syllables. Both children *and* adults were found to be significantly less accurate and also slower when they had to recognize plurals that had undergone a vowel change as a result of the pluralization process versus no such change. In still other research, morphological awareness has been shown to differentially relate to the word recognition and spelling of Dutch first- and sixth-grade children (Rispens, McBride-Chang, & Reitsma, 2008). In first grade, only children's awareness of nominal inflectional morphology related to their word decoding. In sixth grade, in contrast, their awareness of derivational morphology related to both their word decoding and spelling while their awareness of verbal inflectional morphology related to only their spelling. When Keuning and Verhoeven (2008) examined the dimensional structure of spelling development throughout the elementary grades, factor analyses showed that spelling could be conceptualized as a unidimensional ability for second through sixth grade. The children nevertheless showed a tendency to master different types of spelling problems during different – partially overlapping – periods in their development.

4.3   Reading Difficulties in Dutch

4.3.1   Historical and Cultural Context

During the second half of the past century, the term *dyslexia* was commonly used in the Netherlands to refer to any serious reading and spelling problems. Given the emergence of special education as an independent scientific discipline, however, dyslexia gradually became recognized as a *specific* learning problem that thus needed to be studied from the perspective of remediation (Dumont, 1971, 1984, 1991; van der Leij, 1998). The Health Council of the Netherlands came up with the following definition of dyslexia in 1995: "Dyslexia is present when the automatization of word identification (reading) and/or word spelling does not develop or does so very incompletely or with great difficulty." This working definition characterizes dyslexia as severe retardation of reading and spelling, which – when examined more closely – shows very slow and/or inaccurate and easily disturbed word identification and/or word spelling that is not helped by the usual teaching or remedial intervention efforts. This operational definition has been further articulated by the Dutch Dyslexia Foundation (Stichting Dyslexie Nederland, 2008, 2016), and it is still widely recognized in the Netherlands.

Protocols for signaling serious reading and spelling problems were developed to facilitate the early identification of dyslexia in schools (Wentink & Verhoeven, 2001, 2004). At the same time, Blomert (2006) developed separate protocols for the diagnosis and treatment of dyslexia in specialized reading clinics. In these protocols, the pervasiveness of serious reading and spelling problems was determined along with indications of a phonological deficit as evidenced by low performance on tests of phonological awareness, naming speed, and/or letter knowledge. In the diagnostic assessment protocol, severe dyslexia is distinguished from mild dyslexia, other reading problems, and multiple problems based on the severity of the reading and spelling problems but also the underlying cognitive profile, which includes phonological awareness, rapid naming, grapheme–phoneme coupling and verbal short-term memory.

In the intervention protocol developed based on the Blomert (2006) survey results, psycholinguistically motivated intervention guidelines have been formulated for the following: phonological processing, grapheme–phoneme coupling, speed reading, and rule-based spelling. The phonological component focuses on explicit phonics skills with special attention to the different phoneme classes because the different types of phonemes form the basis for the application of spelling rules and for the mastery of grapheme–phoneme correspondence rules. The speed-reading and rule-based spelling components help the words in children's lexicons become more phonologically specified and thus more redundant with respect to their sublexical constituents. Intervention entails a series of weekly one-hour training sessions and homework exercises for a period of one year.

4.3.2   *Identification and Prevalence of Dyslexia*

Dyslexia is diagnosed in the Netherlands when: a child shows *persistent* reading problems as indicated by three consecutive scores in the lowest decile on a standardized word-reading test during the elementary grades; tailored interventions at the school have not produced significant progress; and the diagnosis has been confirmed by assessment in a reading clinic. An attempt was made to estimate the actual number of children with dyslexia in a nationwide survey (Blomert, 2005). It was concluded that around 10 percent of all school-age children could not read efficiently and that about 4 percent of these children could be assumed to suffer from dyslexia. Severe spelling problems were also evidenced for 95 percent of the children who were exhibiting severe reading problems and who had thus been diagnosed as having dyslexia.

In a study by Tilanus, Segers, and Verhoeven (2013), the cognitive profiles of second-grade children who had just been assigned a diagnosis of dyslexia were examined. The speed and accuracy of word and pseudoword decoding as well as the accuracy of word spelling were assessed along with four types of precursors (i.e., rapid naming, verbal working memory, phonemic awareness, and letter knowledge). The group diagnosed as dyslexic indeed lagged significantly behind on all measures, and this explained two thirds of the variance associated with the group difference.

In a nationwide study, Verhoeven and Keuning (2018) examined the speed and accuracy of word and pseudoword decoding for four different lengths of word forms and three types of phonological abilities (i.e., phonological awareness, rapid naming, and phonological working memory) for children from Grades 1 through 6. The results are presented in Figure 4.1. For typical readers, decoding ability levels were found to be largely a matter of increasing speed across grades. For the readers with dyslexia, in contrast, accurate decoding was found to be particularly challenging. Strong lexical status and length effects were evidenced showing that, compared to typical readers, the children with dyslexia had more trouble accurately decoding pseudowords (relative to real words) and decoding longer (as opposed to shorter) words and pseudowords. It can thus be concluded that children with a diagnosis of dyslexia lag behind with regard to both the speed and accuracy of applying the sublexical strategies required for pseudoword decoding and the lexical strategies required for word decoding. Furthermore, the children with dyslexia consistently lagged behind their typical reading peers on all of the phonological measures, although the effect sizes were small. It could thus be tentatively concluded based on this latter finding that children with dyslexia in the intermediate and upper levels of elementary school show only minor problems with their phonological abilities and that these problems only manifest themselves when the phonological recoding of orthographic representations is required.

A series of logistic regression analyses was conducted to assess the diagnostic sensitivity and specificity of word and pseudoword decoding tests, along with tests for phonological awareness, rapid naming, and verbal short-term

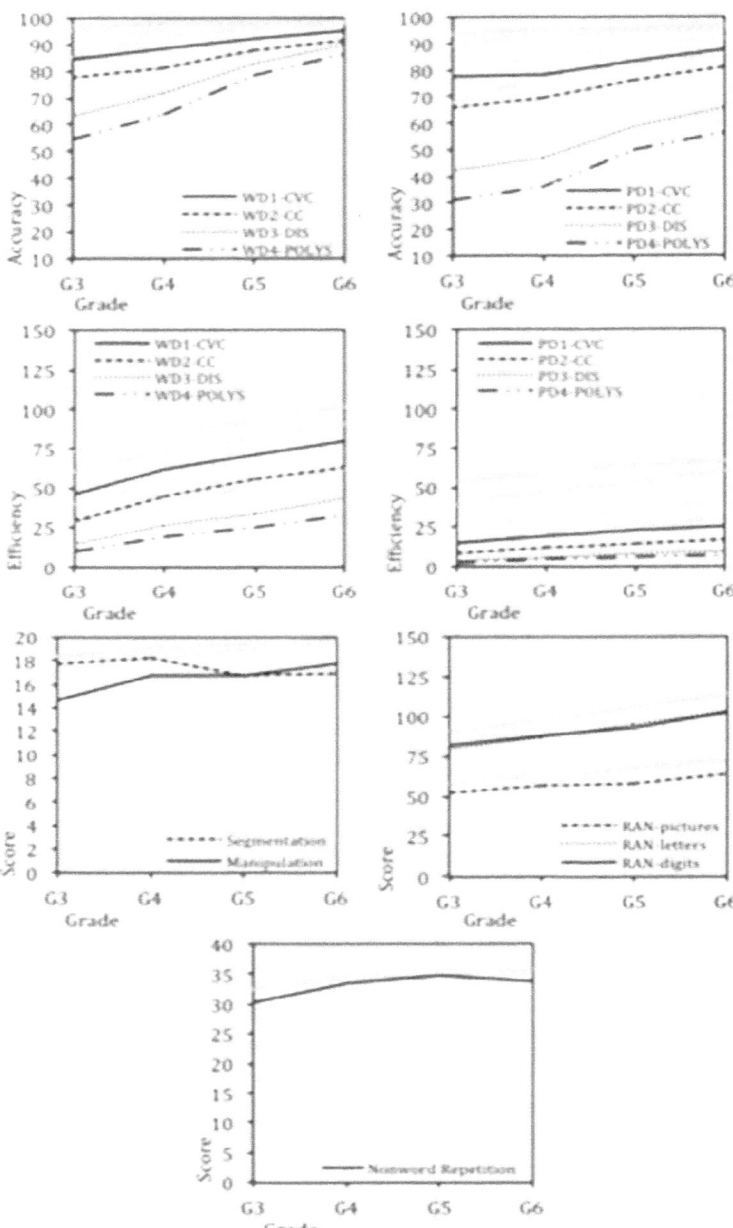

Figure 4.1 Performances on word decoding (WD) and pseudoword decoding (PD) accuracy and efficiency; serial rapid naming (RAN); phonological awareness; and phonological working memory (bottom), for children without dyslexia (gray) versus children with dyslexia (black) according to elementary grade

memory. Sensitivity was high for the speed of pseudoword decoding and moderate for not only the accuracy of pseudoword decoding but also both the speed and accuracy of word decoding. Sensitivity was further found to be moderate for phonological awareness. It thus appears that it is not so much insight into phonological abilities that helps identify dyslexic readers but, rather, insight into the ability to *apply* phonological knowledge during the task of phonological recoding. Phonological abilities measured outside the context of reading did not add to the identification of dyslexia. Even the full model including all phonological measures and decoding measures did not improve the prediction of dyslexia over the inclusion of just word- and pseudo-word-decoding measures. These findings are in keeping with the findings of previous research showing the core of the reading problem encountered in dyslexia to lie in the use of sublexical strategies for phonological recoding or, in other words, the development of fluent word decoding (cf. Ramus, 2004; Ziegler et al., 2008).

4.4   Behavioral and Neurocognitive Evidence

4.4.1   Nature of Reading Problems in Dutch

Research on reading problems in Dutch has been largely predicated on the assumption that one of the main reading problems reflects a deficiency in the language system, particularly at the level of phonological processing (Pugh et al., 2013; Ramus, 2014). The reading and spelling problems of children at risk for dyslexia, for example, have been shown to be associated with problems in the domains of phonological awareness, phonological memory, and rapid naming (see de Bree, Wijnen, & Gerrits, 2010; Gijsel, Bosman, & Verhoeven, 2006; van der Leij et al., 2013).

Several researchers have specifically examined the phonological processing of children at risk for dyslexia in relation to their later reading. When Boets and colleagues (2010) compared the development of phonology and literacy in children with a family risk of dyslexia to that of matched controls, children diagnosed with dyslexia in third grade showed impaired phonological processing and reading performance from kindergarten on; children with a family risk of dyslexia but no diagnosis of dyslexia in third grade also scored more poorly than the control children, suggesting that the family risk for dyslexia is not an all-or-none predictor. When Schaars, Segers, and Verhoeven (2017) recently examined the early word decoding of children at risk of dyslexia with that of matched controls in kindergarten and first grade, they found impaired kinder-garten phonemic awareness to characterize the children at risk of dyslexia. During the first five months of reading instruction, moreover, the children at risk for dyslexia showed less efficient word decoding than the control children and this discrepancy only increased during the first five months of reading instruction. In the period following the children's initial reading instruction, the observed discrepancy continued for simple words and only increased for more complex words. In contrast to the word-decoding measures, the measures of phonemic awareness and lexical retrieval equally predicted the reading development of the children at risk of dyslexia and the control children.

In other research, kindergarten children at risk of dyslexia but with no later diagnosis of dyslexia performed *better* than kindergarten children at risk of dyslexia and a later diagnosis of dyslexia, but *worse* than control children (van Bergen et al., 2011). The intergroup differences for reading development and its precursors in children from kindergarten through fifth grade were found for letter knowledge and rapid naming but not for phonological awareness. The children at risk of dyslexia and a later diagnosis of dyslexia read less fluently than the other groups from first grade on. The reading fluency of the children at risk of dyslexia but no later diagnosis of dyslexia was intermediate between the other groups of children at the start of reading instruction. In a similar line of research, de Jong and van der Leij (2003) also found ongoing phonological impairments (e.g., rapid-naming impairments), to characterize poor readers from kindergarten through sixth grade. The phonological impairments in these children in first grade nevertheless tended to disappear by the end of elementary school, depending on task demands. This finding led the authors to suggest that the different manifestations of phonological awareness and phonological deficits may reflect different developmental reading pathways.

In still other research, van Bergen et al. (2012) highlighted the importance of intergenerational factors in the occurrence of dyslexia. In a longitudinal study, they showed severely impaired performance of children with a family risk of dyslexia on naming, phonology, spelling, and word/pseudoword reading tasks. It was also found that differences in parental word-reading fluency and rapid-naming performance were predictive of differences in the children's reading abilities, even after the predictive capacity of the differences in the children's cognitive skills were taken into consideration. The finding of intergenerational correlations suggests that intertwined genetic and environmental pathways may confer a liability for dyslexia on children based on a phonological deficit.

A number of other studies have attempted to test the hypothesis that the phonological deficit observed in dyslexia might stem from a more general auditory processing deficit. To begin with, Boets et al. (2007) tested the categorical speech perception and speech-in-noise perception of a group of 5-year-old preschool children genetically at risk for dyslexia and compared this to what they found for a group of well-matched control children and a group of adults. As could be expected for such a young age, both groups of children differed significantly from the adult group on all of the speech measures. The group of children genetically at risk for dyslexia showed a slight but significant speech-in-noise perception deficit, particularly in the most difficult listening condition. For categorical speech perception, a marginally significant deficit was observed on the category discrimination but not the category identification task for the children at risk of dyslexia. Speech parameters were significantly related to phonological awareness and low-level auditory measures. The category discrimination and speech-in-noise perception problems of the children at risk for dyslexia are taken as evidence for a causal model in which low-level auditory problems are hypothesized to lead to subtle speech perception problems that can then interfere with the development of children's phonological, reading, and spelling abilities. Noordenbos et al. (2012a) assessed the categorical perception abilities of children at risk of dyslexia both before and after formal reading instruction in first grade. Children at risk of dyslexia showed a shift from an allophonic mode of speech perception to a phonemic mode of speech perception during the course of first grade, while the control group of children showed a phonemic mode of speech perception already in kindergarten. An allophonic mode of speech perception was thus taken on the basis of this research to constitute a clinical marker for potential reading problems. Along these lines, Vandermosten et al. (2011) found evidence for an auditory processing deficit in adults with dyslexia and have argued that the deficit is not specific to speech: Adults with dyslexia showed impaired categorization of speech and nonspeech sounds that differ in terms of rapidly changing acoustic cues (i.e., temporal cues) but accurately categorized steady-state speech and nonspeech sounds). These studies seem to indicate that children with dyslexia may not only have problems with becoming phonologically aware but also with the identification of phoneme boundaries that are pre-requisite for phonological awareness.

Finally, several studies have examined the specific orthographic component of Dutch dyslexia. Bekebrede et al. (2010) tested the phonological-core, variable-orthographic differences model of word reading (van der Leij & Morfidi, 2006) in adults with or without dyslexia. The adults with dyslexia were found to share a core phonological deficit. As predicted, moreover, significantly greater variability was found among the group with dyslexia in orthographic coding relative to phonological coding. Orthographic coding also explained additional variance in word-reading fluency after phonological coding was controlled for. Other studies have shown the orthographic representations of readers with dyslexia tend to be less specified and less redundant than those of typical readers (de Jong & Messbauer, 2011; Marinus & de Jong, 2008, 2011; van den Bos, 2008; van den Bos et al., 2002, 2003). And this has been shown to be particularly the case for the decoding of pseudowords (van den Broeck & Geudens, 2012; van den Broeck, Geudens, & van den Bos, 2010).

4.4.2   Underlying Causes of Reading Problems in Dutch

While it has been shown that phonological processing is vulnerable in Dutch dyslexia, an important question that remains for neurocognitive research is how orthographic representation and its development can be characterized in individuals with dyslexia. Noordenbos et al. (2013) examined event-related potentials in response to auditory word pairs that differed in phonological overlap during a rhyme-judgment task in 6-year-old children at risk of dyslexia and in control children. Both groups exhibited neural responses for the basic rhyme relations versus unrelated targets but only the control children did so for the rhyming versus non-rhyming overlap items. These findings suggest that children at risk base their judgments on comparison of overall sound similarity whereas children not at risk solve the rhyming task in a more analytic manner. In a diffusion MRI study, moreover, Vandermosten et al. (2015) showed the dorsal, left-hemispheric specialization for the phonological aspects of reading, as observed in adults, to be formed differently during the reading development of typical versus dyslexic readers. It is further suggested that the atypical white-matter organization previously found in dyslexic adults may be causal rather than the outcome of a lifetime of reading difficulties, but that the location of the causal deficit may vary throughout development.

In a series of studies, Blomert and colleagues attempted to identify the neural signature for the mapping problems of orthographic and phonological constituents in dyslexia (see Blomert, 2011). It was assumed in this series of studies that beginning readers are quite capable of determining which letters belong to which speech sounds but that it takes much more effort to integrate this information into newly constructed audiovisual units. This extended learning process is taken to correspond to observations that reliable indications of letter- and word-specific activations in the fusiform cortex are observed relatively late in development. From an additional series of electrophysiological and neuroimaging studies of the nature and mechanisms involved in letter–speech sound integration in normal and dyslexic readers (Blomert & Froyen, 2010; Blomert & Willems, 2010), it was concluded that letter–speech sound associations are immediately operative in development for the formation of orthographic–phonological units that stay on to be effective in advanced reading. It was also claimed that ineffective letter–speech sound integration precludes the development of reliable letter recognition in beginning dyslexic readers and is thus responsible for the reading fluency problems found in adult dyslexia. And it was further suggested that similar, integrated audiovisual representations may be effective for larger grain sizes of orthographic representations in the same posterior network as for the orthographic-phonological representations of letters and speech sounds.

In contrast to the above, it may be the case that individuals with dyslexia have intact phonological representations but problems accessing these. In a study by Boets et al. (2013), functional magnetic resonance imaging was combined with multivoxel pattern analysis and both functional and structural connectivity analyses in an effort to resolve whether the phonological deficits observed in dyslexia are caused by poor-quality phonetic representations or difficulties accessing intact phonetic representations. It was found that phonetic representations are hosted bilaterally in the primary and secondary auditory cortices and that their neural quality in terms of robustness and distinctness was intact in adults with dyslexia. However, the functional and structural connectivity between the bilateral auditory cortices and the left inferior frontal gyrus (or a region of the brain involved in higher-level phonological processing) was found to be significantly hampered in the adults with dyslexia, suggesting – indeed – deficient access to otherwise intact phonetic representations.

Neurocognitive studies have provided additional support for the hypothesis that a more general auditory processing deficit underlies dyslexia. Six-year-old beginning readers with a familial risk of dyslexia were found to be more sensitive to acoustic speech properties when compared to beginning readers with no familial risk of dyslexia when the negative markers were mismatched in a categorical perception task (Noordenbos et al., 2012b). Furthermore, van den Bunt and colleagues (2017) examined whether the development of dyslexia could be characterized by deficiencies in the speech-sensory, motor feedforward, and motor feedback mechanisms involved in the modulation of phonological representations. The study participants with dyslexia adapted more strongly during the ramp phase and returned less to baseline when feedback was back to normal when compared to the typical reading group. This finding was taken to be consistent with the notion that the phonological deficit in developmental dyslexia is associated with a weaker sensorimotor magnet for phonological representations.

4.5   Intervention

4.5.1   Early Intervention

In a series of training studies, researchers attempted to enhance the early literacy skills of children known to be at risk of dyslexia (see van der Leij, 2013). Eleveld (2005) used a training program of thirty ten-minute sessions with a focus on heightening the phonemic awareness and letter knowledge of kindergarten children at risk of dyslexia. At post-test, a combined measure of phoneme awareness and letter knowledge showed improvement relative to a control group, but these effects did not transfer to reading at the end of first grade. In a study by van Otterloo, van der Leij, and Henrichs (2009), a home-based intervention of fifty ten-minute sessions was conducted, with a focus on heightening phonemic awareness and letter knowledge in children at risk of dyslexia. At post-test, the experimental group showed greater progress than the control group on several measures of phonemic awareness but not on letter knowledge. Upon follow-up at the end of first grade, no significant differences were found between the two groups on tests of reading and spelling. In a follow-up study, van Otterloo and van der Leij (2009) extended the training program to seventy sessions and now found a significant effect for letter knowledge as well, but no transfer of the effects to tests of reading and spelling at the end of first grade. Another intervention, by Regtvoort and van der Leij (2007), involved seventy computer-based training sessions for phonemic awareness and letter knowledge together with practice on the reading of simple words for children at risk for dyslexia in kindergarten. At post-test, the trained children gained more on a combined measure of phoneme awareness than the controls, but there was no transfer to reading and spelling in first grade. To conclude, these studies show that the early literacy skills of children at risk for dyslexia can be trained in phonological awareness in kindergarten while the generation of transfer effects to word decoding and spelling in first grade, for example, remains difficult.

4.5.2   Reading and Spelling Intervention

More generally, experimental training studies have been conducted to find out how the performance of children with reading and spelling problems can be improved. Steenbeek-Planting, van Bon, and Schreuder (2013) investigated the effects of two training conditions on the reading speed of poor readers using a computer-based word-reading task. One condition focused on words the children read correctly (*successes*), the other on words they read incorrectly (*failures*). Overall, reading speed improved and transferred to untrained, orthographically more complex words. These transfer effects were characterized by an Aptitude-Treatment Interaction. Poor readers with a low initial reading level improved most in the training focused on successes. For poor readers with a high initial reading level, however, it appeared to be more profitable to practice with their failures. This study suggests that the improvement of general reading speed in a transparent orthography is closely related to both the children's initial reading level and the type of words they practice with: common and familiar words when training their successes, and uncommon and less familiar words when training their failures. In another training study, Van Gorp, Segers, and Verhoeven (2017) tested the use of a word-identification game to enhance the word-decoding efficiency of second graders with poor reading skills. The game included elements to enhance engagement and supported word identification (i.e., word reading) with word repetition, corrective feedback, and semantic retrieval. After the brief, five-hour tablet intervention across a period of five weeks, significant increases were found for decoding efficiency. Transfer effects to numerous untrained items were also evidenced.

For spelling, Cordewener, Bosman, and Verhoeven (2015) examined the influences of implicit versus explicit instruction on the acquisition of two types of Dutch spelling rules: a morphological rule and a phonological rule. High- and low-skilled spellers in first grade were assigned to implicit instruction, explicit instruction, and control instruction conditions. The results showed students in the explicit instruction condition to make more progress than students in the control condition for both the morphological and phonological spelling rules. For the morphological rule, the students in the explicit instruction condition also showed higher post-test scores on pseudowords than the students in the implicit instruction condition. The results in the three conditions did not differ for the high- versus low-skilled spellers, however. And both the high- and low-skilled spellers in the implicit and explicit instruction conditions did not fully generalize their knowledge of either the morphological rule or the phonological rule to new words and pseudowords.

4.5.3   Long-Term Intervention Effects

Several attempts have also been made to demonstrate the long-term effectiveness of a special treatment program for children with dyslexia. Tijms et al. (2003) found significant treatment effects for the reading of words, the reading of text, and spelling. The attained level of word reading and text reading was found to be stable across a four-year follow-up period, moreover. Spelling showed a slight decline one year following treatment but remained stable thereafter. In a follow-up study, Tijms (2011) further investigated the clinical effectiveness of the same treatment program, along with the possibly mediating effects of various cognitive factors on treatment success. The treatment group again accrued significantly greater gains than the control group for both reading and spelling. The treatment group obtained levels of reading and spelling accuracy that were comparable to the norm. Post-treatment levels of reading speed were also comparable to the lower bound for the normal reading range. Treatment effectiveness was robust against individual differences, with the exception of mediating effects of phonological memory and rapid automatized naming. In a similar vein, Tilanus, Segers, and Verhoeven (2016) evaluated responsiveness to a twelve-week phonics-based intervention in second-grade Dutch children with dyslexia. To do this, they compared reading and spelling gains to those of a control group of typical readers. The results showed the group of children with dyslexia to make more progress than the typical reading group on speed and accuracy of grapheme–phoneme conversion, word decoding and pseudoword decoding, and spelling accuracy. In addition, direct effects were found for the precursor measures of rapid automatized naming, verbal working memory, and phoneme deletion on the grapheme–phoneme conversion speed progress of the children with dyslexia and indirect effects of the precursor measures of rapid automatized naming and phoneme deletion on word-decoding speed, pseudoword efficiency, and real-word decoding accuracy via the scores on these same tests at pretest.

Finally, van der Kleij et al. (2017) investigated how response to a fifty-week phonics-based intervention, on the one hand, and reading levels before the intervention, on the other, predicted long-term reading outcomes for children with dyslexia in fifth grade. In Grade 5, the children with dyslexia still showed significantly slower word and pseudoword reading than their typically developing peers, which is obviously not surprising. The long-term pseudoword reading results for the children with dyslexia were predicted by their pseudoword reading at pretest and the growth in their pseudoword reading during the intervention, which was itself predicted by their pseudoword reading at pretest. The long-term real-word reading of the children with dyslexia was directly predicted by not only their pretest word reading but also indirectly by their pretest pseudoword reading via growth in both their pseudoword and real-word reading. It can thus be concluded that pseudoword reading is a good indicator of the severity of reading difficulties in children with dyslexia, but also an indicator of who may profit from an intervention in the long run.

4.6   Discussion and Conclusion

The research results reviewed in this chapter make it clear that Dutch orthography can be considered highly consistent, with orthographic complexities occurring in mainly polysyllabic words. Learning to read in Dutch is, accordingly, relatively easy for most children. Dutch children have been found to be highly accurate in their decoding from first grade on, and the further development of this skill is largely a matter of increasing speed (i.e., automatization of word decoding). The basic task confronting children to become fluent readers of Dutch is thus to progress from slow, sequential, grapheme-to-phoneme word decoding to fast, parallel, phonology-based orthographic word decoding.

4.6.1   *Evidence of a Phonological Deficit*

For children with dyslexia, accurate decoding turns out to be quite a challenge, particularly when it comes to longer or unfamiliar Dutch words. Even more problems present themselves when the reading process must be speeded up, as attested by the incremental arrears that manifest themselves in the decoding efficiency of children with developmental dyslexia throughout the elementary school years. The fact that the stagnation in the decoding efficiency of children with dyslexia is found to be greater for pseudowords than for real Dutch words and greater for longer than for shorter Dutch words shows the heart of their reading problems to lie in making fast connections between graphemes and phonemes in the context of decoding (pseudo)words. Nevertheless, initial analyses of the sensitivity and specificity of Dutch phonological processing tasks yielded only moderate markers of dyslexia for children learning to read. The sensitivity of children's decoding substantially increased when pseudo-word decoding was added to the phonological processing tasks, however, and the prediction of the diagnosis of dyslexia improved as a result. Most children with a diagnosis of dyslexia have a phonological deficit that creates a developmental lag for both the accuracy and efficiency of applying sublexical strategies required for pseudoword decoding and lexical strategies used for word decoding (cf. Ziegler, Perry, & Zorzi, 2014).

The large body of behavioral and neurocognitive research on the etiology of dyslexia points in the direction of an intergenerational phonological deficit. Lying at the core of this deficit is a failure to understand that words consist of speech sounds represented by letters. There is consistent evidence that Dutch children with dyslexia have difficulties with the development of efficient routines for the mapping of alphabetic characters onto the phonetic constituents they represent. It is nevertheless important in this light to note that the core phonological deficit appears to be associated with problems with the letter–sound *integration* in words. Neuroimaging studies by Blomert and colleagues suggest that dyslexia is associated with an inferior integration of letters and speech sounds in a specific neural circuit that appears to lack the redundancies and well-connectedness characteristic of audiovisual integration. The result is inferior and more effortful integration of letters and speech sounds.

This recently hypothesized vulnerability in the domain of multisensory integration might already be operational during the first year of life (see Blomert & Froyen, 2010). An alternative explanation for the observed phonological deficit in dyslexia is that the relevant phonological representations are overspecified as opposed to underspecified. In several recent studies, for example, it has been found that children and adults with dyslexia show categorical perception problems. And this finding suggests that individuals with dyslexia may have a so-called allophonic mode of speech perception (Serniclaes, 2011).

To conclude, there is evidence that dyslexia in Dutch is associated with a multifaceted phonological deficit that can be characterized by a reduced sensitivity to the relevant phonological information for the integration of orthographic units into words, by a heightened sensitivity to (often irrelevant) allophonic speech contrasts, and/or by difficulties accessing existing phonological representations (see also Boets et al., 2013; Pugh et al., 2013; Ramus, 2014).

4.6.2   Clinical Implications

Thanks to the widespread acceptance of protocols for the diagnosis and treatment of dyslexia by Dutch health-insurance companies today, children showing reading and spelling problems at school are entitled to referral to a specialized reading clinic for assessment, diagnosis, and intervention as needed. About 5 percent of the school population has qualified for these services in the Netherlands to date.

The present review shows early intervention to be important for the prevention of later reading and spelling problems. Strengthening such pre-reading skills as phonological awareness and letter recognition in preschool and kindergarten nevertheless appears to be promising. But there is still no evidence showing early interventions to facilitate the process of learning to read and spell in first grade, when formal literacy instruction starts. With regard to later interventions for children diagnosed with dyslexia, it has been found that the *accuracy* of their reading can be improved while the *speed* of their reading is proving more difficult to improve. Recent incorporation of motivators into game-based reading interventions, however, appears to be improving reading efficiency during the early years of elementary school and thus seems promising as an intervention for developmental dyslexia. More research is nevertheless needed to better understand these encouraging results.

To close, the present insights into Dutch dyslexia can be generalized to children encountering problems with learning to read and spell in other languages with transparent orthographies. Our main finding – namely that problems with phonological recoding lie at the heart of developmental dyslexia – calls for the initiation of phonological awareness and early literacy training in preschool and kindergarten in addition to well-structured phonics instruction during the early years of elementary school (see de Graaff et al., 2009). Children must be *systematically* taught the inventory of graphic forms that the writing system requires them to master. They must learn to identify the written language units (graphemes) that connect to spoken language units (phonemes) and just how graphemes map onto the phonemes, and vice versa. Children must discover not only the basic orthographic principles underlying the written language but also be given plenty of opportunities to practice linking written and spoken language forms (i.e., encouraged to read). Only then can an inventory of familiar written words be established, thereby creating the foundation for the orthographic lexicon that is needed to make the progression from the slow, sequential, grapheme-to-phoneme recoding to the fast, parallel, phonology-based orthographic decoding of words.

References

Bekebrede, J., van der Leij, A., Plakas, A., Share, D., & Morfidi, E. (2010). Dutch dyslexia in adulthood: Core features and variety. *Scientific Studies of Reading, 14*, 183–210.

Blomert, L. (2005). *Dyslexie in Nederland: Theorie, praktijk en beleid* [Dyslexia in The Netherlands: theory, practice and policy]. Amsterdam: Nieuwezijds Publishers.

Blomert, L. (2006). *Protocol dyslexie diagnostiek en behandeling* [Protocol dyslexia diagnosis and treatment]. Amsterdam: CVZ.

Blomert, L. (2011). The neural signature of orthographic-phonological binding in successful and failing reading development. *Neuroimage, 57*, 695–703.

Blomert, L., & Froyen, D. (2010). Multi-sensory learning and learning to read. *International Journal of Psychophysiology, 77*, 195–204.

Blomert, L., & Willems, G. (2010). Is there a causal link from a phonological awareness deficit to reading failure in children at familial risk for dyslexia? *Dyslexia, 16*, 300–317.

Boets, B., Ghesquière, P., van Wieringen, A., & Wouters, J. (2007). Speech perception in preschoolers at family risk for dyslexia: Relations with low-level auditory processing and phonological ability. *Brain and Language, 101*, 19–30.

Boets, B., Op de Beeck, H. P., & Vandermosten, M. et al. (2013). Intact but less accessible phonetic representations in adults with dyslexia. *Science, 342*, 1251–1254.

Boets, N., De Smedt, B., & Cleuren, L. et al. (2010). Towards a further characterization of phonological and literacy problems in children with dyslexia. *British Journal of Developmental Psychology, 28*, 5–31.

Booij, G. (1977). *Dutch morphology: A study of word formation in generative grammar.* Dordrecht: Foris.

Bosman, A. M. T., & Van Orden, G. C. (1997). Why spelling is more difficult than reading. In C. A. Perfetti, L. Rieben, & M. Fayol (Eds.), *Learning to spell: Research, theory, and practice across languages* (pp. 173–194). Hillsdale, NJ: Lawrence Erlbaum Associates.

Cordewener, K. A. H., Bosman, A. M. T., & Verhoeven, L. (2015). Implicit and explicit instruction: The case of spelling acquisition. *Written Language & Literacy, 18*, 121–152.

de Bree, E. H., Wijnen, F. N. K., & Gerrits, P. A. M. (2010). Non-word repetition and literacy in Dutch children at-risk of dyslexia and children with SLI: Results of the follow-up study. *Dyslexia, 16*, 36–44.

de Graaff, S., Bosman, A. M. T., Hasselman, F., & Verhoeven, L. (2009). Benefits of systematic phonics instruction. *Scientific Studies of Reading, 13*, 318–333.

de Jong, P. F., & Messbauer, V. C. S. (2011). Orthographic context and the acquisition of orthographic knowledge in normal and dyslexic readers. *Dyslexia, 17*, 107–122.

de Jong, P. F., & van der Leij, A. (1999). Specific contributions of phonological abilities to early reading acquisition: Results from a Dutch latent variable longitudinal study. *Journal of Educational Psychology, 91*, 450–476.

de Jong, P. F., & van der Leij, A. (2003). Developmental changes in the manifestation of a phonological deficit in dyslexic children learning to read a regular orthography. *Journal of Educational Psychology, 95*, 22–40.

Dumont, J. J. (1971). *Leerstoornissen* [Learning disabilities]. Rotterdam: Lemniscaat.

Dumont, J. J. (1984). *Lees- en spellingproblemen* [Reading and spelling difficulties]. Rotterdam: Lemniscaat.

Dumont, J. J. (1991). *Dyslexie: Theorie, diagnostiek en behandeling* [Dyslexia: Theory, diagnostics and treatment]. Rotterdam: Lemniscaat.

Eleveld, M. (2005). *At risk for dyslexia: The role of phonological abilities, letter knowledge* (Doctoral dissertation). Groningen: University of Groningen.

Gijsel, M. A. R., Bosman, A. M. T., & Verhoeven, L. (2006). Kindergarten risk factors, cognitive factors, and teacher judgments as predictors of early reading in Dutch. *Journal of Learning Disabilities, 39*, 558–571.

Health Council of the Netherlands. (1995). *Dyslexia: Definition and treatment* (publication no. 1995/15). The Hague: Health Council of the Netherlands.

Keuning, J., & Verhoeven, L. (2007). Screening for word reading and spelling problems in elementary school: An item response theory approach. *Education & Child Psychology*, *24*, 42–56.

Keuning, J., & Verhoeven, L. (2008). Spelling development throughout the elementary grades: The Dutch case. *Learning and Individual Differences*, *18*, 459–470.

Marinus, E., & de Jong, P. F. (2008). The use of sublexical clusters in normal reading and dyslexic readers. *Scientific Studies of Reading*, *12*, 253–280.

Marinus, E., & de Jong, P. F. (2011). Dyslexic and typical-reading children use vowel digraphs as perceptual units in reading. *The Quarterly Journal of Experimental Psychology*, *64*, 504–516.

Noordenbos, M. W., Segers, P. C. J., Serniclaes, W., Mitterer, H. A., & Verhoeven, L. T. W. (2012a). Allophonic mode of speech perception in Dutch children at risk for dyslexia: A longitudinal study. *Research in Developmental Disabilities*, *33*, 1469–1483.

Noordenbos, M. W. Segers, P. C. J., Serniclaes, W., Mitterer, H. A., & Verhoeven, L. T. W. (2012b). Neural evidence of allophonic perception in children at risk for dyslexia. *Neuropsychologia*, *50*, 2010–2017.

Noordenbos, M. W., Segers, P. C. J., Wagensveld, B., & Verhoeven, L. T. W. (2013). Aberrant N400 responses to phonological overlap during rhyme judgements in children at risk for dyslexia. *Brain Research*, *1537*, 233–243.

Nunn, A. (1998). *Dutch orthography*. Utrecht: Center for Language Studies.

Patel, T. K., Snowling, M. J., & de Jong, P. F. (2004). A cross-linguistic comparison of children learning to read in English and Dutch. *Journal of Educational Psychology*, *96*, 785–797.

Perfetti, C. A. (1997). The psycholinguistics of spelling and reading. In C. A. Perfetti, L. Rieben & M. Fayol (Eds.), *Learning to spell: Research, theory, and practice across languages* (pp. 21–38). Mahwah, NJ: Lawrence Erlbaum Associates.

Pugh, K. R., Landi, N., & Preston, J. L. et al. (2013). The relationship between phonological and auditory processing and brain organization in beginning readers. *Brain and Language*, *125*, 173–183.

Ramus, F. (2004). Neurobiology of dyslexia: A reinterpretation of the data. *Trends in Neurosciences*, *27*, 720–726.

Ramus, F. (2014). Neuroimaging sheds new light on the phonological deficit in dyslexia. *Trends in Cognitive Sciences*, *18*, 274–275.

Regtvoort, A. G. F. M., & van der Leij, A. (2007). Early intervention with children of dyslexic parents: Effects of computer-based reading instruction at home on literacy acquisition. *Learning and Individual Differences*, *17*, 35–53.

Rispens, J. E., McBride-Chang, C., & Reitsma, P. (2008). Morphological awareness and early and advanced word recognition and spelling in Dutch: A cross-sectional study. *Reading and Writing*, *21*, 587–607.

Schaars, M. M. H., Segers, E., & Verhoeven, L. (2017). Word decoding development during phonics instruction in children at risk for dyslexia. *Dyslexia*, *23*, 141–160.

Serniclaes, W. (2011). Allophonic perception in dyslexia: An overview. *Escritos de Psicología*, *4*, 25–34.

Steenbeek-Planting, E. G., van Bon, W. H., & Schreuder, R. (2013). Instability of children's reading errors in bisyllabic words: The role of context-sensitive spelling rules. *Learning and Instruction*, *26*, 59–70.

Stichting Dyslexie Nederland. (2008). *Diagnose en behandeling van dyslexie* (4th ed.) [Diagnosis and remediation of dyslexia]. Bilthoven, the Netherlands: Stichting Dyslexie Nederland.

Stichting Dyslexie Nederland. (2016). *Diagnose en behandeling van dyslexie* (5th ed.) [Diagnosis and remediation of dyslexia]. Bilthoven, the Netherlands: Stichting Dyslexie Nederland.

Tijms, J. (2011). Effectiveness of computer-based treatment for dyslexia in a clinical care setting: Outcomes and moderators. *Educational Psychology, 31*, 873–896.

Tijms, J., Hoeks, J. J. W. M., Paulussen-Hoogeboom M. C., & Smolenaars, A. J. (2003). Long-term effects of a psycholinguistic treatment for dyslexia. *Journal of Research in Reading, 26*, 121–140.

Tilanus, E. A. T., Segers, E., & Verhoeven, L. (2013). Diagnostic profiles of children with developmental disabilities in a transparent orthography. *Research in Developmental Disabilities, 34*, 4194–4202.

Tilanus, E. A. T., Segers, E., & Verhoeven, L. (2016). Responsiveness to intervention in children with dyslexia. *Dyslexia, 22*, 214–232.

van Bergen, E., de Jong, P. F., Plakas, A., Maassen, B., & van der Leij, A. (2012). Child and parental literacy levels within families with a history of dyslexia. *Journal of Child Psychology and Psychiatry, 53*, 28–36.

van Bergen, E., de Jong, P. F., Regtvoort, A. et al. (2011). Dutch children at family risk of dyslexia: Precursors, reading development, and parental effects. *Dyslexia, 17*, 2–18.

van den Boer, M., van Bergen, E., & de Jong, P. F. (2015). The specific relation of visual attention span with reading and spelling in Dutch. *Learning and Individual Differences, 39*, 141–149.

van den Bos, K. P. (2008). Word-reading development, the double-deficit hypothesis, and the diagnosis of dyslexia. *Educational and Child Psychology, 25*, 51–69.

van den Bos, K. P., Zijlstra, B. J. H., & lutje Spelberg, H. C. (2002). Life-span data on continuous naming speeds of numbers, letters, colors, and pictured objects, and word-reading speed. *Scientific Studies of Reading, 6*, 25–49.

van den Bos, K. P., Zijlstra, B. J. H., & van den Broeck, W. (2003). Specific relations between alphanumeric-naming speed and reading speeds of monosyllabic and multi-syllabic words. *Applied Psycholinguistics, 24*, 407–430.

van den Broeck, W., & Geudens, A. (2012). Old and new ways to study characteristics of reading disability: The case of the nonword-reading deficit. *Cognitive Psychology, 65*, 414–456.

van den Broeck, W., Geudens, A., & van den Bos, K. P. (2010). The nonword-reading deficit of disabled readers: A developmental interpretation. *Developmental Psychology, 46*, 717–734.

van den Bunt, M., Groen, M., Ito, T. et al. (2017). Increased response to altered auditory feedback in dyslexia: A weaker sensorimotor magnet implied in the phonological deficit. *Journal of Speech, Language, and Hearing Research, 60*, 654–667.

van der Kleij, S. W., Segers, E., Groen, M. A., & Verhoeven, L. (2017). Response to intervention as a predictor of long-term reading outcomes in children with dyslexia. *Dyslexia, 23*, 268–282.

van der Leij, A. (1998). *Leesproblemen en dyslexie* [Reading problems and dyslexia]. Rotterdam: Lemniscaat.

van der Leij, A. (2013). Dyslexia and early intervention: What did we learn from the Dutch dyslexia programme? *Dyslexia, 19*, 241–255.

van der Leij, A., & Morfidi, E. (2006). Core deficits and variable differences in Dutch poor readers learning English. *Journal of Learning Disabilities*, *39*, 74–90.

van der Leij A., van Bergen, E., van Zuijen, T. et al. (2013). Precursors of developmental dyslexia: An overview of the longitudinal Dutch dyslexia programme study. *Dyslexia*, *19*, 191–213

van Gorp, K., Segers, P. C. J. & Verhoeven, L. T. W. (2017). Enhancing decoding efficiency in poor readers via a word identification game. *Reading Research Quarterly*, *52*, 105–123.

van Otterloo, S. G., & van der Leij, A. (2009). Dutch home-based pre-reading intervention with children at familial risk of dyslexia. *Annals of Dyslexia*, *59*, 169–195.

van Otterloo, S. G., van der Leij, A., & Henrichs, L. F. (2009). Early home-based intervention in the Netherlands for children at familial risk of dyslexia. *Dyslexia*, *15*, 187–217.

Vandermosten, M., Boets, B., & Luts, H. et al. (2011). Impairments in speech and nonspeech sound categorization in children with dyslexia are driven by temporal processing difficulties. *Research in Developmental Disabilities*, *32*, 593–603.

Vandermosten, M., Vanderauwera, J., & Theys, C. et al. (2015). A DTI tractography study in pre-readers at risk for dyslexia. *Developmental Cognitive Neuroscience*, *14*, 8–15.

Verhoeven, L. (2017). Learning to read Dutch. In L. Verhoeven & C. Perfetti (Eds.), *Learning to read across languages and writing systems* (pp. 323–346). Cambridge, UK: Cambridge University Press.

Verhoeven, L., & Keuning, J. (2018). The nature of developmental dyslexia in a transparent orthography. *Scientific Studies of Reading*, *22*, 7–23.

Verhoeven, L., Schreuder, R., & Baayen, R. H. (2006). Learnability of graphotactic rules in visual word identification. *Learning and Instruction*, *16*, 538–548.

Verhoeven, L., Schreuder, R., & Haarman, V. (2006). Prefix identification in the reading of Dutch bisyllabic words. *Reading and Writing*, *19*, 651–668.

Verhoeven, L., & van Leeuwe, J. (2009). Modeling the growth of word decoding skills: Evidence from Dutch. *Scientific Studies of Reading*, *13*, 205–223.

Verhoeven, L. & van Leeuwe, J. (2011). Role of gender and linguistic diversity in word decoding development. *Learning and Individual Differences*, *21*, 359–367.

Verhoeven, L., van Leeuwe, J., Irausquin, R., & Segers, E. (2016). The unique role of lexical accessibility in predicting kindergarten emergent literacy. *Reading and Writing*, *29*, 591–608.

Vloedgraven, J. & Verhoeven, L. (2007). Screening of phonological awareness in the early elementary grades: An IRT approach. *Annals of Dyslexia*, *57*, 33–50.

Vloedgraven, J. & Verhoeven, L. (2009). The nature of phonological awareness throughout the elementary grades: An item response theory perspective. *Learning and Individual Differences*, *19*, 161–169.

Wentink, H., & Verhoeven, L. (2001). *Protocol leesproblemen en dyslexie in de onderbouw* [Protocol reading problems in the lower primary grades]. Nijmegen, the Netherlands: Expertisecentrum Nederlands.

Wentink, H., & Verhoeven, L. (2004). *Protocol leesproblemen en dyslexie in de bovenbouw* [Protocol reading problems in the upper primary grades]. Nijmegen, the Netherlands: Expertisecentrum Nederlands.

Ziegler, J. C., Castel, C., Pech-Georgel, C., George, F., Alario, F. X., & Perry C. (2008). Developmental dyslexia and the dual route model of reading: Simulating individual differences and subtypes. *Cognition*, *107*, 151–178.

Ziegler, J. C., Perry, C., & Zorzi, M. (2014). Modelling reading development through phonological decoding and self-teaching: Implications for dyslexia. *Philosophical Transactions of the Royal Society, B: Biological Sciences*, *369*, 20120397.

5 Developmental Dyslexia in Czech and Slovak

Markéta Caravolas, Marína Mikulajová,
and Anna Kuchaská

5.1 Introduction

Two small, closely related countries in Central Europe, the Czech Republic and Slovakia, have enjoyed a recent surge in research activities, at the national and international levels, in the areas of typical and atypical literacy development. Many new and exciting findings are informing developments in diagnosis, assessment, and educational policy regarding the prevention and remediation of literacy problems due to dyslexia. In the present chapter, we review much of this recent work. Despite their historical, geopolitical, cultural, and linguistic connections – having existed as a single country for seventy-five years (1918–1993) – the Czech and Slovak countries and their languages are nevertheless distinct. We therefore take a comparative approach throughout the chapter, contrasting the findings in these languages with each other as well as with findings from English and other languages.

In the sections that follow, we provide a brief overview of each language and orthography, and summarize some of the key features of typical reading and spelling development; for fuller details see Caravolas (2017). We then describe clinical and educational practice related to dyslexia, as it evolved in the historical and cultural contexts of the second half of the twentieth century, in the then unified Czechoslovakia. Next, we focus on research developments on dyslexia in the Czech Republic and Slovakia over the past ten to twenty years, including studies on intervention. In taking a cross-linguistic perspective throughout the chapter, we relate the Czech and Slovak findings to dominant, sometimes competing, theories of the causes and manifestations of dyslexia arising from research in other languages. In particular, we consider the extent to which the Czech/Slovak evidence is consistent with the core phonological deficit account of dyslexia, with the existence of subtypes, the current classifications of distinct literacy disorders, and with the broader outlook on proximal and distal causes of individual differences in a dimensional framework of developmental disorders of literacy (e.g., Snowling & Hulme, 2012).

5.2 Learning to Read Czech and Slovak

5.2.1 Czech and Slovak Languages and Their Orthographies

Czech and Slovak are closely related, mutually intelligible, West Slavic languages. They share many characteristics at the grammatical, morphosyntactic, phonological, and orthographic levels. Details are provided by Caravolas (2017; also Sokolová, Musilová, & Slančová, 2005). Our main focus here being dyslexia, we describe the oral and written languages in terms of the features that are important for literacy acquisition. Although Czech and Slovak have relatively consistent orthographies (Kessler & Caravolas, 2011), several phonological, supraphonological, morphological, and morphosyntactic processes bring about inconsistencies in phoneme–grapheme mappings, which mainly affect spelling. Children are explicitly taught proscriptive rules and strategies for resolving most of these inconsistencies over the primary-school years, as part of a gradual and systematic grammar (i.e. Czech/Slovak language) curriculum. The main causes of difficulty are highlighted below.

Both languages have rich systems of inflectional morphology, which reflect a complex grammar and entail a prevalence of polysyllabic words (three-syllable words being the most frequent), primarily comprised of open syllables. Complex onsets (CCV, CCCV, etc.) are relatively frequent, as compared with other languages (e.g., Kučera & Monroe, 1968). The distributions of word lengths, as well as of simple (C) and complex syllable onset structures, are virtually identical across the two languages (Caravolas, 2017). Thus, from the start of literacy learning, Czech and Slovak children are frequently confronted with long and complex word structures.

Both languages have five short–long vowel pairs and Czech has three, while Slovak has four diphthongs. All of these have relatively consistent letter–sound mappings, with the exception of /i-iː/, which may be spelled ‹i-í› or ‹y-ý› depending on graphotactic and/or grammatical context (see further details in Caravolas, 2017). The number of consonants is similar across languages (Czech: twenty-seven; Slovak: twenty-nine). The use of diacritics on (Latin) letters to mark duration (mainly with the acute accent ʹ) of vowels (e.g., /aː/ ‹á›) (and in Slovak also two consonants) and to mark place of articulation (mainly with the háček ˇ) on non-anterior coronal (e.g., /ʃ/, /ʧ/ ‹š, č›) and palatalized consonants (e.g., / ɟ, c/ ‹ď, ť›), is a special feature of the orthographies and contributes to their consistency.

Like many other alphabetic orthographies, Czech and Slovak retain some aspects of morphology in the spelling system, which cause morphophonological inconsistency. These mainly reflect the assimilation of voicing at morpheme boundaries in the spoken, but not in the written, language (e.g., [potpora] ("support") → ⟨podpora⟩), including word-final devoicing of obstruents (e.g., [met] ("honey") → ⟨med⟩). At the suprasegmental level, both languages have fixed, first-syllable stress, which should make the identification of word boundaries in the speech stream quite predictable. However, the process of affixation of clitics to word onsets (e.g., the two words ⟨do školy⟩ "to school" pronounced as the prosodic word ["doʃkoli"]) often obscures word boundaries.

Morphosyntactic processes, which operate at the phrase level (e.g., for grammatical agreement) cause sound-spelling ambiguity specifically of the inflectional ending /i/ or /iː/, which may be spelled with ⟨i⟩/⟨y⟩ or ⟨í⟩/⟨ý⟩ depending on grammatical context. Moreover, many loan words containing /i/ or /iː/ retain their original spellings (e.g., ⟨dieta⟩, ⟨cyklus⟩) even when in violation of the proscriptive graphotactic rules. Consequently, in both countries, much explicit spelling instruction focuses on the graphotactic (second grade), exception word (third grade) and grammatical (fourth to fifth grade) "disambiguation" of /i-iː/ spellings.

5.2.2   Challenges in Learning to Read Czech and Slovak

As detailed in Caravolas (2017), the contemporary approaches to schooling and literacy instruction in the Czech Republic and Slovakia are highly comparable. Preschool/kindergarten practices, statutory age for start of formal schooling, and the dominant *analytic-synthetic phonics* methods of literacy instruction in the lower primary grades are more or less the same. Most children attend at least one kindergarten year, just prior to formal schooling, during which education focuses on the development of social, physical, and cognitive school-readiness skills, but not on literacy. Language play and phonological awareness activities are included, although usually not as part of a systematic curriculum.

In primary school, the typical milestones of reading development are as follows: Children learn the alphabet and basic phonic skills by mid-first grade; they decode and read simple texts independently by the end of first grade; by the end of second grade, children can read sufficiently fluently (approx. 70–80 words per minute) to underpin effective reading comprehension (Caravolas, 2017; Matějček, 1995). The more gradual spelling/orthographic curriculum spans through to fourth grade in Slovakia and to fifth grade in the Czech Republic (details in Caravolas, 2017). The main milestones for spelling are as follows: by the end of first grade, children can write all letters of the alphabet correctly, and write simple words with phonetic accuracy (i.e., using invented spellings); by the end of second grade, they apply proscriptive graphotactic rules for the spellings of palatalized consonants with/without diacritics, and, for the context-dependent spelling of the vowels /i, iː/ as ⟨i, í⟩ or ⟨y, ý⟩; by the end of third grade, children can systematically apply the explicitly taught assimilation of voicing rules at morpheme boundaries, apply strategies for uncovering word boundaries in prosodic words (clitic + root morpheme), and rote-learn a set of proscribed exception words; by fourth grade and throughout fifth grade, they work on consolidating word-internal voicing assimilation rules, and learn the explicitly taught morphosyntactic agreement rules for the spelling of /i, i:/ as ⟨i, í⟩ or ⟨y, ý⟩. Normative studies of spelling development in Czech (Caravolas & Volín, 2005) and Slovak (Caravolas, Mikulajová, & Vencelová, 2008b) confirm that children's spelling development in both languages largely reflects the teaching curriculum and the above milestones.

Recent cross-linguistic studies of the cognitive underpinnings of reading and spelling development in Czech and Slovak revealed that three core skills – phoneme awareness, letter knowledge, and rapid automatized naming (RAN) – measured in kindergarten, uniquely predicted first-grade children's outcomes in word-reading efficiency and spelling accuracy (Caravolas et al., 2012), as well as growth of silent word reading (Caravolas et al., 2013). These three skills (and the auto-regressors) explained over 60 percent of the variance in word-level literacy not only in Czech- and Slovak-, but also in matched Spanish- and English-speaking groups. The findings resonate with those of Swedish-, Norwegian- (Furnes & Samuelsson, 2011; Lervåg & Hulme, 2009), and English-speaking children in a number of different countries (e.g., Kirby, Parrila, & Pfeiffer, 2003; Schatschneider et al., 2004). Thus, phoneme awareness, letter knowledge, and RAN represent the core *triple foundation* of proximal, code-related skills driving reading and spelling development across the spectrum of alphabetic orthographies. Accordingly, we consider this triple foundation as a language-general framework for investigating disordered literacy development, particularly of a phonological deficit in dyslexia.

5.3   Reading Difficulties in Czech and Slovak

5.3.1   *Historical and Cultural Context*

The first Czech case of dyslexia, documented by the psychiatrist Heveroch, appeared in 1904, coinciding with the earliest observations of similar cases in the English-speaking world (e.g., by Morgan, 1896; Hinshelwood, 1895; Orton, 1925; as cited in Matějček, 1995). However, the more systematic study of dyslexia in the Czechoslovak Republic (1918–1992) began in the 1950s. A pioneering figure contributing to awareness-raising, research, and educational provision in this field during the second half of the twentieth century was child psychologist Zdeněk Matějček (1922–2004). A first important milestone of the 1950s was the recognition of specific difficulties in reading and writing in a subgroup of children with perinatal encephalopathy – later renamed *mild brain dysfunction*. Within this neurological framework, dyslexia was seen as a circumscribed problem of reading, predominantly due to a perceptual-motor deficit, with verbal deficits as peripheral, and not co-occurring systematically (Matějček, 1978). Despite a similar understanding of dyslexia by Czech and Slovak practitioners, some differences in emphasis existed. The Slovak psychologist T. Pardel (1966), in *Written Language, Its Development and Disorders*, inspired by Lurian neuropsychological perspectives, emphasized verbal deficits in dyslexia *and* dysorthographia.

During the Czechoslovak Socialist era, lasting until 1989, the state largely supported the care and education of children with additional learning needs, including dyslexia. During the 1950s, children with diagnoses of learning disorders were under the purview of the medical/psychiatric profession, but their diagnosis and care was undertaken from the start by multidisciplinary teams of physicians, psychologists, and special education teachers. The 1960s saw the integration of pupils with dyslexia and other specific learning disorders into mainstream schools. They attended specialized classes, and were additionally supported by various relevant professionals. During the 1970s, a support network of educational psychology counseling centers began to emerge, which carried out diagnosis, intervention, and counseling of affected children and their families and worked collaboratively with the schools. By the 1980s, this network was fully established (with approximately 100 centers in the Czech Republic, 40 in Slovakia), and was deemed to reflect a very good, systematically upheld standard of care for children with learning difficulties. Since 1989, the system of centers has undergone reorganization but continues to function in support of schools and pupils with significant learning needs.

Research into various aspects of dyslexia was undertaken during the second half of the twentieth century (Matějček, 1959, 1961), with its main emphasis on assessments and remediation of perceptual-motor functions (e.g., Edfeldt, 1968; Frostig, 1972; Míka, 1982). Since 1993, both the Czech Republic and Slovakia have broadened their work on dyslexia nationally, as well as through participation in research, educational projects, and training programs with other European countries. The impacts of these recent and current developments on theory and practice in dyslexia are examined in the ensuing sections.

5.3.2   *Identification and Prevalence of Dyslexia*

Literacy difficulties have traditionally been classified into three main, dissociable problems: dyslexia (specific reading difficulties), dysorthographia (spelling and grammatical problems in writing), and dysgraphia (handwriting deficit). This classification is still applied, and is in line with current educational legislation in the Czech Republic. It partly resonates with the current classification in the *Diagnostic and Statistical Manual of Mental Disorders*

(5th ed.; DSM-V; American Psychiatric Association, 2013), which sees dyslexia ("impairment in reading") and writing difficulties ("impairment in written expression") as two separable specific learning disorders, although unlike in the Czech/Slovak systems, it considers decoding and spelling deficits to be key features of dyslexia; handwriting difficulties are classified as a symptom of developmental coordination disorder.

The prevalence rates for this trio of disorders are currently estimated at 5–8 percent in the Czech Republic, with the most frequently occurring being dyslexia. This relatively high number may reflect the inclusion of a broader spectrum of severity relative to some other countries. In Slovakia, there are no precise statistical prevalence data, but the broad estimates are of 3–5 percent. In both languages, moreover, dyslexia manifests with a high degree of heterogeneity and comorbidity with other disorders, as is the case in other languages (e.g., Goulandris, 2003, Pennington, 2006). A study of 152 Czech children with learning disorders revealed that 20 percent had pure dyslexia, while 63 percent had dyslexia plus writing-related (dysorthographia/dysgraphia) difficulties (Gebhardtová, 1994). The co-occurrence of dyslexia with ADHD has been reported at 18–20 percent (Švancarová & Kucharská, 2001). Comorbid language impairment among children with dyslexia is particularly common, with estimates ranging from 30–36 percent (Kucharská, 2014; Matějček, 1995) up to 51 percent (Mladá, 1996) of dyslexia cases.

A major development of recent years is the recognition of dyslexia and dysorthographia as primarily neurodevelopmental, language-based disorders, marked by a phonological processing deficit, of which certain behavioral markers can be identified across the lifespan. This revision brings the Czech and Slovak definitions closer to those of the DSM-V and the International Dyslexia Association (2002). Accordingly, language-sensitive and code-sensitive skills assessments, which include measures of phoneme awareness, naming speed, reading fluency, and orthographic knowledge, are now in use not only with the primary-school-aged population (e.g., in Slovak: Mikulajová et al., 2012; in Czech: Caravolas & Volín, 2005; Cimlerová, Pokorná, & Chalupová, 2007), but also with preschoolers and post-secondary-school populations. In addition, the benefits of early identification and intervention for children at risk of literacy failure are being recognized. The Czech government has recently enacted a *response to intervention* framework (Mertin, 2008), in which children's literacy development is monitored from late kindergarten/early first grade with the use of screening tools (e.g., Seidlová Málková & Caravolas, 2013; Švancarová & Kucharská, 2001), and those deemed to be at risk receive added learning support in school, including speech therapy services if necessary. In Slovakia, similar trends for early screening (Mikulajová et al., 2012) and intervention are emerging. These new Czech/Slovak models of early detection and intervention are similar to those envisaged for the UK, and the USA.

Alongside these developments, the traditional approach continues of formally diagnosing dyslexia/dysorthographia in the mid-primary-school years, once children have demonstrated significant delays in literacy, despite adequate support and intervention. Moreover, there is a general view that children's literacy profiles do not stabilize until approximately the second grade (e.g., Schöffelová & Mikulajová, 2012). In both countries, the diagnosis is typically made by an educational psychologist on the basis of an IQ–literacy attainment discrepancy.

5.4   Behavioral and Neurocognitive Evidence

The recent proliferation of research and diagnostic tools has generated empirical findings about the nature, causes, and manifestations of dyslexia in Czech and Slovak.[1] These are mainly derived from behavioral studies and many publications exist solely in the native languages (recent compendia include for Slovak: Mikulajová et al., 2012; for Czech: Kucharská et al., 2014). In this section, we first summarize the main and most robust findings regarding the manifestations of dyslexia in the reading and spelling profiles of affected children, and then we turn to studies of the concurrent and longitudinal cognitive markers of the disorder.

5.4.1   *Nature of Reading and Spelling Problems in Czech and Slovak*

5.4.1.1   Reading Problems   Reading difficulties in Czech and Slovak share many characteristics, in particular among the majority of children in each nation (over 80 percent) who have systematically been taught through the analytic-synthetic phonics method (Kucharská & Barešová, 2012). As in other languages, key characteristics of reading among children with dyslexia are slow, effortful, and disfluent word reading. In line with this, Caravolas, Volín, and Hulme (2005) found that Czech children with dyslexia in third to fifth grade (9–12 years of age), read word lists dramatically more slowly than their age-matched typical reader peers (Cohen's $d = 2.31$) and younger, spelling-ability-matched peers ($d = .57$). Moreover, in a study tracking twenty-four children at family risk of dyslexia, who went on to develop the disorder, Kucharská (2014) found that in third grade, the clearest marker of reading difficulty, consistent with a phonological deficit, was these children's nonword reading speed, which set them apart not only from typical readers ($d = .65$) but also age-matched peers with speech and language difficulties (SLD) ($d = .20$).

---

[1]   Note that henceforth, unless otherwise specified, we use the term dyslexia in reference to word-level deficits in reading *and* spelling.

Beyond this, the Czech/Slovak dyslexic reading profile has commonalities with that of peers learning other relatively consistent alphabetic orthographies (e.g., Wimmer, 1993), such that reading accuracy may or may not be significantly impaired, although errors are typically observed when reading phonologically complex words, with long consonant clusters (e.g., ‹štvrtok› – "Thursday," ‹zmrzlina› – "ice cream"). Even in the context of accurate decoding, however, a clinical indicator of difficulty is persisting *double reading* (i.e. quiet sounding out followed by the aloud pronunciation of the identified word), a strategy typical readers abandon before the end of second grade.

Some difficulties in reading comprehension have also been reported among populations with dyslexia. For example, Caravolas et al. (2005) found that the third to fifth graders in their study performed significantly less well on a timed cloze reading test (which required the selection of missing words in short passages) relative to their age-mates ($d = 2.35$); however, in this silent task, it was difficult to disambiguate the contributions of slow decoding from those of weak comprehension. Using the same measure with her third-grade groups, Kucharská's (2014) study sheds some light on the latter question. She found that children with language delay – who also had weak oral comprehension skills, but relatively mild nonword reading difficulties – performed considerably less well on the reading comprehension test than typical readers, and also than children with dyslexia ($d = .51$). The group with dyslexia, in turn, performed less well than their typical reader peers ($d = .43$). These findings suggest that reading comprehension skills may be compromised among children with dyslexia, albeit less profoundly than among children with specific language delay.

It is possible that reading comprehension difficulties may arise among Slovak and Czech dyslexic children not simply due to their slow and inefficient decoding, but also due to certain grammatical and syntactic complexities of the languages. Written texts present many relatively long words, the specific meanings of which are often revealed only upon reading the final inflectional graphemes, and dyslexic children may be more likely to misread these segments; moreover, the relatively free word order does not provide strong cues to comprehension, such as those found in English, for example. It is interesting to note that in a study of text reading with Slovak, fourth-grade average and poor readers, Váryová (2012) found that although poor readers committed word-level errors 4 percent of the time (good readers did so less than 1 percent of the time), approximately 30 percent of their misreadings caused illegal morpho-syntactic changes in words, which in turn altered sentence meanings (this was negligible among the good readers). It remains to be investigated whether these difficulties occur primarily among dyslexic children who have comorbid broader language impairments.

Thus, to date, studies of Czech and Slovak dyslexic children's reading profiles confirm significantly impaired speed and fluency, which, together with less well consolidated blending skills (double reading) and pronounced nonword reading deficits, provide evidence of weakness in phonological processing. The potentially interesting interactions between phonological, morphological, and syntactic characteristics of these languages, and their impacts on reading comprehension among readers with dyslexia, await further research.

5.4.1.2 Spelling Problems Czech and Slovak children with dyslexia experience significant and persistent spelling difficulties. These seem to have their roots in phonological recoding deficits. However, other aspects of spelling that tap broader language processes also appear to be affected. Evidence of phonologically motivated difficulties was reported in Caravolas and Volín's (2001) study, where third- to fifth-grade children (the same as those in Caravolas et al., 2005) with dyslexia produced significantly fewer accurate nonword spellings (70 percent) relative to chronological-age peers (88 percent), and to (word) spelling-ability-matched peers (78 percent), who were at least two years younger. Furthermore, in real-word spellings, the dyslexic group committed more phonologically implausible errors than age-matched peers, and the magnitude of this deficit remained stable, still showing no sign of resolving in fifth grade. Kucharská's (2014) third graders with dyslexia similarly showed significantly weaker nonword and word-spelling skills than their unimpaired agemates.

Caravolas, Mikulajová, and Vencelová (2008a) examined the spelling profiles of forty Slovak third- and fourth-grade children with dyslexia and compared their performance to typical spellers in first to fourth grade. All groups were assessed on a range of spelling patterns that are taught in the primary grades, namely, (1) spelling of letters of the alphabet – including the letters with diacritics marking place of articulation and vowel duration (taught in first grade), (2) graphotactically constrained spellings of /i-i:/ in specific consonantal contexts (taught in second grade), (3) patterns with voicing assimilation at morpheme boundaries (taught in third grade), and (4) clitic + root morpheme sequences testing word-boundary rules (taught in third grade; see the example in Section 5.2.1 and in Caravolas, 2017).

As expected, on the letter-writing task, typical spellers reached mastery (long vowels) or ceiling (all consonants) by the end of first grade. In contrast, while the dyslexic children produced alphabet letters without diacritics (e.g., ⟨s⟩) and those with diacritics marking place of articulation (e.g., ⟨š⟩) just as well as their non-dyslexic counterparts, they failed to mark the diacritic for vowel duration 40 percent of the time in third grade ($d = 1.34$) and 15 percent of the time in fourth grade ($d = 1.03$). Contrary to the widely held assumptions that Czech/Slovak children with dyslexia characteristically omit all types of diacritics due to visual learning and attention, or speed of processing deficits (e.g., Matějček, 1995), these and other findings (Caravolas & Mikulajová,

2008) suggest that their diacritic omissions are not indiscriminate, and are most frequent on segments requiring the phonological analysis of vowel duration.

On all of the other above-mentioned patterns, (2) to (4), the typical spellers reached mastery levels by third grade. The fourth graders with dyslexia tended to perform better than their third-grade dyslexic peers; however, neither group attained grade-appropriate spelling levels, and the severity of their delays depended on the nature of the inconsistency. On the conditional graphotactic spelling patterns, which do not necessitate linguistic analysis, the groups with dyslexia showed improvements relative to each other, and a small yet significant level of impairment relative to typical spellers ($d = .77$). On the patterns involving voicing assimilation rules, they again showed significant gains across grades, but greater impairments relative to typical spellers ($d = 1.22$). On items requiring knowledge of word-boundary rules/strategies, the groups with dyslexia exhibited no significant gains in learning and the largest deficit ($d = 1.43$). Thus, they incorrectly treated clitic prepositions and root morphemes (e.g., *do školy*) as single words (**doškoly*) approximately 55 percent of the time, on a par with first-grade typical spellers (typical third- and fourth-grade spellers respectively attained 87 and 92 percent).

This general pattern of results was replicated in another study comparing fourth graders with dyslexia and same-aged as well as younger (second-grade) reading-ability-matched children (Vencelová & Mikulajová, 2010). Here, the groups did not differ on spellings of the graphotactically conditioned patterns ⟨i/í⟩ and ⟨y/ý⟩, which do not necessitate linguistic analysis, but children with dyslexia showed deficits on morphophonologically motivated spellings. It could be argued that dyslexic children's relative facility with graphotactic knowledge simply reflects its earlier-learned status. However, this is unlikely given their sizeable impairment on the very basic and earliest-learned skill of diacritic marking on long vowels, which clearly requires phonological analysis. Together, our studies of Czech and Slovak children with dyslexia suggest that, in these languages as in English, individuals with dyslexia experience persistent deficits in skills bearing on phonological processing, but seemingly also on broader language skills.

5.4.2   Underlying Causes of Reading and Spelling Problems in Czech and Slovak

5.4.2.1   Cognitive Profiles of Children with Dyslexia   Studies of cognitive profiles of children with dyslexia typically seek to uncover the underlying causes of disordered reading and spelling development. As summarized in Section 5.2.2, three core components, and proximal predictors of individual differences in reading and spelling have been identified across a number of alphabetic orthographies: phoneme awareness, letter knowledge, and RAN (e.g., Caravolas et al., 2012; Furnes & Samuelsson, 2011). Phoneme awareness is assumed to tap the quality and accessibility of phonological representations, letter knowledge presumably taps aspects of orthographic representations, while RAN (still debated) may estimate the efficiency of the connections between phonological (including phonemic) and orthographic (including graphemic) representations (e.g., Kirby et al., 2010; Lervåg & Hulme, 2009). On the view that children with dyslexia rely on the same cognitive architecture as typical readers in learning to read and spell, it follows that the selective or combined impairments of the three core skills constitute the proximal cause(s) of reading and spelling difficulties across alphabetic orthographies. Moreover, the most typical (though not the only) indicator of a phonological processing deficit is considered to be weak phoneme awareness. Letter knowledge, through its close and reciprocal relationship with phoneme awareness, as demonstrated for English and Czech (e.g., Hulme et al., 2005), can also be considered a language-general marker of dyslexia. However, most children, including those with dyslexia, learn their alphabet letters by the second or third grade, and consequently, measures of letter knowledge are often excluded in studies with children beyond the second grade. Nevertheless, in studies using innovative age-appropriate letter-knowledge measures, such as primed letter–sound integration, older children with dyslexia have shown persisting deficits (e.g., Froyen, Willems, & Blomert, 2010). Weakness in RAN should also be a marker of dyslexia across languages, although the exact nature of this relationship, and the extent to which a RAN impairment can be selective is not yet clear (e.g., Georgiou, Parrila, & Liao, 2008; Kirby et al., 2010). While additional skills such as verbal short-term memory and visual attention are associated with alphabetic literacy development, their causal roles in dyslexia are still debated and not observed systematically (e.g., Bosse, Tainturier, & Valdois, 2007; Caravolas et al., 2005; Landerl et al., 2013).

In languages with alphabetic orthographies, the importance of orthographic consistency as a *moderator* of the cognitive profile in dyslexia is still in question. A dominant view (e.g., Share, 2008) is that in English and other inconsistent orthographies, phonological processing (i.e., phoneme awareness) is the most important marker of reading difficulty in dyslexia, because decoding skills develop more slowly and are measured by reading accuracy (to which phoneme awareness measures are sensitive). In contrast, it plays a less important causal role in reading impairments in relatively consistent alphabetic orthographies, where even children with dyslexia are said to master phoneme awareness (and accurate decoding) skills by about the end of second grade; instead, the most robust marker of dyslexia is RAN, which best estimates reading speed (e.g., Kirby et al., 2010; Wimmer, Mayringer, & Landerl, 2000). An alternative view (e.g., Caravolas et al., 2005) is that to the extent that individuals with dyslexia suffer a persistent phonological processing impairment, then phoneme awareness should be a marker of dyslexia across the alphabetic consistency spectrum; and, the roles of phoneme awareness and RAN should not "trade off" in importance as a function of orthographic consistency. The role of the phoneme-awareness deficit as a marker of spelling impairments is less contentious because a robust association has typically been found in relatively consistent (e.g., Wimmer et al., 2000) and inconsistent (Caravolas et al., 2005) orthographies. Finally, RAN has also been found to be a marker of spelling difficulty in dyslexia, albeit weaker than of reading inefficiency (e.g., Moll et al., 2014; Wimmer et al., 2000).

In Caravolas et al.'s (2005) direct comparison of Czech- and English-speaking children with dyslexia, Czech children performed better overall on literacy and phonological skills, as anticipated, relative to their English peers. However, *both* groups exhibited phoneme-awareness impairments, as well as other indicators of weak phonological processing (nonword reading and nonword spelling accuracy), relative to chronological-age controls. Moreover, the Czech dyslexic group showed deficits relative to much younger ability-matched controls, suggesting that phoneme awareness provides an index of a phonological processing deficit in dyslexia regardless of orthographic consistency.

The above study did not include measures of RAN, and so could not fully address the issue of the differential roles of phoneme awareness versus naming speed in Czech versus English. However, a recent cross-linguistic study (Landerl et al., 2013) compared the relative importance of these two measures as predictors of dyslexia status in over 1,000 children from five language groups spanning the orthographic consistency spectrum. Performance on both RAN and phoneme awareness predicted dyslexia, and both skills covaried in strength as a function of orthographic consistency. That is, both skills were more predictive of dyslexia status in relatively inconsistent orthographies than in more consistent ones. However, contrary to earlier claims, phoneme awareness was a *stronger* predictor than RAN within the most consistent *and* the most inconsistent orthographies. On the other hand, RAN was a relatively strong predictor of dyslexia status in comparison to phoneme awareness in moderately consistent orthographies. Thus, the field is beginning to converge on the understanding that *two key cognitive markers of dyslexia* among school-aged learners of alphabetic orthographies are phoneme awareness and naming fluency. Although their relative weightings *within* languages may vary to some extent, the precise determiners of such fluctuations – including attributes of the orthography, characteristics of the measures being used, cultural and educational factors, and/or participant sample details – have yet to be determined.

5.4.2.2 Subtypes and Comorbidities

As stated earlier, in the Czech and Slovak traditions, dyslexia and dysorthographia are considered to be separate, albeit the most frequently co-occurring, disorders of learning (e.g., Gebhardtová,

1994; Matějček, 1995). Whether these should alternatively be considered to be subtypes of dyslexia or two comorbid disorders remains open to empirical investigation. In languages such as English and German, dissociations of reading and spelling skills (e.g., "good reader – poor speller" versus "poor reader – poor speller," and recently also "poor reader – good speller," Moll & Landerl, 2009), are considered to reflect dyslexia subtypes (e.g., Frith, 1980), or dimensional variations in the severity of the disorder (e.g., Bruck & Waters, 1988), but not two separate disorders.

Preliminary data from a study of Slovak third-grade typical readers (TD) and children with a formal diagnosis of dyslexia (Mikulajová & Velecká, 2012) suggest that the traditional dyslexia–dysorthographia distinction may not be warranted, and that spelling – a key aspect of the dysorthographia diagnosis – may constitute a core impairment in dyslexia. While their participants with dyslexia, who were comparable to the TD group on nonverbal ability, could be divided on a measure of reading fluency into disfluent readers and relatively fluent readers, *both subgroups* had significant spelling difficulties. Furthermore, the dyslexic subgroups were indistinguishable from each other (and severely impaired) on measures of phonological, morphological, and syntactic awareness, as well as vocabulary and verbal short-term memory, but they differed on the RAN task, where the relatively fluent dyslexic readers performed similarly to the TD group. These results point to the dissociable role of RAN as a proximal indicator of reading fluency. Notably, however, they also illustrate that, in addition to weak phonological and broader language skills, spelling difficulties are typical among children with dyslexia, regardless of the variations in their reading fluency (cf. Bruck & Waters, 1988).

Another approach to the study of cognitive causes of reading and spelling difficulties within and across languages is the "at-risk" paradigm, in which preschool-aged children are tracked longitudinally into the school years because they are at genetic risk of dyslexia, having at least one affected first-degree relative, or because they exhibit language-acquisition delay (e.g., Pennington & Lefly, 2001; Snowling, Gallagher, & Frith, 2003). One advantage of this design is its potential to reveal not only the proximal causes of literacy difficulties, but also the potentially more distal causes of literacy failure. In a recent study, Czech and Slovak preschool children at risk of reading and spelling difficulties due to familial risk of dyslexia ($n = 38$) or observed speech and language difficulties ($n = 60$) were tracked and compared to a group of children with no known difficulties $n = 100$) for three years from kindergarten until the end of the first grade (Moll et al., 2016). In view of their overall similarities (Caravolas, 2017, Caravolas et al., 2012), the two language groups were combined. Latent variable path models revealed a two-phase trajectory linking these children's early language skills to later reading and spelling skills via the foundational skills of phoneme awareness, letter knowledge, and RAN. Early language skills, marked by poor receptive and expressive grammar and vocabulary impairments predicted the code-related skills of RAN, letter knowledge, and phoneme awareness measured at the start of formal schooling. In turn these precursors predicted individual differences in reading and spelling outcomes in first grade. Moreover, the effects of language in kindergarten on reading and spelling in first grade were fully mediated by the effects of the triple foundation skills. These results are consistent with those of similar at-risk studies of English-speaking children (Moll, Loff, & Snowling, 2013). Nevertheless, a replication of this study with larger groups is necessary, allowing for separate investigations of the children with language delay and family risk of dyslexia. Indicatively, however, it illustrates that, whatever the dampening effects of orthographic consistency may be on the later manifestations of dyslexia in different alphabetic orthographies, a language-general relationship exists between the development of oral language and written language skills, both in typical and in atypical literacy development.

5.5   Intervention

Controlled intervention studies for ameliorating the literacy skills of Czech and Slovak children at risk of or with dyslexia are still lacking, although new efforts to innovate teaching methods in mainstream classes are now in the offing (e.g., Vencelová & Kapalková, 2014). There is, however, a long tradition in both countries of intervention and special education for children with learning difficulties (Matějček, 1995). Specialized support for pupils with a diagnosis of dyslexia has traditionally been delivered based on principles of dynamic assessment (Košč, 1987), explicit scaffolding and training of metacognitive learning strategies (Borkowski & Muthukrishna, 1992), and the training of visual-motor skills (Matějček, 1995). However, well-controlled (e.g., randomized controlled trials) studies of the effectiveness of these approaches with Czech/Slovak dyslexic pupils are still lacking.

With the emerging focus on early identification and prevention of literacy failure, mainstream interventions for children with dyslexia have improved in several key aspects. The importance of early language development in the trajectory of developmental dyslexia, as well as the benefits of early intervention, are now being highlighted. One example of this is a codified thirty-week program of phonological awareness training, based on the original work of D. B. Elkonin and the Russian psychological framework of Vygotsky, which has been adapted and used widely in Czech and Slovak kindergartens over the past decade (Mikulajová et al., 2016; Mikulajová, Tokárová, & Sümegiová, 2014). The program focuses exclusively on the oral phonological domain, and has been found to effectively impact not only children's phonological awareness but also their morphosyntactic skills (Tiefenbacherová, 2014). It is also used and well rated by practitioners in specialist centers for children with language and communication impairments; however, a controlled evaluation of its efficacy with such populations is still awaited.

The trends toward early language-based interventions are reflected in changes in national educational policies. In the Czech Republic they are embedded within the *response to intervention* educational framework (Mertin, 2008). In Slovakia, a new state educational program for kindergartens is coming into force, in which a large emphasis will be placed on preliteracy skills, in particular on the development of phonological awareness skills. These developments are ascribed to the surge in basic research and in the proliferation of evidence-based findings in both countries.

5.6   Discussion and Conclusion

In this chapter, we have reviewed the theoretical perspectives, clinical and educational approaches, and the research findings on dyslexia in Czech and Slovak, from a cross-linguistic perspective. Our comparison of the Czech and Slovak languages, orthographies, and literacy development revealed that the similarities between them far outweigh the differences (Caravolas, 2017), and thus we can be reasonably confident that most findings in one language generalize to the other. The broader cross-linguistic comparisons with other languages (most often, but not only, with English) also indicated that the similarities outnumbered the differences, at least across alphabetic orthographies. Together, the findings contribute important information to the building of an accurate language-general understanding of literacy development, typical and atypical.

In the Czechoslovak context, the view of dyslexia that emphasized defective visual-motor and attentional functions (although also noting the role of language functions in the syndrome) endured throughout the second half of the twentieth century (Matějček, 1995; Mikulajová, 2010). During this time, the English-speaking world saw a boom in dyslexia research, and the emphasis shifted to the language domain, and specifically to the potential causal role of impaired phonological processing. Over the past fifteen years, the focus in the Czech and Slovak states has also turned to language as the likely basis of difficulties in dyslexia.

Our review of the reading and spelling profiles, as well as cross-sectional and longitudinal studies examining cognitive profiles, concurs that Czech and Slovak children at risk of or with dyslexia reliably manifest difficulties in phoneme awareness and other measures of phonological processing. In contrast, evidence of *core* difficulties in other areas, such as visual attention and visual and verbal short-term memory has not been found (although research specifically targeting nonverbal skills has received little attention to date). Direct cross-linguistic comparisons of Czech and Slovak children's profiles also revealed that they are highly similar not only to each other, but also to those of children learning other languages, including English (Caravolas et al., 2005; Moll et al., 2016).

More specifically, the Czech/Slovak findings concur with a growing evidence base from numerous languages with alphabetic orthographies, which indicates that reading and spelling development is underpinned by three core, code-related skills of phoneme awareness, letter knowledge, and RAN (Caravolas et al., 2012; Furnes & Samuelsson, 2011), and that impairments in these skills represent the proximal causes of reading and spelling difficulties observed in dyslexia (e.g., Caravolas et al., 2005; Landerl et al., 2013; Moll et al., 2016; Snowling et al., 2003; Torppa et al., 2006). We suggest that these three skills represent language-general proximal causes of dyslexia, and that they exert their effects in much the same way across alphabetic orthographies.

Moll et al.'s (2016) study of Czech and Slovak children at risk of dyslexia, as well as studies of spelling and cognitive profiles of older Slovak groups with dyslexia (Caravolas et al., 2008a; Mikulajová & Velecká, 2012) have moreover revealed that these children experience weak broader language skills, including grammar and vocabulary. These findings, too, resonate with recent reports in other languages, including English (e.g., Snowling et al., 2003; Torppa et al., 2010), suggesting that underlying the code-related deficits of children who develop dyslexia and the more distal cause of the manifest phonological deficits may be impairments in broader language skills.

Beyond the many similarities between features of dyslexia in Czech, Slovak, and other languages, differences also exist. First, the diagnostic classifications in the Czech and Slovak contexts assume that reading (dyslexia) and spelling (dysorthographia) impairments represent separate disorders. In contrast the English-based DSM-V and other definitions, such as the International Dyslexia Association's, consider impaired reading *and* spelling (and their associated behavioral difficulties) to constitute dyslexia. Whether the more specific classifications in the Czech and Slovak context simply reflect historical tradition, or whether in clinical practice there is truly a significant incidence of these singular impairments is not clear. However, the Czech prevalence data (e.g., Gebhardtová, 1994) and the profiles of children with dyslexia reviewed here suggest that poor word-reading efficiency and poor spelling go hand in hand, although reading fluency can vary considerably, while spelling and associated oral language skills tend to be more systematically impaired (Mikulajová & Velecká, 2012). Further investigation into the role(s) of potential comorbidities such as ADHD and Developmental Coordination Disorder (DCD) in driving these reading–spelling dissociations is also needed.

One clear difference with the English profile is that, as in other languages with relatively consistent orthographies (e.g., Landerl, Wimmer, & Frith, 1997), Czech and Slovak children with dyslexia acquire alphabetic skills, basic reading, and spelling skills relatively quickly. However, as we have pointed out here and elsewhere, the faster rate of development need not entail significant differences in the architecture or the cognitive drivers of that development. Indeed, the patterns of cognitive impairments associated with reading and spelling impairments in dyslexia appear to be very similar across a wide range of alphabetic orthographies. Together the above studies suggest that, despite the impact of orthographic consistency on the *rate* of acquisition of word-level literacy and code-related skills, the underlying cognitive architecture is the same (Caravolas & Samara, 2015). Moreover, the relative importance of phoneme awareness and RAN as markers of deficits in dyslexia must be considered in terms of the persisting lag between dyslexic and typical readers within languages, rather than through comparisons of relative performance across languages, as illustrated in the study by Caravolas et al. (2005). It will also be informative to examine, over and above the unique contributions of each of the three foundation skills, how their shared variance might fluctuate in relation to reading and spelling outcomes between languages. An interesting challenge for future studies will be to tease apart the role of letter knowledge relative to phoneme awareness and RAN as an additional marker of dyslexia among children beyond the first year or two of schooling, using novel tasks appropriate for older children (e.g., Froyen et al., 2010) and longitudinal designs tracking dyslexic children's literacy development from the earliest stages (e.g., Torppa et al., 2006).

An important question for clinical and educational practice is whether, in conjunction with a faster rate of growth in literacy skills, the negative impacts of dyslexia are less severe for learners of Czech, Slovak, and other consistent orthographies. It is true after all, that mid-primary-school-aged English-speaking children with dyslexia attain significantly lower scores on literacy and code-related skills than their counterparts learning Czech (Caravolas et al., 2005) or German (Landerl et al., 1997). However, such direct cross-language comparisons may be misleading. In most of the studies cited here, Czech and Slovak children with dyslexia lagged behind their age-mates by, on average, two years by mid-primary school, and Caravolas and Volín (2001) found this discrepancy to remain stable at least to fifth grade. Thus, relative to the norm in their countries, the impairments of children with dyslexia are indeed often severe and potentially as handicapping in the longer term as in languages like English. This issue, along with a future program of scientifically validated intervention studies, deserves further investigation using broader measures of academic, health, and socioeconomic outcomes in direct cross-linguistic comparisons of populations with dyslexia.

References

American Psychiatric Association. (2013). *Diagnostic and statistical manual of mental disorders* (5th ed.). Washington, DC: American Psychiatric Association.

Borkowski, J., & Muthukrishna, N. (1992). Moving metacognition into the classroom: "Working models" and effective strategy teaching. In M. Pressley, K. R. Harris, &

J. T. Guthrie (Eds.), *Promoting academic competence and literacy in school* (pp. 477–501). Orlando, FL: Academic Press.

Bosse, M.-L., Tainturier, M.-J., & Valdois, S. (2007). Developmental dyslexia: The visual attention span deficit hypothesis. *Cognition, 104,* 198–230.

Bruck, M., & Waters, G. (1988). An analysis of the spelling errors of children who differ in their reading and spelling skills. *Applied Psycholinguistics, 9,* 77–92.

Caravolas, M. (2017). Learning to read Czech and Slovak. In L. Verhoeven & C. Perfetti (Eds.), *Learning to read across languages and writing systems* (pp. 371–392). Cambridge, UK: Cambridge University Press.

Caravolas, M., Lervåg, A., Defior, S., Seidlová Málková, G., & Hulme, C. (2013). Different patterns, but equivalent predictors, of growth in reading in consistent and inconsistent orthographies. *Psychological Science, 24,* 1398–1407.

Caravolas, M., Lervåg, A., & Mousikou, P. et al. (2012). Common patterns of prediction of literacy development in different alphabetic orthographies. *Psychological Science, 23,* 678–686.

Caravolas, M., & Mikulajová, M. (2008). Effects of letter-sound consistency, letter-form complexity, and frequency in learning canonical and contextually conditioned letter spellings in Slovak. *Phonetica Pragensia, 11,* 21–30.

Caravolas, M., Mikulajová, M., & Vencelová, L. (2008a). *Spelling of Slovak children with dyslexia.* Paper presented at the International Conference of the British Dyslexia Association, Harrogate, UK.

Caravolas, M., Mikulajová, M., & Vencelová, L. (2008b). *Súbor testov na hodnotenie pravopisných schopností pre škoslkú a klinickú prax* [Battery of tests for the assessment of spelling skills for school and clinical practice]. Bratislava, Slovakia: Slovenská asociácia logopédov.

Caravolas, M., & Samara, A., (2015). Learning to read and spell words in different writing systems. In A. Pollatsek & R. Treiman (Eds.), *The Oxford handbook of reading.* Oxford: Oxford University Press. doi: http://dx.doi.org/10.1093/oxfordhb/9780199324576.013.21.

Caravolas, M., & Volín, J. (2001). Phonological spelling errors among dyslexic children learning a transparent orthography: The case of Czech. *Dyslexia, 7,* 229–245.

Caravolas, M., & Volín, J. (2005). *Baterie diagnostických testů gramotnostních dovedností pro žáky 2. až 5. ročníků ZŠ* [Battery of diagnostic tests of literacy skills for pupils in 2nd *to* 5th grade]. Prague: IPPP ČR.

Caravolas, M., Volín, J., & Hulme, C. (2005). Phoneme awareness is a key component of alphabetic literacy skills in consistent and inconsistent orthographies: Evidence from Czech and English children. *Journal of Experimental Child Psychology, 92,* 107–139.

Cimlerová, P., Pokorná, D., & Chalupová, E. (2007). *Diagnostika specifických poruch učení u adolescentů a dospělých osob* [Diagnosis of specific reading disorders in adolescents and adults].Prague: IPPP ČR.

Edfeldt, W. A. (1968). *Reverzní test* [Reversals test]. Bratislava: Psychodiagnostika.

Frith, U. (1980). Unexpected spelling problems. In U. Frith (Ed.), *Cognitive processes in spelling.* London: Academic Press.

Frostig, M. (1972). *Vývojový test zrakového vnímání* [Developmental test of visual perception]. Bratislava: Psychodiagnostika.

Froyen, D., Willems, G., & Blomert, L. (2010). Evidence for a specific cross-modal association deficit in dyslexia: An electrophysiological study of letter-speech sound processing. *Developmental Science, 14,* 635–648.

Furnes, B., & Samuelsson, S. (2011). Phonological awareness and rapid automatized naming predicting early development in reading and spelling: Results from a cross-linguistic longitudinal study. *Learning and Individual Differences, 21*, 85–95.

Gebhardtová, D. (1994). Výsledky výzkumu dětí se specifickými vývojovými poruchami v oblasti čtení a psaní [Results of research on children with specific developmental disorders in reading and spelling]. In Kucharská, A., Slavíková, I., & Lepová, R. (Eds.), *Specifické poruchy učení a chování* [Specific disorders of learning and behavior]. Prague: IPPP ČR.

Georgiou, G. K., Parrila, R., & Liao, C. H. (2008). Rapid naming speed and reading across languages that vary in orthographic consistency. *Reading and Writing, 21*, 885–903.

Goulandris, N. (2003). *Dyslexia in different languages: Cross-linguistic comparisons.* London: Whurr.

Hulme, C., Caravolas, M., Málková, G., & Brigstocke, S. (2005). Phoneme isolation ability is not simply a consequence of letter-sound knowledge. *Cognition, 97*, B1–B11.

International Dyslexia Association. (2002). *Definition of dyslexia.* http://eida.org/definition-of-dyslexia/.

Kessler, B., & Caravolas, M. (2011). Weslalex: West Slavic lexicon of child-directed printed words. http://spell.psychology.wustl.edu/weslalex.

Kirby, J. R., Georgiou, G. K., Martinussen, R., & Parrila, R. (2010). Naming speed and reading: From prediction to instruction. *Reading Research Quarterly, 45*, 341–362.

Kirby, J. R., Parrila, R. K., & Pfeiffer, S. L. (2003). Naming speed and phonological awareness as predictors of reading development. *Journal of Educational Psychology, 95*, 453–464.

Košč, L. (1987). *Patopsychológia učenia a jej neuropsychologické základy* [Pathology of learning and its neuropsychological foundations]. Bratislava: SPN.

Kučera, H., & Monroe, G. K. (1968). *A comparative, quantitative phonology of Russian, Czech, and German.* New York: Elsevier.

Kucharská, A. (2014). *Rizika vzniku dyslexie* [Risks of developing dyslexia]. Habilitační práce. Prague: PedF UK v Praze.

Kucharská, A., & Barešová, P. (2012). Vývojová dynamika čtení v analyticko-syntetické metodě čtení a metodě genetické v 1. a 2. třídě a její uplatnění v poradenské diagnostice [The dynamics of reading development in the analytic-synthetic versus the genetic methods in 1st and 2nd grade, and their validity for clinical diagnosis]. *Pedagogika, 62* (1–2), 65–80.

Kucharská, A., Seidlová, M., Sotáková, H. et al. (2014). *Porozumění čtenému I. Typický vývoj porozumění čtenému – východiska, témata, zdroje (kritická analýza)* [Reading Comprehension I. Typical development of reading comprehension – perspectives, themes, tools (critical analysis)]. Prague, Czech Republic: Pedagogical Faculty – Charles University.

Landerl, K., Ramus, F., & Moll, K. et al. (2013). Predictors of developmental dyslexia in European orthographies with varying complexity. *Journal of Child Psychology and Psychiatry, 54*, 686–694.

Landerl, K., Wimmer, H., & Frith, U. (1997). The impact of orthographic consistency on dyslexia: A German-English comparison. *Cognition, 63*, 315–334.

Lervåg, A., & Hulme, C. (2009). Rapid automatized naming (RAN) taps a mechanism that places constraints on the development of early reading fluency. *Psychological Science, 20*, 1040–1048.

Matějček, Z. (1959) Klinický obraz dyslektického dieťaťa [Clinical profile of the dyslexic child] Psychológia a patopsychológia dieťaťa, 1(2), 83–86.

Matějček, Z. (1961) Školní selhání některých dětí normálního nadání [Scholastic failure of some children with normal abilities]. Československá pediatrie, 16(10), 877–882.

Matějček, Z. (1978) Vývojové poruchy čtení [Developmental disorders of learning]. Prague: SPN

Matějček, Z. (1995) Dyslexie: specifické poruchy čtení [Dyslexias: specific disorder of reading]. Jinočany: Czech Republic: H&H.

Mertin, V. (2008) Reakce na intervenci – nové kritérium při diagnostice specifických poruch učení [Response to intervention – New criteria in diagnosing specific disorders of learning] Pražské sociálně vědní studie, Psychologická řada PSY-22. Prague: FSV UK a FF UK.

Míka, J. (1982) Orientační test dynamické praxe [Orientational test of dynamic practice] Bratislava: Psychodiagnostika.

Mikulajová, M. (2010) Metódy diagnostiky dyslexie [Methods of diagnosing dyslexia]. CD nosič. Bratislava: Mabag.

Mikulajová, M. Horňáková Schöffelová, M., Tokárová, O., & Dostálová, A. (2016). Tréning jazykových schopností podle D. B. Elkonina [Training of language abilities according to D B Elkonin]. 2nd ed. Prague: Centrum Rozum, V.O.S.

Mikulajová, M. Tokárová, O., & Sümegiová, Z. (2014). Tréning fonematického uvedomovania podľa D B Eľkonina [Training of phoneme awareness according to D.B. Elkonin]. 2nd ed Bratislava: Dialóg, spol. s r.o.

Mikulajová, M Vágnerová, B., Vencelová, L., Caravolas, M., & Škrabáková, G. (2012). Čítanie, písanie a dyslexia (s testami a normami) [Reading, writing and dyslexia (with tests and norms)] Bratislava: Slovenská asociácia logopédov.

Mikulajová, M & Velecká, A. (2012). Profil slovenských dětí s „dyslexií" z pohledu jejich čtenárských schopností. Pedagogika, 62(1–2), 137–149.

Mladá, P. (1996) Zbývá jen málo – chtít pochopit, aneb dyslexie na 2. stupni ZŠ. [All that remains is to want to understand, or, dyslexia in the second grade of elementary school]. In A. Kucharská (red) Specifické poruchy učení a chování 1996 (pp. 61–64.). Prague: Portál

Moll, K., & Landerl, K. (2009). Double dissociation between reading and spelling deficits. Scientific Studies of Reading, 13, 359–382.

Moll, K., Loff, A & Snowling, M. (2013). Cognitive endophenotypes of dyslexia. Scientific Studies of Reading, 17, 385–397. doi: http://dx.doi.org/10.1080/10888438 .2012.736439

Moll, K , Ramus F & Barding et al. (2014). Cognitive mechanisms underlying reading and spelling development in five European orthographies. Learning and Instruction, 29, 65–77 doi http //dx doi.org/10.1016/j.learninstruc.2013.09.003.

Moll, K., Thompson P A., & Mikulajová, M. et al. (2016). Precursors of reading difficulties in Czech and Slovak children at-risk of dyslexia. Dyslexia, 22, 120–136. doi: http //dx doi org/doi:10.1002/dys.1526.

Pardel, T. (1966) Písaná reč, jej vývin a poruchy u detí [Written language, its development and disorders] Bratislava: SPN.

Pennington, B F (2006) From single to multiple deficit models of developmental disorders Cognition, 101, 385–413.

Pennington, B. F., & Lefly, D. L. (2001). Early reading development in children at family risk for dyslexia. *Child Development*, *72*, 816–833. doi: http://dx.doi.org/10.1111/1467-8624.00317 .

Schatschneider, C., Fletcher, J. M., Francis, D. J., Carlson, C. D., & Foorman, B. R. (2004). Kindergarten prediction of reading skills: A longitudinal comparative analysis. *Journal of Educational Psychology*, *96*, 265–282.

Schöffelová, M., & Mikulajová, M. (2012). Vývoj různých aspektů čtení ve slovenštině [The development of various aspects of reading in Slovak]. *Pedagogika*, *1–2*, 111–125.

Seidlová Málková, G., & Caravolas, M. (2013). *Baterie testů fonologických schopností, BTFS* [Battery of tests of phonological abilities]. Prague: Národní ústav pro vzdělávání.

Share, D. (2008). On the Anglocentricities of current reading research and practice: The perils of overreliance on an "outlier" orthography. *Psychological Bulletin*, *134*, 584–615.

Snowling, M. J., Gallagher, A., & Frith, U. (2003). Family risk of dyslexia is continuous: individual differences in the precursors of reading skill. *Child Development*, *74*, 358–373. doi: http://dx.doi.org/10.1111/1467-8624.7402003.

Snowling, M. J., & Hulme, C. (2012). Annual research review: The nature and classification of reading disorders – A commentary on proposals for DSM-5. *Journal of Child Psychology and Psychiatry*, *53*, 593–607.

Sokolová, M., Musilová, K., & Slančová, D. (2005). *Slovenčina a čeština (Synchrónne porovnanie s cvičeniami)* [Slovak and Czech (Synchronic comparison with exercises)]. Bratislava: FF UK.

Švancarová, D., & Kucharská, A. (2001). *Test rizika poruch čtení a psaní pro rané školáky* [Test of risk of disorders in reading and writing for young school children]. Prague: Scientia.

Tiefenbacherová, B. (2014). *Možnosti stimulácie morfo-syntaktických schopností v predškolskom veku* [Approaches to the stimulation of morphosyntactic abilities in the preschool years]. Master's thesis. Bratislava: Pedagogical Faculty, Comenius University.

Torppa, M., Lyytinen, P., Erskine, J., Eklund, K., & Lyytinen, H. (2010). Language development, literacy skills, and predictive connections to reading in Finnish children with and without familial risk for dyslexia. *Journal of Learning Disabilities*, *43*, 308–321. doi: http://dx.doi.org/10.1177/0022219410369096.

Torppa, M., Poikkeus, A.-M., Laakso, M.-L., Eklund, K., & Lyytinen, H. (2006). Predicting delayed letter knowledge development and its relation to grade 1 reading achievement among children with and without familial risk for dyslexia. *Developmental Psychology*, *42*, 1128–1142.

Váryová, B. (2012). Skúšky čítania pre mladší školský vek [Tests of reading for the younger school years]. In Mikulajová, M., Váryová, B., Vencelová, L., Caravolas, M., & Škrabáková, G. (Eds.). *Čítanie, písanie a dyslexia (s testami a normami)* [Reading, writing and dyslexia (with tests and norms)] (pp. 126–159). Bratislava: Slovenská asociácia logopédov.

Vencelová, L., & Kapalková, S. (2014). Východiská tvorby novej inovatívnej metodiky výučby slovenského jazyka v 1. ročníku základnej školy [The scope of the new innovative method in Slovak language arts curriculum for grade 1]. *Logopaedica* XVII, 105–117.

Vencelová, L., & Mikulajová, M. (2010). Čítanie a pravopis po slovensky hovoriacich dyslektických detí – porovnávacia štúdia [Reading and spelling of Slovak-speaking children with dyslexia – Comparative study]. *Psychológia a patopsychológia diet'at'a, 45 (3)*, 215–228.

Wimmer, H. (1993). Characteristics of developmental dyslexia in a regular writing system. *Applied Psycholinguistics, 14*, 1–33.

Wimmer, H., Mayringer, H., & Landerl, K. (2000). The double-deficit hypothesis and difficulties in learning to read a regular orthography. *Journal of Educational Psychology, 92*, 668–680.

6   Developmental Dyslexia in Finnish

Heikki Lyytinen, Ulla Richardson, and Mikko Aro

6.1   Introduction

Written Finnish and the Finnish literacy culture provide an exceptional context for an interesting separation of the various processes associated with reading acquisition. The orthography of Finnish is relatively optimally wired to give young learners an easy time acquiring basic decoding skills. Finnish orthography has full transparency in both reading and writing. After learning the limited set of sounds connected consistently with specific graphemes, learners usually learn to decode accurately, even those with learning difficulties in reading.

The high status of literacy in Finland, which dates from the early stages of its writing system, has led to additional benefits. The written language of Finnish was established in the mid-sixteenth century. The first book published in Finnish was an ABC-book, a primer for reading and a catechism. As early as the seventeenth century, literacy started to become more common with the influence of the church. People were instructed and encouraged to learn to read, because they were given permission to marry only if they were able to read Luther's Small Catechism. This was one of the central factors that incentivized people to learn reading skills. Prior to this, the use of writing was restricted to the learned and those of high social status. In contrast, today reading is universal in Finland and there is practically no illiteracy.

The high status of literacy in Finnish is related also to the general use of a standardized spoken language form. This standard form clearly differs from the typical colloquial speech, specifically in its more complex syntactical forms. In general, speakers can use the standard form or at least a modified version of it, and experience it in formal communication situations including television and radio (even in children's programs), public speeches, and in schools. In turn, standard Finnish closely follows the established written form of the language. In fact, one of the specific duties of the Institute for the Languages of Finland is to provide guidance for the correct use of standard Finnish including its written language forms, and in general compliance with these guidelines is high. The dominance of the standard language form in the written text is obvious since almost all published texts (including subtitles on foreign TV programs) use the standard language form instead of colloquial expressions. There is no reason why colloquial expressions could not be used in a written format, since they also can be written using the language's consistent grapheme–phoneme correspondence rules. However, currently these colloquial expressions are used in a written format mainly for personal communication, especially by the younger generations of Finnish speakers. Thus, learners are usually well accustomed to the written text form (standard Finnish) that represents the standard spoken language that is still widely used in Finnish society. This in turn facilitates the learning of the main point of decoding skills; that is the connection between spoken language units and the corresponding written language units.

In this writing context the learning burden required in order to attain accurate decoding skills is low. Following optimal instruction in the basics of reading, learning to read is a matter of practicing twenty-four letter–sound connections (occurring in Finnish words) and the organization of these sounds into words. But even in this system, some children struggle. More than 20 percent of Finnish children get organized remedial support in school. That some children need more time to learn is understood as a natural phenomenon. This has meant that dyslexia has not had a very visible role in the nomenclature used by Finnish educators (nor that of medical experts). In fact, it was only very recently (in the year 2006) that individuals who continue to struggle with reading and writing were officially granted special arrangements in the matriculation examination, which is a national exam, taken at the end of the student's high-school education.

Compromised reading in the Finnish context (and in any transparent orthography) tends to mean difficulties becoming sufficiently fluent that cognitive/memory resources are spared expending considerable effort on comprehending long and difficult written sentences. Struggling readers focus their attention on single letters and are unable to read with the fluency needed for learning. It has been observed (PIAAC, 2012, see Malin, Sulkunen, & Laine, 2013, p. 38) that even today around 370,000 Finnish adults are not fully literate. They do not comprehend what they read at the expected level. The most likely reason is that they did not continue to practice reading after leaving school.

6.2   Learning to Read Finnish

6.2.1   Finnish Language and Its Orthography

The Finnish language does not belong to the Indo-European group of languages, but to the small Fenno-Ugric language family. The basic Finnish vocabulary is quite distinct as compared to major European languages, although there are a large number of loan words, both old and more recent, from especially

Germanic and Baltic languages. It is different from the more prominent languages of reading research with respect to its morphology and orthographic transparency. Thus, Finnish offers an interesting contrast especially with English, in revealing universal and more language-specific aspects of reading acquisition and its problems. Here, we aim to describe briefly the basic aspects of linguistic and writing systems of Finnish, as well as the basic findings concerning reading acquisition (for more details on the topic, see Aro, 2017).

Finnish has eight vowel sounds and thirteen native consonant sounds. In addition there are three consonant sounds that are used in recent loan words only. Finnish also has many diphthongs that combine two distinct vowel sounds. The vowel harmony means that there can be only either front or back vowels in a word, and this also affects endings. One important feature of the Finnish phonological system is that all vowels and most consonants can have two lengths: short and long. The length distinction affects meaning, and the length of vowels and consonants can vary independently. This means that words like *tuli* [fire], *tuuli* [wind], and *tulli* [customs] differ only with respect to phoneme lengths. The syllable structure is relatively simple, with a lot of open syllables. Consonant clusters are rare, and in the initial position exist only in recent loan words.

The Finnish morphology is agglutinative and relatively complex. Nouns, adjectives, verbs, numerals, and pronouns are inflected based on their grammatical role within the sentence, and words can have several affixes. For example, nouns can have fifteen cases expressed with inflections, and on top of that possessive suffixes and various clitics. Thus, a single word can carry a lot of morphological information. For example, a question like "Would you believe?" can be expressed as "Uskoisitko?" in Finnish. A noun can have over 2,000 different forms depending on its inflections, and this number is even higher for verbs. On top of this rich inflectional system, the use of derivative suffixes is common in word formation, and compounding is frequent. From the point of view of reading, this means that words with one morpheme are less common in texts than words with several morphemes.

Finnish writing system uses the twenty-six letters of the Latin alphabet with the addition of <å>, <ä>, and <ö>. All Finnish phonemes have a distinct corresponding grapheme, with the exception of /ng/, which is marked with the letter <n(+k)> and with a digraph <ng> as a long sound. The long phonemic sound is in all other cases systematically marked in writing by doubling the corresponding letter. Thus, although the morphological system is complex, the orthography reflects a rather strict phonemic principle. Each letter reliably represents a single sound, and each phoneme is reliably represented with a corresponding letter, independent of the context. The words in a text tend to be long (averaging between seven and eight letters), due to compounding, derivations, and inflections.

6.2.2   Challenges in Learning to Read Finnish

For the learner, the orthographic principle is easy to master, and phonemic assembly on the level of single letters is sufficient for decoding. The challenges for decoding (and spelling) relate to marking the length of the phoneme and long words. Correspondingly, the early instruction of reading and spelling emphasizes the syllable as a substage in decoding, and syllables are marked with hyphens in early reading materials. Due to the transparency of the orthography, most children acquire basic decoding skills rather effortlessly and often with fairly little instructional support. Around one third of children are already able to decode when they start school, and typically, close to perfect reading accuracy is reached quite early. The individual differences in reading skill are reflected mostly in reading speed, although children struggling with reading also make more errors in reading and especially spelling as compared to typically developing peers. Reading instruction is based on synthetic phonics, and attempts at reading are based rather uniformly on decoding; there are no indications of a *logographic stage* in reading development. The correlation between word and pseudoword reading in the early years of reading development is reported as close to perfect. Since grapheme–phoneme correspondences are regular and symmetrical, spelling instruction starts hand in hand with reading instruction, and typically early spelling development closely follows development in reading.

The studies focusing on development of phonological awareness have indicated development from large (syllables) to small (phonemes) units. The awareness of phonemes seems intertwined with letter knowledge and early reading skills, since the orthography is transparent at the level of single-letter graphemes and the letter names consistently include the letter sounds. The role of morphological awareness in reading development is still largely unstudied. That is a direction of research that is especially interesting from the point of fluency development, the stage after the acquisition of basic accurate decoding skills.

6.3   Reading Difficulties in Finnish

6.3.1   Historical and Cultural Context

Soon after Finnish orthography was defined by Bishop Agricola (1510–1557; his ABC-book was published in 1543), carefully following the Latin model, the religious authorities invented an effective way to motivate people to learn to read. To be allowed to marry in a Christian church in Finland, people had to learn the Vähä katekismus, the Small Catechism (published in Finnish in 1529), which contained the core Lutheran religious messages. Motivation for reading continues to be high in modern Finland. If one were to ask children starting school what they wish to learn there, most will mention reading as the most important target. More than a third of Finnish children have learned to read before they enter school at the age of seven.

6.3.2   Identification and Prevalence of Dyslexia

In the Finnish school system formal diagnosis of a disability is not necessary in order to receive extra support at school. Learning support is built on three levels (general, intensified, and specific support) with the individualization, intensity, means of support, and involvement of special education teachers increasing with the levels. The need for support is assessed by the teachers, and the means of that support are usually planned by the classroom teacher and special education teacher, working together. In more severe cases of learning difficulty, multidisciplinary expertise is involved in planning and follow-up, including that of psychologists or physicians. Typically, dyslexic problems are dealt with within the school context. In every Finnish school special educational support is available. For dyslexia, support is carried out typically at the levels of general or intensified support in the form of part-time special education. This means that the child has one or more lessons per week either individually or in a small group with a special education teacher. More than one fifth of the children at grade levels 1–9 receive part-time special education at some point of the school year, this figure being highest for children in the first two grades (Official Statistics of Finland, 2014).

Typically, children struggling with skill development are identified early. The special education teachers screen the children for poor reading skills, letter knowledge, and relevant prereading skills at school entry. On the basis of screening results, the need for extra support is evaluated, and it is typically offered in the form of part-time special education. The first months of reading instruction might also be carried out in flexible groups, where a special education teacher is responsible for teaching the children that seem most at risk of problems in skill development. Also, co-teaching is becoming more common. At later grade levels, the reading problems are generally supported via part-time special education and individualized pedagogical arrangements in various learning situations, like tests.

A formal medical diagnosis of dyslexia in children is quite rare, and is mainly given to children who have encountered medical professionals due to especially severe or comorbid problems. It is clear, however, that the prevalence of developmental reading problems, or dyslexia, is unrelated to diagnostic practices. Prevalence estimates are always dependent on the criteria used, but also on the level of skill that is considered age-appropriate. The early curriculum is more or less based on the assumption that children acquire the ability to read independently during the first school year, or at the latest, second grade from third grade on the schoolchildren are expected to use their reading skill fluently to meet the demand of school subjects and longer texts. Although it is hard to give an objective estimate of the prevalence of dyslexia in Finnish, it is safe to assume that it does not differ markedly from other languages. Reading accuracy in Finnish generally develops rather quickly after early reading instruction and even children struggling with decoding master it during the first or second grade. Dyslexic children, however, have long-lasting and marked problems in reading speed and sometimes also in spelling accuracy. Thus, the tests used for identification of reading problems are typically measures of reading efficiency, combining accuracy and speed in the test score.

While the majority of dyslexic children do not get support outside the school setting, the children can be referred for an assessment by a school psychologist, who can usually be found in cities and large rural municipalities, or psychologists at the municipality's family guidance center. This consultation is used to plan and tailor the support that is built into the school and classroom setting.

6.4   Behavioral and Neurocognitive Evidence

The development of readiness to learn to read has been examined in detail in the Jyväskylä Longitudinal study of Dyslexia (JLD; for the most recent review of the results see Lyytinen et al., 2015). This study of children at familial risk for dyslexia has now followed 100 such individuals from birth to puberty along with a comparable group of individuals without risk. The earliest predictive signs of dyslexia were observed at the age of 3 to 5 days old, using brain event related potentials to both sinusoidal sounds (Leppänen et al., 2010) and syllables (da-ba-ga; Guttorm et al., 2010). Both studies revealed event related potential (ERP) features which had significant correlations to reading acquisition. Surprisingly the significant prediction was observed not only from responses to speech sounds but also the so-called mismatch negativity (MMN) response to pitch differences. Possibly the most surprising result was that within the group with familial risk the children who did and did not end up developing dyslexia differed the following way: children who went on to develop dyslexia failed to show MMN response to a pitch change (1000 vs 1100 Hz), which suggests the possibility of auditory insensitivity as the initial problem. ERPs to syllables differed between risk and non-risk groups at that very early age and these differences had significant predictive correlations to a large number of reading-related measures years later. These are purely empirical predictions that show that something in the brain's activity reflected in processing sounds behaves differently depending on the occurrence of dyslexia, which obviously is only observable later on when children attempt to learn to read.

To gain some understanding of how this may happen, we consider another discovery: that speech perception of phonemic duration is compromised from the very beginning. This difficulty is the most distinctive feature of dyslexia in Finnish and is observable in the spelling of almost all children with dyslexia at reading age. It is also typical for children to tend to make spelling errors associated with phonemic length when first learning to write. Most Finnish phonemes can occur in short and long form, and this is also reflected in the writing: The short phonemes are written with one letter, but long phonemes are written with two identical letters. Infants become sensitive to and perceive these differences from a very early age. We observed (Richardson et al., 2003) that at 6 months, categorical perception of phonemic length (measured through head-turn conditioning) reveals differences between children with and without familial risk. The at-risk children need a longer silence in the context of the *t*-consonant in order to perceive it as long than that required by the non-risk children.

Thus, it appears that the brains of children with a genetic predisposition to dyslexia do not respond to language input in the same way as those of typical children. These children may fail to perceive the distinctive features of speech that differentiate between similar phonemes. In transparent writing environment learners have to be able to differentiate very small units – phonemes, including their short and long forms – from each other to connect them to their written form. Perceptual difficulties thus form an understandable bottleneck compromising typical reading acquisition.

This all means learners' readiness to learn to differentiate between and store the sounds of letters forms a natural basis of basic reading acquisition, which can be observed in how children first learn letter names and then their sounds. In Finnish the names given to letters provide an effective cue for the sounds of the letters. This means that children who have learned the names of letters without difficulties – as most do – are most likely also not to face any difficulties in learning the sounds of letters if instructed in an appropriate way. This is why it was no surprise that letter-name knowledge proved to be an extremely effective predictor of reading acquisition among the JLD participants, as shown in Figure 6.1, which displays the predictive associations of developmental measures, from the early preschool years to reading acquisition, among children who faced severe problems in learning to read. Practically all had difficulties in storing letter names, and this was a far more reliable predictor than any other. This has led to the adaptation of a very easy to use and practical measure with which to identify children who need preventive help and ensure that they receive such help to a sufficient degree. This type of prevention saves them from being affected by the experience of failing to learn to read in a context (Finnish) in which the vast majority attain perfect decoding skills.

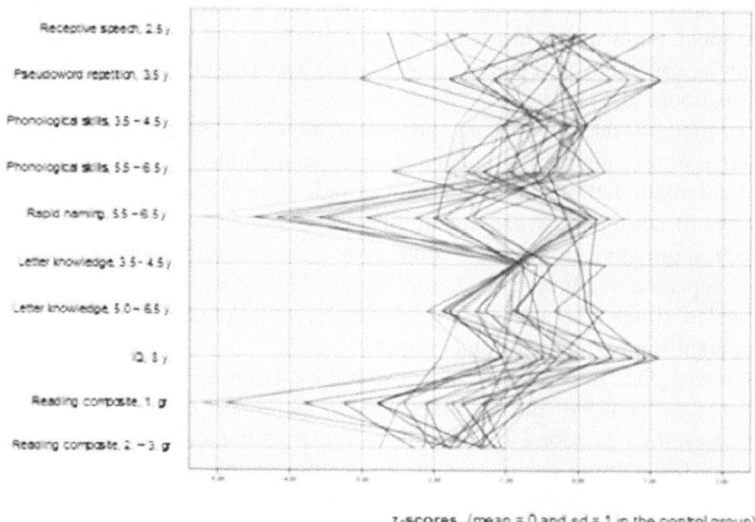

z-scores, (mean = 0 and sd = 1 in the control group)

Individual profiles of all JLD children showing compromised reading at the end of the 2nd grade

Figure 6.1 The JLD follow-up from birth to school age of reading-related development: Individual profiles of the prediction measures of the children whose reading acquisition was most severely compromised (modified from Lyytinen et al., 2009, p. 670)

6.5   Intervention

6.5.1   Focus on Specific Skills

Training and intervention methods used in Finnish schools to support the reading development of struggling learners typically involve individual or small-group training led by special education teachers. Such training is usually provided once or twice a week, maximally for one lesson (forty-five minutes) and typically for a limited period of time (one school term or such) but sometimes for a much longer period.

6.5.1.1   Training Phonological Skills   The tendency is to provide the bulk of interventions during the early stages of school (first to third grade, i.e., 7–9 years) when children are taking their first steps in learning to read; learners with persistent and more severe deficits also attend specific training sessions in the later stages of their formal schooling, with the same relatively low intensity rate (typically once a week face-to-face meetings with special education teachers or other experts). As of the year 2009, 19 percent of first graders received part-time special education due to problems in reading and spelling development; at ninth grade the percentage was 1.5 percent (Kirjavainen, Pulkkinen, & Jahnukainen, 2013).

The methods used in training and intervention studies typically involve tasks aimed at improving phonological awareness and phonological sensitivity (e.g., segment manipulations involving either single sound/letter segments, syllables, or parts of compound words), auditory–visual connections (e.g., transcribing speech segments into written counterparts), reading and spelling exercises (e.g., repeated reading and shared reading sessions), and language games (syllables, rimes, phonemes). A mix of different tasks is often used to achieve significant improvements in reading skills.

In many of the intervention studies, training focuses on one linguistic/auditory factor as the center of the exercises. Due to the almost perfect[1] consistency of letter–sound connections in both dimensions (reading and spelling) in Finnish, much of the training has focused on these connections. However, increasingly syllables are also used as training units. In Finnish, primary stress (with a lengthening of sound durations and higher fundamental frequency, *tone*) provides a strong perceptual cue to word beginnings. Cues to syllable segmentation also come from the system of lexical stress. As a rule, the primary stress systematically falls on the first syllable and the secondary stress falls on every other syllable; the last syllable is never stressed. Because stress patterns are relatively systematic and predictable, thus facilitating syllable detection, syllables are used in school instruction as well as in intervention studies.

6.5.1.2 Training Reading Skills   Next, we provide a brief account of the findings of intervention studies with Finnish-speaking dyslexic and/or poor readers at different stages of reading development. Several intervention studies have investigated the efficacy of training phonological (awareness) skills or phonological sensitivity in improving accuracy in reading and spelling for struggling readers. Poskiparta, Niemi, & Vauras (1999) conducted an intervention study with 7- to 8-year-old children attending their first year at school (twenty-minute intervention sessions in small groups, three to four times a week for forty-seven sessions altogether). The at-risk readers, whose phonological skills were assessed as being specifically poor at the beginning of the school year, were divided into three matched groups: One group attended phonological awareness intervention, the second received training in a normal special education group, and the third group received no extra

---

[1] The only exception for the letter–sound correspondence in Finnish is the fact that for the voiced velar nasal sound there is no unique letter that represents only that specific sound. This sound is represented by the letter ⟨n⟩ in front of the unvoiced velar stop sound /k/ and when the sound is geminated it is marked with the letter combination of /ng/.

support. The results show that the group who received specific training in phonological awareness skills using nursery rhymes performed significantly better than the other groups at word recognition, spelling, and listening comprehension. The children's skills were reassessed at the end of the first grade and the intervention group's achieved gains remained. Thus, it seems that training in phonological awareness skills clearly benefits Finnish-speaking at-risk readers. However, in the follow-up study, the same children's reading-related skills were reassessed again in the third grade and the results showed that the children who had been in the intervention group did not perform any better than the children in the control groups. It should be noted that the predictive value of phonological awareness skills on decoding skills in Finnish seems to diminish after children learn the basics of decoding skills (Holopainen, Ahonen, & Lyytinen, 2001). Instead the predictive power of orthographic skills (letter knowledge) is very high in Finnish. It could be that once children learn Finnish letter–sound correspondences they can utilize this knowledge to perform better in phonological awareness tasks, thus reducing the predictive value of phonological awareness skills in reading skills.

Ketonen (2010) conducted a phonological intervention study of six treatment-resistant dyslexic children taking part in the JLD study who at the beginning of the intervention had familial risk for dyslexia and poor letter knowledge at preschool. The twenty-week intervention (one hour per week) focusing on phonological skills and letter–sound knowledge was conducted at preschool or during the first year at school. The children's development was followed until the seventh grade (12–13 years). The study found that although phonological awareness skills and letter knowledge improved after the intervention period, this improvement was not reflected in children's reading and spelling skills. Thus, although the intervention was successful in improving certain reading-related skills, this was not enough to significantly support children who had severe learning difficulties specifically in reading.

Apart from intervention studies focusing on improving reading accuracy, Finnish intervention studies have targeted reading speed (fluency). This is particularly relevant in the Finnish-language context due to the fact that even struggling readers can often read accurately, but slowly. Heikkilä et al.'s (2013) intervention study of fluency skills was conducted with poor readers from the second and third grades (8- to 9-year-olds). Children were trained with a computerized repeated reading task for two to three weeks for about fifteen minutes at a time, three to five times a week. The training material included both short and long syllables. After the intervention, children's reading speed increased significantly for the trained syllables. The transfer effect to reading words including the syllables was significant only in reading words with infrequent syllables.

Huemer et al. (2010) conducted a crossover design intervention study in which poor readers from fourth to sixth grade (10- to 12-year-old children) participated in ten training sessions over a two-week period while the other group of poor readers waited to participate in the second part of the intervention. The children were trained to read a set of low-frequency syllables (thirty syllables) with altogether fifty presentations each during the intervention period. The results show that reading speed of the trained syllables increased after the intervention. Also, reading speed of pseudowords containing the trained syllables increased significantly. There was no transfer of the increased speed to reading a text that included only a very small portion (below 0.5 percent) of the trained infrequent syllables, which suggests the effects of the training were item-specific. The intervention studies on fluency skills show that it seems to be possible to increase the speed of reading the specific trained items. The findings suggest that at a certain stage of skill development, poor reading fluency might be supported by practicing syllables as sublexical units larger than single phonemes/letters.

6.5.1.3 Training Perceptual Skills   Apart from phonological and repeated reading training, Finnish intervention studies of poor readers have also been conducted involving auditory perception tasks. The intervention study by Oksanen (2012) included auditory training, training on connecting auditory and visual stimuli, and reading and spelling training. All training tasks occurred in a separate period devoted to the intervention study. The training groups were further divided by the type of training stimuli used in the intervention: either speech or non-speech stimuli with computerized tasks. The participating poor readers were third graders (9-year-olds). Children with matched reading skills from the same school classes served as non-training controls. The results of the different training periods showed that training with non-speech stimuli benefited children in the auditory–visual connection tasks significantly more than the children who were trained with speech stimuli. Training with speech stimuli, on the other hand, improved reading accuracy skills significantly more than when children were trained with non-speech stimuli.

The training of auditory–visual matching skills alone has also been studied in the Finnish-language context. The Audilex computer program was used in an intervention by Kujala et al. (2001). Audilex uses various nonverbal sound patterns together with visual symbols (rectangles), the aim being to match presented sound patterns with the corresponding visually presented patterns of symbols. Seven-year-old poor readers participated in the seven-week intervention including fourteen ten-minute training sessions once or twice per week. Both behavioral and brain measures were used in the assessments. The positive effects of training were shown on reading scores. Importantly, the results also showed observable plastic changes in the auditory cortex after training, indicated with increased MMNs as well as faster reaction times to changes of speed.

6.5.2   Effects of GraphoLearn

For over a decade now the computerized training and assessment environment, GraphoLearn (GL; previously known as GraphoGame; known as Ekapeli in Finnish), has been used in intervention studies that focus on connecting units of speech directly with corresponding written language units. (For a summary of results associated with GL, see Richardson & Lyytinen, 2014.) The rationale for the game environment originally came from research findings that indicated that learners who struggle in reading find it difficult to learn the connections between speech sounds and letters. This led to the adaptation of a very easy to use and practical means of identifying children who need extra support to prevent their being affected by the experience of failing to learn to read during the first few months of reading instruction, when the vast majority of others attain accurate reading skills. The game adapts to each individual player's skills by providing training content that is sufficiently challenging but at the same time enables even struggling learners to succeed in finding correct correspondences between spoken and written items.

Following this failure-prevention logic, Mönkkönen et al. carried out a GraphoLearn intervention study with preschool-aged children (6- to 7-year-olds) who had poor letter–sound knowledge at the end of preschool and prior to starting school.[2] A crossover design was used in which children played first either GraphoLearn during the first six weeks of the intervention, for on average 3.5 hours altogether in short ten-to-fifteen-minute playing sessions, or a similar game with math content for the same period of time. After six weeks, the groups switched to playing the game that they had not played during the first intervention period. In addition, the study design included a matched group of children who did not participate in any intervention training sessions. The results show that even after this short but relatively intensive training period with GraphoLearn, children's letter knowledge as well as pseudoword reading skills had improved significantly in comparison to those of the children playing the math game or those not participating in training.

A study conducted by Saine et al. (2011) followed children's development after a relatively long and intensive GraphoLearn intervention period (twenty-eight weeks with fifteen-minute training sessions with GraphoLearn, plus thirty minutes of regular reading support for four times a week). The study design included two control groups: matched level poor readers at the start of the first grade (7-year-olds) who received regular reading support similarly to the GraphoLearn intervention group for forty-five minutes at each training session but without the fifteen-minute GraphoLearn training. Second, the classmates of the intervention group children participated in the study as typically reading

---

[2] A. Mönkkönen, S. Bach, & S. Brem et al. (manuscript in preparation). Technology-enhanced training of basic decoding skills in preschool age children.

controls who did not need any extra support for learning to read. Children's reading skills were assessed immediately after the end of the intervention period as well as when they were in third grade at school (9-year-olds). The results showed that the long and intensive training period with GraphoLearn had a significant effect on the poor readers' reading skills in comparison to those of the children attending regular remedial support. Significantly, the GraphoLearn intervention was sufficient to increase poor learners' reading skills up to the level of their nonintervention mainstream peers when their reading skills were assessed almost two years after the intervention period. This finding seems very encouraging in terms of the efficiency of training reading skills of poor readers in Finnish. It seems that in a language like Finnish with shallow orthography, training that directly matches speech sounds to written language units in intensive and motivating learning sessions is sufficient to significantly support poor learners' reading skills.

Interestingly GraphoLearn has motivated a number of brain-related studies. For example, Brem et al. (2010) used several concomitant imaging methods to observe the associative learning occurring after a short (3–4-hour) playing time of GraphoLearn and observed the results of learning in specific brain areas, including the so-called Visual Word Form Area of the brain. These promising findings have motivated researchers in many countries to carry out similar intervention studies based on the success in Finland, where educational authorities have facilitated applications of the interventions. The website www .lukimat.fi supports both reading and math skills via Ekapeli and provides an information database to help teachers and parents understand how best to support struggling learners. Today it is thought that over 10,000 Finnish children may play these learning games within the space of one day; hundreds of thousands have benefited from this support after became freely available to learners via the Internet in 2006.

6.6   Discussion and Conclusion

In the Finnish-language context, learners have a relatively easy job of accessing the first important steps of learning to read. This is largely because the Finnish language has a very straightforward system in which there is one-to-one correspondence between speech sounds and letters in both reading and writing. However, struggling learners of Finnish orthography find it difficult to learn even this simple system of connections. It takes them significantly longer to learn letter–sound correspondences and this is reflected in the speed in which they learn how to combine units to make larger units such as syllables and words. In general, however, even individuals with dyslexia learn to accurately decode Finnish writing. Also, they may make spelling mistakes especially in reproducing the phonemic length accurately in writing. The factor that seems to be both a cause and a consequence of dyslexia is that reading tends to stay slow. This is at least partly due to a compromised interest in reading for leisure, a practice which could help in automatizing decoding skills.

The intervention methods used in Finland to support dyslexic and poor readers have been proven to be effective in improving their reading accuracy and even speed of reading. Importantly, the Finnish-language context facilitates identification of poor learners at the age before they start to learn to read. This makes it possible to provide preventive training which in turn is important for learners' motivation and learning careers. As with any severe learning difficulty, early identification, appropriate content for training, and sufficiently intensive and long-lasting training support is urgently needed. As the intervention studies reviewed here indicate, providing an engaging learning environment such as GraphoLearn for individually adaptive training, with endless opportunities to repeat the speech–sound connections and to increase the speed of these connections – can be the key for supporting the reading development of poor learners.

References

Aro, M. (2017). Learning to read Finnish. In L. Verhoeven & C. Perfetti (Eds.), *Learning to read across languages and writing systems* (pp. 416–436). Cambridge, UK: Cambridge University.

Brem, S., Bach, S., & Kucian, K. et al. (2010). Brain sensitivity to print emerges when children learn letter–speech sound correspondences. *Proceedings of the National Academy of Sciences, 107*, 7939–7944.

Guttorm, T., Leppänen, P., Hämäläinen, J., Eklund, K., & Lyytinen, H. (2010). Newborn event-related potentials predict poorer pre-reading skills in children with dyslexia. *Journal of Learning Disabilities, 43*, 391–401.

Heikkilä, R., Aro, M., Närhi, V., Westerholm, J., & Ahonen, T. (2013). Does training in syllable recognition improve reading speed? A computer-based trial with poor readers from second and third grade. *Scientific Studies of Reading, 17*, 398–414.

Holopainen, L., Ahonen, T., & Lyytinen, H. (2001). Predicting delay in reading achievement in a highly transparent language. *Journal of Learning Disabilities, 3*(4), 401–413.

Huemer, S., Aro, M., Landerl, K., & Lyytinen, H. (2010). Repeated reading of syllables among Finnish speaking children with poor reading skills. *Scientific Studies of Reading, 14*, 317–340.

Ketonen, R. (2010). Jyväskylä Studies in Education, *Psychology and Social Research, 0075-4625, 404.* Jyväskylä: University of Jyväskylä.

Kirjavainen, T., Pulkkinen, J., & Jahnukainen, M. (2013). *Erityisopetuksen muutostrendit perusopetuksessa 2000-luvulla* [The trends of change in special education after year 2000] Valtiontalouden tarkastusvirasto [National Audit Office of Finland]. https://docplayer.fi/10162284-Erityisopetuksen-muutostrendit-perusopetuksessa-2000-luvulla.html. Accessed January 25, 2015.

Kujala, T., Karma, K., & Ceponiene, R. et al. (2001). Plastic neural changes and reading improvement caused by audiovisual training in reading-impaired children. *Proceedings of the National Academy of Sciences, 98*, 10509–10514.

Leppänen, P. H. T., Hämäläinen, J. A., & Salminen, H. et al. (2010). Brain event-related potentials reveal atypical processing of sound frequency and the subsequent association with later literacy skills in children with familial dyslexia. *Cortex, 46*, 1362–1376.

Lyytinen, H., Erskine, J., Hämäläinen, J., Torppa, M., & Ronimus, M. (2015). Dyslexia – Early identification and prevention: Highlights from the Jyväskylä Longitudinal Study of Dyslexia. *Current Developmental Disorders Reports, 2*, 330–338.

Lyytinen, H., Erskine, J., Kujala, J., Ojanen, E., & Richardson, U. (2009). In search of a science-based application: A learning tool for reading acquisition. *Scandinavian Journal of Psychology, 50*, 668–675.

Malin, A., Sulkunen, S., & Laine, K. (2013). *PIAAC 2012. Kansainvälisen aikuistutkimuksen ensituloksia [PIAAC 2012. The survey of adult skills]*. Helsinki: Opetus- ja kulttuuriministeriön julkaisuja, 19.

Official Statistics of Finland. (2014). *Special education. Share of students having received special support diminished* [e-publication]. Helsinki: Statistics Finland. www .tilastokeskus.fi/til/erop/2013/erop_2013_2014–06-12_tie_001_en.html. Accessed January 25, 2015.

Oksanen, A.-M. (2012). *Auditiivisen ja kielellisen harjoittelun vaikutus kolmannella luokalla olevien heikkojen lukijoiden lukutaitoon*. Jyväskylä Studies in Education, Psychology and Social Research, *443*. Jyväskylä: University of Jyväskylä.

Poskiparta, E., Niemi, P., & Vauras, M. (1999). Who benefits from training in linguistic awareness in the first grade, and what components show training effects? *Journal of Learning Disabilities, 32*, 437–446.

Richardson, U., Leppänen, P. H. T., Leiwo, M., & Lyytinen, H. (2003). Speech perception of infants with high familial risk for dyslexia differ at the age of 6 months. *Developmental Neuropsychology, 23*, 385–397.

Richardson, U., & Lyytinen, H. (2014). The GraphoGame method: The theoretical and methodological background of the technology-enhanced learning environment for learning to read. *Human Technology, 10*, 39–60.

Saine, N. L., Lerkkanen, M.-K., Ahonen, T., Tolvanen, A., & Lyytinen, H. (2011). Computer-assisted remedial reading intervention for school beginners at-risk for reading disability. *Child Development, 82*, 1013–1028.

7 Developmental Dyslexia in Russian

Marina Zhukova and Elena Grigorenko

7.1 Introduction

This chapter provides an overview of studies of (a)typical reading acquisition in Russian. Although it is titled "Developmental Dyslexia in Russian" by the editors of the volume, its scope is much wider; this is due to the circumstance that there is no consensus definition of dyslexia in Russian scientific studies of reading, nor are such studies voluminous. Russians have been referred to as "the most reading nation on Earth" (Voice of America, 2010), based on the levels of literacy in the general population, the time spent by an average person reading, and the promotion of reading as a cultural activity. That is one of the reasons why, perhaps, the problem of atypical reading acquisition has not been at the forefront of cognitive and educational psychology in Russia. However, there is nonetheless a tradition of relevant research, of which this chapter provides an overview.

7.2 Learning to Read in Russian

7.2.1 Russian Language and Its Orthography

Russian orthography is based on the Cyrillic /sɪ'rɪlɪk/ alphabet. This alphabet was derived from the Glagolitic alphabet – the first alphabet created by Saints Cyril and Methodius (Кѵриллъ и Меѳодїи in Old Church Slavonic) to transcribe Old Church Slavonic – through the systematic efforts of writers and scholars of the First Bulgarian Empire. The Cyrillic alphabet has experienced multiple transformations, responding to geographic segmentation, political stratification, and regional variation, and adapting to changes in spoken language; it has been academically reformed and politically decreed. The Russian alphabet is a variation of the Cyrillic alphabet, which was reformed into thirty-three letters (compared to forty-one in the Glagolitic and forty-four in the Old Cyrillic alphabets), grouped into three categories: vowels, consonants, and auxiliary letters (Cubberley, 2002). There are disagreements on whether Russian has forty-one or forty-two phonemes (Bondarko, 1998). The linguistic system of Russian (i.e., its phonology, morphology, and orthography) is described in detail elsewhere (Rakhlin, Kornilov, & Grigorenko, 2017).

It has been observed that Russian is uneven in terms of its letter-to-sound and sound-to-letter mappings (Grigorenko, 2005), with the former being much more transparent than the latter. Whereas the characteristics of the former mapping are explained by the original effort to match an existing (Greek) alphabet onto the spoken Slavic languages, the characteristics of the latter mapping are attributed to its low phoneme-to-grapheme conversion, which is attributed to the large number of phonological principles that change the spelling (Boulware-Gooden, Joshi, & Grigorenko, 2015).

Russian has ten vowels, twenty-one consonants, and two auxiliary letters. The vowel letters in Russian (*а, о, э, и, у, ы, е, ё, ю, я*) are heterogeneous. Four of them (*е, ё, ю, я*) are represented by complex sounds, as they are formed by two phonemes $е = j+э, ё = j+о, ю = j+u, я = j+a$. This phenomenon is called jotation, as the sound formation has a formula of "$j + ...$" Moreover, Russian vowels can be divided into two subgroups: those that indicate the hardness of the following consonants (*а, о, э, у, ы*); and those that designate the softness of the following consonants (*е, ё, ю, я, и*). In primary school, children are taught to distinguish vowels from consonants by singing them or calling them out. Vowels are sonorous, as the air is not blocked during vowel formation. Importantly, vowel pronunciation depends on a linguistic stress (linguistic accent, i.e., a relative emphasis or prominence given to a certain syllable in a word); therefore, it is challenging to figure out the spelling based solely on the pronunciation. Unstressed vowels are subject to vowel reduction, which can appear in the root, prefix, or suffix of a word. For example, the word *вода́* [vada], 'water' in English, has an unstressed ‹o› in its root. In order to determine the right spelling, one should find a related word, where the vowel in question is in the stressed position (*во́дный* [vodniy], "aquatic"). However, not all vowels are subject to that rule, so beginning readers need to memorize several irregular cases, i.e., spellings of words that are not verifiable by the stress rule; for example, the word "weather" is pronounced as *pagoda*, but spelled as *погода*; the word "sparrow" is pronounced as *varabey*, but spelled as *воробей*. When a vowel reduction appears in the affix rather than a root, spelling is mostly memorized and beginning spellers are taught to perform a morphological decomposition of the word to determine the position of the vowel, then utilize their knowledge of Russian morphology to survey, for example, permissible prefixes, suffixes, and endings. A word in Russian has only one stress; however its position is arbitrary and must be learned, creating another complication for language learners.

The consonant group is prevalent in Russian as it contains twenty-one letters. They can be divided into subgroups based on their palatalization and voicing. Palatalized consonants are followed by vowels of soft-series or by a soft sign.

Some consonants exist only in soft form, such as *ч, щ*. Some consonants cannot be palatalized as they are hard consonants by default, i.e., *ж, ш, ц*. The major complication for beginning readers and spellers is that soft and hard consonants are typically grouped with vowels of soft- and hard-series (i.e. soft consonants are grouped with soft vowels and hard consonants are grouped with hard vowels), but there are multiple exceptions (i.e. soft consonants are groups with hard vowels and hard consonants are groups with soft vowels). Voicing is another characteristic of Russian consonants. In primary school children learn the consonants in pairs: *г-к, д-т, б-п, в-ф, з-с*. The main difference between voiced and voiceless consonant sounds is the vibration of vocal cords. When voiced and voiceless consonants are adjacent to each other the second consonant takes the characteristic of the former. For example: *когти* "claws," in which ⟨г⟩ is a voiced consonant followed by a voiceless ⟨т⟩, is thus pronounced [ko̲kti]. Similarly, when a voiceless ⟨т⟩ is followed by a voiced ⟨б⟩, the word *отбой* ("bedtime" in one of its meanings) is pronounced [a̲dboi]. In consonant clusters, consonants are often muted, such as in: *солнце* [so̲ntse], "sun"; and *звездный* [zvyo̲zniy], "starry." The traditional curriculum in Russian language is phonetically based, so children learning to read and spell in Russian are taught to perform a phonetic decomposition of words and blend them back together (Elkonin, 1988).

Auxiliary letters do not form independent sounds and serve grammatical and phonological purposes only. There are only two auxiliary letters: ⟨ь⟩ (soft sign) and ⟨ъ⟩ (hard sign). Usually the soft sign is written after a consonant, indicating its palatalization (*конь* – "horse," *моль* – "moth," *кольцо* – "ring"). Apart from the softening function, it can indicate the separation between a consonant and a vowel (*семья* [sem'ja]); without the soft sign, the word would be pronounced [sem'a]. A soft sign can also have grammatical functions; it is written after a final consonant in singular nouns of the third declension (*тушь* – "mascara," *рожь* – "rye", *мышь* – "mouse") or in particular verb forms (*поднять* – "lift," *подняться* – "get oneself up"). A hard sign indicates separation and is most often placed between a prefix and a root. It precedes soft vowel letters (*я, ю, ё, е*): *подъезд* – "entrance" is [padjest], *объем* – "volume" [ab'jom], *съёжиться* – "shrivel" [sjozhitsa].

Importantly, Russian orthography does not reflect changes in the sound quality of vowels and consonants due to palatalization, positional (de)voicing, and/or stress fluctuations. That is why reading (i.e., the mapping of graphemes to phonemes) is easy and spelling (i.e., the mapping of phonemes to graphemes) is difficult.

7.2.2 Challenges in Learning to Read and Spell Russian

Modern compulsory education in the Russian Federation is comprised of eleven years (divided into four years in primary school, four years in middle school, and three years in high school: see https://fgos.ru/). Of note is that reading as a subject is taught only in elementary school, in most programs, for the first three years of education, whereas grammar, spelling, and literature are taught through all eleven years of education (Ministerstvo Obrazovaniya i Nauki Rossijskoj Federacii, 2011).

In general, reading in Russian is taught analytically-synthetically, phonetically, alphabetically, and syllabically, where phonemes and letters are presented individually and then blended into syllables, and syllables are then combined into words (and, later, words are split into their syllabic components). A popular version of this general approach is the syllabic-phonic method, utilizing CV syllables as basic reading units (Beten'kova, Goreckij, & Fonin, 2004). It is based on the syllabic principles of Russian orthography: namely, the phonemic quality (softness/hardness) of the consonant is determined by the choice of the vowel following it. Ideally, the unity of subsyllabic elements should be contextualized by their content. In reality, Russian syllables are often characterized by complex onsets and codas, and the instruction to break up consonant clusters separating CV units is not effective. Thus, early acquisition of reading in Russian is speeded up by the special cohesion of CV units in Russian orthography, but is slowed down by the instability of syllabic boundaries (Kerek & Niemi, 2012). In fact, one of the most challenging steps in acquiring reading in Russian is achieving fluency in reading multisyllabic words (Starzhinskaya, 1988).

Although not explicated in the Federal Standards of Education (Ministerstvo Obrazovaniya i Nauki Rossijskoj Federacii, 2011), the timeline assumes that the alphabet and syllables are mastered in Grade 1, where accurate reading may be accomplished, whereas Grades 2 and 3 are aimed at the development of reading fluency and reading comprehension. Similarly, the Standards do not specify achievement expectations, but it is assumed that by the end of Grade 1, children in Russia will already be able to demonstrate accurate whole-word reading of words with simple syllable structure and accurate syllabic reading (i.e., pronouncing words syllable by syllable) of words with complex syllable structure, with a reading speed of at least 35–40 words per minute during oral text reading and a target of 120–150 words per minute, that is, the average tempo of speech (Rakhlin, Cardoso-Martins, & Grigorenko, 2014). The limited data available in the literature seem to substantiate these numbers; it has been observed that the average reading speed in Grade 1 is 48 words per minute, whereas in Grade 10 it is 138 words per minute, with only about 10 percent of students in Grades 4–8 reading slower than 60 words per minute (Kuznetsov & Khromov, 1983).

Spelling and grammar are taught, explicitly and implicitly, throughout all years of schooling. Language arts lessons are delivered every day and are focused on the development of spoken and written literacy, knowledge of the

Russian language, and exposure to literature, both national and international. Yet, due to the non-transparent mapping of phonemes onto graphemes in Russian, spelling and grammaticality remain quite challenging for both children and adults, rendering them a reliable source of individual differences among Russian speakers.

The Russian educational system, despite the fact that it consumes less than the OECD average both per student and as a share of gross domestic product, or GDP (OECD, 2016), has proven to be effective. It is estimated that 99.7 percent of the population (99.7 percent males and 99.6 percent females) are literate.[1] Russian school-aged children have scored variably on international assessments (e.g., Progress in International Reading Literacy study, PIRLS, and the Program for International Student Assessment, PISA). For example, in the most recently published (2016) PIRLS report (Mullis et al., 2017), the Russian fourth graders took one of the leading positions in reading performance along with children from Singapore, which has consistently been a top-performing country. The 2016 results are similar, but better than the 2011 results (Thompson et al., 2012). In 2011, the Russian Federation was listed second out of fifty-seven participating countries. On average girls performed better than boys, with this discrepancy taking place for all countries, except Colombia; this difference in average reading scores for Russian children was 18 points. Reading skills among Russian children were defined as *advanced* for 19 percent of the participating students, *high* for 44 percent, *intermediate* for 29 percent, and *low* for 7 percent; only 1 percent of all participants from the Russian Federation did not meet the minimum benchmark in reading. Interestingly, Russian fourth graders were equally successful in reading fiction and scientific texts (there was no significant difference between children's performance on these two genres). The most typical mistakes included failure to answer the question based on the text rather than on personal experience – 30 percent, inaccurate retrieval of information – 20 percent; and the biggest difficulty was articulating their own thoughts in written form even when the reading material was well understood – 40 percent (Kovaleva et al., 2013).

In 2016, the Russian Federation was ranked first in reading out of fifty participating countries. Russian fourth graders outperformed all other countries on reading achievement except for Singapore. Analysis of the general trend in reading performance suggests linear growth for the Russian Federation, with a steady increase in reading scores from 528 in 2001 to 581 in 2016. The difference in average reading scores for Russian children was 15 points, favoring girls. In terms of reaching international benchmarks for reading in 2016, 26 percent of Russian students were ranked as *advanced*, 70 percent were ranked as *high*, 94 percent as intermediate, and ninety-nine students reached the *low*

---

[1] See www.cia.gov/library/publications/the-world-factbook/fields/2103.html.

benchmark; only 1 percent of all participants from the Russian Federation did not meet the minimum benchmark in reading. Compared to the results from previous assessments the Russian Federation has increased its percentage of students reaching international reading benchmarks (Kovaleva et al., 2013). The PIRLS 2016 Assessment Framework focuses on two overarching purposes for reading that account for most of the reading done by young students both in and out of school: for literary experience, and to acquire and use information. Russian fourth graders had the highest literary and information scores, compared to other participating countries, with significantly higher scores in acquiring and using information compared to their overall PIRLS average score.

The latest published data from the PISA administration is from 2015. PISA features 15-year-old students (i.e., ninth graders), and those students scored just above the OECD average (495 compared to 493), ranking 26 among 70 country-participants.[2]

The observed discrepancy between the reading levels of fourth and ninth graders in the Russian Federation has been discussed in the literature. Experts argue, based on the nature and specifics of PIRLS assessments, that the Russian educational system lacks whatever is needed to help students map the material they learn from textbooks into real-life practice (Zukerman, Kovaleva, & Kuznetsova, 2007, 2011). That is, Russian secondary-school students seem to fail at tasks in which they need to apply academic knowledge to real-life problems. The pluralism of information (captured via multiple points of view of multiple correct answers) confuses Russian students and leads to poorer performance. Traditionally, Russian students are taught to comprehend and retell complex fiction texts. However, problem-solving is not part of their acquired skill set (Kornev, Rakhlin, & Grigorenko, 2010).

7.3   Reading Difficulties in Russian

7.3.1   Historical and Cultural Context

The diagnosis of dyslexia (and/or any other category labeling difficulties in reading acquisition) is not typically used in the Russian Federation. This is a historical artifact which is due, in large part, to two distinct characteristics of the educational system of Soviet Russia. First, in Soviet Russia, there was a very strong system of preventive language-based services (provided by speech and language pathologists, *logoped* in Russian) that was received by virtually every child exhibiting difficulties in language acquisition in pre-school, and in reading acquisition in elementary school (Chirkina & Grigorenko, 2014). Although no longer universal, this system, or rather the

---

[2] See https://nces.ed.gov/surveys/pisa/pisa2015/pisa2015highlights_4.asp.

elements of that system, is still present in various educational structures in the Russian Federation. Second, the Soviet system of education had multiple junctions for diversification at the end of middle school (formally Grade 9); at this point, students whose academic performance was below average were counseled into technical schools, where they completed their compulsory education while training in professional skills (Grigorenko, 1998). In conjunction with the specifics of grapheme–phoneme mapping in Russian, these two characteristics of the Soviet educational system – an intense preventive effort and a diversion of children with academic difficulties into skill-based professions early on (with multiple subsequent opportunities to continue their education after receiving a profession) – resulted in a certain degree of negligence of the phenomenon in the Soviet Russia. The disruption of these preventive language-based services and other critical changes to the educational system in the 1990s resulted in an increased number of children who manifested and experienced difficulties in reading acquisition. It is not that the phenomenon had not been documented and researched in Russia before. Quite the contrary; observations and discussions of dyslexia have been present in the Russian literature since the 1930s (Chirkina & Grigorenko, 2014; Kornev et al., 2010; Karpova, Granik, & Kabardov, 2013). Yet, as a public health issue, dyslexia is just coming to be recognized; this recognition is driven both by professionals (e.g., the Russian Dyslexia Association was formed in 2004) and parents (e.g., publicly recognizable figures openly sharing their experiences with dyslexia[3]).

7.3.2   Identification and Prevalence of Dyslexia

Despite the current pressure from both practitioners and parents, dyslexia in Russian is severely understudied. First, it is understudied theoretically. Currently, in the Russian scientific literature, there is no unified definition of dyslexia and classification of its forms. One of the most used (and taught) classifications of dyslexia belongs to Raisa Lalaeva (Lalaeva, 1983). She differentiated phonematic (characterized by poor phoneme awareness), semantic (characterized by mechanical reading with no understanding of the context), ungrammatical (characterized by poor grammatical awareness), mnestical (characterized by poor verbal memory), optical (characterized by poor recognition of grapheme), and tactile (associated with blindness) forms of dyslexia. This classification, however, is primarily descriptive and is not substantiated by a body of empirical literature. Second, the existing estimates of the prevalence rates of dyslexia and related conditions such as dysgraphia (which have been found to co-occur significantly with dyslexia in Russian, Kornev, 2003) among

---

[3] See http://dyslexiarf.com/2017/06/07/radi-kogo-doch-direktora-ermitazha-brosila-bankovskuyu-kareru.

school-aged children in Russia are contradictory. They vary from 5–10 percent (Zavadenko, Roumyantseva, 2008; Kornev, 2007) to 53 percent (Paramonova, 2006). There are multiple reasons for this dispersion of estimates, including disagreements on definitions, varying age ranges of the assessed children, and small sample sizes.

The international literature suggests that in languages with high orthographic transparency, which Russian exemplifies, at least in its grapheme-to-phoneme mappings, children mostly experience problems with fluency rather than with accuracy of reading. However, this assumption has been challenged by a study showing that many accuracy-related errors may occur when words with unpredictable stress patterns are encountered (Grigorenko et al., 2011).

7.4   Behavioral and Neurocognitive Evidence

7.4.1   *Nature of Reading and Spelling Problems in Russian*

Relatively speaking, there is a dearth of empirical research on problems encountered when learning to read Russian. Few available studies focus on specific reading difficulties, both for emergent literacy and subsequent challenges related to reading comprehension and spelling. In the Russian literature, signs of reading difficulties can be divided into five major behavioral manifestations (Grigorenko, 2010). *Immature reading* is characterized by difficulties in transitioning from letter-by-letter to syllable-by-syllable reading, and then to whole-word reading. Children with immature reading skills lag behind their age peers in their reading performance. Notably, educators do not use standardized assessments when determining reading mastery; they commonly rely on so-called age expectancy reading rates (Kornev & Ishimova, 2010). *Low reading speed* is often accompanied by immature reading. This type of reading difficulty is also characterized by a lack of prosodic components. It is common for children with reading difficulties to exhibit *monotonous reading*, with no pitch contrast. *Lack of accuracy when reading out loud* can be manifested in letter omissions or substitutions. It is reported that vowel substitutions are more common than consonant substitutions. Moreover, paired consonants are often confused (⟨к⟩ and ⟨г⟩, ⟨д⟩ and ⟨т⟩). Another common problem in reading accuracy is a substitution of graphemes that look alike (⟨ш⟩, ⟨щ⟩, and ⟨ц⟩; ⟨б⟩ and ⟨в⟩). Reported reading difficulties can be highly inconsistent within one reader (the same word may be read differently when encountered multiple times in the text). Depending on its severity, the lack of reading accuracy may result in either real-word substitutions or in nonword formations that make no sense to the listener. The phenomenon of *repeated reading* (reading a word multiple times first silently than aloud) is yet another common characteristic of Russian-speaking children with reading difficulties. Silent reading is performed on a letter-by-letter or syllable-by-syllable basis. When reading out loud a child might recognize only a part of the word and guess the whole word based on the context or randomly. A child who lacks understanding might understand separate words in the text, but fail to integrate them into the context. This leads to verbal substitutions, ungrammatical phrases, and loss of the general meaning of the text.

In addition to this mostly descriptive work, there is a cluster of studies that utilize a number of constructs commonly used in Western literature, although some of them, arguably, originated in studies of (a)typical reading acquisition in Russian (Chirkina & Grigorenko, 2014). These constructs connect the acquisition of spoken and written language, both holistically, correlating the specifics of mastering speaking with those of reading (Lyakso & Frolova, 2013; Lyakso et al., 2012), and componentially, identifying cognitive processes that are characteristic and predictive of both spoken and written language acquisition. Among these processes are phonemic awareness (i.e., the child's capacity to manipulate spoken units of language, phonemes) and rapid naming (i.e., the child's capacity to rapidly sequentially name letters, numbers, objects, and colors). It has been shown that both phonemic awareness and rapid naming can serve as important predictors of reading at the prereading stage. A longitudinal study that tracked children's reading progress from kindergarten to the end of primary school showed that accuracy and fluency of single-word identification are strongly related to the development of phonemic awareness (Grigorenko, 2011c).

Another study demonstrated that, in elementary and middle school, accuracy of reading is primarily associated with performance on phonemic awareness tasks, whereas fluency of reading is primarily associated with performance on rapid-naming tasks (Grigorenko, 2011b). Another observation that is of interest is that performance on rapid-naming tasks might also be a predictor of generalized learning difficulties, rather than difficulties specific to reading acquisition (Akhutina & Pronina, 2015). A study that investigated an overlap of difficulties in the acquisition of spoken and written language in a sample of Russian-speaking children found that these types of difficulties are characterized by impoverished performance on both phoneme awareness and rapid automatized naming tasks, although the difficulties in phonemic awareness appeared to be more strongly associated statistically with difficulties in both language and reading acquisition (Rakhlin et al., 2014). Similarly, componential processes have been shown to be predictive of indicators of reading comprehension (Grigorenko, 2012). Moreover, spelling deficits have been associated with poor accuracy in orthographic and morphological awareness and pseudoword repetition (Rakhlin et al., 2013). There is a significant overlap between poor reading and poor spelling in Russian. The typical pattern of spelling errors demonstrated by Russian-speaking high-school students are morphological, although, remarkably, phonology-based errors are also made, even though it is assumed that phonemic mapping is mastered by the end of primary school (Grigorenko, 2003). Finally, it is important to recognize that neither Russian teachers nor Russian students themselves appear to be sensitive to the difficulties demonstrated by students on maximum performance assessments, such as assessments of phonemic awareness or rapid naming (Grigorenko, 2011a). As teachers' ratings are key to the academic success of students, this finding underscores the necessity for the development of standardized assessments of reading and its componential processes in Russian; currently such assessments do not exist.

7.4.2   *Underlying Causes of Reading Problems in Russian*

Little work has been done on understanding neurocognitive foundations of (a)typical reading in Russian. These studies can be classified into two groups – studies of brain activity that is either predictive or characteristic of (a)typical reading; and studies that utilize genetically informative designs to elicit the etiological bases of (a)typical reading.

With regard to the first group of studies, there are two types. The first stream of research uses quantitative EEG and eye-tracking techniques to investigate neurobiological bases of speech and language disorders, including dyslexia. One EEG study established an association between changes in EEG patterns and the type of writing problems in children with dyslexia. Specifically, it has been shown that reading difficulties are associated with such neurophysiological markers as altered resting-state EEG patterns (Kornev, 2003). Moreover, research has demonstrated that children with spelling difficulties showed abnormal activation in frontal regions of the left hemisphere, whereas phonological and morphological difficulties were associated with atypical activation in temporal and parietal regions of the right hemisphere (Dmitrova et al., 2005). These results point to the complex nature of dyslexia and the shared contribution of both hemispheres to language skills. Another study demonstrated the dominant pattern of activation in the right hemisphere and the late maturation of cortical structures in struggling and beginning readers while performing reading tasks (Sokolova, 2005). Notably, most of the empirical literature on the neurocognitive bases of dyslexia in Russian uses neuropsychological approaches to the identification and characterization of the disorder (Akhutina, 2006; Vizel, 2005). This approach is rooted in the work of Alexander Luria (Luria, 1969) and continues to be the most prevalent type of assessment in research and clinical settings (Zabozlaeva, Suprun, & Lugovyh, 2010). Eye-tracking has been also used in dyslexia research. One study demonstrated that struggling readers are characterized by a deficiency of visual perception, which hinders grapheme–phoneme decoding (Vasil'eva & Rozhkova, 2011). Other researchers have also emphasized the importance of visual skills in reading tasks and shown that beginning readers have different ocular motor activity compared to experienced readers. They found that beginning readers are characterized by longer fixation, a low amplitude of saccades, and an increased number of regressions while performing reading tasks (Bezrukikh, Adamovskaya, & Ivanov, 2017). An intervention aimed at enhancing binocular skills in struggling readers has been argued to help to improve reading speed in poor readers (Vasil'eva, 2011), which, according to the author, demonstrates the importance of developed binocular vision for the acquisition of reading in Russian. The observations from these isolated studies need to be replicated and compared to the international literature on the role of vision in the (a)typical acquisition of reading.

The second stream of research does not directly investigate dyslexia, but focuses on the neurophysiological underpinnings of developmental language disorder (DLD). There is a debate around the etiological overlap between DLD and developmental dyslexia; however it is generally agreed that reading difficulties and DLD have shared phonological deficits (Ramus et al., 2013). In this context, it is important to mention the following DLD studies that were conducted with a geographically isolated Russian-speaking population with an atypically high prevalence of DLD (Rakhlin et al., 2013). The first study demonstrated that unlike their typically developing peers, children with combined DLD and reading disabilities demonstrate large incongruity-related N4 components in both mismatch and match conditions (Kornilov et al., 2015). The second study reported attenuated attentional processing (a reduced P3 component) along with a reduced N4 effect in response to mismatch conditions (Kornilov et al., 2014). Authors attributed this effect to overactivation and reduced inhibitory reactions in the language processing of children with DLD.

With regard to the utilization of genetically informative designs, two studies will be illustrated here. The first study (Naples et al., 2009) attempted to investigate the psychological and genetic bases of reading ability and disability, and to evaluate the plausibility of a variety of psychological models of reading involving phonological awareness and rapid naming, both hypothesized to be principal components in such models. A large sample of unselected families were assessed with indicators of both processes to investigate familial aggregation and to obtain estimates of both the number and effect-magnitude of the genetic loci involved in the transmission of these traits. The results of these analyses indicated the presence of genetic effects in the etiology of individual differences for both phonemic awareness and rapid naming, and pointed to both the shared and unique sources of this genetic variance, which appeared to be exerted by multiple (3–6 for phonemic awareness and 3–5 for rapid naming) genes. In the second study, using the same set of families, the researchers (Naples, Katz, & Grigorenko, 2012) evaluated whether lexical decision can be viewed as a putative endophenotype for reading comprehension. Heritability estimates and segregation analyses parameter estimates were obtained for both of these phenotypes. Specifically, in a segregation analysis it was established that there is little to no overlap between genes contributing to lexical decision and reading comprehension, and that the genetic mechanism behind lexical decision, derived from this analysis, appears to be more complex than that for reading comprehension. It was concluded that in this sample of unselected Russian families, lexical decision was not a good candidate as an endophenotype for reading comprehension, despite previous suggestions from the literature.

Thus, studies of the neurocognitive foundations of (a)typical reading in Russian are limited both in number and in scope, and more work needs to be done to substantiate the generic assumption that these foundations are universal for all languages (Grigorenko & Elliot, 2012).

7.5   Intervention

Although severely diminished, challenged with financial problems, and deemed non-prestigious for young professionals to work in, the system of early language intervention (and prevention of reading difficulties) is still strong in Russia. This system is available to most children from the age of 2, with some geographic variation. It is federally mandated that children in all state kindergartens are screened for signs of speech and language impairments and, if these are identified, the child and his/her family are referred to remediation with a speech-language pathologist (*logoped*) free of charge, or (if available) the child can be placed into a group for children with learning and language disabilities (often referred to as a "special child group"). In cases where language disorders are severe, families are offered a transfer to a correctional (*logopedic*) kindergarten, free of charge (Kornev et al., 2010), although the number of these institutions is declining as a result of a federal law mandating the inclusion of children with special needs into mainstream schooling. Clearly, there has been and is a large amount of variation both in interventions (and how they are delivered) and in each child's response (and recovery).

Previously, in the Soviet Union, there was no legislation for inclusive education. Correspondingly, children with speech and language disorders (i.e., children for whom early intervention had not been effective for a variety of reasons) were placed in special schools. The segregation of children with special educational needs has a complex historical background. At one point, the Soviet government proclaimed all standardized psychological assessments to be pedagogical perversions (CK VKP, 1936) and psychological tests were banned on a legislative level; all forms of intelligence testing were forbidden, as the propaganda declared that all children should be given the same educational rights, regardless of their individual differences in intellectual capacity (Grigorenko & Kornilova, 1997). Initially, under this declaration, all children were assigned to mainstream schooling; however, this disregard for individual learning needs led to academic problems in a substantial number of children. As standardized assessments were banned, schoolchildren were differentiated by an ill-defined concept of educability. This concept, in conjunction with a list of manifested developmental disabilities, resulted in the formation of a system of special education. Although substantially reformed and challenged by an inclusive education law recently ratified by the Russian government (Ministerstvo Obrazovaniya i Nauki Rossijskoj Federacii, 2012) that mandates a general course for the inclusion and integration of children with special educational needs, the system of special education still exists. There are eight types of special correctional schools: (1) for children who are deaf; (2) for children with hearing impairments; (3) for children who are blind; (4) for children with visual problems; (5) for children with severe speech and language disabilities; (6) for motor development problems accompanying brain injuries (e.g., cerebral palsy); (7) for children with developmental delays and minimal brain dysfunction (labeled *задержка психического развития* – zaderzhka psihicheskogo razvitija – in Russian, developmental delay); and (8) for children with an intellectual disability. The schools for children with special educational needs are called *correctional schools* as they are aimed at the correction and remediation of a child's disorder.

Schools of the fifth type are designed to support and remediate children with severe forms of various speech-language disorders (dysarthria, stuttering, and aphasia, among others). The academic program of these schools is designed to promote speech and language development. Until the implementation of the inclusive education federal law in 2012, children with severe dyslexia were typically placed in the fifth type of correctional school. In 2017, depending on the severity of the language disorder, children can either attend mainstream classroom (receiving services from a *logoped*), be placed in a special classroom with an adapted curriculum, or attend special educational institutions, similar to the fifth type of correction schools.

Placement depends on the decision made by the local psychological-medical-pedagogical-committee (PMPC), which is assembled based on specific federal and local regulations, meets on a regular basis and aims at evaluating numerous child cases in a single session. The PMPC also recommends remediation services and monitors the child's progress. The committee usually consists of a psychiatrist, a special educator, a psychologist, and a speech-language pathologist (*logoped*, see above). Children with speech and language difficulties typically attend special education schools until the PMPC rules that a student has improved enough to attend a mainstream school. The first stage of special education is aimed at correcting speech–sound pronunciation deficits (if there are any), and enhancing phoneme awareness, grammaticality, and the coherence of speech. The second stage is aimed at maintaining the appropriate level of oral and written communication that is necessary for adaptive functioning in society. Students with dyslexia are typically asked to fill in the gaps after they have read a text once. Gaps can contain missing words, i.e., a semantic task, or missing syllables, i.e., a morphological task (Barabanova, 2014). To receive a school diploma, students, whether in special or mainstream education, need to pass a federally instituted final examination. There are accommodations available to children with special educational needs when they take this examination. However, there is a caveat to this regulation: Since there is no official list of medical conditions that make students eligible for special accommodations during examinations, this decision strongly relies on the PMPC.[4]

There are also some targeted programs that are aimed both at the prevention of reading difficulties, in elementary school (Zukerman & Shkolyarenko, 1997), and their remediation, in after-school programs (Akhutina & Pylaeva, 2008; Chirkina, Rusetskaya, & Rossijskaya, 2009, 2011), but these programs are few and their empirical foundation is not extensive.

7.6   Discussion and Conclusion

Revisiting the above, let us highlight the most prominent lines of this discussion. The properties of the Russian language are such that reading (i.e., the mapping of graphemes to phonemes) the language is easy, and spelling (i.e., the mapping of phonemes to graphemes) its words is more difficult. Therefore, the mastery of accurate (but not necessarily fluent) word-level reading in Russian is widespread and generally achieved by middle school, although difficulty with spelling, especially in individuals with language and reading difficulties, may be lifelong. The Russian pedagogical tradition of teaching reading was founded by Konstantin Ushinski (Константин Ушинский) in the middle of the nineteenth century and was substantiated and verified in empirical linguistic, psychological, and pedagogical studies carried out in the late nineteenth and early twentieth centuries. Based on Ushinski's scientific pedagogy and a large collection of relevant empirical studies, reading in Russian in the Russian Empire, Soviet Union, and Russian Federation has always been taught analytically-synthetically, phonetically, alphabetically, and syllabically, whereby phonemes and letters are presented individually and then blended into syllables, and syllables are then combined into words. Due to the existence of a very strong language-based preventive approach to the manifestation of problems in the acquisition of reading, as well as to the system of education that diverted a large number of not-so-academically able children after nine years of compulsory education into vocational training, dyslexia was not recognized as a public health challenge

---

[4] See: www.ege.edu.ru/ru/classes-11/participant/.

until the early twenty-first century, when the preventive system of early language intervention had weakened and the structure of education had changed. Now dyslexia has become the focus of a number of parent-advocacy and professional groups, a development which, in turn, has stimulated the field of empirical research on dyslexia in Russia. This field is still relatively small, with only a limited number of studies focused on issues pertaining to the characterization of dyslexia in Russian, its identification and diagnosis, and its etiology and remediation. In that regard, Russian science is in the curious position of being highly influential in forming the parameters of world research into (a)typical acquisition of reading in the early twentieth century, although it was practically absent from this research for decades, into the late twentieth century. The social, political, educational, and scientific dynamics of the early twenty-first century indicate an increased interest in research on (a)typical reading acquisition. Let us hope that these dynamics continue.

Author Note

The writing of this chapter was supported by grant no. 14.Z50.31.0027 from the Government of the Russian Federation. Grantees undertaking such projects are encouraged to express their professional judgment freely. The chapter, therefore, does not necessarily reflect the position or policies of the above-mentioned funding agency, and no official endorsement should be inferred. We thank the volume editors for their invitation to contribute. We are also grateful to Ms. Mei Tan from the University of Houston for her editorial assistance. All correspondence should be addressed to Elena L. Grigorenko at elena.grigorenko@times.uh.edu.

References

Akhutina, T. V. (2006). Nejropsihologicheskij podhod k izucheniyu trudnostej pis'ma i chteniya [Neuropsychological approach to analyzing reading and writing difficulties]. Paper presented at the conference "Rannyaya diagnostika, profilaktika i korrekciya narushenij pis'ma i chteniya: materialy II mezhdunarodnoj konferencii Rossijskoj associacii disleksii."

Akhutina, T. V., & Pronina, E. A. (2015). Ocenka sostoyaniya regulyacii aktivacii u pervoklassnikov s pomoshch'yu metodiki RAN/RAS [Assessment of brain activation regulation in first-graders via RAN/RAS test]. *Nacional'nyj psihologicheskij zhurnal, 1*, 61–69.

Akhutina, T. V., & Pylaeva, N. M. (2008). *Preodolenie trudnostej ucheniya: nejropsihologicheskij podhod [Overcoming learning disabilities: the neuropsychological approach]*. St Petersburg: Piter.

Barabanova, S. YU. (2014). Psihologo-pedagogicheskie osnovy po okazaniyu pomoshchi detyam v formirovanii navyka beglogo chteniya [Psychological-pedagogical foundations of intervention for reading fluency in children]. *Municipal'noe obrazovanie: innovacii i eksperiment, 3,* 24–27.

Bezrukikh, M. M., Adamovskaya, O. N., & Ivanov, V. V. (2017). Osobennosti zritel'nogo vospriyatiya i okulomotornoj aktivnosti u pervoklassnikov pri chtenii tekstov razlichnoj slozhnosti [Characteristics of visual perception and oculomotor activity in first-graders while reading texts of various difficulty]. *Fiziologiya cheloveka, 43,* 56–65.

Beten'kova, N., Goreckij, V., & Fonin, D. (2004). *Azbuka. Dlya pervogo klassa chetyrekhletnej nachal'noj shkoly [Alphabet. For the first grade of primary school]* (3rd ed.). St Petersburg: SpecLit, Planeta znanij.

Bondarko, L. V. (1998). *Fonetika sovremennogo russkogo yazyka [Phonetics of modern Russian language].* St Petersburg: St Petersburg State University.

Boulware-Gooden, R., Joshi, R. M., & Grigorenko, E. L. (2015). The role of phonology, morphology, and orthography in English and Russian spelling. *Dyslexia, 21,* 142–161.

Chirkina, G. V., & Grigorenko, E. L. (2014). Tracking citations: A science detective story. *Journal of Learning Disabilities, 7,* 366–373. doi: http://dx.doi.org/10.1177/0022219412471995.

Chirkina, G. V., Rusetskaya, M. N., & Rossijskaya, E. N. (Eds.). (2011). *Kognitivnoe i kommunikativnoe razvitie shkol'nikov s disleksiej: integral'nyj podhod [Development of cognition and communication in students with dyslexia: integration approach].* Moscow: Nacional'nyj knizhnyj centr.

Chirkina, G. V., Rusetskaya, M. N., & Rossijskaya, E. N. (Eds.). (2009). *Variativnye strategii soprovozhdeniya uchashchihsya s narusheniyami pis'ma i chteniya [Various strategies of intervention for students with reading and writing disabilities].* Moscow: RDA, MGPU, URAO IKP.

CK VKP. (1936). *Postanovlenie CK VKP(b) ot 04.07.1936 o pedologicheskih izvrashcheniyah v sisteme NARKOMPROSOV (Act on pedological perversions in the system of NARKOMPROS).* Moscow. http://pravo.levonevsky.org/baza/soviet/sssr6510.htm.

Cubberley, P. (2002). *Russian: A linguistic introduction.* Cambridge, MA: Cambridge University Press.

Dmitrova, E. D., Dubrovinskaya, N. V., Lukashevich, I. P., Machinskaya, R. I., & Shklovskij, V. M. (2005). Osobennosti mozgovogo obespecheniya verbal'nyh processov u detej s trudnostyami pis'ma i chteniya [Features of cerebral support of verbal processes in children with dysgraphia and dyslexia]. *Fiziologiya cheloveka, 31,* 5–12.

Elkonin, D. B. (1988). How to teach children to read. *Advances in Psychology, 49,* 387–426.

Grigorenko, E. L. (1998). Russian "defectology": Anticipating perestroika in the field. *Journal of Learning Disabilities, 31,* 193–207.

Grigorenko, E. L. (2003). Matryoshka, matryozhka, or motryoshka: The difficulty of mastering reading and spelling in Russian. In N. Goulandris (Ed.), *Dyslexia in different languages: A cross-linguistic comparison* (pp. 92–111). London: Whurr Publishers.

Grigorenko, E. L. (2005). If John were Ivan: Would he fail in reading? In R. M. Joshi & P. G. Aaron (Eds.), *Handbook of orthography and literacy* (pp. 303–320). Mahwah, NJ: Lawrence Erlbaum Associates.

Grigorenko, E. L. (2010). Report on the Russian language for the World Dyslexia Forum. www.dyslexia-international.org/WDF/Files/WDF2010-Grigorenko-paper.pdf.

Grigorenko, E. L. (2011a). Gramotnost' shkol'nika; eyo ocenka uchitelem, samim shkol'nikom i ob"ektivnymi testami [Literacy of students: its evaluation provided by a teacher, student and direct testing]. *Mir Obrazovaniya*, *3*, 119–125.

Grigorenko, E. L. (2011b). Universal'nye prediktory gramotnosti. Universal'ny li oni i dlya russkogo yazyka? [Universal predictors of literacy. Are they universal in the context of Russian language?] *Novoe v Psihologo-pedagogicheskih Issledovaniyah*, *4*, 63–68.

Grigorenko, E. L. (2011c). Etap «dochteniya», ego harakteristiki i ih rol' v ovladenii chteniem [The stage of "pre-reading," its characteristics and their role in mastering reading]. *Voprosy psihologii*, *6*, 122–130.

Grigorenko, E. L. (2012). Ponimanie prochitannogo shkol'nikami i ego prediktory [Pupils' reading comprehension its predictors]. *Psihologicheskaya nauka i obrazovanie*, *1*, 65–74.

Grigorenko, E. L., & Elliott, D. D. (2012). *Chtenie o chtenii [Reading about reading]*. Voronezh: Ayist.

Grigorenko, E. L., Kornev, A. N., Rakhlin, N., & Krivulskaya, S. (2011). Reading-related skills, reading achievement, and inattention: A correlational study. *Journal of Cognitive Education and Psychology*, *10*, 140–156.

Grigorenko, E. L., & Kornilova, T. V. (1997). The resolution of the nature-nurture controversy by Russian psychology: Culturally biased or culturally specific? In R. J. Sternberg & E. L. Grigorenko (Eds.), *Intelligence, heredity, and environment* (pp. 393–439). New York, NY: Cambridge University Press.

Karpova, N., Granik, G., & Kabardov, M. (Eds.). (2013). *Issledovaniya chteniya i gramotnosti v Psihologicheskom institute za 100 let: Hrestomatiya [Studies of reading and literacy carried out at the Psychological Institute of the Russian Academy of Education in a hundred years]*. Moscow: Russkaya shkol'naya bibliotechnaya associaciya.

Kerek, E., & Niemi, P. (2012). Grain-size units of phonological awareness among Russian first graders. *Written Language & Literacy*, *15*, 80–113. doi: http://dx.doi.org/10.1075/wll.15.1.05ker.

Kornev, A. N. (2003). *Narusheniya chteniya i pis'ma u detej [Reading disabilities in children]*. St Petersburg: Rech'.

Kornev, A. N. (2007). Uzlovye voprosy disleksii. *Defektologiya [Main issues in Defectology]*, *1*, 59–66.

Kornev, A. N., & Ishimova, O. (2010). *Metodika diagnostiki disleksii u detej [Method of diagnosing dyslexia]*. St Petersburg: Izdatel'stvo Politekhnicheskogo instituta.

Kornev, A. N., Rakhlin, N., & Grigorenko, E. L. (2010). Dyslexia from a cross-linguistic and cross-cultural perspective: The case of Russian and Russia. *Learning Disabilities: A Contemporary Journal*, *8*, 41–69.

Kornilov, S. A., Landi, N., Rakhlin, N., Fang, S. Y., Grigorenko, E. L., & Magnuson, J. S. (2014). Attentional but not pre-attentive neural measures of auditory discrimination are atypical in children with developmental language disorder. *Developmental Neuropsychology*, *39*, 543–567.

Kornilov, S. A., Magnuson, J. S., Rakhlin, N., Landi, N., & Grigorenko, E. L. (2015). Lexical processing deficits in children with developmental language disorder: An event-related potentials study. *Development and Psychopathology*, *27*, 459–476.

Kovaleva, G. S., Koshelenko, N. G., Kuznetsova, M. I., Loginova, O. B., & Zukerman, G. A. (2013). *Osnovnye rezul'taty mezhdunarodnogo issledovaniya chitatel'skoj gramotnosti*

PIRLS-2011: Analiticheskij otchet [Main results of international research on readers' literacy PIRLS-2011: Analytical report]. Moscow: MAKS Press.

Kuznetsov, O. A., & Khromov, L. N. (1983). *Tekhnika bystrogo chteniya [Speed reading technique].* Moscow: Kniga.

Lalaeva, R. I. (1983). *Narushenie processa ovladeniya chteniem u shkol'nikov [Reading disabilities in students].* Moscow: Prosveshchenie.

Luria, A. R. (1969). *Vysshie korkovye funkcii cheloveka [Human higher order cortical functions].* Moscow.

Lyakso, E. E., & Frolova, O. V. (2013). Razvitie rechi i formirovanie navyka chteniya u detej: Longityudnoe issledovanie ot rozhdeniya do 7 let. [Speech development and reading skills formation in children: longitudinal study from birth to 7 years.] *Psihologicheskij Zhurnal, 34*(3), 24–35.

Lyakso, E. E., Frolova, O. V., Smirnov, A. G. et al. (2012). Uroven' rechevogo razvitiya detej na ehtape formirovaniya navyka chteniya [Level of language development of children at the stage of reading development]. *Psihologicheskij Zhurnal, 33*(1), 73–87.

Ministerstvo Obrazovaniya i Nauki Rossijskoj Federacii. (2011). *Federal'nye gosudarstvennye obrazovatel'nye standarty [Federal educational standards].* Moscow: Ministerstvo Obrazovaniya i Nauki Rossijskoj Federacii.

Ministerstvo Obrazovaniya i Nauki Rossijskoj Federacii. (2012). *Ob obrazovanii v Rossijskoj Federacii. (Federal'nyj zakon ot 29.12.2012 N 273-FZ (red. ot 01.05.2017, s izm. ot 05.07.2017)) (Federal law N 273-FZ of 29/12/2012 on education).* Moscow: Ministerstvo obrazovaniya i nauki Rossijskoj Federacii.

Mullis, I. V. S., Martin, M. O., Foy, P., & Hooper, M. (2017). *PIRLS 2016 international results in reading.* Chestnut Hill, MA: TIMSS & PIRLS International Study Center, Lynch School of Education, Boston College and International Association for the Evaluation of Educational Achievement (IEA).

Naples, A. J., Chang, J. T., Katz, L., & Grigorenko, E. L. (2009). Same or different? Insights into the etiology of phonological awareness and rapid naming. *Biological Psychology, 80,* 226–239. doi: http://dx.doi.org/10.1016/j.biopsycho.2008.10.002.

Naples, A. J., Katz, L., & Grigorenko, E. L. (2012). Lexical decision as an endophenotype for reading comprehension: An exploration of an association. *Development and Psychopathology, 24,* 1345–1360.

OECD. (2016). Russian Federation. *Education at a glance 2016: OECD indicators.* Paris, France: OECD Publishing. doi: http://dx.doi.org/10.1787/eag-2016-76-en.

Paramonova, L. (2006). *Disgrafiya: diagnostika, profilaktika, korrekciya [Dysgraphia: assessment, prevention, intervention].* St Petersburg: Detstvo-Press.

Rakhlin, N., Cardoso-Martins, C., Kornilov, S. A., & Grigorenko, E. L. (2013a). Spelling well despite developmental language disorder: What makes it possible? *Annals of Dyslexia, 63,* 253–273.

Rakhlin, N., Cardoso-Martins, C., & Grigorenko, E. L. (2014). Phonemic awareness is a more important predictor of orthographic processing than rapid serial naming: Evidence from Russian. *Scientific Studies of Reading, 18,* 395–414.

Rakhlin, N., Kornilov, S. A., & Grigorenko, E. L. (2017). Reading acquisition in Russian. In L. T. V. Verhoeven & C. Perfetti (Eds.), *Learning to read across languages and writing systems* (pp. 393–415). Cambridge, UK: Cambridge University Press.

Rakhlin, N., Kornilov, S. A., & Palejev, D. et al. (2013b). The language phenotype of a small geographically isolated Russian-speaking population: Implications for genetic and clinical studies of developmental language disorder. *Applied Psycholinguistics, 34*, 971–1003.

Ramus, F., Marshall, C. R., Rosen, S., & van der Lely, H. K. (2013). Phonological deficits in specific language impairment and developmental dyslexia: towards a multidimensional model. *Brain, 136*, 630–645.

Sokolova, L. V. (2005). *Psihofiziologicheskie osnovy formirovaniya navyka chteniya: Diss. d-ra biologichekih nauk* [Psychophysiological foundations of reading development: PhD dissertation] 03.00. 13, 19.00. 02/Sokolova Lyudmila Vladimirovna.-Arhangel'sk, 2005.-284 s. RGB OD, 71, 06-3.

Starzhinskaya, N. S. (1988). Formirovanie sinteticheskogo chteniya u detej 6 let [Development of synthetic reading skills in 6-year-old children]. *Voprosy psihologii, 5*, 54–62.

Thompson, S., Provasnik, S., Kastberg, D., Ferraro, D., Lemanski, N., & Roey, S. (2012). *Highlights from PIRLS 2011: Reading achievement of US fourth-grade students in an international context.* Washington, DC: NCES. https://nces.ed.gov/p ubs2013/2013010rev.pdf.

Vasil'eva, N. N. (2011). Korrekciya trudnostej formirovaniya navyka chteniya u mladshih shkol'nikov v processe razvitiya binokulyarnyh zritel'nyh funkcij [Correction of reading difficulties in primary school students in the process of development of binocular vision functions]. *Tekhnicheskie nauki, 19*, 5–15.

Vasil'eva, N. N., & Rozhkova, G. I. (2011). Trenirovka binokulyarnyh zritel'nyh funkcij u mladshih shkol'nikov s trudnostyami v chtenii kak faktor korrekcionnoj raboty [Training of binocular vision functions intervention in primary school students with reading disabilities]. *Novye issledovaniya, 1*, 5–17.

Vizel, T. G. (2005). *Osnovy nejropsihologii [Foundations of neuropsychology].* Moscow: Astrel.

Voice of America. (2010). *Russkiye – samaya chitayushchaya natsiya v mire: mif ili real'nost'? [Russians – the most reading nation in the world: Myth or reality?]* www .golos-ameriki.ru/a/russia-books-2010–08-18–101018824/187666.html.

Zabozlaeva, I. V., Suprun, S. A., & Lugovyh, N. A. (2010). Kliniko-patogeneticheskie osobennosti smeshannyh rasstrojstv razvitiya shkol'nyh navykov [Clinico-patogeneticals pecularities of the mixed school skills disorders]. *Ural'skij medicinskij zhurnal, 9*, 35–38.

Zavadenko, N. N., & Roumyantseva, M. (2008). Disleksiya: mekhanizmy razvitiya i principy lecheniya [Dyslexia: underlying mechanisms and treatment principles]. *Russkij zhurnal detskoj nevrologii, 3*, 3–9.

Zukerman, G. A., Kovaleva, G. S., & Kuznetsova, M. I. (2007). Horosho li chitayut rossijskie shkol'niki? [Do Russian pupils read well?] *Voprosy obrazovaniya, 4*, 240–267.

Zukerman, G. A., Kovaleva, G. S., & Kuznetsova, M. I. (2011). Pobeda v PIRLS i porazhenie v PISA: sud'ba chitatel'skoj gramotnosti 10–15-letnih shkol'nikov [Winning the PIRLS and losing PISA: Destiny of readers' literacy in 10–15-year-old students]. *Voprosy obrazovaniya, 2*, 123–150.

Zukerman, G. A., & Shkolyarenko, E. K. (1997). *Kak Vinni-Puh i vse-vse-vse nauchilis' chitat' [How Winnie the Pooh and friends learned how to read].* Moscow: INTOR.

8   Developmental Dyslexia in Hebrew

David L. Share, Michal Shany, and Orly Lipka

8.1   Introduction

Research on Hebrew-speaking dyslexics, in many ways, is a microcosm of dyslexia research in the mainstream English-language literature. Familiar universal themes are evident, such as phonology and morphology, together with the current "race" to identify basic underlying perceptual and brain mechanisms of dyslexia, which has yet to reach consensus. Less familiar language-specific/script-specific issues are also apparent, such as diacritics and homography. Several original, "homegrown" theories have emerged regarding the underlying mechanisms of dyslexia as well as a novel sub-typing scheme. We begin by outlining the characteristics of the Hebrew language and writing system before sketching the process of learning to read. A third section provides a brief historical survey of the legislative and service-delivery frameworks that have evolved over the years since the establishment of the State of Israel in 1948. Identification and assessment of dyslexia are then considered, followed by a review of a second genera-tion of behavioral and neurocognitive research published since a previous review (Share, 2003). A final section summarizes the handful of research-based interventions that have been undertaken in this country in recent years. We conclude by recapping several of the broader universal themes shared by most of the chapters in this volume.

8.2   Learning to Read Hebrew

8.2.1   Hebrew Language and Its Orthography

Hebrew, the language of the Jewish Bible, the Christian Old Testament, has been in continual use since biblical times and today is the official language of the modern State of Israel. Native speakers of Hebrew number only some 10 million but Semitic languages (e.g., Hebrew and Arabic) are spoken today by over 400 million. Furthermore, the consonantal scripts (abjads) first created by Semitic speakers are the ancestors of writing systems used today by billions

(Daniels & Bright, 1996; Diringer, 1948) including alphabets and akshara-based Brahmi-derived scripts (abugidas/alphasyllabaries).

Structurally, Hebrew is a heavily inflected synthetic (S)VO language, permitting flexible word order, with word formation via nonlinear (root-and-pattern) morphology and linear structures, and direct borrowings becoming increasingly common (Berman, 1985; Ravid, 1990, 2012). The core of Hebrew word formation is the uniquely Semitic root-and-pattern system consisting of polymorphemic combinations of tri-consonantal roots interwoven with a vowel pattern (infixes with or without CV affixes). These morphophonemic vowel patterns convert an unpronounceable and discontinuous consonantal root (e.g., ד . ג. ב B, G, D) into a pronounceable word BeGeD (בֶּגֶד "article of clothing"). The consonantal root is the semantic core of most content words; hence, it is a fundamental unit of processing in both the spoken and written language. The root-and-pattern infrastructure is the key to understanding the Hebrew writing system and reading and writing development. The polymorphemic nature of many words and extensive affixation of many grammatical morphemes requires considerable morphemic unpacking but, as we see below, the architecture of the writing system excels in making the morphology transparent.

Phonologically, a once extensive inventory of both vowels and consonants (such as long and short vowels, emphatics, and pharyngeals) has been neutralized in modern Hebrew to a small set of five vowels, three diphthongs, and nineteen consonantal phonemes. Unfortunately for the speller, Hebrew orthography preserves all the once-distinct phonemes: no fewer than six of Hebrew's nineteen consonantal phonemes are represented by two or more letters (Ravid, 2012). This polygraphy is the main challenge for the developing writer.

The Hebrew writing system is an abjad or consonantal writing system (Daniels, 1990); consonants are full-fledged letters linearly arrayed from right to left: Vowels are either omitted or have subordinate status. Furthermore, despite numerous opportunities to become a full alphabet, Hebrew has never abandoned its consonantal architecture. Following the post-biblical demise of spoken Hebrew, however, the introduction of vowel signs became a necessity. Two systems of vowel marking evolved. The earliest, called the *mothers-of-reading*, provides partial vowel specification using four consonantal letters (AHVY, אהוי) to denote vowels as well as consonants. The second system consists of diacritic-like extra-linear dots or points that provide exhaustive vowel identity. For example; דִ /di/, דֻ /du/, דָ /da/, דֶ /dɛ/ etc. Each of these consonant-vowel combinations forms a graphically integral CV syllable block (*tseruf*). These same units are the basic phonic building blocks of pointed Hebrew taught in initial instruction in most Israeli schools. Thus, beginning readers learn to read fully vocalized *pointed* Hebrew before transitioning to *unpointed* Hebrew (around Grade 3) which retains the mothers-of-reading, and hence is partly vocalized.

8.2.2   *Challenges in Learning to Read Hebrew*

Share and Bar-On (2017) discuss three challenges in learning to read Hebrew. Their *Triplex* model postulates three phases of Hebrew reading development, each corresponding to one of the three successive challenges; a progression from sequential (*sublexical*) spelling-to-sound translation characteristic of the Phase 1 (Grade 1) challenge of mastering the fully pointed Hebrew script, to higher-order word-level (*lexical*) lexico-morpho-orthographic processing (Phase 2, Grade 2) necessary for the phonologically underspecified unpointed script, and, in the upper elementary grades, a *supra-lexical* contextual level essential for dealing with the pervasive homography of unpointed script.

In the initial sublexical phase (Grade 1), children typically achieve high levels (between 80 percent and 90 percent) of reading accuracy in the phonologically transparent pointed (fully vocalized) Hebrew script taught to beginning readers. In this beginning phase, children normally translate print to sound in a serial CV (+ C) by CV (+ C) fashion referred to as *kriya metsarefet*, loosely translatable as "combining" or "joining-up"-style reading. The only (minor) stumbling blocks in this initial phase are certain low-frequency vowel points, and the occasional divergence between spoken and written forms. This initial phase is not only *sub*-lexical but also *non*-lexical in the sense that words and matched pseudowords are read with the same speed and accuracy (i.e., there is no word superiority effect) and orthographic learning is minimal (Share, 2004). During this foundational phase, the child's phonological awareness is crucial, although the critical units appear to be CV conglomerates (*tserufim* or "core syllables") and extra-core (preceding or subsequent – (C) CV(C)) consonants. Early in Grade 2, the curriculum switches from a learning-to-read to a reading-to-learn mode.

The next major challenge confronting the developing reader is the transition to unpointed script, which poses two challenges. The first is determining the identity of phonologically underspecified (i.e., incompletely vocalized) letter strings (Phase 2), and second (Phase 3 of the Triplex model), resolving the ambiguity created by pervasive homography. Converging evidence indicates that Grade 2 is a crucial turning point in Hebrew reading development as the young reader gradually relies less on low-level sublexical phonology and more on higher-order lexical and morpho-orthographic knowledge. Word reading becomes less labored and faster. Children now begin showing reliable evidence of the acquisition of word-specific and morpheme-specific orthographic representations that signal the growth of the orthographic lexicon. Henceforth, the accuracy of pure phonological decoding of pseudowords actually *declines* after Grade 1, alongside growing sensitivity to higher-order (word-level) morphological and lexical constraints. These developments in Grade 2 provide the platform for negotiating the transition from pointed text to unpointed text – the standard script from Grade 3 onwards. At this point, typical readers no longer need the points and are able to rely on a growing lexicon of familiar words and roots, and their knowledge of familiar morpho-phonological patterns. At this point, the unpointed script ceases to be an obstacle.

Hebrew readers in second and third grades gain fluency as their lexico-morpho-orthographic knowledge (sight vocabulary) expands, but still struggle with the problem of extensive homography. Accurate pronunciation of homographic (unpointed) text demands reliance on higher-level context, which is the focus of the third, supra-lexical phase. Bar-On and Ravid (2011) found that the ability to benefit from supportive context develops more gradually and over a longer period than the lexico-morpho-orthographic word identification discussed above in Phase 2. The authors suggested that, compared to morpho-orthographic identification, morpho-*syntactic* identification makes greater demands on integrative top-down contextual processes. In a study of lexical ambiguity resolution using garden-path sentences, Bar-On and Ravid (2011) found that only in the upper elementary grades (between Grades 4 and 7) were Hebrew readers able to recover from the preceding misleading (garden-path) context by exploiting information from subsequent context.

8.3   Reading Difficulties in Hebrew

8.3.1   Historical and Cultural Context

Following the founding of the State of Israel in 1948, special education policy was based on segregation; children with special educational needs were assigned to separate schools designed to serve their needs (Gumpel & Sharoni, 2007). A turning point was marked by the Special Education Law (SEL) of 1988 (Yunay, 1992) which mandated integration of this population via services provided within the general education framework (Avishar & Layser, 2000). All children receiving special education services are divided into twelve different eligibility categories based on their primary disability with learning disability (LD) being the largest category numerically (Gumpel, 1999). This was the first formal recognition of learning disability in Israel. In 2002, the SEL (2002) was amended in order to accelerate inclusion (Avishar & Layser, 2000; Gumpel & Sharoni, 2007). These revisions changed the wording in the law from a "handicapped child" to an "included child" and this amendment guided additional teaching and learning as well as special services (Al-Yagon & Margalit, 2001).

The last two decades have witnessed a growing awareness of the specific needs of the learning-disabled child within the special education population and the need for educational intervention. Subsequently, two committees headed by Professor Malka Margalit were appointed by the Ministry of Education in order to examine two aspects of the integration of students with

LD: the effectiveness of treatment/intervention (Margalit, 1997) and the degree of SEL's implementation (Margalit, 2000). Both committees highlighted the importance of effective intervention and equality of opportunities for students with LD. These committees also pointed to the relevance of early detection and diagnosis, the need for professionals able to determine the optimal treatment for LD students, and the need for public centers to supply diagnoses and monitor progress. Today, special education services for individuals with LD are provided either in noninclusive settings that are detached from mainstream education (special kindergartens or special schools) or in self-contained special classes within mainstream schools. Within mainstream schools, individuals with LD are eligible to receive individual support in the classroom or in a *pull-out* program (Avissar, 2012).

Every student with special needs in Israel is entitled to the Individualized Education Program (IEP). The IEP takes into account the current educational performance of the student, his or her strengths and weaknesses, and a variety of goals – educational, behavioral, emotional, sensory-motor, communicative, and life skills. In addition, the IEP stipulates educational service needs and the distribution of responsibilities of relevant staff. Parents' involvement during the decision-making process is encouraged.

In practice, a student with LD enrolled in a special education school or class receives a personal curriculum *(tal'a)*. This curriculum, designed by a multidisciplinary team, includes instructional goals that derive from relevant assessment or evaluation based on the learner's profile. A student who is integrated in a regular class, also receives a unique individualized curriculum *(techi)*. It specifies expected standards, tools, and implementation time, based on instructional goals that derive from the general curriculum. Methods of feedback and evaluation for monitoring educational progress are also mentioned.

Since the early 2000s in Israel, the IEP has been standards-based; criteria are oriented to achievement goals. Accordingly, the standards define what students should know and what they should be able to do. Thus, every subject of study, in theory, is specified in terms of content and required skills, from kindergarten through elementary school, junior high school, and senior high school (Friedman & Philosoph, 2001). Over the years, various types of standards have been developed (e.g., content, performance, learning opportunities, and assessment standards) (Friedman & Philosoph, 2001).

It is essential to note that there are standards of language and literacy that refer to each of the following; speaking, writing, reading, and listening proficiency, at each of three time points; the end of second, fourth, and sixth grade. Individuals with LD in elementary school usually receive support from the "integration teacher" *(mora meshalevet)* who is (often) a specialist in LD. This support is delivered either in the classroom or individually in a pull-out program.

In high-school settings, there are multidisciplinary teams (school counselors and teachers) that have pedagogical responsibility for LD students. These teams are responsible for customizing testing methods and simultaneously ensuring adequate support and assistance throughout secondary schooling. Periodically, meetings take place in order to monitor students' progress and make necessary adjustments.

Following the Margalit Report's (1997) recommendations, there is special training for *"Matal"* teachers in middle and high school aimed at developing LD professionals. In practice, a *Matal* teacher serves as a resource and consultant in the field of learning, promoting processes of detection, diagnosis, and adaption of teaching methods to the LD student's various needs in the regular classroom. The *Matal* teacher deals with assessments and the development of intervention plans for children with LD by developing individual inclusion plans and learning strategies, and promoting discussion with general education teachers about possible allowances and appropriate accommodations (Gumpel & Sharoni, 2007).

Within high schools, a new kind of support, Mahut Centers ("Essence Centers") was established in recent years following the model being implemented in post-secondary education in Israel. These new centers assist LD students in a variety of areas including emotional, educational, and technical support. Specifically, these centers aim to broaden understanding of the student and his or her environment with regard to the disability and its impact on all aspects of a student's life, providing emotional and instructional support for both students and their teachers. Another recent reform with regards to intervention for middle-school LD (Ministry of Education, 2016) is based on the recommendations of the Margalit II Report, and focuses on system learning and teaching processes rather than on diagnosis and testing accommodations. Additionally, the new reform concentrates on strengthening teaching staff knowledge and know-how about the difficulties of students with learning difficulties and is mainly based on the Response to Intervention model (RTI).

With regard to post-secondary education, a law concerning the rights of students with LD in higher-education institutions was enacted in 2009. This law states that the LD student is entitled to adjustments during the process of admission and study. It further mandated the establishment of learning centers within higher-education institutions. These centers are charged with the mission of assisting students to gain admission to academic study, learn, and complete their studies successfully, and with empowering them (Meltzer, 2003), and, simultaneously, to increase awareness among the teaching and administrative staff regarding the integration of LD students within the institution (Dahan, Melzer, & Finkelstein, 2011).

These post-secondary learning centers offer a range of support services, primarily in areas of academic study, but also in the emotional and social spheres (Dahan & Russak, 2005; Vogel et al., 2003). Professionals provide assistance in reading and academic writing, promotion of academic skills, support in English as a second language, providing strategies for statistics, using assistive technologies, as well as coaching, tutoring, mentoring, and social-emotional support. In addition, based on the assessment's recommendations, students receive accommodations in testing situations.

8.3.2   Identification and Prevalence of Dyslexia

When the topic of learning disabilities first came to the attention of the general public in Israel (1980s), the accepted theoretical basis of word-reading difficulties was that word reading was related to visual perception (Simpson, 1983). Alongside these measures of visual perception, evaluation of reading abilities included reading syllables, single words, sentences, and texts, all written with vowels. With the ascendance of cognitive research into reading in North America in the 1980s and the recognition that the basis of most reading difficulties was linguistic (and specifically phonological) rather than visual-perceptual, a new generation of research in Israel confirmed the phonological basis of dyslexia (e.g., Ben-Dror, Frost, & Bentin, 1995; Bentin & Leshem, 1993; for a review, see Share, 2003). This led to assessment practices that included measures of phonological awareness and pointed pseudoword reading. Since the mid-1990s, deficits in morphological knowledge have also been shown to be a basis for reading difficulties (Ben-Dror, Bentin, & Frost, 1995; Schiff & Raveh, 2007; Schiff & Ravid, 2004, 2007, 2013). This work has become instrumental in analyzing reading and spelling errors among struggling readers. A new line of research (e.g., Bar-On & Ravid, 2011) emphasizing the role of morpho-syntactic and semantic-pragmatic knowledge in disambiguating the many homographs in unpointed text is now seeing new assessment tools added to the reading specialist's diagnostic toolkit (e.g., decoding of unpointed pseudowords by utilizing morpho-phonological knowledge). Furthermore, Beidas, Khateb, and Breznitz (2013) tested the executive functions (EF) of adult dyslexics at university using a composite EF score based on planning, shifting, and inhibition. Dyslexics were found to be *superior* to controls. Their reading comprehension was also comparable to that of matched normal readers. The latest focus of dyslexia research in this country into the perceptual and neuro-biological basis of dyslexia reviewed in the following section, has yet to influence assessment practices, probably due to the lack of convergence of findings from multiple competing theories and models as discussed in Section 8.4 below.

Consistent with the ecological approach to assessment (D'Amato et al., 2005), current assessment procedures in Israel typically include collection and integration of data from multiple sources (parents, teachers, and other professionals), including: developmental and familial history (language, motor skills, emotional regulation, history of parental reading and of reading difficulties among family members), academic functioning (early reading acquisition, subjects in which there are difficulties), educational environment (relationships with teachers, teaching methods), and behavioral-social-emotional aspects.

Reading skills are evaluated on the basis of multiple indicators: accuracy and rate while reading different orthographic structures: consonant and vowel combinations (*tserufim*), pointed and unpointed pseudowords in morphologically admissible (legal) and non-admissible structures (only in pointed pseudowords), pointed and unpointed texts; recognition and production of spelling structures; reading comprehension; and written expression. Four basic reading-related abilities are generally included in assessment: phonological awareness, naming speed (RAN), working memory, and attention.

In Israel, both clinical training protocols at institutions of higher learning and assessment procedures in practice align well with the criteria delineated in DSM-5 (American Psychiatric Association, 2013). As in several other countries, the diagnosis of developmental dyslexia is based on deficits in accuracy and/or rate in reading isolated orthographic structures including consonant and vowel (CV) combinations (*tserufim*), words, and pseudowords, as well as on the basis of abnormal representation of written structures (Shany et al., 2006). Diagnosis, as in other languages, relates abnormal reading rate and accuracy to basic linguistic processes.

Although the cutoff point for diagnosis is arbitrary, by convention, it is often set at or below the 16th percentile among children on the aforementioned reading tasks (Breznitz, 2002b; Shany et al., 2006). In Israel, there is only a single standardized reading test with national norms for the elementary years (Shany et al., 2006), and none for ages 12–18. Reading disability is therefore diagnosed based on low performance on tests designated for younger age groups and on clinical evaluation. There is a standardized test for assessing adults, with a diagnostic cutoff below the 3rd percentile (Ben-Simon & Inbar-Weiss, 2013; MATAL, 2007). Tests are accompanied by a clinical intake to rule out sensory deficits, developmental disorders, instructional deficits, and neurological damage. If reading functions are abnormal at the time of assessment, diagnosis of reading disability is not ruled out even if no evidence is presented of difficulties in reading acquisition at an early age.

Despite DSM-5's assertion that diagnosis of reading disability should not be based on intelligence-test results, the Israeli Ministry of Education requires that assessments rule out low intelligence before providing testing accommodations, such as having directions read aloud or reduction of the material covered. Severity level may also be addressed in reading disability assessments, based on documentation of behavioral expressions, level of deviation from the norm (when norms are available), and comorbidity with additional conditions such as deficits in attentional or executive functions, language difficulties, or substantial emotional problems.

8.4   Behavioral and Neurocognitive Evidence

This section opens with a brief synopsis of the work on deficits in phonology and morphology followed by a summary of a second generation of more recent work investigating the basic perceptual and brain mechanisms underlying dyslexia. The bulk of this work, understandably, has focused on the most prominent and broadly debated Anglophone theories, including Tallal's temporal processing hypothesis, Nicolson and Fawcett's automatization-cerebellar -proceduralization hypothesis, and Stein's magnocellular hypothesis. We also review two original theories of dyslexia developed in this country – Zvia Breznitz's *asynchrony* theory and Merav Ahissar's *anchoring deficit* hypothesis, as well as a novel dyslexia subtyping scheme developed by Michal Shany. Yet another new line of research, led by Tami Katzir, has examined affective factors such as reading self-concept (Kasperski, Shany, & Katzir, 2016; Katzir, Lesaux, & Kim, 2009), reading anxiety (Meer, Breznitz, & Katzir, 2016), and self-confidence and self-regulation (Katzir et al., 2018).

8.4.1   *The Nature of Reading Problems in Hebrew*

8.4.1.1   Phonological and Morphological Deficits   The first generation of modern cognitive research into dyslexia in Israel resoundingly confirmed the phonological deficit theory of dyslexia (for reviews of this work, see Share, 2003). At the same time, morphology (and morpho-syntax) was also being brought to the attention of dyslexia researchers by Ram Frost, Shlomo Bentin, and Avital Deutsch (e.g., Ben-Dror, Frost, & Bentin, 1995; Bentin, Deutsch, & Liberman, 1990; Frost & Bentin, 1992; Frost, Forster, & Deutsch, 1997), and Ravid (1990, 1996), and has since been firmly established by many dyslexia researchers to be another *independent* source of difficulty for dyslexics.

Confirming earlier studies investigating explicit morphological knowledge among dyslexics (summarized in Share, 2003), a number of studies among children and adults has shown that dyslexics are consistently poor on a variety of tasks assessing explicit knowledge of both derivational and inflectional morphology (Leikin & Even-Zur, 2006; Schiff et al., 2016; Schiff & Ravid, 2004, 2007, 2013; Schiff, Schwartz-Nahshon, & Nagar, 2011). Adult dyslexics often perform at the level of young children (e.g., Schiff & Ravid, 2004, 2007) and also make an unusual number of semantic responses (Schiff & Ravid, 2007; Schiff et al., 2016; Ram-Tsur, Faust, & Zivotofsky, 2006), cf. Share, 1995). These deficits, furthermore, are not accounted for by either phonological deficits or working memory (Leikin & Even-Zur, 2006; Schiff et al., 2016; Shalev-Leifer, 2016). It is noteworthy that, in some circumstances, morphological priming, including masked priming, has been found to be comparable to that of typically developing readers (Leikin & Even-Zur, 2006; Raveh & Schiff, 2008; Schiff et al., 2016) suggesting that, despite their weaknesses, Hebrew dyslexics are relying heavily on morphology, probably because this is an inescapably core feature of linguistic competence in Semitic languages, as discussed in Section 8.1 above. Further confirmation of the importance of morphology comes from the first morphological training study in Hebrew (Bar-Kochva, 2016) showing (mostly) positive post-training reading and spelling outcomes for her brief (two-session) morpheme-based training with adult dyslexics.

Leikin and Assayag-Bouskila (2004) examined syntactic processing in fifth-grade dyslexics using measures of spoken sentence-picture matching, syntactic judgment, and sentence correction. Dyslexics were consistently slower and less accurate in sentence-processing tasks, reinforcing earlier findings by Bentin and Deutsch.

8.4.1.2 Temporal Processing Deficit Hypothesis Inspired by Paula Tallal's groundbreaking work, a number of Israeli investigators have examined temporal processing among Hebrew dyslexics. In general, this work has been supportive of Tallal's hypothesis.

In three separate samples, Fostick and colleagues (Ben-Artzi, Fostick, & Babkoff, 2005; Fostick, Bar-El, & Ram-Tsur, 2012; Fostick et al., 2014) found adult dyslexics to be less accurate and slower on the standard (pure-tone) Repetition Test (Tallal, 1980). These investigations ruled out the possibility that performance differences were due to frequency-based spectral/holistic pattern processing rather than temporal order judgments per se. Two identical pure tones were presented dichotically and the participants required to indicate in which ear, right or left, a pure tone was first heard. Fostick et al. (2014) found no overall (group-averaged) deficit on a non-temporal (intensity-discrimination) task (see also Amitay et al., 2002, see below in Section 8.4.1.4) Following up these correlational findings with an experimental training study, dyslexic and normal students were compared on phonological awareness before and after short-term training in either temporal processing, non-temporal auditory processing (intensity discrimination), or no training. Only the temporal training condition evinced significant improvement in phoneme deletion and pseudoword reading.

Cohen-Mimran (2006) also compared Hebrew dyslexic and normal children on discrimination of spoken syllables /ba/ /pa/, distinguished by a temporal cue – voice onset time, using short (50 msec) and long (500 msec) inter-stimulus intervals. Dyslexics were less accurate and slower on the syllable discrimination at both short and long inter-stimulus intervals (ISIs). Electrophysiologically, the dyslexics' P300 latencies were significantly delayed. Both P300 latencies and TOJ (temporal order judgment) scores correlated significantly with phonological awareness and pseudoword reading at the short but not long ISI.

Another new line of research, also originally inspired by Tallal's auditory temporal processing deficit hypothesis, has appeared, led by Merav Ahissar and her colleagues. They proposed that dyslexics have difficulties forming perceptual anchors (for a review, see Ahissar, 2007). In the first anchoring study, Ahissar et al. (2006) presented a sequence of two pure tones to adult dyslexics asking them to decide which had the higher pitch. In the "standard" "anchored" condition, a 1000-Hz tone was presented in every trial as either the first or second of the two stimuli; the other tone was always higher. In the no-standard unanchored condition, there was no standard tone. Ahissar et al. argued that in the standard condition, subjects could form a perceptual anchor based on the repeated tone which was always the lower of the two. The no-standard or unanchored condition required subjects to actively compare the two tones using high-level executive operations of working memory. Ahissar et al. found that the critical interaction between group and condition was significant; controls, but not the dyslexics, were better in the "anchored" condition. Furthermore, the degree of failure to form a perceptual anchor correlated with their difficulties in phonological and working-memory tasks. Ahissar's group has extended this finding to speech-sound discrimination, syllable span, pseudoword span with either repeated or non-repeated syllables, and even serial (RAN-style) naming of printed pseudowords with repeated or non-repeated stimuli (Oganian & Ahissar, 2012).

However, attempts to replicate the anchoring effect by other researchers using group-averaged data have not met with success (Badcock et al., 2013; Conner, 2013; Di Filippo, Zoccolotti, & Ziegler, 2008; Willburger & Landerl, 2010; Ziegler, 2008). However, looking at anchoring effects on a case-by-case basis, Badcock et al. (2013) found a subgroup of dyslexics with anchoring deficits (I return to this issue below in Section 8.6). At this point, therefore, it seems too early to make a call regarding the viability of the anchoring deficit hypothesis.

8.4.1.3 Procedural Learning-Deficit Hypothesis Inspired by Nicolson and Fawcett's automatization/cerebellar/procedural learning-deficit hypothesis of dyslexia, Gabay and colleagues (Gabay, Schiff, & Vakil, 2012a, 2012b, 2012c) investigated skill learning and consolidation among adult dyslexics using the serial reaction time (SRT) task – involving implicit learning of a repeated sequence of visual stimuli appearing at different spatial locations. Initial ("on-line") learning was less effective among dyslexics than typical readers and more prone to interference; dyslexics also showed poorer consolidation (overnight "off-line" gains). This pattern of findings was interpreted as support for an automatization deficit and Nicolson & Fawcett's cerebellar hypothesis; but the authors also conceded that their data were also consistent with impaired attention, which was controlled only by self-reported ADHD signs – a selection procedure which can leave significant between-group differences in attention (see, e.g., Sela & Karni, 2012). Gabay et al., (2012a) also compared motor-sequence learning and procedural learning of letter names. Contrary to the two earlier studies, motor-sequence learning was intact, but specific linguistic (letter-name) procedural learning was deficient.

Seeking to specify the nature of the link between the procedural learning deficits and phonological impairment, Gabay and Holt (2015) went on to test the hypothesis that impaired procedural learning affects phonological processing by interfering with phonetic category learning. Dyslexics and controls were compared on incidental auditory category learning for artificial non-speech sounds in the context of an action videogame. Dyslexics were poorer on all measures and category-learning scores correlated with poorer pseudo-word decoding and phonological awareness.

A related study, also focusing on the Nicolson and Fawcett automatization-cerebellar-procedural learning hypothesis, was carried out by Sela and Karni (2012), who aimed to determine whether dyslexic students' controls show a deficit in manual procedural learning or a dysfunction of the posture and balance-control system, or both. Adult dyslexic and control groups practiced a novel sequence of cued manual (touch) movements (with feedback) on a touch-sensitive screen while standing on a force plate that monitored posture and balance. Overall, the dyslexics were reliably slower to initiate the first touch in response to the "go" cue, but learning (reaction time speedup) was similarly robust in both groups. As regards posture, the skilled readers, but not dyslexics, showed reliable training effects in the form of reduced variance.

Sela and Karni concluded that dyslexics' unimpaired learning and retention of the movement sequence was not consistent with Nicolson and Fawcett's general procedural (motor) learning or automatization deficit, but that dyslexics' greater postural sway during learning was "not inconsistent" with the notion of a cerebellar deficit. The two sets of studies therefore do not provide compelling support for a general procedural (non-linguistic) learning or automatization deficit, although the Sela and Karni sway data are consistent with the Nicolson and Fawcett cerebellar hypothesis.

Gabay, Thiessen, and Holt (2015) examined statistical learning among English-speaking dyslexics. Dyslexics and controls heard a continuous stream of syllables or sine-wave tones containing sequences of three items with either high or low transitional probabilities. Participants were subsequently asked to select the more familiar triplet from a high- and a low-probability pair.

Dyslexics were significantly poorer in both speech and non-speech tasks, and performance correlated with sight-word-reading fluency and decoding fluency.

Kahta and Schiff (2016) compared implicit and explicit sequential learning among dyslexics within the context of artificial grammar learning. Participants were first exposed to "grammatical" strings of (English) letters and then presented with novel strings that either conformed or did not conform to the rules of the grammar. In an implicit version of the task, participants were informed that the strings shared a set of rules only *after* seeing the training strings. In the explicit version of the task participants were told that all strings shared a common set of rules *before* seeing the training strings; they were then asked to try and figure out the underlying rules. The performance of dyslexics was inferior to controls in the implicit but not explicit version of the task.

To summarize, these studies point to impaired procedural learning in the speech-auditory and linguistic domain, but not in the motor domain; however, samples were small and doubts linger about the role of inattention.

8.4.1.4 Magno-Cellular Deficit Hypothesis   A series of studies by Ahissar, Ben-Yehuda, and colleagues, together with related work by several other investigators, have obtained evidence at odds with the magnocellular theory. Ben-Yehuda et al. (2001) found dyslexic adults had significantly impaired sensitivity for drifting and flickering visual gratings in a temporal (sequentially presented) forced-choice task, but not when these were presented simultaneously in a spatial forced-choice task. Ben-Yehuda and Ahissar (2004) later extended this result to spatial frequency discrimination (see also Ram-Tsur, Faust, & Zivotsky, 2006, 2008). A related finding by Kaminsky, Eviatar, and Norman (2002) found that fifth- and sixth-grade dyslexics performed as well as control children on a non-linguistic (visual) non-sequential task, but more poorly when sequential order became crucial.

Amitay et al. (2002) administered a battery of magnocellular (e.g., flicker, drift, coherent motion) and non-magnocellular tasks (visual spatial frequency discrimination, auditory intensity, and frequency discrimination) to a group of thirty adult dyslexics. Only a small proportion (six out of thirty) of the dyslexics were reliably poor on the magnocellular tasks, but this subgroup was also poor on the non-magnocellular tasks. Chase and Stein (2003) criticized the criterion for poor performance as unrealistically conservative, but a re-analysis of the data by Amitay et al. (2003) added only a single subject to the magnocellular subgroup.

Ram-Tsur et al. (2006) also tested the magnocellular theory using contrast detection thresholds. Several temporal and non-temporal, spatial magnocellular tasks were administered to adult dyslexics. Replicating Ben-Yehudah and Ahissar, impaired performance was found only for the temporal-sequential but not spatial magnocellular tasks.

On the whole then, it appears that, with the possible exception of Heth and Lavidor's training study (presented below in Section 8.4), the magnocellular hypothesis has not fared particularly well in the handful of Hebrew investigations conducted to date.

8.4.1.5 Accuracy versus Speed Deficits An original accuracy-versus-rate-based subtyping framework, developed by Michal Shany (Shany & Breznitz, 2011; Shany & Share, 2011) classifies dyslexics into three groups each representing around one third of the dyslexic group; rate-disabled, accuracy-disabled and doubly disabled. In a nationally representative sample of fourth graders, the two selectively disabled subgroups displayed intact reading achievement on the non-disabled dimension, demonstrating a true double dissociation (Shany & Share, 2011). Validating this subdivision, the rate-specific disability appeared to reflect a rapid naming (RAN) deficit; the accuracy-only disability subgroup displayed selective deficits in phonological awareness and morphological knowledge. These findings were replicated in a large clinical sample of over 300 dyslexic university students and 200 controls (Shany & Breznitz, 2011). Slightly under half of the dyslexics were classified as rate-disabled or accuracy-disabled, and only 10 percent of the dyslexic group as accuracy-plus-rate-disabled.

Unlike most subtyping frameworks which have been developed in English (e.g., the dual-route distinction between phonological and surface dyslexia), which are routinely based on word-reading accuracy alone, Shany's framework considers both accuracy and speed, and consequently has potentially universal applicability. Shany's approach also has the potential to clarify the controversial "double-deficit" hypothesis of Wolf and Bowers (1999); see also Katzir et al. (2008).

8.4.1.6 The Asynchrony Deficit Hypothesis Yet another original Israeli theory has been developed by Zvia Breznitz (2002a, 2002b) who claimed that dyslexics show speed of processing problems which may point to a cross-modal integration ("synchrony") deficit. In a sample of young people with dyslexia, Breznitz (2002a) assessed speed of processing (SOP) using a large number of non-linguistic and linguistic, auditory and visual low-level tasks (light flashes and pure tones) and higher-level orthographic and phonological tasks (letters and words). Both behaviorally (response reaction time differences) and electro-physiologically (the raw difference in milliseconds (i.e., "temporal gap") between mean P300 latencies recorded at CZ (central brain) sites during low-level visual versus auditory tasks as well as higher-level orthographic versus phonological tasks) was significantly wider among dyslexics. Furthermore, these temporal "gaps" (in particular the linguistic, orthographic-phonological gap) explained much of the variance in word recognition. Breznitz and Misra (2003) followed up these findings with a larger sample (n = 40) of compensated adult dyslexics. Once again, the critical cross-modal gap between P300 latencies in the auditory-phonological versus visual-orthographic tasks was significantly greater for dyslexics than controls.

8.4.2   Underlying Causes of Reading Problems in Hebrew

At the outset, it is important to note that each and every one of these studies of basic perceptual and neurobiological mechanisms in (Hebrew) dyslexia has, *without exception*, confirmed the primacy of phonological processing deficits among dyslexics, usually in the course of validating group identity. In some cases, there is no overlap whatsoever in phonological skills such as pseudo-word reading (see, e.g., Gabay et al., 2013; Shovman & Ahissar, 2006). Typically, too, the phonological gaps tend to widen over age (Miller-Shaul, 2005). As such, the Hebrew literature seems to be a microcosm of the far larger mostly English research literature, although almost all the dyslexia research undertaken in Israel has used convenience samples of undergraduate ("compensated") dyslexics, who may not be representative of the general population of dyslexics. Among high-functioning dyslexics, difficulties may be masked by compensatory mechanisms or strategies (see, e.g., Lum, Ullman, & Conti-Ramsden, 2013; Shaul, 2014).

Turning to the search for additional deficits or basic underlying mechanisms, the findings, like those of the English-language literature, remain inconclusive, although Tallal's temporal processing or sequential processing deficit hypothesis has attracted the most attention and seems the most viable candidate. The other candidate theories have yet to be consistently replicated in labs other than those in which they originated. Many of the studies reviewed in this section suffer from small sample sizes and/or marginal statistical results, but the biggest problem is comorbidity, especially the attentional impairments that are very common among dyslexics. Another issue that has not always received due consideration in this literature is where these basic non-phonological (or pre-phonological) deficits stand in relation to phonological deficits? Are they (1) *in addition to,* (2) *instead of, or* (3) *the "root cause(s)" of phonological deficits*? We return to this important point later on.

Comorbidity is a big problem in almost all these studies which (with the exception of Faust and colleagues (Faust, Dimitrovsky, & Shacht, 2003; Faust & Sharfstein-Friedman, 2003) who controlled both SLI *and* ADHD) typically focus on a single dimension of comorbidity – either SLI or ADHD but not both. Attentional deficits, for example, are often treated as categorical, with arbitrary cutoffs applied using self-reported signs. However, inattention is a graded continuum, hence cutting points often retain dyslexics who do not strictly qualify as ADHD but have mild attentional impairments. Given that subjects in these studies are performing highly repetitive psychophysical tasks that place a premium on distractibility and sustained attention, objective measurement of inattention is imperative. The question of group-averaged means as opposed to subgroup analyses, or case-by-case examination of outcomes, is taken up in Section 8.6.

8.5   Intervention

In addition to Fostick et al.'s (2014) auditory temporal training study mentioned earlier, there have been several other promising evidence-based training/intervention studies with Hebrew dyslexics. Most have been tailored to a single specific component skill or basic mechanism presumed to underlie dyslexia; only one program has taken a more comprehensive, multi-componential approach to intervention.

The Breznitz reading acceleration program (RAP) (summarized in detail in Breznitz, 2006, chapter 6) has repeatedly demonstrated reliable gains in decoding accuracy, rate, and reading comprehension in multiple samples of normal and dyslexic readers. These studies have furnished evidence that multiple factors appear to explain the training effects (e.g., reduced distractibility, attenuated working-memory limitations, enhanced synchronization of brain systems, and reduced reliance on frontal areas). Since this earlier work, the acceleration effect has now been replicated in multiple languages and among adult and adolescent Hebrew-speaking dyslexics (e.g., Breznitz et al., 2013; Dai, Zhang, & Liu, 2016; Horowitz-Kraus et al., 2014). Furthermore, Horowitz-Kraus and Breznitz (2014) reported that rate and comprehension gains were maintained six months after training (Breznitz et al., 2013).

Heth and Lavidor (2015) employed transcranial direct current stimulation (tDCS) to test whether the magnocellular-dominant dorsal (V5) stream has a causal role in dyslexia. Visual extra-striate area left-MT/V5 was stimulated in five sessions over a period of two weeks. Reading was assessed before, immediately after, and one week later ($n = 10$) and compared to matched controls ($n = 9$) undergoing sham treatment. Significant gains appeared in text-reading speed in the treatment group but not the control (sham) group one week later. Heth and Lavidor argued that gains selective to letter and number-naming speed (RAN), but not symbol-search, indicate orthography-specific gains consistent with the magnocellular deficit hypothesis.

In contrast to an intervention targeting one specific aspect of reading, often in the quest to establish the causal status of a basic mechanism hypothesized to underlie dyslexia, the OR program (meaning "light" in Hebrew) is a broad-based Tier 2 intervention founded on the idea that reading is a multifaceted construct (Katzir et al., 2009); hence to be effective and durable, intervention must be multi-componential. This three-pronged program focuses on specific

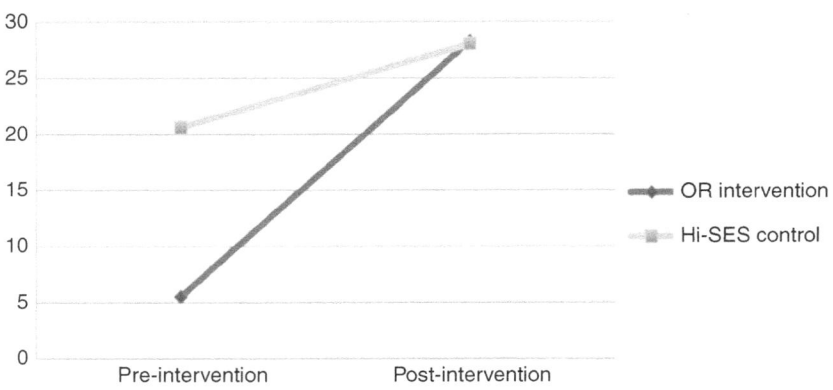

Figure 8.1 Number of real words correctly read in 45 secs pre-intervention (beginning of Grade 1) and post-intervention (at the end of Grade 1) at two schools (the OR intervention program compared to a higher-SES control school)

literacy skills such as phonological awareness (PA), general memory and executive functions, and emotion. Two entire first-grade classes ($n = 43$) from a low-SES school with many language-minority children received whole-class and small-group intervention twice a week (forty-five minutes) for three months. The intervention groups were compared to children from a neighboring higher-SES school using the standard curriculum. Preliminary data showed that despite lower pre-intervention cognitive and reading levels, the OR children had closed the gap in word-reading fluency by the end of the program (see Figure 8.1). Furthermore, the training group maintained their gains over the summer and began second grade significantly *ahead* of the control group. Self-efficacy and motivation were also higher in the trained group. This program is currently being adapted to the dyslexic population.

8.6   Discussion and Conclusion

Dyslexia research and practice among Israeli Hebrew speakers in many ways mirrors the current general zeitgeist. The phonological and, more recently, morphological underpinnings of many, if not most, reading difficulties are now beyond dispute. Efforts to uncover the basic underlying brain mechanisms, by contrast, have made only meager headway, as they have elsewhere, with disparate and non-convergent findings that raise the usual concerns regarding task-specificity and comorbidity confounds, especially attention (ADHD) and language impairment (SLI) that are rarely taken seriously via objective measurement. If we take the classical "winner-takes-all," unitary-deficit approach that typically employs group-averaged data, then it would be fair to say that Tallal's temporal processing hypothesis has gained the most mileage in Hebrew, with inconclusive findings for the other competing theories. But if our model emphasizes heterogeneity, dimensionality, and comorbidity (Clark et al., 2017; Pennington, 2006) then the task ahead will be poorly served by omnibus whole-group comparisons. Instead, the dyslexia mosaic will need to be mapped in a bottom-up, case-by-case fashion, aggregating like cases into subgroups. Furthermore, if heterogeneity and especially comorbidity are the norm, then the general population of dyslexics from which researchers recruit their samples is likely be made up of multiple subpopulations with varying combinations of deficits (see, e.g., Ramus et al., 2003) – an idea consistent with the polygenic basis of dyslexia (Bishop, 2015). Varying participant recruitment procedures, participant attrition, and data-pruning practices could create subtle biases toward one or the other subpopulation: discrepancies between experimental outcomes would be a natural consequence. It may be that each of the current "contenders" – magnocellular, cerebellar, proceduralization, anchoring, asynchrony (and accounts yet to come) are each true causes for at least some dyslexics.

Yet another concern is the tendency to seek domain-general learning mechanisms (procedural, implicit, or statistical learning) that do not align well with the notion of dyslexia as a *specific* learning disorder. Researchers need to give more thought to *how* the hypothesized mechanisms impact learning to read, for example, by asking whether a given deficit contributes to dyslexia via phonological (or non-phonological) language skills, in addition to it, or both.

On the applied front, the notion of learning disability as an undifferentiated category of specific learning disorders, or as a family of variant disabilities with a common basis, remains firmly entrenched in legislation, professional training, and service-delivery practices in Israel. Scientific progress in recent decades has rendered this approach too coarse-grained; different disorders such as dyslexia and dyscalculia have little in common either cognitively, neurobiologically, or genetically (Rubinsten & Henik, 2006). Above all, assessment and intervention practices must be differentiated. It may be time for the LD field to redefine itself.

References

Ahissar, M. (2007). Dyslexia and the anchoring-deficit hypothesis. *Trends in Cognitive Sciences, 11*, 458–465.

Ahissar, M., Lubin, Y., Putter-Katz, H., & Banai, K. (2006). Dyslexia and the failure to form a perceptual anchor. *Nature Neuroscience, 9*, 1558–1564.

Al-Yagon, M., & Margalit, M. (2001). Special and inclusive education in Israel. *Mediterranean Journal of Educational Studies, 6*, 93–112.

American Psychiatric Association. (2013). *Diagnostic and statistical manual of mental disorders* (5th ed.). Arlington, VA: American Psychiatric Publishing.

Amitay, S., Ben-Yehudah, G., Banai, K., & Ahissar, M. (2002). Disabled readers suffer from visual and auditory impairments but not from a specific magnocellular deficit. *Brain, 125*, 2272–2285.

Amitay, S., Ben-Yehudah, G., Banai, K., & Ahissar, M. (2003). Reply to: Visual magnocellular deficits in dyslexia. *Brain, 126*, e3.

Avishar, G., & Layser, Y. (2000). Evaluating values in special education as change in education [in Hebrew]. *Halacha veMa'ashe b'Tichnun Limudim, 15*, 97–124.

Avissar, G. (2012). Inclusive education in Israel from a curriculum perspective: An exploratory study. *European Journal of Special Needs Education, 27*, 35–49.

Badcock, N., Ewing, L., Preece, K., Jeffery, L., Rhodes, G., & McArthur, G. (2013, June). *Reading and language abilities are related to auditory perceptual anchoring in children with learning difficulties.* Poster session presented at the Language in Developmental and Acquired disorders: Future directions, The Royal Society at Chicheley Hall, Chicheley, United Kingdom.

Bar-Kochva, I. (2016). An examination of an intervention program designed to enhance reading and spelling through the training of morphological decomposition in word recognition. *Scientific Studies of Reading, 20*, 163–172.

Bar-On, A., & Ravid, D. (2011). Morphological analysis in learning to read pseudowords in Hebrew. *Applied Psycholinguistics, 32*, 553–581.

Beidas, H., Khateb, A., & Breznitz, Z. (2013). The cognitive profile of adult dyslexics and its relation to their reading abilities. *Reading and Writing, 26*, 1487–1515.

Ben-Artzi, E., Fostick, L., & Babkoff, H. (2005). Deficits in temporal-order judgments in dyslexia: Evidence from dichotic stimuli differing spectrally and from dichotic stimuli differing only by perceived location. *Neuropsychologia, 43*, 714–723.

Ben-Dror, I., Bentin, S., & Frost, R. (1995). Semantic, phonologic, and morphologic skills in reading disabled and normal children: Evidence from perception and production of spoken Hebrew. *Reading Research Quarterly, 30*, 876–893.

Ben-Dror, I., Frost, R., & Bentin, S. (1995). Orthographic representation and phonemic segmentation in skilled readers: A cross-language comparison. *Psychological Science, 6*, 176–181.

Ben-Simon, A., & Inbar-Weiss, N. (2013). *MATAL: A computer-based test battery for the diagnosis of learning disabilities: User guide.* Jerusalem: National Institute for Testing and Evaluation NITE.

Bentin, S., Deutsch, A., & Liberman, I. Y. (1990). Syntactic competence and reading ability in children. *Journal of Experimental Child Psychology, 49*, 147–172.

Bentin, S., & Leshem, H. (1993). On the interaction between phonological awareness and reading acquisition: It's a two-way street. *Annals of Dyslexia, 43*, 125–148.

Ben-Yehudah, G., & Ahissar, M. (2004). Sequential spatial frequency discrimination is consistently impaired among adult dyslexics. *Vision Research, 44*, 1047–1063.

Ben-Yehudah, G., Sackett, E., Malchi-Ginzberg, L., & Ahissar, M. (2001). Impaired temporal contrast sensitivity in dyslexics is specific to retain-and-compare paradigms. *Brain, 124*, 1381–1395.

Berman, R. (1985). The acquisition of Hebrew. In D. I. Slobin (Ed.), *The cross-linguistic study of language acquisition* (pp. 255–371). Hillsdale, NJ: Erlbaum.

Bishop, D. V. M. (2015). The interface between genetics and psychology: Lessons from developmental dyslexia. *Proceedings of the Royal Society B, 282*(1806), 20143139.

Breznitz, Z. (2002a). Asynchrony of visual-orthographic and auditory-phonological word recognition processes: An underlying factor in dyslexia. *Reading and Writing, 15*, 15–42.

Breznitz, Z. (2002b). *The frequency of reading difficulties and characterization of reading disability in students from the fourth grade in the Jewish population in the state of Israel.* Report to the chief scientist of the Ministry of Education.

Breznitz, Z. (2006). *Fluency in reading: Synchronization of processes.* Mahwah, NJ: Lawrence Erlbaum.

Breznitz, Z., & Misra, M. (2003). Speed of processing of the visual–orthographic and auditory–phonological systems in adult dyslexics: The contribution of "asynchrony" to word recognition deficits. *Brain and Language, 85*, 486–502.

Breznitz, Z., Shaul, S., Horowitz-Kraus, T., Sela, I., Nevat, M., & Karni, A. (2013). Enhanced reading by training with imposed time constraint in typical and dyslexic adults. *Nature Communications, 4*, 1486.

Chase, C., & Stein, J. (2003). Visual magnocellular deficits in dyslexia. *Brain, 126*, e2.

Clark, L. A., Cuthbert, B., Lewis-Fernández, R., Narrow, W. E., & Reed, G. M. (2017). Three approaches to understanding and classifying mental disorder: ICD-11, DSM-5, and the National Institute of Mental Health's Research Domain Criteria (RDoC). *Psychological Science in the Public Interest, 18*, 72–145.

Cohen-Mimran, R. (2006). Temporal processing deficits in Hebrew speaking children with reading disabilities. *Journal of Speech, Language, and Hearing Research, 49*, 127–137.

Conner, P. S. (2013). *Novel spoken word learning in adults with developmental dyslexia.* Unpublished doctoral dissertation. The City University of New York.

Dahan, O., Melzer, Y., & Finkelstein, G. (2011). Changes in the integration of students with learning disabilities in higher education in Israel. In G. Avishar, Y. Laizer, & S. Reiter (Eds.), *Shiluvim (Integration): Education and society systems* (pp. 315–343). Haifa, Israel: Achva.

Dahan, O., & Russak, S. (2005). A support center for students with learning disabilities – community partnership. *Issues in Special Education and Rehabilitation, 20*(2), 85–92.

Dai, L., Zhang, C., & Liu, X. (2016). A special Chinese reading acceleration training paradigm to enhance the reading fluency and comprehension of Chinese children with reading disabilities. *Frontiers of Psychology, 7*, 1937.

D'Amato, R. C., Crepeau-Hobson, F., Huang, L. V., & Geil, M. (2005). Ecological neuropsychology: An alternative to the deficit model for conceptualizing and serving students with learning disabilities. *Neuropsychology review, 15*, 97–103.

Daniels, P. T. (1990). Fundamentals of grammatology. *Journal of the American Oriental Society, 110*, 727–731.

Daniels, P. T., & Bright, W. (Eds.). (1996). *The world's writing systems.* New York, NY: Oxford University Press.

Di Filippo, G., Zoccolotti, P., & Ziegler, J. C. (2008). Rapid naming deficits in dyslexia: A stumbling block for the perceptual anchor theory of dyslexia. *Developmental Science, 11*(6), 40–47.

Diringer, D. (1948). *The alphabet: A key to the history of mankind.* London: Thames & Hudson.

Faust, M., Dimitrovsky, L., & Shacht, T. (2003). Naming difficulties in children with dyslexia: Application of the tip of the tongue paradigm. *Journal of Learning Disabilities, 36*, 203–216.

Faust, M., & Sharfstein-Friedman, S. (2003). Naming difficulties in adolescents with dyslexia: Application of the tip-of-the-tongue paradigm. *Brain and Cognition, 53*, 211–217.

Fostick, L., Bar-El, S., & Ram-Tsur, R. (2012). Auditory temporal processing and working memory: Two independent deficits for dyslexia. *Psychology Research, 2*, 308–318.

Fostick, L., Eshcoly, R., Shtibelman, H., Nehemia, R., & Levi, H. (2014). Efficacy of temporal processing training to improve phonological awareness among dyslexic and normal reading students. *Journal of Experimental Psychology: Human Perception and Performance, 40*, 1799–1807.

Friedman. I., & Philosoph, S. (2001). *Standards in education systems* [in Hebrew]. Jerusalem: Henrietta Szold Institute.

Frost, R., & Bentin, S. (1992). Processing phonological and semantic ambiguity: Evidence from semantic priming at different SOAs. *Journal of Experimental Psychology: Learning, Memory, and Cognition, 18*, 58–68.

Frost, R., Forster, K. I., & Deutsch, A. (1997). What can we learn from the morphology of Hebrew? A masked-priming investigation of morphological representation. *Journal of Experimental Psychology: Learning, Memory, and Cognition, 23*, 829–856.

Gabay, Y., Gabay, S., Schiff, R., Ashkenazi, S., & Henik, A. (2013). Visuospatial attention deficits in developmental dyslexia: evidence from visual and mental number line bisection tasks. *Archives of Clinical Neuropsychology, 28*, 829–836.

Gabay, Y., & Holt, L. L. (2015). Incidental learning of sound categories is impaired in developmental dyslexia. *Cortex, 73*, 131–143.

Gabay, Y., Schiff, R., & Vakil, E. (2012a). Attentional requirements during acquisition and consolidation of a skill in normal readers and developmental dyslexics. *Neuropsychology, 26*, 744–757.

Gabay, Y., Schiff, R., & Vakil, E. (2012b). Dissociation between online and offline learning in developmental dyslexia. *Journal of Clinical and Experimental Neuropsychology, 34*, 279–288.

Gabay, Y., Schiff, R., & Vakil, E. (2012c). Dissociation between the procedural learning of letter names and motor sequences in developmental dyslexia. *Neuropsychologia, 50*, 2435–2441.

Gabay, Y., Thiessen, E. D., & Holt, L. L. (2015). Impaired statistical learning in developmental dyslexia. *Journal of Speech, Language, and Hearing Research, 58*, 934–945.

Gumpel, T. P. (1999). Special education towards the second millennium: Where have we come from and where are we going? [in Hebrew]. *Issues in Special Education and Rehabilitation, 14*(2), 71–82.

Gumpel, T. P., & Sharoni, V. (2007). Current best practices in learning disabilities in Israel. *Learning Disabilities Research & Practice, 22*, 202–209.

Heth, I., & Lavidor, M. (2015). Improved reading measures in adults with dyslexia following transcranial direct current stimulation treatment. *Neuropsychologia, 70*, 107–113.

Horowitz-Kraus, T., & Breznitz, Z. (2014). Can reading rate acceleration improve error monitoring and cognitive abilities underlying reading in adolescents with reading difficulties and in typical readers? *Brain Research, 1544*, 1–14.

Horowitz-Kraus, T., Cicchino, N., Amiel, M., Holland, S. K., & Breznitz, Z. (2014). Reading improvement in English and Hebrew-Speaking children with reading difficulties after reading acceleration training. *Annals of Dyslexia, 64*(3), 183–201.

Kahta, S., & Schiff, R. (2016). Implicit learning deficits among adults with developmental dyslexia. *Annals of Dyslexia, 66,* 235–250.

Kaminsky, M., Eviatar, Z., & Norman, J. (2002). The timing deficit hypothesis of dyslexia and its implications for Hebrew reading. *Brain and Cognition, 48,* 394–398.

Kasperski, R., Shany, M., & Katzir, T. (2016). The role of RAN and reading rate in predicting reading self-concept. *Reading and Writing, 29,* 117–136.

Katzir, T., Kim, Y. S., Wolf, M., Morris, R., & Lovett, M. W. (2008). The varieties of pathways to dysfluent reading: Comparing subtypes of children with dyslexia at letter, word, and connected text levels of reading. *Journal of Learning Disabilities, 41,* 47–66.

Katzir, T., Lesaux, N. K., & Kim, Y. S. (2009). The role of reading self-concept and home literacy practices in fourth grade reading comprehension. *Reading and Writing, 22,* 261–276.

Katzir, T., Markovich, V., Tesler, E., & Shany. M. (2018). Self-regulation and reading comprehension: Self-perceptions, self-evaluations, and effective strategies for intervention. In L. Meltzer (Ed.), *Executive function in education: From theory to practice* (pp. 240–262). New York, NY: The Guilford Press.

Leikin, M., & Assayag Bouskila, O. (2004). Expression of syntactic complexity in sentence comprehension: A comparison between dyslexic and regular readers. *Reading and Writing, 17,* 801–822.

Leikin, M., & Even-Zur, H. (2006). Morphological processing in adult dyslexia. *Journal of Psycholinguistic Research, 35,* 471–490.

Lum, J. A., Ullman, M. T., & Conti-Ramsden, G. (2013). Procedural learning is impaired in dyslexia: Evidence from a meta-analysis of serial reaction time studies. *Research in Developmental Disabilities, 34,* 3460–3476.

Margalit, M. (1997*). Report of the public committee to explore the advancement of abilities among Students with learning disabilities.* Report submitted to the Ministry of Education, Culture, and Science. Jerusalem: Ministry of Education, Culture and Science.

Margalit, M. (2000). *Report of a committee for examination of implementation of the law for special education (Margalit Report).* Jerusalem: Ministry of Education.

MATAL. (2007). *A computer-based test battery for the diagnosis of learning disabilities (2007).* Jerusalem: National institute for Testing and Evaluation and the Council of Higher Education in Israel.

Meer, Y., Breznitz, Z., & Katzir, T. (2016). Calibration of self-reports of anxiety and physiological measures of anxiety while reading in adults with and without reading disability. *Dyslexia, 22,* 267–284.

Meltzer, Y. (2003). *A plan of Renovation and equipping a support center building for Learning Disabilities students* (unpublished). Jerusalem: National Insurance Institute. Fund for developing services for disabled people.

Miller-Shaul, S. (2005). The characteristics of young and adult dyslexics readers on reading and reading related cognitive tasks as compared to normal readers. *Dyslexia, 11,* 132–151.

Ministry of Education. (2016). *From disabilities to learning. System plan for intervention for students with learning disabilities and ADHD.* Jerusalem: Ministry of Education.

Oganian, Y., & Ahissar, M. (2012). Poor anchoring limits dyslexics' perceptual, memory, and reading skills. *Neuropsychologia, 50,* 1895–1905.

Pennington, B. F. (2006). From single to multiple deficit models of developmental disorders. *Cognition, 101*, 385–413.

Ram-Tsur, R., Faust, M., & Zivotofsky, A. Z. (2006). Sequential processing deficits of reading disabled persons is independent of inter-stimulus interval. *Vision Research, 46*, 3949–3960.

Ram-Tsur, R., Faust, M., & Zivotofsky, A. Z. (2008). Poor performance on serial visual tasks in persons with reading disabilities impaired working memory? *Journal of Learning Disabilities, 41*, 437–450.

Ramus, F., Rosen, S., Dakin, S. C., Day, B. L., Castellote, J. M., White, S., & Frith, U. (2003). Theories of developmental dyslexia: insights from a multiple case study of dyslexic adults. *Brain, 126*, 841–865.

Raveh, M., & Schiff, R. (2008). Visual and auditory morphological priming in adults with developmental dyslexia. *Scientific Studies of Reading, 12*, 221–252.

Ravid, D. (1990). Internal structure constraints on new-word formation devices in Modern Hebrew. *Folia Linguistica, 24*(3–4), 289–346.

Ravid, D. (1996). Accessing the mental lexicon: Evidence from incompatibility between representation of spoken and written morphology. *Linguistics, 34*, 1219–1246.

Ravid, D. (2012). *Spelling morphology.* New York, NY: Springer.

Rubinsten, O., & Henik, A. (2006). Double dissociation of functions in developmental dyslexia and dyscalculia. *Journal of Educational Psychology, 98*, 854–867.

Schiff, R., Cohen, M., Ben-Artzi, Sasson, A., & Ravid, D. (2016). Auditory morphological knowledge among children with developmental dyslexia. *Scientific Studies of Reading, 20*, 140–154.

Schiff, R., & Raveh, M. (2007). Deficient morphological processing in adults with developmental dyslexia: Another barrier to efficient word recognition? *Dyslexia, 13*, 110–129.

Schiff, R., & Ravid, D. (2004). Representing written vowels in university students with dyslexia compared with normal Hebrew readers. *Annals of Dyslexia, 54*, 39–64.

Schiff, R., & Ravid, D. (2007). Morphological analogies in Hebrew-speaking university students with dyslexia compared with typically developing grade schoolers. *Journal of Psycholinguistic Research, 36*, 237–253.

Schiff, R., & Ravid, D. (2013). Morphological processing in Hebrew-speaking students with reading disabilities. *Journal of Learning Disabilities, 46*, 220–229. doi: http://dx .doi.org/10.1177/0022219412449425.

Schiff, R., Schwartz-Nahshon, S., & Nagar, R. (2011). Effect of phonological and morphological awareness on reading comprehension in Hebrew-speaking adolescents with reading disabilities. *Annals of Dyslexia, 61*, 44–63.

Sela, I., & Karni, A. (2012). Differences in learning volitional (manual) and non-volitional (posture) aspects of a complex motor skill in young adult dyslexic and skilled readers. *PLoS One, 7*(9): e43488. doi: http://dx.doi.org/10.1371/journal .pone.0043488.

Shalev-Leifer, C. (2016). *On the link between developmental dyslexia and specific language impairment in Hebrew: Cognitive and psycholinguistic aspects.* Unpublished doctoral dissertation. University of Haifa.

Shany, M., & Breznitz, Z. (2011). Rate- and accuracy-disabled subtype profiles among adults with dyslexia in the Hebrew orthography. *Developmental Neuropsychology, 36*, 889–913.

Shany, M., Lachman, D., Shalem, Z., Bahat, A., & Zeiger, T. (2006). *"Aleph-Taph" – a test for the diagnosis of reading and writing disabilities, based on national Israeli norms*. Tel Aviv: Yesod Publishing.

Shany, M., & Share, D. L. (2011). Subtypes of reading disability in a shallow orthography: A double dissociation between accuracy-disabled and rate-disabled reading in Hebrew. *Annals of Dyslexia, 61*, 64–84.

Share, D. L. (1995). Phonological recoding and self-teaching: Sine qua non of reading acquisition. *Cognition, 55*, 151–218.

Share, D. L. (2003). Dyslexia in Hebrew. In N. Goulandris (Ed.), *Dyslexia in different languages: Cross-linguistic comparisons* (pp. 208–234). London: Whurr.

Share, D. L. (2004). Orthographic learning at a glance: On the time course and developmental onset of self-teaching. *Journal of Experimental Child Psychology, 87*, 267–298.

Share, D. L., & Bar-On, A. (2017). Learning to read a Semitic Abjad: The Triplex model of Hebrew reading development. *Journal of Learning Disabilities. Advance online publication.* doi: http://dx.doi.org/10.1177/0022219417718198.

Shaul, S. (2014). Visual, auditory and cross modal lexical decision: A comparison between dyslexic and typical readers. *Psychology, 5*, 1855–1869. doi: http://dx.doi.org/10.4236/psych.2014.516191.

Shovman, M. M., & Ahissar, M. (2006). Isolating the impact of visual perception on dyslexics' reading ability. *Vision Research, 46*, 3514–3525.

Simpson, S. (1983). *Dyslexia theory and practice, assessment and enhancement of reading disability.* Tel Aviv: Ramot Publication.

Special Education Law. (2002). *Instructions, chapter D1 for Special Education Law, 4763* [Correction number 7 for Special Education Law, 1988].

Tallal, P. (1980). Auditory temporal perception, phonics, and reading disabilities in children. *Brain and language, 9*, 182–198.

Vogel, S. A., Vogel, G., Sharoni, V., & Dahan, O. (Eds.). (2003). *Learning disabilities in higher education and beyond: An international perspective.* Baltimore, MD: York Press.

Willburger, E., & Landerl, K. (2010). Anchoring the deficit of the anchor deficit: Dyslexia or attention? *Dyslexia, 16*, 175–182.

Wolf, M., & Bowers, P. G. (1999). The double-deficit hypothesis for the developmental dyslexias. *Journal of Educational Psychology, 91*, 415–438.

Yunay, Y. (1992). The 1988 National Special Education Law. *Education of special education students.* Jerusalem: Ministry of Education and Culture.

Ziegler, J. C. (2008). Better to lose the anchor than the whole ship. *Trends in Cognitive Sciences, 12*, 244–245.

9 Developmental Dyslexia in Japanese

Taeko N. Wydell

9.1 Introduction

In this chapter, language universality and language specificity of reading processes especially in Japanese are discussed with a special focus given to typical and atypical literacy acquisition/development by Japanese children. First, a brief introduction to the Japanese writing systems is provided: the syllabic Hiragana and Katakana and the morphographic Kanji. Second, research into the cognitive processes involved in reading Kana and Kanji is introduced, including a discussion on how whole-word-level and sub-word-level processes contribute to the computation of phonology from Kana and Kanji from a language-universality perspective. Third, the prevalence of reading impairments amongst Japanese children is discussed, including how their reading impairments (dyslexia) are manifested in reading Kana and Kanji, drawing attention to the fact that different orthographies manifest children's reading difficulties differently, linking this to the language specificity. Finally, differences in the neural correlates of reading in different orthographies as well as in dyslexic and normal readers are discussed.

9.2 Learning to Read Japanese

9.2.1 Japanese Language and Its Orthographies

Japanese is an S-O-V syllabic language with limited numbers of subtle pitch accents; e.g., the pitch accent on the first mora (syllable-like unit), /**ha**-shi/ (chopsticks) versus the pitch accent on the second mora, /ha-**shi**/ (bridge). It has a simple sound system that consists of five vowels and sixteen consonants. From this small inventory of phonemes a limited number (110) of simple rhythmic syllabic units (morae) can be built up with constant durations of uttering. Given that Japanese phonology does not discriminate tonal differences in Sino-Japanese words, dependence on Kanji, which is derived from Chinese characters, emerged.

As a result, Japanese orthography consists of two qualitatively different writing systems: logographic, morphographic Kanji, derived from Chinese characters, and two forms of syllabic Kana, Hiragana and Katakana, whose visual forms are derived from Kanji characters (see Sampson, 1985; Wydell & Butterworth, 1999; Wydell, Butterworth, & Patterson, 1995; Wydell, Patterson, & Humphreys, 1993, for more details). Chinese and Japanese contrast linguistically in several ways. Chinese is tonal, with a Subject-Verb-Object (SVO) ordering.

Kana characters were thus derived from Kanji characters in order to transcribe the Japanese language effectively (Takebe, 1979). The Kana characters can encode all Japanese words; however, each Kana transcribes different classes of words.

9.2.1.1 Hiragana and Katakana   Hiragana characters are used mainly for function words, e.g., し か し /shi-ka-shi/ (but); そ し て /so-shi-te/ (and) as well as the inflections of verbs, e.g., 働 く /hatara-ku/ (work), adjectives, e.g., 美 し い / utsuku-shi-i/ (beautiful), and adverbs, e.g., 忙 し く /isoga-shi-ku/ (busily). Also, some nouns with uncommon Kanji representations, i.e., exception words analogous to *yacht* in English – e.g., か か し /ka-ka-shi/ (scarecrow) written in Kanji as 案山子 /an-san-shi/, where the correct reading of this particular Kanji word has to be learned as a whole word – are often transcribed in Hiragana.

Katakana characters are used for the large number of foreign loan words in contemporary Japanese, e.g. テ レ ビ /te-re-bi/ (TV); カ メ ラ /ka-me-ra/ (camera), and for transcribing onomatopoetic words, e.g., ワ ン ワ ン /wa-n-wa-n/ (dog's bark); ニ ャ ー ニ ャ ー /nya-a-nya-a/ (cat's meowing).

Both forms of Kana have an almost perfect one-to-one relationship between character and pronunciation. That is, one Kana character always represents one particular mora/syllable of the Japanese language, and its sound value does not change whether the character appears in the first position, the middle position, or at the end of a multisyllable word. Hence, the relationship between character and pronunciation is very transparent. This is different from English, where orthographic units not only map onto sub-syllabic phonological units, but the mapping will also depend on context, i.e. the location within the word.

For both Hiragana and Katakana, there are forty-six basic Kana characters (Takebe, 1979) but with diacritical marks, either " or o, e.g., は ・ ハ /ha/ → ば ・ パ /pa/ → ば ・ バ /ba/ and others e.g., **Yoon** (contracted sounds) き ゃ ・ キ ャ /kya/; し ゅ ・ シ ュ /shu/, and **Sokuon** (germinations) き っ て ・ キ ッ テ / kitte/. Thus all the 110 moraic sounds which exist in the Japanese language can be transcribed.

9.2.1.2 Kanji   Kanji characters are used for nouns, which are not inflected in Japanese e.g., 机 /tsukue/ (desk); 大学 /dai-gaku/ (university) and for the root morphemes of inflected verbs, adjectives, and adverbs e.g., 働く /hatara-ku/ (work), 美しい /utsuku-shi-i/ (beautiful), and 忙しく /isoga-shi-ku/ (busily) respectively.

In contrast to Kana, Kanji characters are at the other extreme end of the transparency continuum. That is, the relationship between character and pronunciation in Kanji is very opaque. This is because each Kanji character is a morphographic element that cannot phonetically be decomposed in the way that an alphabetic word can be. There are no separate components of a character that correspond to the individual phonemes (see Wydell et al., 1995, for a further discussion). Words in Kanji have 1–5 characters, with 2 being the modal number, and 2.4 the mean (Yokosawa & Umeda, 1988).

Further, most Kanji characters have one or more ON-readings (pronunciations that were imported from the spoken Chinese language along with their corresponding characters) as well as a KUN-reading from the original Japanese spoken language. Some characters have no KUN-reading, but for those which have, the KUN-reading is almost always the correct reading when this character constitutes a word on its own. For example, the character 花, pronounced as /hana/ in KUN-reading, is a single-character word (flower). Also, the same KUN-reading can be seen in two-character words such as 花束 /**hana**-taba/ (bouquet), or 花屋 /**hana**-ya/ (florist). However, the same character is also pronounced as /ka/ in ON-reading as in 花瓶 /**ka**-bin/ (vase) or 花粉 /**ka**-fun/ (pollen). Note that the majority of the Japanese words are multi-morae (syllable) words.

Moreover, the Chinese words, once introduced into the Japanese language, lost their original Chinese accents/tones, because Japanese is not a tonal language. Consequently there are many homophones in ON-reading Kanji characters/words, which in the original Chinese could be distinguished from each other by tones/accents. For example, the character pronunciation, /**ka**/ has at least fourteen different ON-reading homophonic characters: 火, 化, 可, 香, 家, 課, 科, 蚊, 架, 貨, 歌, 加, 華, 価, and so on.

As with Chinese characters, some Kanji characters contain phonetic or semantic radicals. However, the phonetic radicals are not necessarily an accurate guide to the correct pronunciation. For example, the phonetic radicals give no clue at all to KUN-reading, and in a sample of 1668 commonly used Kanji characters analysed by Saito, Kawakami, and Matsuda (1995), only 32 per cent have ON-readings identical to their phonetic radicals. Similarly, semantic radicals do not necessarily lead to the actual meanings of characters (as is true in Chinese). For example, the character, 魚 meaning 'fish' (/sakana/ in KUN-reading and /gyo/ in ON-reading) can be a semantic radical seen in many fish-related Kanji words, e.g., 鯛 /tai/ (sea bream), 鱸/Suzuki/ (sea bass), or 鯵/ aji/ (horse mackerel). It is clear from these examples that these characters are all something to do with 'fish', but they cannot lead us to the retrievals of the correct names of the fish.

9.2.2   Learning to Read in Japanese

Given the syllabic/moraic Kana and morphographic Kanji link to spoken Japanese through different mappings, it is reasonable to assume Kana and Kanji require different weightings for the whole-word-level and the sub-word-level contributions in the computation of phonology from the respective writing systems.

9.2.2.1   Learning to Read Kana
In the first year of primary-school education (aged 7), Hiragana is taught first and then Katakana. Because of the transparent Kana character-to-pronunciation relationship, i.e., one character represents a whole syllable/mora, children master both Kana writing systems very quickly. Most children learn the Hiragana even before they start primary-school education (Gibson & Levin, 1975; Makita, 1968; Muraishi, 1972; Sakamoto & Makita, 1973).

Cognitive behavioural studies of Kana reading with adult participants revealed that both whole-word lexical reading and sequential character-by-character sub-lexical reading processes are taking place (e.g., Besner & Hilderbrandt, 1987; Rastle et al., 2009) in reading Kana. For example, Besner and Hilderbrandt (1987) showed a significant lexicality effect in reading Katakana. Reaction times (RTs) for Katakana real words were significantly shorter than pronounceable Katakana non-words, showing word-level processing in Kana reading. Similarly, Rastle et al. (2009) showed both lexicality and word-frequency effects in reading Hiragana and Katakana words and non-words, thus showing a word-level familiarity effect in both Hiragana and Katakana reading. RTs for real words in Hiragana and Katakana were significantly shorter than those for Hiragana transcriptions of Katakana words and Katakana transcriptions of Hiragana words, and RTs for high-frequency words were shorter than those for low-frequency words in reading Hiragana and Katakana respectively.

Further, Rastle et al. (2009) also found significant length effects for both word and Katakana/Hiragana transcription stimuli in reading Hiragana and Katakana. The stimuli were divided into equal groups of 3, 4, 5, or 6 morae for two word conditions (i.e., Hiragana, Katakana) and two pseudo-word conditions (i.e., Hiragana transcriptions of Katakana words and Katakana transcriptions of Hiragana words respectively). The length effect was substantially larger in Katakana or Hiragana transcriptions than Hiragana or Katakana real words. Rastle et al. noted that some research suggested that sub-lexical processing may be particularly strong in languages with shallower orthographies (e.g., Frost, Kats, & Bentin, 1987; Wydell et al., 2003), adding that if the length effect arose because of a serial character-by-character sub-lexical process, this could explain why a particularly strong length effect for words was also observed.

Because of the transparent relationship between Kana and pronunciation, it is reasonable to assume that reading Kana leads to the use of sub-word syllabic processing, which is reliable and requires no orthographic segmentation or phonological blending (Wydell & Butterworth, 1999). Therefore, it is also reasonable to assume that Japanese children will not show reading difficulties in Kana, as the research shows. This will be discussed further later in this chapter.

9.2.2.2 Learning to Read Kanji   Given the characteristics of Kanji described earlier, it is reasonable to assume that Kanji character learning is at the level of whole characters, if not at the whole-word level. Kanji learning is essentially by rote: Children are introduced to new Kanji characters in texts. The learning method commonly in use at school is repeated writing (Kusumi, 1992) or rehearsal by writing (Naka & Naoi, 1995) including Kusho, which literally means 'write in the air' (see Sasaki, 1987, for a more detailed account of Kusho). Repeated writing allows children to develop a motor memory of the correct sequence of strokes for any given Kanji character. This strategy is often observed amongst the Japanese, especially amongst Japanese children learning new Kanji characters (e.g., Mann, 1985; Onose, 1987, 1988).

Importantly, Japanese children are not taught to analyse the components of Kanji characters, phonetic radicals, and semantic radicals, until they are at junior high school level (age 13 to 15). This is partly because the children learn simple characters first, and these do not contain phonetic or semantic radicals. Moreover, as described above, even when they learn complex Kanji characters, which contain both phonetic and semantic radicals, these radicals are not necessarily an accurate guide to the correct pronunciation or the correct meaning of a Kanji word (Saito et al., 1995).

During the six years of primary-school education, children are introduced to 996 different Kanji characters, which are prescribed in the Gakunenbetsu kanji haito hyo (the list of Kanji characters to be learned by Japanese primary-school children for each grade from Grade 1 to Grade 6) by the Japanese Ministry of Education (now the Japanese Ministry of Education and Science). By the end of compulsory education (aged 16), a total of slightly more than 2,000 Kanji characters have been learned, always from context. It should be noted, though, that adults need some 3,000 characters for most everyday literacy activities, e.g. reading a national newspaper (National Language Research Institute, 1976).

Cognitive behavioural studies of Kanji reading by adults also revealed both whole-word lexical and character-level sub-lexical processing, although the effect size of the latter is substantially smaller than the former (e.g., Kondo & Wydell, 2011). For example, Kanji word-naming or semantic-judgement experiments invariably showed significant word-frequency or word-familiarity effects, indicating the involvement of whole-word lexical processes (e.g., Fushimi et al., 1999; Kondo & Wydell, 2011; Patterson, Suzuki, & Wydell, 1996; Patterson et al., 1995; Shibahara et al., 2003; Wydell, Butterworth, & Patterson, 1995; Wydell et al., 1993).

Shibahara et al. (2003) found not only a significant word-frequency effect but also a significant *imageability effect* during naming of two-character Kanji words. Both effects are indicative of whole-word level processes in the computation of Kanji word phonology. Shibahara et al. also reported a similar experiment in English, following Strain, Patterson, and Seidenberg (1995). Similar to the experiment with Kanji words, the results showed a significant imageability effect in reading English. However, this effect was significantly stronger in Kanji compared to English.

Furthermore, Patterson et al. (1995) reported a case study of progressive aphasia due to Alzheimer's disease, revealing Legitimate Alternative Reading of Component (LARC) errors in naming two-character Kanji words, whereby the pronunciation of one or more components is inappropriate for the target word but is nonetheless legitimate, and often more typical for words containing the character. Similar LARC errors in another progressive aphasic patient were reported by Fushimi and colleagues (2003). These LARC errors thus indicate character-by-character sub-lexical reading processes, although neither Patterson et al. (1995) nor Fushimi et al. (2003) interpreted the data in terms of the lexical versus sub-lexical reading-processing dichotomy.

Moreover, following Wydell et al.'s (1995) report on the null effect of print-to-sound consistency during reading of Kanji words, Fushimi et al. (1999) showed a small but significant consistency effect in naming Kanji words. Namely, consistent Kanji words, i.e., those two-character Kanji words for which each constituent character of Kanji has only a single ON-reading, yielded shorter naming latencies, and lower error rates than inconsistent Kanji words, i.e., those two-character words for which either one or both characters have a KUN-reading, but a target word takes an ON-reading. The results indicated that sub-word level of constituent character plays a major role in computing the pronunciation of Kanji words. Consistency in two-character Kanji words in these studies was defined as follows: Consistent Kanji words were those in which neither constituent character had an alternative ON-reading or a KUN-reading, hence there could be no pronunciation ambiguity for these words. The inconsistent Kanji words were ON-reading words composed of characters that had KUN-readings that were appropriate to other words in which the characters occur, hence there would be some ambiguity about the pronunciation of the constituent characters (see Wydell et al., 1995 or Fushimi et al., 1999, for further details).

These studies with Japanese Kanji words as stimuli were prompted by many studies in English that have addressed this question, i.e. the effects of spelling-to-sound regularity/consistency in reading (e.g., Andrews, 1982; Glushko, 1979; Jared, 2002; Stanhope & Parkin, 1987; Taraban & McClelland, 1987). According to Glushko (1979), in English, ' . . . consistency rather than rule-defined regularity, provided a better account of empirical results. Although *five* may be a regular word "by rule," its spelling-sound relationship is inconsistent with orthographically similar words such as *give . . . .*' (as cited in Wydell et al., 1995, p. 1155). The fact that inconsistent English words produced longer RTs and were more prone to errors during naming than consistent words suggests that sub-lexical processing plays a significant role in the computation of word pronunciation.

Thus, it appears that the computation of a word's pronunciation in both Japanese Kanji and English has contributions from both whole-word and sub-word levels. The whole-word-level effect is demonstrated by the fact that the consistency effect is modulated by word frequency; i.e., when the frequency of the stimulus words was high, naming latencies were more or less the same regardless of whether the stimuli were consistent or inconsistent.

The presence (Fushimi et al., 1999) or the absence (Wydell et al., 1995) of consistency effects in reading two-character Kanji words may result largely from differences in the experimental paradigms and subsequent statistical analyses. The significant consistency effects in Fushimi et al. (1999) emerged only when the analyses were conducted on the difference of RTs as well as error rates between the immediate-naming task and the delayed-naming task. More recently, the discrepancy between the results obtained by Fushimi et al. (1999) and Wydell et al. (1995) has been resolved by Kondo and Wydell (2011), who conducted immediate and delayed-naming experiments similar to those of Fushimi and colleagues (1999), but with 1,000 two-character Kanji word stimuli as opposed to the 120 two-character Kanji word stimuli used by Fushimi et al. (1999), varying the degree of word familiarity and consistency amongst several other variables. The stimuli were carefully constructed with the use of the NTT Psycholinguistic Database Series (Amano & Kondo, 1999). Similar to the results obtained by Fushimi et al. (1999), a small but statistically significant consistency effect in the latencies as well as the error rates was observed. However, more importantly, the results also revealed that the effect size of word-level contribution, e.g., word familiarity and frequency, was far greater than that of sub-word level contribution in reading Kanji words.

Thus, reading logographic Kanji may require a greater weighting for the whole-word-level contribution in the computation of phonology from orthography, as the relationship between orthography (Kanji) and phonology (pronunciation) is opaque. Learning to read in Kanji appears to be more laborious, and cognitively more demanding than that in Kana. This is further discussed later.

9.3   Developmental Dyslexia in Japanese

9.3.1   Historical and Cultural Context

Having to master not just one but two different writing systems, namely Kanji and Kana (Hiragana and Katakana), possibly three if Romanji (the Roman alphabet) is included, it might be reasonable to assume that Japanese children would experience greater difficulty in learning to read (and write) than English-speaking children learning to read in English using the English alphabet. However, in Japan it was initially reported, in the early days of dyslexia research, that the prevalence of reading difficulties or dyslexia was low, and did not warrant special educational support. In fact, the concept of dyslexia was relatively unknown in Japan until ten to fifteen years ago.

It was Makita (1968) who first claimed through his nationwide survey that, in Japan, less than 0.1 per cent of children had a reading disability. Similarly, several researchers (e.g., Muraishi, 1972; Sakamoto & Makita, 1973) presented evidence for the ease with which the Japanese writing systems are learned. These researchers all attributed the high rate of literacy to the characteristics of Japanese orthography. A more recent longitudinal nationwide survey across 325 primary schools in Japan conducted by the Japanese National Research Institute of Special Education (1996) also revealed that less than 2 per cent of the children showed reading delay/impairment by the time they reached sixth grade (aged 12), the final grade in primary-school education. The survey revealed that for reading, the percentage of children with reading delay (at least by 24 months) decreased as they progressed to higher grades, i.e., 2.28, 1.80, 1.56, 1.39, and 1.08 per cent for Grade 2, 3, 4, 5, and 6, respectively.[1] These figures are higher than those found in the earlier studies, but still lower than that reported (10–12 per cent) in the English-speaking world (e.g., Shaywitz et al., 1990; Snowling, 2000). It should however be pointed out that these studies were based on questionnaires on children's reading and writing attainments completed by their teachers, and hence lacked objectivity.

In contrast, some studies objectively measured reading ability in Japanese children. Stevenson et al. (1982), tested Grade 5 primary-school children's reading abilities in the USA, Japan, and Taiwan. Children in all three countries showed performance of at least two grades below that of average Grade 5 children, and the percentage of these children in the USA, Japan, and Taiwan were 6.3 per cent, 5.4 per cent, and 7.5 per cent respectively. Similarly, Hirose

---

[1] For writing, these were 4.45, 3.13, 2.85, 2.19, and 1.81 per cent for Grade 2, 3, 4, 5, and 6 respectively. Thus, more children had difficulty in writing than reading (cited by Wydell, 2003). This is the same as normal adults: according to Morton and Sasanuma (1984), a Japanese adult's ability to write Kanji characters/words is up to 30 per cent lower than their ability to read the same characters/words.

and Hatta (1985) tested 250 children (aged 8.5 to 13.4) in Japan using Kitao's (1984) standardised test for the reading ability of 8 to 13 years old. It was found that 16.5 per cent of the cohort showed a 12-month delay, and 15.2 per cent showed more than a 24-month delay.

9.3.1.1   Identification and Prevalence of Dyslexia   The above studies are, however, typically concerned with children's reading comprehension, and the test items did not include any single-word-reading tests where no contextual information can be utilised when reading. As Wydell and colleagues pointed out (Wydell & Butterworth, 1999; Wydell & Kondo, 2003), single-word-reading tests are generally used as a diagnostic tool to identify children with reading difficulties, and, therefore, Stevenson et al.'s (1982) or Hirose and Hatta's (1985) study do not provide conclusive evidence for the prevalence of reading difficulties or dyslexia amongst Japanese children.

In order to rectify the shortcomings of these previous studies, Uno et al. (2009) employed an objective paradigm and tested nearly 500 Japanese primary-school children, from Grades 2 to 6, not only for their abilities to read and write single characters/words in Hiragana, Katakana, and Kanji as well as for their vocabulary, but also for other cognitive abilities including arithmetic, visual-spatial, and phonological processing skills. This study led to the development of the first standardised Screening Test of Reading and Writing for Japanese primary-school children, STRAW (Uno et al., 2006–2016).[2] Following other studies (e.g., Shaywitz et al., 1990) in this study the children whose reading or writing test scores were below –1.5 SD[3] were considered as reading disabled (RD) children or writing disabled (WD) children. There was no difference in IQ measured by Raven's Coloured Progressive Matrices (Raven, 1976) between the normal readers' group and the reading disabled and writing disabled (RWD) children's group.

Uno and colleagues (2009) found that the percentage of RD children in the cohort differed greatly according to the writing system –0.4 per cent for Hiragana, 1.4 per cent for Katakana, and 6.9 per cent for Kanji respectively, and that the percentage of WD children similarly differed –1.6 per cent for Hiragana, 3.8 per cent for Katakana, and 6.1 per cent for Kanji. Note that the Kanji stimulus words for each grade were chosen from those that the children

---

[2] The 'STRAW' was developed based on over 1,000 children's data, and is a systematic/comprehensive tool for diagnosing children with dyslexia across primary schools in Japan. The test also identifies areas of cognitive deficits, enabling appropriate intervention programmes to be tailored for each dyslexic child's needs. As the first and only standardised test available, nearly 9,000 institutions in Japan use STRAW, including educational authorities, primary schools, schools for special-needs education, local children's welfare centres, hospitals, clinics, and universities.

[3] Because we used the –1.5SD as the cut-off, statistically speaking, 6.7 per cent of the children in the cohort should be expected to be RD or WD for any given reading/writing tests, if the data are normally distributed.

had learned 12 months earlier. These figures were higher than those found in the earlier studies, but still lower than that reported in the English-speaking world (e.g., Shaywitz et al., 1990; Snowling, 2000).

Thus, Uno, and colleagues (2009) were the first researchers to show the occurrence of RD (and WD) amongst Japanese children across the three different writing systems used in Japan through objective measures.[4] The data are also indicative of the fact that reading Kanji may require different reading strategies, e.g., word-level rather than sub-word-level of reading processes, as discussed earlier, or even different cognitive skills to those required for reading Kana.

9.4   Behavioural and Neurocognitive Evidence

9.4.1   Nature of Reading Problems in Japanese

The majority of children in Japan who are classified as having a learning disability (LD) have both reading and writing difficulties, and often the writing impairment is more severe than the reading impairment. Significantly, there are very few reported cases of children with reading impairments only. The Japanese researchers usually attribute these reading and writing impairments amongst children to 'visual' or 'visuospatial' processing problems rather than phonological processing problems (e.g., Kaneko et al., 1997; Uno, Kaga, & Inagaki, 1995; Uno & Kamibayashi, 1998).

Wei et al. (2014) investigated the relationship between Chinese (another morphographic writing system) reading skills and metalinguistic awareness skills e.g., phonological, morphological, and orthographic awareness skills, with a large cohort of normally developing preschool and Grades 1, 2, and 3 children in mainland China. Their results were that all three metalinguistic awareness skills significantly predicted reading success. In addition, orthographic awareness played a dominant role in the early stages of reading acquisition, and its influence was reduced with age, while the opposite was true for the morphological awareness. Indeed, several studies argued that the major cause of developmental dyslexia in Chinese is a deficit in orthographic processing skills, rather than in phonological processing skills (e.g., Chan et al., 2006; Ho et al., 2004). These results contrast with the many studies in English (reviewed elsewhere in this volume) that find phonological awareness to be the single most potent variable in literacy acquisition.

---

[4] It is also worth noting that for RD and WD children together, the ratio between the boys and girls in the cohort was 2.7:1, which is consistent with the results of other studies in English (Halpern, 1992; Share et al., 1987), but inconsistent with the ratio between adult males and females showing a more even distribution of dyslexia (e.g., National Working Party on Dyslexia in Higher Education, 1999; Richardson & Wydell, 2003).

The Uno et al. (2009) study included a series of regression analyses on the data from the normal and the RWD (RD and WD children combined) groups separately, in order to ascertain which tests, including the Standardised Comprehension Test of Abstract Words (SCTAW) developed by Haruhara and Kaneko (2003) were more closely related to Kanji word-reading or -writing performance. Table 9.1 shows the results of step-wise regression analyses with reading Kanji words as the dependent variable, when the normal reader's data were dichotomised as younger children (Grades 2 & 3, and Grades 2, 3, & 4, respectively) and older children (Grades 4, 5, & 6, and Grades 5 & 6, respectively).

It is clear from Table 9.1 that, in general, vocabulary development (SCTAW) was closely related to performance on reading Kanji words – an increase in vocabulary size led to an improved performance in Kanji word reading. This was in accordance with a view that reading is a secondary linguistic skill (e.g., Mattingley, 1972), and that reading is acquired through spoken language

Table 9.1 *Results of multiple regression analyses for normal readers: Younger versus older children – Reading Kanji words as a dependent variable*

Grades-2 & 3			Grades-4, 5, & 6		
(N=135)	R^2	(p<.05)	(N=296)	R^2	(p<.05)
(h)	0.29		(h)	0.14	
(k)	0.43		(f)	0.19	
(b)	0.46		(k)	0.22	
(f)	0.49		(c)	0.23	
(n)	0.50				
Grades-2, 3 & 4			Grades-5 & 6		
(N=235)	R^2	(p<.05)	(N=196)	R^2	(p<.05)
(k)	0.29		(k)	0.13	
(g)	0.41		(g)	0.23	
(b)	0.45		(h)	0.26	
(j)	0.48		(f)	0.27	
(h)	0.49				
(f)	0.50				
(j)	0.51				

The above table is recreated from Uno et al. (2009).
(b) R.Kata.1CHR = reading single Katakana characters; (c) R.Hira.Word = reading Hiragana words; (f) W.Hira.Word = writing Hiragana words; (g) W.Kata.Word = writing Katakana words; (h) R.Kanji.Word = reading Kanji words; (i) Arithmetic = additions/subtractions; (j) RCPM = Raven's Coloured Progressive Matrices; (k) SCTAW = Standardised Comprehension Test for Abstract Words; (n) RCFT Immed = Reys Complex Figure Test – Immediate Recall.

development (e.g., Bowey & Patel, 1988). This is probably more notably an indication of how Kanji is read.

Moreover, the results of Uno et al. (2009) also revealed that the children in sixth grade (aged 12) showed a strong link between phonological processing skills (i.e., non-word repetition) and Kanji word reading. Many studies in English have established the strong link between phonological development and the acquisition of literacy – better phonological awareness leads to better literacy skill. However, this relationship was seen only in the oldest children in the Uno et al. cohort (2009). Interestingly, the data from the literate Japanese adults showed that phonological processing also takes place early on in Kanji word reading along with lexical and semantic processing (Sakuma et al., 1998; Wydell et al., 1993, for more details). This could mean that the reading system in the Grade 6 children is maturing, and only with this maturation does phonological processing become important.

Similar to Uno et al. (2009), the results from Wei et al.'s (2014) study revealed that the role of phonological awareness became more important in the later stages (children aged 8) in the development of reading skills in Chinese. Wei and colleagues suggested that because each Chinese character has a one-to-one correspondence with a single Chinese syllable, and the syllable is a salient unit in spoken Chinese, children seldom need to analyse the syllable into smaller phonological units (such as phonemes) during their earlier years of literacy acquisition. Consequently, they need more time and practice to develop phonological awareness.

These findings also lend support to the view that some orthographies show a significantly higher incidence of dyslexia than others, especially phonological dyslexia. Researchers (e.g., Landerl, Wimmer, & Frith, 1997; Paulesu et al., 2001; Paulesu et al., 2000; Wydell & Butterworth, 1999) have argued that the discrepancy in the prevalence of dyslexia in the different languages might be primarily due to the differences inherent in how orthographies map onto phonology. In the alphabetic languages where a finer orthography-to-phonology mapping is required such as, for example, English or Danish (Elbro, Møller, & Nielsen, 1995), developmental dyslexia forms a large minority group. Landerl et al. (1997), for example, comparing English and German, pointed out that the different organisation of phonological recoding might be triggered by the key orthographic feature distinguishing the two orthographies, i.e., the difference in the 'consistency/transparency' of grapheme–phoneme relations for vowels. In German such relations are highly consistent, which allows for the immediate on-line assembly of syllables. In contrast, in English or Danish these relations are less consistent. Treiman et al. (1995) commented that for monosyllabic CVC words with the same vowel graphemes in English, the consistency between the vowel graphemes and phonemes was only about 60 per cent (e.g., 'ea' in beak/bread/learn). Therefore, correct pronunciations of the vowels in English are determined by graphemic context, which prevents immediate on-line assembly of syllables.

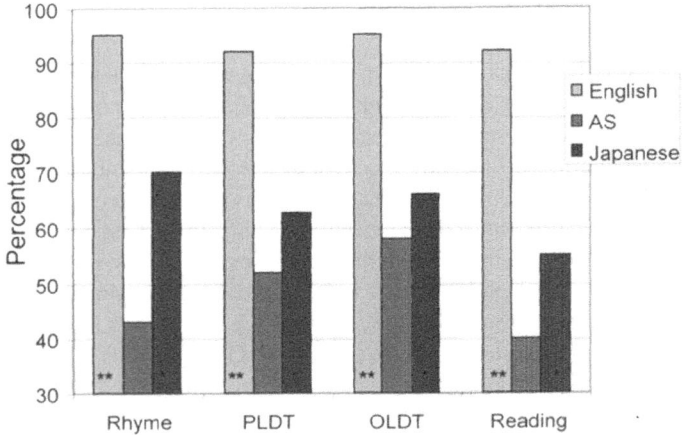

Figure 9.1 Comparing the performances of AS and his English and Japanese controls over rhyme judgments (rhyme), phonological lexical decisions (PLDT, respond yes to 'brane'), orthographic lexical decision (OLDT), and reading in English.
Note: * = p<.05; ** = P<.01 (This figure was recreated based on data from Wydell and Kondo, 2003.)

These orthographic influences suggest that it is theoretically possible to see good reading skills in Japanese but poor reading skills in English in an English–Japanese bilingual individual. Indeed, Wydell and Butterworth (1999) found such an individual named AS. AS's reading skills in Japanese (Kana and Kanji) aged 16 were as good as those of Japanese university students. In contrast, his performance in reading as well as phonological tasks in English was significantly below the mean of not only his English but also his Japanese contemporaries. Figure 9.1 compares the performances of AS and his English and Japanese controls over rhyme judgements, phonological lexical decisions (to respond Yes to 'brane'), orthographic lexical decisions, and reading in English. Having tested AS extensively for his reading and reading-related skills both in English and Japanese, Wydell and Butterworth concluded that AS could be described as a phonological dyslexic in English, while he was a superior reader in Japanese.

A follow-up study was conducted on AS by Wydell and Kondo (2003), which found that his fundamental phonological deficit, which led to his phonological dyslexia in English, still persisted despite his successfully taking a BSc course in an English-speaking country.

Wydell and Butterworth maintained that learning to read English is essentially to acquire complex mappings of sub-syllabic phonological components (i.e. phonemes) to the letter level (i.e. graphemes). Failure to acquire appropriate sub-syllabic skills is characteristic of developmental phonological dyslexia. This is precisely what happened to AS in English.

In contrast, it is not necessary to learn complex mappings between graphemes and phonemes when learning to read syllabic Kana. The computation of phonology from Kana is simple and easy, as the orthography–phonology relationship in Kana is 'transparent'. Hence AS has no problem in learning/reading Kana. Further, as described earlier, each Kanji character is a morphographic element that cannot phonetically be decomposed in the way that an alphabetic word can be. The smallest orthographic unit or 'grain size' for Kanji is a whole character or word, which is larger than a grapheme in English. Hence AS has no problem in learning/reading Kanji. It can therefore be speculated that had AS been a German–Japanese bilingual he might not have been (phonologically) dyslexic in German, and that had he been a Finnish/Italian/Spanish–Japanese bilingual he could not have been (phonologically) dyslexic in any of these languages.

In order to account for the dissociation between reading in English and Japanese shown by AS, Wydell and Butterworth put forward the hypothesis of granularity and transparency, which is illustrated in Figure 9.2.

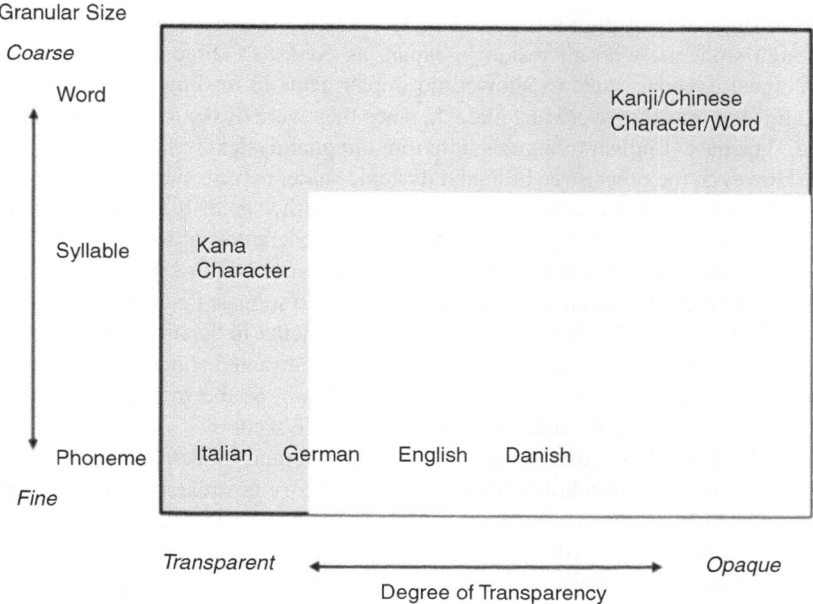

Figure 9.2 Hypothesis of granularity and transparency. (This figure was recreated based on data from Wydell and Butterworth, 1999.)

The hypothesis postulates that orthographies can be described in two dimensions: *transparency* and *granularity*. Wydell and Butterworth argued that (i) any orthography where the print-to-sound mapping is one-to-one or transparent will not produce a high incidence of phonological dyslexia regardless of the level of translation, be it phoneme, syllable, character, etc. (this is the transparency dimension), and (ii) even when this relationship is opaque and not one-to-one, any orthography whose orthographic grain size for the print-to-sound mapping is larger, such as a whole character or whole word, will not produce a high incidence of phonological dyslexia (this is the granularity dimension). Therefore, Wydell and Butterworth suggested that any orthography used in any language can be placed in the transparency–granularity orthogonal dimension as shown in Figure 9.2, and any orthography that falls into the shaded area in the figure should not produce a high incidence of phonological dyslexia.

Recently, Haruhara et al. (2014) reported six cases of Japanese–English bilingual postgraduate students with dyslexia in English from a postgraduate art college in the UK. They had all been educated in Japan until their undergraduate degrees. Their dyslexia in English was diagnosed at this college in the UK. Haruhara et al. (2014) conducted a series of tests (including reading English, Kana, and Kanji as well as phonological awareness and other cognitive skills) on these bilingual dyslexic postgraduate students as well as 202 Japanese senior-high-school pupils (aged 18) and a small number of postgraduate art/design students, who all reside in Japan, as controls. Three out of these six bilingual dyslexic students showed no impairments in reading Japanese Kana/Kanji, and thus they were just like AS, since they were dyslexic only in English; i.e., Japanese–English bilinguals with monolingual dyslexia in English.

However, the other three bilingual dyslexic students were significantly poorer at RAN (Rapid Automatized Naming) than even the senior-high-school pupils. Moreover, two out of these three bilingual dyslexic students took significantly longer in reading Hiragana and Katakana than the senior-high-school pupils. The data from these bilingual dyslexic students seem to suggest that they might have some phonological deficit. The reading impairments in Japanese Kana manifested in these two bilinguals appear not to have warranted concern for remediation while they were at school/university in Japan, as the impairments might have been rather subtle, and thus have been overlooked.

At least the latter two Japanese–English bilingual students with dyslexia would fit with the psycholinguistic grain size theory postulated by Ziegler and Goswami (2005), who were in disagreement with the *transparency* (consistency) dimension of Wydell and Butterworth's (1999) hypothesis of granularity and transparency. They argued that 'If it is accepted that reading is founded in phonology, then children with dyslexia will experience difficulties in acquiring even consistent orthographies. This is because of their reduced phonological sensitivity' (Ziegler & Goswami, 2005, p. 20). They may be right in the case of

Table 9.2 *Mean cycle (naming latencies) and correct rate of normal and dyslexia networks in pronouncing Hiragana, Katakana, and Kanji characters at 40,000 epochs*

		Hiragana (n=71)		Katakana (n=71)		Kanji (n=218)	
Normal model	Cycle	5.51	(0.07)	5.51	(0.07)	4.87	(0.02)
Dyslexia model	Cycle	7.17	(0.04)	7.17	(0.04)	7.41	(0.06)
	Correct rate	0.69	(0.02)	0.69	(0.02)	0.86	(0.02)

Note: Standard error of the mean is in parentheses ().
Source: The above table is recreated from Ijuin and Wydell (2018).

these particular Japanese–English bilingual dyslexic students. However, the fact remains that the other three Japanese–English bilingual students had dyslexia only in English, just like AS, who was an English–Japanese bilingual with monolingual dyslexia in English.

Recently Ijuin and Wydell (2018) successfully developed a computer-simulation model of reading Kana and Kanji in order to verify the validity of the *granularity dimension* of the hypothesis of granularity and transparency with a training corpus of 142 Kana (71 Hiragana and 71 Katakana) and 218 Kanji characters. The model was based on the simulation model developed by Harm and Seidenberg (1999) for reading in English. As shown in Table 9.2, it was revealed that both the *normal model* and the *phonological dyslexia* model showed a better reading performance on Kanji (coarser grain) than Kana (finer grain). In the *normal* model, the reading cycle for Kanji was faster than that for Kana, while in the *dyslexia* model, Kanji had a higher reading accuracy than Kana, but the reading cycle for correctly pronounced Kanji was longer than that for Kana, thus showing a speed–accuracy trade-off. Thus, the model successfully simulated the granularity dimension of the hypothesis of granularity and transparency.

9.4.2   Underlying Causes of Reading Problems in Japanese

One of the most influential studies on the neural correlates of reading in different orthographies was conducted by Paulesu et al. (2000). During a PET (positron emission tomography) scan, English and Italian university students were asked to read words and non-words. Their ingenious five differ-ent word and non-word stimuli in 'opaque' English and 'transparent' Italian consisted of (1) words either in English for English participants or in Italian for Italian participants, (2) non-words from Italian, (3) non-words from English, (4) international words conforming to Italian (e.g., pasta), and (5) international words conforming to English (e.g., business).

Paulesu and colleagues (2000) found a common distributed brain network of activation across the two languages including inferior frontal and premotor cortex, superior middle and inferior temporal gyri and fusiform gyrus on the left, and superior temporal gyrus on the right, thus showing the *language-universality* aspect of reading. Moreover, Italian showed greater activation in the left superior temporal regions, which are often implicated with (*sub-word processing*) phonological processing, while English participants showed greater activations in the left posterior inferior temporal and anterior inferior frontal gyrus, which are known to be associated with word retrieval *(whole-word processing)* during reading, thus showing the *language-specificity aspect of reading.*

Another influential neuroimaging study with fMRI (functional magnetic resonance imaging) conducted by Siok et al. (2004) in Chinese (morpho-graphic orthography) revealed *a language-specific aspect* of neural correlates. It was found that the L-MFG (left middle frontal gyrus) was crucial to successful Chinese reading. They argued that the L-MFG functions as a 'centre for fluent Chinese reading' (p. 71) where typical reading processes in Chinese are mediated; i.e., the conversion of a Chinese character to a syllable, and mapping orthography (Chinese character) to semantics. Furthermore, when compared to Chinese normal readers, Chinese dyslexics showed reduced activation in the L-MFG, and instead greater activation in the left inferior prefrontal gyrus. Siok and colleagues further pointed out that previous fMRI research in English using a similar design to theirs consistently show reduced activation in left temporoparietal areas amongst dyslexics (e.g., Aylward et al., 2003), which is different from the results of research on Chinese. They thus challenged *the biological unity theory of dyslexia* advocated by Paulesu et al. (2001), and instead proposed that 'the biological abnormality of impaired reading is dependent on culture' (p. 71), thus showing the *language-specificity aspect of reading/dyslexia.*

Interestingly, Wydell and Kondo (2015) revealed *neural unity and behavioural dissociation* in the before-mentioned English–Japanese bilingual AS. They recorded the neural activation using magnetoencephalography (MEG) when AS and English/Japanese controls made lexical decisions in English pseudo-homophones (e.g., YES to 'brane') and in Japanese pseudo-homophones in Katakana (e.g., YES to 'エンピツ' for '鉛筆' /enpitsu/ (pencil)) respectively.

AS's initial activation up to 200 ms from the stimulus-onset in the occipital cortex was normal; however, AS revealed significantly weaker cortical activation in the left superior temporal gyrus (L-STG) after 200 ms for both English and Japanese. This area is often implicated in grapheme-to-phoneme conversions in alphabetical languages (e.g., Wydell et al., 2003). His MEG also revealed significant activation in the left supramarginal gyrus (L-SMG) for Kana at 220 ms, not observed with the controls. Other imaging studies showed that this area is often associated with phonological processing when reading real words (e.g., Stoeckel et al., 2009). Wydell and Kondo (2015) therefore argued that with the reduced L-STG activation augmented by the L-SMG, AS was still able to read Kana, because the cognitive demand for Kana character–pronunciation conversion (larger grain size) is less than that for English grapheme–phoneme conversion (smaller grain size). They suggested that the L-SMG appeared to be able to process whole syllables with a coarser grain size as well as words, and can assist an impaired L-STG for reading Kana pseudo-homophones but not English pseudo-homophones, where the smaller grain size requires the finer processing capability of the L-STG, thus indicating the existence of *neural/biological unity but behavioural dissociation* within one bilingual individual.

As discussed earlier, the successful development of Chinese reading primarily depends on orthographic processing skills (Ho et al., 2004; Wei et al., 2014) rather than phonological processing skills, which are considered to be critical for reading alphabetic languages (e.g., Hulme, 1988; Ramus, 2003; Wimmer, Mayringer, & Landerl, 2000). In order to further ascertain neuronally which of these processing skills (orthographic or phonological processing skills) are more critical in reading Chinese, Wang et al. (2010) employed a visual and auditory event-related potential (ERP) experiment, eliciting mismatch negativity (MMN) to investigate the link between dyslexia in Chinese and magnocellular functional abnormality in the visual system (orthographic processing) as well as in the auditory system (phonological processing). The research rationale was based on Stein's (2001) assertion that most reading problems have a fundamental magnocellular deficit, be it auditory or visual modality. [5] The results showed that there was no difference in the auditory MMN between the dyslexic and the two control groups. However, the mean amplitude of visual MMNs in the dyslexic group was smaller (i.e., smaller mismatch negativity ERPs to moving gratings) than that of both of the controls, indicating that the visual magnocellular system was compromised in the Chinese dyslexic group compared to both of the control groups (see Qian et al.'s (2015) fMRI study for similar results), thus showing *the language-specificity of reading/dyslexia.*

In Japanese, neuroimaging research investigating neural correlates of reading in Kana and Kanji in normal readers have started to emerge (e.g., Koyama et al., 2011; Nakamura et al., 2005); however, not many published studies on

---

[5] While there are studies which lend support to the hypothesis of a visual magnocellular deficit in developmental dyslexia, in alphabetic languages not all of the individuals with developmental dyslexia exhibit the deficit in the visual magnocellular pathway, and instead most of these dyslexics consistently showed the phonological deficit (e.g., Ramus et al., 2003).

developmental dyslexia in Japanese are currently available. It will be interesting to see the results from further neuroimaging research, which should be able to further contribute to the scientific debates on various aspects of dyslexia in different orthographies.

9.5   Discussion and Conclusion

This chapter has shown that universality and specificity of reading processes are involved in different languages, focusing on a comparison between Japanese and English. The influence of language and writing system on reading can explain differences in the incidence of phonological dyslexia between the two languages, as hypothesised by the hypothesis of granularity and transparency. Further, the granularity dimension of the hypothesis was successfully implemented in a computer-simulation model.

Additionally, the nature of the phonological dyslexia manifested in the two languages are qualitatively different; i.e., some Japanese (phonological) dyslexic children may be slow at reading, but can achieve comparable reading accuracy to that of normally developing children, whereas English dyslexic children's reading difficulties persist into their adulthood. It can tentatively be concluded that the level of cognitive demand placed by reading Japanese is lower than that of reading English, a conclusion supported not only by the behavioural but also the neuroimaging data.

Finally, it is important to note that the study of dyslexia in Japanese has only recently received much attention. In order to ensure that Japanese children with reading difficulties are optimally served, there is an urgent need for fundamental research on behavioural and neurocognitive underpinnings of developmental dyslexia. Research should not only focus on the identification and prevalence of dyslexia in Japanese, but also on its prevention and early intervention.

References

Amano,S., & Kondo, T. (1999). *Nihongo no goitokusei* [Lexical properties of Japanese] (Vols. 1–6, NTT Psycholinguistic Database Series). Tokyo: Sanseidō.

Andrews, S. (1982). Phonological recoding: Is the regularity effect consistent? *Journal of Memory and Cognition*, *10*, 565–575.

Aylward, E. H., Richards, T. L., Berninger, V. W. et al. (2003). Instructional treatment associated with changes in brain activation in children with dyslexia. *Neurology*, *61*, 212–219.

Besner, D., & Hildebrandt, N. (1987). Orthographic and phonological code in the oral reading of Japanese Kana. *Journal of Experimental Psychology: Learning, Memory and Cognition*, *13*, 335–343.

Bowey, J. A., & Patel, R. K. (1988). Metalinguistic ability and early reading achievement. *Applied Psycholinguistics*, *9*, 367–383.

Chan, D. W., Ho, C. S. H., Tsang, S. M., Lee, S. H., & Chung, K. K. H. (2006). Exploring the reading–writing connection in Chinese children with dyslexia in Hong Kong. *Reading and Writing*, *19*, 543–561.

Elbro, C., Møller, S., & Nielsen, E. M. (1995). Functional reading difficulties in Denmark. A study of adult reading of common text. *Reading and Writing*, *7*, 257–276.

Frost, R., Katz, L., & Bentin, S. (1987). Strategies for visual word recognition and orthographic depth: A multilingual comparison. *Journal of Experimental Psychology: Human Perception and Performance*, *13*, 104–115.

Fushimi, T., Ijuin, M., Patterson, K., & Tatsumi, I. F. (1999). Consistency, frequency, and lexicality effects in naming Japanese Kanji. *Journal of Experimental Psychology: Human Perception and Performance*, *25*, 382–407.

Fushimi, T., Komori, K., & Ikeda, M. et al. (2003). Surface dyslexia in a Japanese patient with semantic dementia: Evidence for similarity-based orthography-to-phonology translation. *Neuropsychologia*, *41*, 1644–1658.

Gibson, E. J., & Levin, H. (1975). *Psychology of reading*. Cambridge, MA: MIT Press.

Glushko, R. J. (1979). The organization and activation of orthographic knowledge in reading aloud. *Journal of Experimental Psychology: Human Perception and Performance*, *5*, 674–691.

Halpern, D. F. (1992). *Sex differences in cognitive abilities* (2nd ed.). Hillsdale, NJ: Erlbaum.

Harm, M. W., & Seidenberg, M. S. (1999). Phonology, reading acquisition, and dyslexia: Insights from connectionist models. *Psychological Review*, *106*, 491–528.

Haruhara, N., & Kaneko, M. (2003). *The standardized comprehension test of abstract words*. Edited by A. Uno. Tokyo: Intelna-Shuppan,

Haruhara, N., Uno, A., Rankin, Q., & Wydell, T. N. (2014, March). *Cognitive abilities and reading/writing attainment in Japanese of Japanese-English bilinguals with monolingual dyslexia in English*. Paper presented at the British Dyslexia Association International Conference, Guildford, UK.

Hirose, T. & Hatta, T. (1985). Reading disabilities in Japan: Evidence against the myth of rarity. *International Journal of Neuroscience*, *26*, 249–252.

Ho, C. S. H., Chan, D. W. O., Lee, S. H., Tsang, S. M., & Luan, V. H. (2004). Cognitive profiling and preliminary subtyping in Chinese developmental dyslexia. *Cognition*, *91*, 43–75.

Hulme, C. (1988). The implausibility of low-level visual deficits as a cause of children's reading difficulties. *Cognitive Neuropsychology*, *5*, 369–374.

Ijuin, M., & Wydell, T. N. (2018). A reading model from the perspective of Japanese orthography: Connectionist approach to the hypothesis of granularity and transparency. *Journal of Learning Disabilities*, *51*(5), 490–498. doi: http://dx.doi.org /10.1177/0022219417718200.

Japanese National Research Institute of Special Education. (1996). *Report C-28: Categorization of primary school children with LD and a study on remediation methods*. Tokyo: Japan.

Jared, D. (2002). Spelling-sound consistency and regularity effects in word naming. *Journal of Memory and Language*, *46*, 723–750.

Kaneko, M., Uno, A., Kaga, M. et al. (1997). Developmental dyslexia and dysgraphia: A case report [in Japanese]. *No To Hattatsu [Brain and Child Development]*, *29*, 249–253.

Kitao, N. (1984). *Reading Ability Test TK-1*. Tokyo: Taken Press.

Kondo, T., & Wydell, T. N. (2011). *Syllable effects during reading 1000 2-Character Kanji words: comparing ON-reading and KUN-reading words*. Paper presented at the

14th Japanese Cognitive Neuropsychology Society Annual Conference (24th September 2011), Nagoya, Japan.

Koyama, M. S., Stein, J. F., Stoodley, C. J., & Hansen, P. C. (2011). Functional MRI evidence for the importance of visual short-term memory in logographic reading. *European Journal of Neuroscience, 33*, 539–548.

Kusumi, T. (1992). Meta-memory. In Y. Anzai, S. Ishizaki, Y. Otsu, G. Hatano, & H. Mizogushi (Eds.), *Handbook of cognitive science*. Tokyo, Japan: Kyoritsu Shuppan.

Landerl, K., Wimmer, H., & Frith, U. (1997). The impact of orthographic consistency on dyslexia: A German–English comparison. *Cognition, 63*, 315–334.

Makita, K. (1968). The rarity of reading disability in Japanese children. *American Journal of Orthopsychiatry, 38*, 599–614.

Mann, V. A. (1985). A cross-language perspective in the relation between temporary memory skills and early reading ability. *Remedial and Special Education, 6*, 37–42.

Mattingley, I. G. (1972). Reading, the linguistic process, and linguistic awareness. In J. F. Kavanagh & I. G. Mattingley (Eds.), *Language by ear and by eye*. Cambridge, MA: MIT Press.

Morton, J. & Sasanuma, S. (1984). Lexical access in Japanese. In L. Henderson (Ed.), *Orthographies and Reading: Perspectives from Cognitive Psychology, Neuropsychology and Linguistics (25–42)*. London: Lawrence Erlbaum Associates.

Muraishi, S. (1972). *Acquisition of reading Japanese syllabic characters in pre-school children in Japan*. Paper presented at the Twentieth International Congress of Psychology, Tokyo.

Naka, M., & Naoi, H. (1995). The effect of repeated writing on memory. *Journal of Memory and Cognition, 23*, 201–212.

Nakamura, K., Oga, T., Okada, T. et al. (2005). Hemispheric asymmetry emerges at distinct parts of the occipitotemporal cortex for objects, logograms and phonograms: A functional MRI study. *Neuroimage, 28*, 521–528

National Language Research Institute. (1976). Gendai Shinbun no Kanji [A study of Chinese characters in modern newspapers], *The National Language Research Institute Report, 56*, Tokyo, Japan: Shuei-shuppan.

National Working Party on Dyslexia in Higher Education. (1999). *Dyslexia in higher education: Policy, provision and practice*. Hull, UK: University of Hull.

Onose, M. (1987). The effect of tracing and copying practice on handwriting skills of Japanese letters in preschool and first grade children. *The Japanese Journal of Educational Psychology, 35*, 9–16.

Onose, M. (1988). Effect of the combination of tracing and copying practices on handwriting skills of Japanese letters in preschool and first grade children. *The Japanese Journal of Educational Psychology, 36*, 129–134.

Patterson, K., Suzuki, T., & Wydell, T. N. (1996). Interpreting a case of Japanese phonological alexia: The key is in phonology. *Cognitive Neuropsychology, 13*, 803–822.

Patterson, K., Suzuki, T., Wydell, T. N., & Sasanuma, S. (1995). Progressive aphasia and surface alexia in Japanese. *Neurocase, 1*, 155–165.

Paulesu, E., Demonet, J. F., Fazio, F. et al. (2001). Dyslexia – Cultural diversity and biological unity. *Science, 291*, 2165–2167.

Paulesu, E., McCrory, E., Fazio, F. et al. (2000). A cultural effect on brain function. *Nature Neuroscience, 3*, 91–96.

Qian, Y., Deng, Y., Zhao, J., & Bi, H. Y. (2015). Magnocellular-dorsal pathway function is associated with orthographic but not phonological skill: fMRI evidence from skilled Chinese readers. *Neuropsychologia, 71*, 84–90. doi: http://dx.doi.org/10.1016/j.neuropsychologia.2015.03.024.

Ramus, F. (2003). Developmental dyslexia: Specific phonological deficit or general sensorimotor dysfunction? *Current Opinion in Neurobiology, 13*, 212–218.

Ramus, F., Rosen, S., Dakin, S. C. et al. (2003). Theories of developmental dyslexia: insights from a multiple case study of dyslexic adults. *Brain, 126*, 841–865.

Rastle, K., Havelka, J., Wydell, T. N., Coltheart, M., & Besner, D. (2009). The cross-script length effect: Further evidence challenging PDP models of reading aloud. *Journal of Experimental Psychology: Learning, Memory and Cognition, 35*, 238–246.

Raven, J. C. (1976). *Coloured progressive matrices: SETS A, AB, B*. Oxford, UK: OPP.

Richardson, J. T. E., & Wydell, T. N. (2003). The representation and attainment of students with dyslexia in UK higher education. *Reading and Writing, 16*, 475–503.

Saito, H., Kawakami, M., & Matsuda, H. (1995). Kanji kousei ni okeru buhin (bushu)-on'in taiouhyou [Variety of phonetic components of radical types in complex left-right Kanji]. *Jouhou Kagaku Kenkyu, 2*, 89–115.

Sakamoto, T., & Makita, K. (1973). Japan. In J. Downing (Ed.), *Comparative reading* (pp. 440–465). New York: Macmillan.

Sakuma, N., Sasanuma, S., Tatsumi, I. F., & Masaki, S. (1998). Orthography and phonology in reading Japanese Kanji words: Evidence from the semantic decision task with homophones. *Journal of Memory and Cognition, 26*, 75–87.

Sampson, G. (1985). *Writing systems*. Stanford, CA: Stanford University Press.

Sasaki, M. (1987). Why do Japanese write characters in space? *International Journal of Behavioural Development, 10*, 135–149.

Share, D. L., McGee, R., McKenzie, D., Williams, S. M., & Silva, P. A. (1987). Further evidence relating to the distinction between specific reading retardation and general reading backwardness. *British Journal of Developmental Psychology, 5*, 35–44.

Shaywitz, S. E., Shaywitz, B. A., Feltcher, J. M., & Escobar, M. D. (1990). Prevalence of reading disability in boys and girls: Results of the Connecticut longitudinal study. *Journal of the American Medical Association, 264*, 998–1002.

Shibahara, N., Zorzi, M., Hill, M. P., Wydell, T. N., & Butterworth, B. (2003). Semantic effects in word naming: Evidence from English and Japanese Kanji. *Quarterly Journal of Experimental Psychology, 56A*, 263–286.

Siok, W. T., Perfetti, C. A., Jin, Z., & Tan, L. H. (2004). Biological abnormality of impaired reading is constrained by culture. *Nature, 431*, 71–76.

Snowling, M. (2000). *Dyslexia* (2nd ed.). London: Blackwell.

Stanhope, N., & Parkin, A. J. (1987). Further explorations of the consistency effect in word and nonword pronunciation. *Journal of Memory and Cognition, 15*, 169–179.

Stein, J. (2001). The magnocellular theory of developmental dyslexia. *Dyslexia, 7*, 12–36.

Stevenson, H. W., Stigler, J. W., Lucker, G. W. et al. (1982). Reading disabilities: The case of Chinese, Japanese, and English. *Child Development, 53*, 1164–1181.

Stoeckel, C., Gough, P. M., Watkins, K. E., Devlin, J. T. (2009). Supramarginal gyrus involvement in visual word recognition. *Cortex, 45*(9), 1091–1096.

Strain, E., Patterson, K., & Seidenberg, M. (1995). Semantic effects in single-word naming. *Journal of Experimental Psychology: Learning, Memory, and Cognition, 21*, 1140–1154.

Takebe, T. (1979). *Nihongo no hyoki* [The Japanese orthography]. Tokyo, Japan: Kadokawa.

Taraban, R., & McClelland, J. L. (1987). Conspiracy effects in word pronunciation. *Journal of Memory and Language, 26*, 608–631.

Treiman, R., Mullennix, J., Bijeljac-Babic, R., & Richmond-Welty, E. D. (1995). The special role of rimes in the description, use and acquisition of English orthography. *Journal of Experimental Psychology: General, 124*, 107–136.

Uno, A., Haruhara, N., Kaneko, M. & Wydell, T. N. (2006–2016). *Shougakusei no Yomi kaki Screening Kensa – Screening test of reading and writing for Japanese primary school children (STRAW)*. Tokyo, Japan: Interuna Shuppan.

Uno, A., Kaga, M., & Inagaki, M. (1995). A specific disorder of Kanji writing observed in a learning-disabled child: Cognitive psychological and neuropsychological analysis. *No To Hattatsu* [The Brain and Child Development], *27*, 395–400.

Uno, A., & Kamibayashi, Y. (1998). Learning disabled child showing writing disorders with ADHD: Cognitive neuropsychological investigation about writing disorders. *Shouji No Seishin To Shinkei [Developmental Neuropsychiatry]*, *38*(2), 117–123.

Uno, A., Wydell, T. N., Haruhara, N., Kaneko, M., & Shinya, N. (2009). Relationship between reading/writing skills and cognitive abilities among Japanese primary-school children: Normal readers versus poor readers (dyslexics). *Reading & Writing, 22*, 755–789.

Wang, J.-J., Bi, H.-Y., Gao, L.-Q., & Wydell, T. N. (2010). The visual magnocellular pathway in Chinese-speaking children with developmental dyslexia. *Neuropsychologia, 48*, 3627–3633.

Wei, T.-Q., Bi, H.-Y., Chen, B.-G. et al. (2014). Developmental changes in the role of different metalinguistic awareness skills in Chinese reading acquisition from pre-school to third grade. *PLoS One, 9*(5), e96240.

Wimmer, H., Mayringer, H., & Landerl, K. (2000). The double-deficit hypothesis and difficulties in learning to read a regular orthography. *Journal of Educational Psychology, 92*, 668–680.

Wydell, T. N. (2003). Dyslexia in Japanese and the 'Hypothesis of Granularity and Transparency'. In A. Goulandris (Ed.), *Dyslexia in different languages: Cross-linguistic comparisons*. London: Whurr Publishers.

Wydell, T. N., & Butterworth, B. (1999). A case study of an English–Japanese bilingual with monolingual dyslexia. *Cognition, 70*, 273–305.

Wydell, T. N., Butterworth, B., & Patterson, K. (1995). The inconsistency of consistency effects in reading: The case of Japanese Kanji. *Journal of Experimental Psychology: Learning, Memory, and Cognition, 21*, 1155–1168.

Wydell, T. N., & Kondo, T. (2003). Phonological deficit and the reliance on orthographic approximation for reading: A follow-up study on an English–Japanese bilingual with monolingual dyslexia. *Journal of Research in Reading, 26*, 33–48.

Wydell, T.N. & Kondo, T. (2015). Behavioral and neuroimaging research of reading: a case of Japanese. *Current Developmental Disorders Reports, 2*(4), 339–345.

Wydell, T., Patterson, K., & Humphreys, G. (1993). Phonologically mediated access to meaning for Kanji: Is a ROWS still a ROSE in Japanese Kanji? *Journal of Experimental Psychology: Learning, Memory, and Cognition, 19*, 491–514.

Wydell, T. N., Vuorinen, T., Helenius, P., & Salmelin, R. (2003). Neural correlates of letter string length and lexicality during reading in a regular orthography. *Journal of Cognitive Neuroscience, 15*, 7, 1052–1062.

Yokosawa, K., & Umeda, M. (1988). Process in human Kanji word recognition. *Proceedings of the 1988 IEEE International Conference on Systems, Man, and Cybernetics* (pp. 377–380). Beijing: IEEE.

Ziegler, J. C., & Goswami, U. (2005). Reading acquisition, developmental dyslexia, and skilled reading across languages: A psycholinguistic grain size theory. *Psychological Bulletin, 131*, 3–29.

10 Developmental Dyslexia in Chinese

Min Xu, Li Hai Tan, and Charles Perfetti

10.1 Introduction

Developmental dyslexia is characterized by unexpectedly low reading ability in people who have adequate nonverbal intelligence, have acquired typical schooling, and have experienced sufficient sociocultural opportunities (Gabrieli, 2009; Peterson & Pennington, 2012). It is a recognized disorder in many literate societies and has been studied in a large variety of languages (Caravolas, 2005). The Chinese writing system presents sharp contrast to the alphabetic writing system in terms of how the graphic unit maps onto phonology and semantics. Thus, the investigations into the mechanisms for Chinese reading disability are important to the understanding of the universal and language-specific mechanisms of developmental dyslexia. The behavioral and neural correlates of Chinese developmental dyslexia have been studied extensively in the past twenty years or so, providing us with a rich understanding of Chinese developmental dyslexia. Genetic studies have been emerging. In what follows, we first introduce the critical features of spoken and written Chinese, and then review previous research that provides behavioral, neurocognitive, and genetic evidence on Chinese dyslexia and discuss how the characteristics of the writing systems may influence the underlying deficits that are associated with dyslexia.

10.2 Learning to Read Chinese

10.2.1 Chinese Language and Its Orthography

Chinese represents a group of related, but in some cases mutually unintelligible language varieties. Based on shared geographic and linguistic features, Chinese is commonly classified as seven dialect families, including Mandarin, Xiāng, Gàn, Wú, Yuè, Kèjiā, and Mǐn (Handel, 2015). Among the seven dialect families in China, the Mandarin family is the largest, with over 70 percent of the speakers (X. Chen & Pasquarella, 2017). Standard Chinese, also known as Standard Mandarin or simply Mandarin, is the official language of mainland

China and Taiwan. It serves as the medium of instruction at all educational levels. Cantonese, the traditional prestige variety of Yuè, is spoken in Hong Kong, Macau, Guangdong, and Guangxi in South China. Cantonese is the medium of instruction in many schools in Hong Kong and Macau, whereas Mandarin has been the medium of instruction in Guangdong and Guangxi, due to the spread of Standard Mandarin after the mid-twentieth century.

Chinese is a tonal language in which different pitches of the voice can convey different meanings of words. There are four tones in Mandarin Chinese; i.e., high-level, rising, dipping, and falling. The four symbols {¯ ′ ˇ `} placed above the vowel of a Pinyin written syllable indicate the relative pitch contours of the four tones. For example, the syllable /yi/ in Mandarin Chinese has different meanings with different tone: /yī / 一, "one"; /yí/, 姨, "aunt"; /yǐ/, 倚, "to lean on"; /yì/, 益, "benefit." In the tradition of Chinese research and Chinese reading instruction, the syllables are parsed into two sub-syllabic parts, the onsets and the rimes. The onsets, representing the beginning of syllables, are single consonants and the rimes represent the final, vocalic center of the syllables that exclude the onsets. Along with twenty-two onsets, Chinese has a small number of rimes – thirty-seven – severely limiting the number of syllables in modern Chinese (C. N. Li & Thompson, 1981). There are about 400 different syllables in Mandarin Chinese, but with tone taken into account, the number of syllables increases to about 1300 (Taylor & Taylor, 1995).

The result of these facts for written Chinese is that it is unavoidable to have a considerable number of characters sharing the same syllables (i.e., homophonic heterographs). Furthermore, about 15 percent of the 2,500 most frequently used Chinese characters have more than one pronunciation (Lu, 2011). Different pronunciations of the character can vary in consonants, vowels, or tones, and they are associated with different meaning or meanings. For example, the character 乐 can be pronounced as /lè/ (meaning happy/laugh/cheerful/surname), or /yuè/ (meaning music).

Starting from the assumption that writing systems differ in how the graphic unit maps onto the phonological unit of language (Perfetti, 1992), Chinese can be characterized as a morphosyllabic system in which graphic units (characters) map to morphemes and syllables, rather than phonemes. This means that there is no stroke or component in a character (e.g., 动, /dòng/, "to act/to move") that corresponds to a specific phoneme (e.g., /d/) in the syllable. About 85 percent of Chinese characters are phonetic compounds that contain a semantic radical and a phonetic radical, which, respectively, provide semantic and phonological information on the characters (Perfetti & Tan, 1998). For example, in the character 枫 (/fēng/, "maple"), the semantic radical 木 (/mù/, "wood") suggests that it is related to wood, and the phonetic radical 风 (/fēng/, "wind") suggests its pronunciation. However, only 26 to 39 percent of phonetic compounds serve the sound-cueing function effectively (Fan, Gao, & Ao,

1984; Zhou, 1978). This inconsistency, to some extent, results from the evolution of the spoken and written languages (Harbaugh, 1998). Therefore, Chinese reading has only very limited support from the sub-lexical phonology.

The basic graphic units of Chinese are characters, which provide visually salient graphs formed with intricate strokes formed into square configurations. Their forms contrast sharply with the linear structure of alphabetic words. Strokes are grouped into identifiable stroke patterns or components, which are arranged in appropriate positions relative to one another in the characters. The spatial relations of the components vary to produce different types of character graphic structures, i.e., simple characters with one component (e.g., 木, /mù/, "wood"), left–right structure (e.g., 枫, /fēng/, "maple"), top–down structure (e.g., 思, /sī/, "to think"), half-enclosure structure (e.g., 迁, /qiān/, "to move") and enclosure structure (e.g., 国, /guó /, "country").

Chinese is written in two major scripts. The traditional Chinese script is used in Hong Kong and Taiwan, while mainland China uses a simplified script. Table 10.1 shows examples of the two scripts. The two vary in complexity, with possible consequences for reading (Chang, Chen, & Perfetti, 2017). In addition, the strong tradition of writing by hand produces variations in appearance. In all scripts, characters are separated by spaces but words are not. Because multisyllable words are common (and two-syllable words are the most frequent), this means that a given character may be a single-morpheme word or part of a multi-morpheme/multisyllable word. Indeed, the spacing conventions of written Chinese have raised the question of whether the character or the word is the basic unit of identification in reading (X. Li et al., 2013).

10.2.2   Challenges in Learning to Read Chinese

Chinese children in mainland China begin formal instruction with an alphabetic system, Hanyu Pinyin. Pinyin uses the twenty-six Roman letters to phonetically spell the syllables of characters, with tone marks placed over the syllable nucleus. This instruction provides a phonetic foundation prior to the introduction of Chinese characters and helps children establish the association of a visual character form and its pronunciation. In Taiwan, Zhu-Yin-Fu-Hao,

Table 10.1 *Examples of the traditional script and simplified script*

Traditional	Simplified	English translation
麵包	面包	bread
發現	发现	discover/discovery

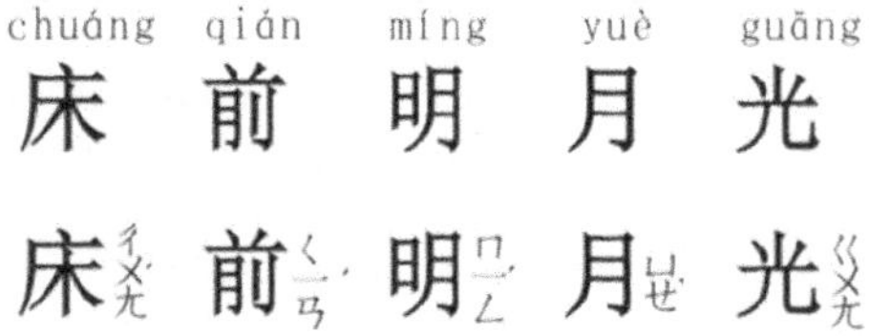

chuáng   qián   míng   yuè   guāng

床   前   明   月   光

床ㄔㄨㄤˊ 前ㄑㄧㄢˊ˙ 明ㄇㄧㄥˊ 月ㄩㄝˋ 光ㄍㄨㄤ

Figure 10.1 A line of an old Chinese poem with Pinyin (above) and Zhu-Yin-Fu-Hao (below) representing the pronunciations of each character. The Pinyin appears immediately above the character and Zhu-Yin-Fu-Hao symbols appear to the right of the characters

a phonetic system using thirty-seven symbols for transcribing Mandarin, is taught to help children learn to read. Zhu-Yin-Fu-Hao is based on syllable onset and rime, rather than on consonants and vowels. Figure 10.1 shows examples of Pinyin and Zhu-Yin-Fu-Hao. The Pinyin appears immediately above the character in the mainland language textbooks, whereas in the Taiwanese textbooks, Zhu-Yin-Fu-Hao symbols appear to the right of the characters. In Hong Kong, no such phonetic system is used, so children must learn whole words and characters.

Writing in Chinese requires thousands of characters, and it takes students 6 years to master about 3,000 characters. The challenging properties of Chinese characters (no phonemic constituents and visually complex forms) have led to a prevalent strategy of learning to read through repeatedly writing the characters. Children are taught to write the characters following a set of pre-specified sequence rules. Through writing, children learn how to deconstruct characters into strokes and stroke patterns and then regroup these stroke patterns into a square unit, and, with practice, to establish long-term motor memory of Chinese characters (McBride-Chang, Chung, & Tong, 2011; Tan, Spinks et al., 2005). We have found that children's reading ability is positively correlated with the time they spent on writing in a large sample of primary school children (Tan et al., 2013).

10.3   Reading Difficulties in Chinese

10.3.1   Historical Context

The arbitrary script–sound relationship in written Chinese led some early researchers to speculate whether there would be very low prevalence of developmental dyslexia in China (e.g., W. F. Kuo, 1978), because the reading of Chinese script did not require alphabetic skills. However, Stevenson and colleagues (1982) found that the prevalence of dyslexia was comparable among American, Japanese, and Chinese children.

10.3.2   *Identification and Prevalence of Chinese Dyslexia*

The prevalence of developmental dyslexia in China is estimated to range from about 2 to 12 percent, depending on the diagnostic criteria (Chan et al., 2007; Stevenson et al., 1982; C. F. Zhang et al., 1996). For example, Stevenson et al. (1982) reported that the prevalence of dyslexia in Taiwan was 2 percent, using the criterion of expected grade levels in which reading-disabled children were identified as such if they had a reading performance of two grades behind the expected reading level. The prevalence rate was 7.5 percent if using the definition of low reading ability (1 SD below the mean) together with average or near-average IQ. In another study, C. F. Zhang et al. (1996) reported that the prevalence rate of dyslexia in mainland China was 4.55 percent using the criterion of low reading ability (i.e., 2 SD below the average of reading scores), and the prevalence rate was 7.96 percent using a regression-based discrepancy approach. With the regression-based approach, a difference score is calculated between the predicted reading score (predicted by IQ) and the actual reading achievement score. A child was considered dyslexic if his or her difference score exceeded a predetermined critical value (e.g., 2 SD). In Hong Kong, Chan et al. (2007) reported that the prevalence rate of dyslexia was estimated to be between 9.7 percent and 12.6 percent based on the composite score profile in the Hong Kong Test of Specific Learning Difficulties in Reading and Writing (HKT-SpLD).

The Chinese character-reading tests have been widely used to measure children's reading abilities. The tests were constructed by including 100–300 characters selected from Chinese-language textbooks (e.g., Cao et al., 2017; Siok et al., 2008; Song et al., 2015). Some studies used a composite score of character-reading tests and comprehension tests to index children's reading abilities (Stevenson et al., 1982; C. F. Zhang et al., 1996). In Hong Kong, a widely used standardized test for the diagnosis of dyslexia is the HKT-SpLD (Ho et al., 2000). Dyslexic children are identified as such if they have normal intelligence, and their literacy composite scores and at least one of their cognitive composite scores are at least 1 SD below their respective age means in the HKT-SpLD (e.g., Chan et al., 2003; Ho et al., 2007).

10.4   Behavioral and Neurocognitive Evidence

10.4.1   *Nature of Reading Problems in Chinese*

It is well documented that phonological skills are strong predictors of reading acquisition (Bradley & Bryant, 1983; Wagner et al., 1997; Ziegler & Goswami, 2005). In the 1970s, Liberman and colleagues proposed a phonological-deficit hypothesis of dyslexia. According to this hypothesis, dyslexic readers have difficulties with mapping the continuous acoustic signal of spoken language onto the discrete symbols of written languages (Liberman, 1971; Liberman et al., 1974). The phonological-deficit hypothesis has been the leading explanation for the cause of dyslexia in alphabetic languages in the past few decades. In written Chinese, the graphic units (characters) correspond to specific morphemes (as part of a multi-morpheme word or as a single character mono-morphemic word). The character maps onto a whole syllable and phonemes are not represented. With this writing system difference, it is possible that phoneme-level awareness is not important for developing Chinese reading skill. The question of whether Chinese dyslexia can be traced to phonological deficits is another matter.

Evidence supporting the phonological-deficit hypothesis shows that Chinese dyslexic children performed significantly poorer than both age-matched and reading-level-matched children in tasks measuring phonological awareness (e.g., onset/rime detection tasks; Ho, Law, & Ng, 2000), Zhu-Yin-Fu-Hao synthesis (Lee, Hung, & Tzeng, 2006), and also tasks tapping phonological memory (e.g., word and nonword repetition tasks; Ho & Lai, 1999; Ho, Law, & Ng, 2000). However, the role of different levels of phonological awareness in reading seems to vary across languages (McBride-Chang et al., 2004; Ziegler & Goswami, 2005). For instance, phoneme awareness is a better predictor of early reading skills than onset/rime awareness in alphabetic languages (Hulme et al., 2002; Nation & Hulme, 1997), but phonological awareness at the onset /rime and syllable levels are more important in Chinese reading acquisition (McBride-Chang et al., 2004; Siok & Fletcher, 2001). This may be accounted for by the differences in the mapping of graphic symbols to spoken language in different writing systems, with the syllable level in Chinese compared with the phoneme level in alphabetic writing.

Nevertheless, it remains unclear whether phonological deficits are the core deficits of Chinese dyslexia. It appears not to be the only factor. Research has found that other factors, such as rapid naming (Ho et al., 2004), knowledge of orthography (Ho et al., 2004) and morphology (Shu et al., 2006), have significantly contributed to reading difficulties in Chinese dyslexics.

Naming speed, often measured by Rapid Automatized Naming tasks that require subjects to name a series of high-frequency stimuli (e.g., objects, colors, letters, or digits) as quickly as they can, is strongly related to reading abilities in both alphabetic languages (Compton, 2003; Lervåg & Hulme, 2009) and Chinese (Tan, Spinks et al., 2005). Children with Chinese reading disability are found to be slower than normal readers at rapid naming of digits, colors, pictures, and Chinese characters (Ho et al., 2002; Ho et al., 2004; Ho & Lai, 1999; Penney et al., 2005; Yan et al., 2013; Zhao et al., 2014; Zhou et al., 2014). Ho et al. (2002) found that rapid naming was the most dominant deficit among several cognitive skills including rapid naming, visual, phonological, and orthographic skills in Chinese dyslexics. Rapid naming may involve several componential skills that are crucial in the development of Chinese reading, such as general processing speed, phonological process, and speed-sensitive visual and visual-motion processes (Tan, Spinks et al., 2005). Yan et al. (2013), in an eye-tracking experiment, found that Chinese dyslexic children showed a reduced perceptual span and extracted less parafoveal information compared with control children during rapid naming of digits. The authors suggested that the dyslexic children might recruit more resources to foveal processing due to their difficulty in converting visual symbols to their phonological forms, as required by the naming task, thereby causing a reduction of the perceptual span.

Dyslexic individuals have been frequently reported to show visual processing impairments, leading to the suggestion that phonological deficits are secondary to these more fundamental sensory deficits (e.g., Eden et al., 1996). In fact, there has been a long tradition that views a visual processing deficit as the core cause of dyslexia (Hinshelwood, 1917; Morgan, 1896). A modern instantiation of this tradition is the magnocellular deficit hypothesis, which proposes that a deficit arises in the visual magnocellular pathway. This pathway handles visual input at low frequencies and low luminance and is particularly sensitive to visual motion, and direction of movement and gaze (Stein, 2001; Stein & Walsh, 1997). Postmortem studies by Galaburda and colleagues also showed decreased magnocellular neuron size in dyslexic brains (Geschwind and Galaburda, 1985; Livingstone et al., 1991).

The morpho-syllabic nature of characters and their visually complex structures have led to the speculation that reading Chinese makes great demands on the visual systems; thus, visual skills should play a more important role in the reading of Chinese than alphabetic languages. An early study conducted by Woo and Hoosain (1984) reported that Chinese dyslexic children showed dysfunction of visual but not auditory processing. Some research has shown that visual skills are closely related to Chinese children's reading abilities (Huang & Hanley, 1995; Siok & Fletcher, 2001). Recent studies have used tasks targeted to specific dynamic aspects of visual processing: the coherent-motion detection task (X. Meng et al., 2011; Qian & Bi, 2014), texture discrimination task (X. Meng et al., 2014; Z. Wang et al., 2014), the moving grating task (J. J. Wang et al., 2010), the temporal order judgment task (Chung et al., 2008), and the global/local decision task (Zhao et al., 2014). Results from these tasks suggest that Chinese dyslexics, like some of their alphabetic counterparts, have deficits in the magnocellular pathway. For example, X. Meng et al. (2011) found that Chinese dyslexic children showed reduced coherent-motion detection relative to their age- and IQ-matched controls, but were comparable to the controls in a static pattern perception task. They further found that children's motion detection threshold accounted for 11 percent variance in the speed of the orthographic similarity judgment task, suggesting that the development of dynamic visual perception might be specifically related to orthographic processing during Chinese reading. Nonetheless, the question as to the exact mechanism by which these visual deficits may impede reading remains unaddressed.

Due to the close orthography–meaning relationship in written Chinese, morphological processing has attracted great attention in the research on Chinese reading development. Morphological awareness, which is referred to as awareness of and access to morphemes in words, has been found to be a critical contributor to reading-skill acquisition and to be associated with reading disability (Chung et al., 2010; McBride-Chang et al., 2003; Shu et al., 2006). For example, Shu and colleagues (2006) found that morphological awareness could most accurately discriminate dyslexic readers from age-matched controls among a series of variables including phonological aware-ness, morphological awareness, rapid naming, and vocabulary, and it was the strongest predictor of reading-related skills across both normal and dyslexic groups. In this study, morphological awareness was measured using a morpheme production task and a morpheme judgment task. In the morpheme production task, the subjects heard a two-syllable Chinese word and they were asked to produce two words with a target morpheme. In the morpheme judg-ment task, the subjects were presented with two two-morpheme words and they judged whether the syllable common to both words had a similar or different meaning. Moreover, morphological-awareness deficit was also found in Chinese preschool children at risk of dyslexia (McBride-Chang, Lam et al., 2011; McBride-Chang et al., 2008).

The research as a whole shows that a great variety of behavioral manifesta-tions occur in Chinese dyslexia. This variety suggests that there may be multi-ple deficits without a core cause, or alternatively, a core cause leads to different manifestations. To get a better understanding of dyslexia, we need to integrate information across multiple levels of analysis, from genetics to brain and to behavior. Recent advances in brain imaging and genetics hold promise for shedding new light on the cause of dyslexia.

10.4.2   Neural Correlates of Chinese Developmental Dyslexia

Evidence from neuroimaging studies has also supported a multiple-deficit view for Chinese dyslexia. These studies have revealed atypical patterns of brain activation associated with specific reading processes in Chinese dyslexia, including phonological (Cao et al., 2017; Siok et al., 2008; Siok et al., 2004; Xu et al., 2015), semantic (Hu et al., 2010; L. Liu et al., 2012; Siok et al., 2004), morphological (L. Liu, Tao et al., 2013), visuospatial processing (Siok et al., 2009) and implicit motor learning (Y. Yang et al., 2013). To examine whether there are significant convergent patterns of brain activity associated with Chinese dyslexia, we carried out a quantitative meta-analysis using the

Table 10.2 *Neuroimaging studies of Chinese dyslexia included in the meta-analysis*

Study	Year	Task	No. of subjects (Dys, Nor)	Mean age (Dys, Nor)
Siok et al.	2004	homophone judgment	8, 8	10.9, 11.1
		lexical decision	8, 8	10.9, 11.1
Siok et al.	2008	rhyme judgment	16, 16	11.0, 11.0
Siok et al.	2009	physical size judgment	12, 12	10.9, 11.0
Hu et al.	2010	semantic word matching	8, 8	14.1, 14.5
L. Liu et al.	2012	rhyme and semantic judgment	16, 16	12.0, 11.6
L. Liu, You et al.	2013	morphological processing	14, 14	11.9, 11.7
Y. Yang et al.	2013	implicit motor learning	9, 12	12.1, 12.8
Xu et al.	2015	phonological working memory	12, 12	10.6, 10.2
Cao et al.	2017	auditory rhyming judgment	17, 14	11.1, 11.2

Dys: dyslexic; Nor: normal.

activation likelihood estimation (ALE) method for neuroimaging studies that have reported coordinates of differential activation between dyslexic readers and controls. A total of ten experiments from nine articles were selected (Table 10.2 lists the selected articles).

In Figure 10.2A, we showed the coordinates reported in these studies for the contrast of controls>dyslexics. Because the number of studies is not large enough, we used a relatively liberal threshold for the analysis (p <0.001 uncorrected, with a minimum cluster size of $200mm^3$). We found that brain areas that were most consistently reported across studies were located in the left middle frontal gyrus (MFG) at BA 9 and inferior frontal gyrus (IFG) at BA 45/47 (as shown in Figure 10.2B). Other peaks of convergence were found in the left precentral gyrus at BA 4, cingulate gyrus at BA32/24, and the left fusiform gyrus at BA 37. For the meta-analysis of the contrast of dyslexics>controls, there was no convergence of activity.

Children with dyslexia exhibited reduced activation in the left MFG compared to the normal controls when performing phonological tasks, such as deciding whether two characters have an identical pronunciation or whether or not two characters rhyme. This has been interpreted as suggesting that Chinese readers with dyslexia may manifest a deficit in mapping orthography to phonology (Siok et al., 2004, 2008). By using a phonological working-memory task, we found that Chinese dyslexic children exhibited reduced dominance of the left-hemispheric regions including MFG (Xu et al., 2015). Moreover, a phonological deficit was found to coexist with a visuospatial deficit in Chinese dyslexics (Siok et al., 2009). Dyslexic children showed

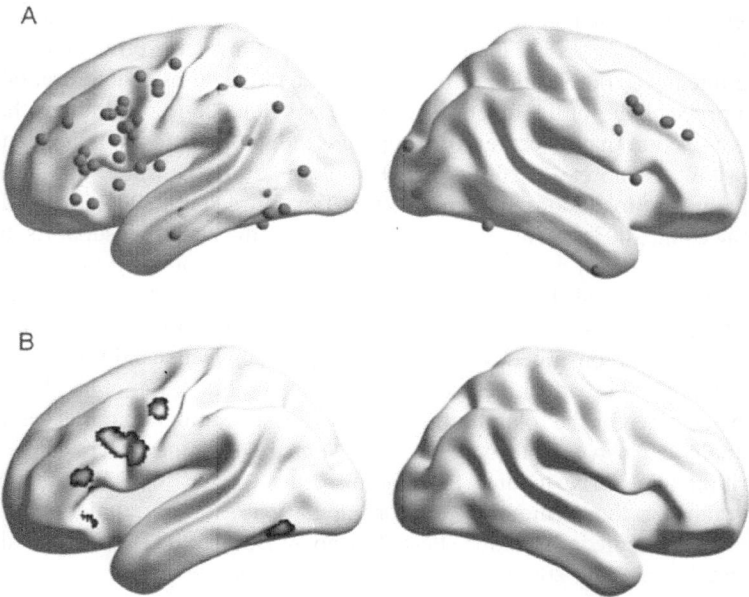

Figure 10.2 (A) Peak activation for the contrast of controls>dyslexics reported in previous studies. Each red circle represents a coordinate of the peak activation. (B) ALE map generated to assess the convergent patterns of brain activity associated with Chinese dyslexia (threshold at p<0.001 uncorrected, a minimum cluster size of 200 mm^3)

reduced activation in the left MFG during a phonological task and reduced activation in the left intraparietal sulcus for visuospatial processing during a physical size judgment task. However, no correlation was observed between activation of the left MFG and the left intraparietal sulcus or between behavioral performance of phonological and visuospatial tasks, indicating that the phonological and visuospatial deficits are independent.

Hypoactivation of the left MFG is also evident when dyslexic children are compared with typically developing readers during orthographic and semantic tasks (Hu et al., 2010; Siok et al., 2004). In Siok et al.'s (2004) study, children with dyslexia and normal children judged whether a viewed stimulus was a real Chinese character; in Hu et al. (2010) the subjects performed a word-matching task in which the correct choice was determined by a semantic relationship between two words. Reduced activity in the left MFG during these tasks may suggest a deficit in coordination, and integration of visual-orthographic and semantic processes in Chinese dyslexics.

Processing Chinese characters requires intensive visual-orthographic analysis and the arbitrary association between visual forms and pronunciations demand intensive coordination of different linguistic features. Therefore, one explanatory account for the function of the left MFG in Chinese reading is that it serves as a coordination center for mapping orthography onto phonology and meaning (W. J. Kuo et al., 2001; W. J. Kuo et al., 2003; L. Liu et al., 2009; Perfetti, Tan, & Siok, 2006; Siok et al., 2008; Tan, Laird et al., 2005; Tan et al., 2001; Tan et al., 2003). An alternative account is that the left MFG supports the motoric representation and visual-motor activity for phonological processing (W. J. Kuo et al., 2004; Perfetti & Tan, 2013; Perfetti et al., 2006; Tan, Laird et al., 2005; Tan, Spinks et al., 2005). This account was supported by behavioral studies, which demonstrated a robust correlation between handwriting and children's ability to read Chinese (Tan, Spinks et al., 2005; Tan et al., 2013). The two accounts for the role of left MFG in Chinese reading are not necessarily mutually exclusive. Instead, the learning strategy of Chinese characters by handwriting may serve to tune the reading center in the left MFG that is spatially close to the premotor cortex for integration of orthographic, phonological, and semantic information (Perfetti, Cao, & Booth, 2013; Perfetti et al., 2006; Tan, Laird et al., 2005; Tan, Spinks et al., 2005).

Abnormal activation of the left IFG is also commonly reported in Chinese dyslexics (Cao et al., 2017; L. Liu et al., 2012; Siok et al., 2004). Using a rhyming judgment task and a semantic association judgment task, L. Liu et al. (2012) found that dyslexic children showed reduced activation compared with normal children in both tasks in the left dorsal IFG, the right visual cortex and left ventral occipitotemporal cortex. Significant correlation was observed between activation in the IFG and in the cuneus in normal children during the semantic task, whereas such correlation was absent in dyslexic children, indicating a visual-orthographic deficit and a connectivity deficit in dyslexics. In a more recent study, Cao et al. (2017) used an auditory rhyming judgment task and found reduced activation in the left dorsal IFG in Chinese dyslexic children compared to both age-matched controls and reading-matched controls, suggesting phonological processing deficits of dyslexia in this region that are independent of reading ability and task performance (Cao et al., 2017). Activation level in the left dorsal IFG was positively correlated with reading skills in dyslexic children, indicating that phonological deficits in this region may be associated with the severity of dyslexia. However, in another study, Siok et al. (2004) have reported increased rather than reduced activation in the left IFG during a phonological task, which may reflect a compensatory mechanism for the phonological deficit. Similarly, neuroimaging studies of alphabetic languages have also reported inconsistent results as to whether dyslexics showed hypoactivity (Paulesu et al., 1996; B. A. Shaywitz et al., 2002) or hyperactivity (Hoeft et al., 2007; S. E. Shaywitz et al., 1998) in the left

IFG. This may be partly due to the nature of variation in dyslexia, and the differences of reading processes involved in the in-scanner tasks.

Liu et al. examined the neural basis for morphological processing deficit in Chinese dyslexics (L. Liu, Tao et al., 2013). They used a semantic relatedness judgment task and manipulated the relations between semantic relatedness and the morphemic overlap of the two words, such that there were congruent and incongruent conditions. In the congruent condition, the two words were either semantically related with a common morpheme or unrelated without morpheme overlap. In the incongruent condition, the two words were either related without morpheme overlap or unrelated with a common morpheme. It was found that normal children manifested greater activation for incongruent than congruent conditions in the left dorsal and ventral IFG (BA 9 and BA 47), whereas dyslexic children did not show such an incongruent effect, which may reflect less sensitivity to morphological information in the dyslexic readers.

Dyslexia in alphabetic languages has been found to be associated consistently with reduced activation in the left temporoparietal cortex. This suggests that the neural basis for dyslexia in Chinese is at least partly different from that of alphabetic languages. Indeed, Siok et al. (2008) found activation and graymatter volume decreases in children with dyslexia in the left MFG, but failed to find any functional or structural difference between dyslexic and normal groups in the regions that were previously found to show structural and functional abnormalities in dyslexic readers of alphabetic languages. However, Hu et al. (2010) found some common neuroanatomical correlates for English and Chinese dyslexia. Both Chinese and English dyslexics showed weaker activation than normal subjects in the left angular gyrus, left MFG, posterior temporal, and occipitotemporal regions during a semantic matching task. Hu et al. (2010) suggested the common pattern of reduced activation in the two groups of dyslexics might reflect the effect of weak phonological and visuospatial working memory in the access of semantic information.

Brain structural abnormalities have also been reported in Chinese dyslexic readers compared with normal readers (L. Liu, You et al., 2013; Qi et al., 2016; Siok et al., 2008; Y.-H. Yang et al., 2016). For example, Siok et al. (2008) found a gray-matter volume decrease in children with dyslexia that corresponded to the key area of functional under-activation in the left MFG. Liu et al. found reduced gray-matter volume in dyslexic children in a wide range of regions including the bilateral ventromedial prefrontal cortex, the left IFG, right inferior occipital gyrus and so on (L. Liu, You et al., 2013).

Recent MRI studies used a structural network-based analysis to explore the topological organization characteristics of the brain in Chinese dyslexics (K. Liu et al., 2015; Qi et al., 2016). K. Liu et al. (2015) recruited twenty-five dyslexic children and twenty-five typically developing children and constructed the structural networks based on the pairwise correlation of gray-matter volume from ninety brain regions. Results showed that the structural network of dyslexic children exhibited significantly increased local efficiency combined with a tendency of decreased global efficiency, reflecting a more locally specialized topological organization. The authors explained that the increased regional network property perhaps compensates for the dilatory establishment of long-range connections in dyslexic readers. In another study by Qi et al. (2016), structural imaging data from seventeen Chinese dyslexic children and seventeen age-matched controls were used to construct cortical thickness and surface area networks. Cortical thickness is sensitive to postnatal development and the surface area is sensitive to prenatal development. They found that dyslexic children showed atypical structural connectivity in terms of both the thickness network (reduced nodal network properties in the left hemisphere and enhanced nodal properties in the right hemisphere) and the surface network (lower nodal properties in the posterior brain regions and higher nodal properties in the anterior brain regions). As the authors suggest, the aberrant structural connectivity in the dyslexic individuals may be due to both a late developmental effect reflected in the altered thickness network as well as a congenital effect during prenatal development, reflected in the altered surface network.

The investigation of white-matter structural connectivity in Chinese dyslexia remains scarce. A recent study conducted by Cui et al. (2016) used machine learning to discriminate between dyslexic and normally reading children on multiple white-matter features at a regional level, including white-matter volume, fractional anisotropy, mean diffusivity, axial diffusivity, and radial diffusivity. They found that using a combination of these white-matter features yielded a classification accuracy of 83.6 percent. The most discriminative features that contributed to the classification were primarily within three networks; i.e., the putative reading network involving the superior longitudinal fasciculus and inferior fronto-occipital fasciculus, the limbic system involving the cingulum and fornix, and the motor system involving the cerebellar peduncle, corona radiata, and corticospinal tract. The finding supports the disconnection hypothesis of Chinese dyslexia and has important implication for using brain imaging as a diagnostic tool to identify children with dyslexia.

To summarize, neuroimaging studies of Chinese dyslexics suggest deficits in visuospatial, visual-orthographic, phonological, semantic, and morphological processing of written Chinese. Results from functional and structural neuroimaging studies attempting to characterize the cortical abnormalities in Chinese dyslexics are only partly consistent, but they have converged to highlight the important role of the left prefrontal cortex in Chinese dyslexics. Moreover, atypical brain structural networks have recently been revealed in Chinese dyslexics.

10.4.3 Genetic Studies on Chinese Dyslexia

Research suggests that dyslexia runs in families. Family and twin studies have demonstrated that up to 75 percent of the phenotypic variance in developmental dyslexia can be explained by genetic factors (Poelmans et al. 2011). Developmental dyslexia is multifactorial and has been shown to be associated with multiple genes that may control how the brain develops. The past few years have seen an increase of genetic studies on Chinese reading development and dyslexia (H. Chen et al., 2014; Chow et al., 2011; Lim et al., 2011; Sun et al., 2014; G. Wang et al., 2015; Y. Zhang et al., 2012). For instance, Lim et al. (2011) genotyped 8 genetic variants in 393 individuals from 131 Chinese families with dyslexia. The study found a significant association between the single nucleotide polymorphisms (SNP) rs3743205 of the "dyslexia susceptibility" gene DYX1C1 and Chinese dyslexia. Quantitative traits analyses showed that this SNP was significantly associated with reading, digit rapid naming, phonological memory, and orthographic skills. Another study by Y. Zhang et al. (2012) used a longitudinal design in examining the association of DYX1C1 and reading abilities over multiple time points. They used the data from a general population cohort of 284 unrelated children aged 5 to 11 years who were participating in a longitudinal study of Chinese reading development. Three SNPs (rs3743205, rs11629841, and rs57809907) that showed significant association in previous studies were genotyped. Results showed that rs11629841 was associated with children's orthographic judgments at ages 7 and 8 years, and associated with Chinese character dictation at ages 9, 10, and 11 years. These two studies may suggest a universal effect of DYX1C1 on reading abilities in both dyslexic children and the general population, but they are limited by small sample size and limited DYX1C1 marker coverage.

Studies have repeatedly implicated the DYX2 locus, where two susceptible genes KIAA0319 and DCDC2 showed significant association (Cope et al., 2005; H. Meng et al., 2005). However, Sun et al. (2014) failed to find significant association of these two genes with developmental dyslexia in Chinese population. They selected 60 SNPs that were frequently reported by previous studies and performed high-density genotyping on DCDC2 and KIAA0319 in a large unrelated Chinese cohort with 502 dyslexic children and 522 healthy controls. Several SNPs showed weak associations with Chinese dyslexia, but none of these results survived Bonferroni correction for multiple comparisons. Given the substantial differences of linguistic and genetic backgrounds between Chinese and other Western populations, the findings of this study suggest caution when considering the generalization of genetic findings related to developmental dyslexia among different populations.

It also should be emphasized that external environments can affect the expression or function of genes, either strengthening or weakening the effect of genes on phenotypes (Pennington et al., 2009). Su et al. (2015) investigated the interactions of genetic (DCDC2) and environmental (home literacy) factors on orthographic processing of Chinese characters at the behavioral and neural level, with the N170 as a neural marker for orthographic processing (Su et al., 2015). They found that there was a significant interaction effect between SNP rs1091047 in DCDC2 and home literacy on the differential N170 between real words and nonword stroke combination in the left hemisphere. The results suggested that home literacy might modulate the role of DCDC2 in the neuro-electrophysiology of orthographic processing.

10.5   Intervention

Remediation studies have undoubtedly rekindled the hope of individuals who suffer from developmental dyslexia. Recent intervention studies for Chinese dyslexics have focused on using non-phonological intervention protocols, such as visual-perceptual (X. Meng et al., 2014), visual-motor (Qian & Bi, 2015), and working-memory training (Luo et al., 2013), to help improve reading performance in dyslexics. For example, X. Meng et al. (2014) gave a four-week visual-perceptual training session using a texture discrimination task, in which dyslexic children and normal controls were asked to discriminate the orientation of target bars. They found that Chinese dyslexic children improved reading performance after the training, whereas the normal children and the non-training dyslexic children did not show any improvement in reading. In addition, the training-induced improvement in reading fluency was maintained in follow-up tests two months post training.

In another study, Qian and Bi (2015) used magnocellular-based visual-motor intervention, which contained three training projects, i.e., (i) a coherent-motion detection task that aimed to train magnocellular function directly, (ii) visual search and visual tracking tasks that focused on eye movement, object localiza-tion, and visual spatial attention, and (iii) juggling used to train visual percep-tion and spatial anticipation of moving objects. After ten sessions of training within five weeks, dyslexic children improved magnocellular function and phonological awareness to normal level as age-matched controls, whereas the non-training dyslexics did not. These findings suggest that Chinese dyslexics who have visual deficits may also have correctable impairments of visual word processing

Ho and her colleagues (2014) have developed and implemented a more comprehensive intervention program with a core reading instruction curricu-lum in Hong Kong primary schools. Following the framework of the Response-to-Intervention (RIT) model, they provided three tiers of instruction, i.e., whole-class quality instruction, small-group supplemental instruction, and individualized intensive instruction. Those who fall below the benchmarks receive more intensive intervention. The curriculum emphasizes three levels of skill building, including oral language skills (oral vocabulary and morphological skills), word-level skills (orthographic skills and word recognition), and text-level skills (reading fluency, syntactic skills, reading comprehension, and writing strategies). Results showed that the whole-class quality instruction was effective in enhancing the literacy and cognitive-linguistic skills of children in the program school, as compared to the control school. Importantly, they found that 18 to 58 percent of poor readers receiving small-group supplemental instruction and 7 percent of dyslexic readers receiving individualized intensive instruction reached the benchmark of Chinese literacy after 1–2 years of intervention. Because the intervention program is comprehensive, covering the major important cognitive-linguistic components for reading, specific component causes for the improvements cannot be specified. However, the authors suggest that instructions of the orthographic skills and morphological awareness are crucial to Chinese reading instructions, whereas phonological training may be more important for learning to read English (Ho et al., 2014).

10.6   Discussion and Conclusion

Developmental dyslexia is a severe and specific difficulty in reading acquisition, with neurological and genetic bases. To understand the mechanisms underlying dyslexia, it is important to elucidate the pathways among genetics, developmental brain changes, and cognitive deficits associated with the disorder (Galaburda et al., 2006). In the past two decades, research into the behavioral, neuroimaging, and genetic studies have greatly advanced our understanding of Chinese dyslexia. The findings of these studies have practical and theoretical implications for the diagnosis and treatment of the disorder.

A great variety of symptoms have been observed in Chinese developmental dyslexics, including deficits in phonological awareness, rapid naming, visual skills, morphological processing, and so on. No single theory can account for the full range of difficulties in dyslexic individuals. The Chinese writing system differs from the alphabetic writing system in terms of visual-orthographic features and how the written symbols map onto phonology and semantics, which may entail different contributions of different cognitive components to reading development across writing systems. Furthermore, the dynamic nature of reading development may have complicated the interpretation of results in different studies, since the relationships between the variables proposed in these theories and various reading skills may depend on age (Goswami, 2003). Indeed, research using cross-sectional or longitudinal design has demonstrated that the role of certain cognitive abilities in Chinese reading changes across age groups (Lei et al., 2011; Siok & Fletcher, 2001; Zhou et al., 2014). Furthermore, functional neuroimaging studies have demonstrated abnormalities in the left inferior and middle frontal cortices, left posterior parietal cortex, and the occipitotemporal regions in the processing of Chinese words.

These findings are only partly consistent with those from studies of dyslexics in alphabetic languages, indicating that language and writing system factors can influence the weighting of the various challenges of reading and thus the neural expression of reading difficulties. Successful reading requires both efficient processing in cortical areas and information transmission among these areas. From a developmental point of view, the spatially distinct neural systems crucial for reading may have been well established before children learn to read, and the learning process adjusts the functional connections among these systems, enabling efficient mapping between visual word forms and phonological or semantic representations (Johnson, 2011; Schlaggar & McCandliss, 2007). Previous studies of alphabetic languages have generally suggested that developmental dyslexia was associated with reduced connectivity among left-hemisphere regions, including the left IFG, left temporoparietal regions, and left occipitotemporal cortex, and excessive connection among the right-hemisphere regions that might be due to compensatory mechanisms for the disruption of left-hemisphere connectivity (Boets et al., 2013; Cao, Bitan, & Booth, 2008; Horwitz, Rumsey, & Donohue, 1998; L. Liu et al., 2010; Pugh et al., 2000; Quaglino et al., 2008; van der Mark et al., 2011). However, our knowledge is especially lacking on the patterns of functional integration of neural systems associated with Chinese dyslexia. It also remains elusive as to whether and how the connectivity patterns in dyslexics vary across different languages.

Evidence from genetic studies is accumulating, aiming at identifying candidate genes and examining the relationship between genetic variations and behavioral manifestations in Chinese dyslexia. For a more comprehensive understanding of the mechanisms underlying dyslexia, it is important to elucidate how the genes that alter expression of the proteins give rise to the change in brain functions and structure that underlie cognitive deficits in dyslexia. Because the effects of the genes are not expressed directly at the behavioral level, but rather are mediated by their molecular effects on the brain (Eicher & Gruen, 2013), neuroimaging correlates of dyslexia can provide the intermediate biologic phenotypes to explain the neurobiological mechanisms by which gene variants can affect behavior. Moreover, imaging genetics holds great promise of identifying new candidate genes that contribute to functional and structural variations in brain circuitry with much smaller samples (Bigos & Weinberger, 2010).

The heritability estimates indicate a strong effect of genetics on developmental dyslexia, but there are also important environmental influences. Environmental factors, such as home literacy, parent education, socioeconomic status, and so on, have been shown to influence the development of reading abilities (Evans, Shaw, & Bell, 2000; Noble, Farah, & McCandliss, 2006). In a recent study with a large sample of primary school children in mainland China, we have demonstrated that children's reading performance significantly decreases with their utilization of the Pinyin input method, but increases with their time spent on handwriting (Tan et al., 2013). The Pinyin input method does not require the users to construct the characters by combining strokes, as one would do in writing Chinese characters. Therefore, increasing reliance on electronic modes over handwriting for communications makes learning to read even more challenging in the information age.

Finally, there is an urgent need to help dyslexics to enhance their reading abilities. Studies about using behavioral remediation to alleviate reading difficulties in Chinese dyslexics are still lacking, particularly those that compare the intervention effects of different training programs on dyslexic readers in a way that allows the cause of treatment effects to be attributed to a specific intervention component. In addition, future studies will need to validate the effects of remedial intervention using neuroimaging techniques. In alphabetic languages, many neuroimaging studies have demonstrated improved reading ability and brain plasticity in individuals with dyslexia in response to instructional interventions, bringing their brain activation closer to the level of normal readers (e.g., Eden et al., 2004; Olulade, Napoliello, & Eden, 2013; Spironelli et al., 2010; Temple et al., 2003).

Early identification of children at risk of dyslexia is the key to facilitating effective intervention and preventing reading problems in these children. Current approaches using reading tests to identify dyslexia have a major limitation in the form of the minimum age at which the tests can be administrated. A study conducted by McBride-Chang et al. (2008) found that tone-detection and morphological-awareness tasks can best distinguish Chinese kindergarten children at family risk of reading problems from those who are not at risk. An alternative potential approach to identifying dyslexics at an early age is to use neuroimaging data. Based on the variation in brain function and structure, previous studies have discriminated dyslexic children from normal controls (Cui et al., 2016) and predicted long-term reading improvement in children with dyslexia (Bach et al., 2013; Hoeft et al., 2011; Myers et al., 2014). Nonetheless, validation studies are still needed to optimize the sensitivity, specificity, and accuracy of using neuroimaging as diagnosis tools of dyslexia.

In conclusion, Chinese and alphabetic writing make different demands on reading. Investigations of Chinese dyslexia thus provide an excellent opportunity to understand the universal and language-specific aspects of reading development and reading disability. Findings from studies at the levels of behavior, neurology, and genetics suggest that the deficits associated with developmental dyslexia are only partly universal. These findings motivate further studies on the early screening, diagnosis, and intervention of dyslexia from a language-specific perspective.

References

Bach, S., Richardson, U., Brandeis, D., Martin, E., & Brem, S. (2013). Print-specific multimodal brain activation in kindergarten improves prediction of reading skills in second grade. *NeuroImage*, *82*, 605–615.

Bigos, K. L., & Weinberger, D. R. (2010). Imaging genetics – days of future past. *NeuroImage*, *53*, 804–809.

Boets, B., Op de Beeck, H. P., & Vandermosten, M. et al.(2013). Intact but less accessible phonetic representations in adults with dyslexia. *Science*, *342*, 1251–1254.

Bradley, L., & Bryant, P. E. (1983). Categorizing sounds and learning to read – a causal connection. *Nature*, *301*, 419–421.

Cao, F., Bitan, T., & Booth, J. R. (2008). Effective brain connectivity in children with reading difficulties during phonological processing. *Brain and Language*, *107*, 91–101.

Cao, F., Yan, X., Wang, Z., Liu, Y., Wang, J., Spray, G. J., & Deng, Y. (2017). Neural signatures of phonological deficits in Chinese developmental dyslexia. *NeuroImage*, *146*, 301–311.

Caravolas, M. (2005). The nature and causes of dyslexia in different languages. In M. J. Snowling & C. Hulme (Eds.), *The science of reading: A handbook* (pp. 336–355). Cambridge, MA: Blackwell Publishing.

Chan, D. W., Ho, C. S.-H., Tsang, S.-M., Lee, S.-H., & Chung, K. K. H. (2003). Reading-related behavioral characteristics of Chinese children with dyslexia: The use of the teachers' behavior checklist in Hong Kong. *Annals of Dyslexia*, *53*, 300–323.

Chan, D. W., Ho, C. S.-H., Tsang, S.-M., Lee, S. H., & Chung, K. K. H. (2007). Prevalence, gender ratio and gender differences in reading-related cognitive abilities among Chinese children with dyslexia in Hong Kong. *Educational Studies*, *33*, 249–265.

Chang, L.-Y., Chen, Y. C., & Perfetti, C. A. (2017). GraphCom: A multi-dimensional measure of grapheme complexity: A comparison of 131 written languages. *Behavior Research Methods*, *50*, 427–449.

Chen, H., Wang, G., & Xia, J. et al. (2014). Stuttering candidate genes DRD2 but not SLC6A3 is associated with developmental dyslexia in Chinese population. *Behavioral and Brain Functions*, *10*, 29.

Chen, X., & Pasquarella, A. (2017). Learning to read Chinese. In L. Verhoeven & C. A. Perfetti (Eds.), *Learning to read across languages and writing systems* (pp. 31–56). Cambridge, MA: Cambridge University Press.

Chow, B. W.-Y., Ho, C. S.-H., Wong, S. W.-L., Waye, M. M. Y., & Bishop, D. V. M. (2011). Genetic and environmental influences on Chinese language and reading abilities. *PLoS One*, *6*(2), e16640.

Chung, K. K. H., Ho, C. S.-H., Chan, D. W., Tsang, S.-M., & Lee, S.-H. (2010). Cognitive profiles of Chinese adolescents with dyslexia. *Dyslexia*, *16*, 2–23.

Chung, K. K. H., McBride-Chang, C., Wong, S. W. L. et al. (2008). The role of visual and auditory temporal processing for Chinese children with developmental dyslexia. *Annals of Dyslexia*, *58*, 15–35.

Compton, D. L. (2003). Modeling the relationship between growth in rapid naming speed and growth in decoding skill in first-grade children. *Journal of Educational Psychology*, *95*, 225 239.

Cope, N., Harold, D., Hill, G. et al. (2005). Strong evidence that KIAA0319 on chromosome 6p is a susceptibility gene for developmental dyslexia. *The American Journal of Human Genetics*, *76*, 581–591.

Cui, Z., Xia, Z., Su, M., Shu, H., & Gong, G. (2016). Disrupted white matter connectivity underlying developmental dyslexia: A machine learning approach. *Human Brain Mapping*, *37*, 1443–1458.

Eden, G. F., VanMeter, J. W., Rumsey, J. M., & Zeffiro, T. A. (1996). The visual deficit theory of developmental dyslexia. *NeuroImage*, *4*, S108–S117.

Eden, G. F., Jones, K. M., & Cappell, K. et al. (2004). Neural changes following remediation in adult developmental dyslexia. *Neuron*, *44*, 411–422.

Eicher, J. D., & Gruen, J. R. (2013). Imaging-genetics in dyslexia: Connecting risk genetic variants to brain neuroimaging and ultimately to reading impairments. *Molecular Genetics and Metabolism*, *110*, 201–212.

Evans, M. A., Shaw, D., & Bell, M. (2000). Home literacy activities and their influence on early literacy skills. *Canadian Journal of Experimental Psychology*, *54*(2), 65–75

Fan, K. Y., Gao, J. Y., & Ao, X. P. (1984). Pronunciation principles of the Chinese character and alphabetic writing scripts. *Chinese Character Reform*, *3*, 23–27.

Gabrieli, J. D. E. (2009). Dyslexia: A new synergy between education and cognitive neuroscience. *Science*, *325*, 280–283.

Galaburda, A. M., LoTurco, J., Ramus, F., Fitch, R. H., & Rosen, G. D. (2006). From genes to behavior in developmental dyslexia. *Nature Neuroscience*, *9*, 1213–1217.

Geschwind, N., & Galaburda, A. M. (1985). Cerebral lateralization: Biological mechanisms, associations, and pathology: II. A hypothesis and a program for research. *Archives of Neurology*, *42*, 521–552.

Goswami, U. (2003). Why theories about developmental dyslexia require developmental designs. *Trends in Cognitive Sciences*, *7*, 534–540.

Handel, Z. (2015). The classification of Chinese: Sinitic (the Chinese language family). In W. S.-Y. Wang & C. Sun (Eds.), *The Oxford handbook of Chinese linguistics* (pp. 34–44). New York, NY: Oxford University Press.

Harbaugh, R. (1998). *Chinese characters: A genealogy and dictionary*. New Haven, CT: Yale University Press.

Hinshelwood, J. (1917). *Congenital word-blindness*. London, United Kingdom: Lewis.

Ho, C. S.-H., Chan, D. W., Chung, K. K., Lee, S. H., & Tsang, S. M. (2007). In search of subtypes of Chinese developmental dyslexia. *Journal of Experimental Child Psychology*, *97*, 61 83.

Ho, C. S.-H., Chan, D. W.-O., Lee, S.-H., Tsang, S.-M., & Luan, V. H. (2004). Cognitive profiling and preliminary subtyping in Chinese developmental dyslexia. *Cognition*, *91*, 43–75.

Ho, C. S.-H., Chan, D. W., Tsang, S.-M., & Lee, S.-H. (2000). *The Hong Kong test of specific learning difficulties in reading and writing (HKT-SpLD)*. Hong Kong, China: Chinese University of Hong Kong & Education Department, HKSAR Government.

Ho, C. S.-H., Chan, D. W.-O., Tsang, S.-M., & Lee, S.-H. (2002). The cognitive profile and multiple-deficit hypothesis in Chinese developmental dyslexia. *Developmental psychology*, *38*, 543 553.

Ho, C. S.-H., & Lai, D. N.-C. (1999). Naming-speed deficits and phonological memory deficits in Chinese developmental dyslexia. *Learning and Individual Differences, 11*, 173–186.

Ho, C. S.-H., Law, T. P.-S., & Ng, P. M. (2000). The phonological deficit hypothesis in Chinese developmental dyslexia. *Reading and Writing, 13*, 57–79.

Ho, C. S.-H., Wong, Y.-K., Lo, C.-M. et al. (2014). Helping children with reading disability in Chinese: The response to intervention approach with effective evidence-based curriculum. In X. Chen, Q. Wang, & Y. Luo (Eds.), *Reading development and difficulties in monolingual and bilingual Chinese children* (pp. 103–124). Dordrecht: Springer.

Hoeft, F., McCandliss, B. D., Black, J. M. et al. (2011). Neural systems predicting long-term outcome in dyslexia. *Proceedings of the National Academy of Sciences of the United States of America, 108*, 361–366.

Hoeft, F., Meyler, A., Hernandez, A. et al. (2007). Functional and morphometric brain dissociation between dyslexia and reading ability. *Proceedings of the National Academy of Sciences of the United States of America, 104*, 4234–4239.

Horwitz, B., Rumsey, J. M., & Donohue, B. C. (1998). Functional connectivity of the angular gyrus in normal reading and dyslexia. *Proceedings of the National Academy of Sciences of the United States of America, 95*, 8939–8944.

Hu, W., Lee, H. L., Zhang, Q. et al. (2010). Developmental dyslexia in Chinese and English populations: dissociating the effect of dyslexia from language differences. *Brain, 133*, 1694–1706.

Huang, H. S., & Hanley, J. R. (1995). Phonological awareness and visual skills in learning to read Chinese and English. *Cognition, 54*, 73–98.

Hulme, C., Hatcher, P. J., Nation, K. et al. (2002). Phoneme awareness is a better predictor of early reading skill than onset-rime awareness. *Journal of Experimental Child Psychology, 82*, 2–28.

Johnson, M. H. (2011). Interactive specialization: A domain-general framework for human functional brain development? *Developmental Cognitive Neuroscience, 1*, 7–21.

Kuo, W. F. (1978). A preliminary study of reading disability in the Republic of China. *Bulletin of Educational Research, 20*, 57–78.

Kuo, W. J., Yeh, T. C., Duann, J. R. et al. (2001). A left-lateralized network for reading Chinese words: A 3 T fMRI study. *Neuroreport, 12*, 3997–4001.

Kuo, W. J., Yeh, T. C., Lee, C. Y. et al. (2003). Frequency effects of Chinese character processing in the brain: an event-related fMRI study. *NeuroImage, 18*, 720–730.

Kuo, W. J., Yeh, T. C., Lee, J. R. et al. (2004). Orthographic and phonological processing of Chinese characters: An fMRI study. *NeuroImage, 21*, 1721–1731.

Lee, J. R., Hung, D. L., & Tzeng, O. J. (2006). Cross-linguistic analysis of developmental dyslexia – Does phonology matter in learning to read Chinese? *Language and Linguistics, 7*, 573–594.

Lei, L., Pan, J., Liu, H. et al. (2011). Developmental trajectories of reading development and impairment from ages 3 to 8 years in Chinese children. *Journal of Child Psychology and Psychiatry, 52*, 212–220.

Lervåg, A., & Hulme, C. (2009). Rapid automatized naming (RAN) taps a mechanism that places constraints on the development of early reading fluency. *Psychological Science, 20*, 1040–1048.

Li, C. N., & Thompson, S. A. (1981). *Mandarin Chinese: A functional reference grammar*. Berkeley, CA: University of California Press.

Li, X., Gu, J., Liu, P., & Rayner, K. (2013). The advantage of word-based processing in Chinese reading: Evidence from eye movements. *Journal of Experimental Psychology: Learning, Memory, and Cognition, 39*, 879–889.

Liberman, I. Y. (1971). Basic research in speech and lateralization of language: Some implications for reading disability. *Bulletin of the Orton Society, 21*, 71–87.

Liberman, I. Y., Shankweiler, D., Fischer, F. W., & Carter, B. (1974). Explicit syllable and phoneme segmentation in the young child. *Journal of Experimental Child Psychology, 18*, 201–212.

Lim, C. K., Ho, C. S., Chou, C. H., & Waye, M. M. (2011). Association of the rs3743205 variant of DYX1C1 with dyslexia in Chinese children. *Behavioral and Brain Functions, 7*, 16.

Liu, K., Shi, L., Chen, F. et al. (2015). Altered topological organization of brain structural network in Chinese children with developmental dyslexia. *Neuroscience Letters, 589*, 169–175.

Liu, L., Deng, X., Peng, D. et al. (2009). Modality-and task-specific brain regions involved in Chinese lexical processing. *Journal of Cognitive Neuroscience, 21*, 1473–1487.

Liu, L., Tao, R., Wang, W. et al. (2013). Chinese dyslexics show neural differences in morphological processing. *Developmental Cognitive Neuroscience, 6*, 40–50.

Liu, L., Vira, A., Friedman, E. et al. (2010). Children with reading disability show brain differences in effective connectivity for visual, but not auditory word comprehension. *PLoS One, 5*(10), e13492.

Liu, L., Wang, W., You, W. et al. (2012). Similar alterations in brain function for phonological and semantic processing to visual characters in Chinese dyslexia. *Neuropsychologia, 50*, 2224–2232.

Liu, L., You, W., Wang, W. et al. (2013). Altered brain structure in Chinese dyslexic children. *Neuropsychologia, 51*, 1169–1176.

Livingstone, M. S., Rosen, G. D., Drislane, F. W., & Galaburda, A. M. (1991). Physiological and anatomical evidence for a magnocellular defect in developmental dyslexia. *Proceedings of the National Academy of Sciences of the United States of America, 88*, 7943–7947.

Lu, W. (2011). Structure of multiple-pronunciation characters in modern Chinese (In Chinese). *Journal of Jiangsu Institute of Education (Social Science), 27*, 120–124.

Luo, Y., Wang, J., Wu, H., Zhu, D., & Zhang, Y. (2013). Working-memory training improves developmental dyslexia in Chinese children. *Neural Regeneration Research, 8*, 452–460.

McBride-Chang, C., Bialystok, E., Chong, K. K., & Li, Y. (2004). Levels of phonological awareness in three cultures. *Journal of Experimental Child Psychology, 89*, 93–111.

McBride-Chang, C., Chung, K. K., & Tong, X. (2011). Copying skills in relation to word reading and writing in Chinese children with and without dyslexia. *Journal of Experimental Child Psychology, 110*, 422–433.

McBride-Chang, C., Lam, F., Lam, C. et al. (2011). Early predictors of dyslexia in Chinese children: Familial history of dyslexia, language delay, and cognitive profiles. *Journal of Child Psychology and Psychiatry, 52*, 204–211.

McBride-Chang, C., Lam, F., Lam, C. et al. (2008). Word recognition and cognitive profiles of Chinese pre-school children at risk for dyslexia through language delay or familial history of dyslexia. *Journal of Child Psychology and Psychiatry, 49*, 211–218.

McBride-Chang, C., Shu, H., Zhou, A., Wat, C. P., & Wagner, R. K. (2003). Morphological awareness uniquely predicts young children's Chinese character recognition. *Journal of Educational Psychology, 95*, 743–751.

Meng, H., Smith, S. D., Hager, K. et al. (2005). DCDC2 is associated with reading disability and modulates neuronal development in the brain. *Proceedings of the National Academy of Sciences of the United States of America, 102*, 17053–17058.

Meng, X., Cheng-Lai, A., Zeng, B., Stein, J. F., & Zhou, X. (2011). Dynamic visual perception and reading development in Chinese school children. *Annals of Dyslexia, 61*, 161–176.

Meng, X., Lin, O., Wang, F., Jiang, Y., & Song, Y. (2014). Reading performance is enhanced by visual texture discrimination training in Chinese-speaking children with developmental dyslexia. *PLoS One, 9*(9), e108274.

Morgan, W. P. (1896). A case of congenital word blindness. *British Medical Journal, 2* (1871), 1378.

Myers, C. A., Vandermosten, M., Farris, E. A. et al. (2014). White matter morphometric changes uniquely predict children's reading acquisition. *Psychological Science, 25*, 1870–1883.

Nation, K., & Hulme, C. (1997). Phonemic segmentation, not onset-rime segmentation, predicts early reading and spelling skills. *Reading Research Quarterly, 32*, 154–167.

Noble, K. G., Farah, M. J., & McCandliss, B. D. (2006). Socioeconomic background modulates cognition-achievement relationships in reading. *Cognitive Development, 21*, 349–368.

Olulade, O. A., Napoliello, E. M., & Eden, G. F. (2013). Abnormal visual motion processing is not a cause of dyslexia. *Neuron, 79*, 180–190.

Paulesu, E., Frith, U., Snowling, M. et al. (1996). Is developmental dyslexia a disconnection syndrome? Evidence from PET scanning. *Brain, 119*, 143–157.

Penney, T. B., Leung, K. M., Chan, P. C., Meng, X., & McBride-Chang, C. A. (2005). Poor readers of Chinese respond slower than good readers in phonological, rapid naming, and interval timing tasks. *Annals of Dyslexia, 55*, 9–27.

Pennington, B. F., McGrath, L. M., & Rosenberg, J. (2009). Gene × environment interactions in reading disability and attention-deficit/hyperactivity disorder. *Developmental Psychology, 45*, 77–89.

Perfetti, C. A. (1992). The representation problem in reading acquisition. In P. B. Gough, L. C. Ehri, & R. Reiman (Eds.), *Reading acquisition* (pp. 145–174). Hillsdale, NJ: Lawrence Erlbaum Associates.

Perfetti, C., Cao, F., & Booth, J. (2013). Specialization and universals in the development of reading skill: How Chinese research informs a universal science of reading. *Scientific Studies of Reading, 17*, 5–21.

Perfetti, C. A., & Tan, L. H. (1998). The time course of graphic, phonological, and semantic activation in Chinese character identification. *Journal of Experimental Psychology: Learning, Memory, and Cognition, 24*, 101–118.

Perfetti, C. A., & Tan, L. H. (2013). Write to read: The brain's universal reading and writing network. *Trends in Cognitive Sciences, 17*, 56–57.

Perfetti, C. A., Tan, L. H., & Siok, W. T. (2006). Brain-behavior relations in reading and dyslexia: Implications of Chinese results. *Brain and Language, 98*, 344–346.

Peterson, R. L., & Pennington, B. F. (2012). Developmental dyslexia. *The Lancet, 379*, 1997–2007.

Poelmans, G., Buitelaar, J. K., Pauls, D. L., & Franke, B. (2011). A theoretical molecular network for dyslexia: Integrating available genetic findings. *Molecular Psychiatry, 16*, 365–382.

Pugh, K. R., Mencl, W. E., Shaywitz, B. A. et al. (2000). The angular gyrus in developmental dyslexia: task-specific differences in functional connectivity within posterior cortex. *Psychological Science, 11*, 51–56.

Qi, T., Gu, B., Ding, G. et al. (2016). More bilateral, more anterior: Alterations of brain organization in the large-scale structural network in Chinese dyslexia. *NeuroImage, 124*, 63–74.

Qian, Y., & Bi, H. Y. (2014). The visual magnocellular deficit in Chinese-speaking children with developmental dyslexia. *Frontiers in Psychology, 5*, 692.

Qian, Y., & Bi, H. Y. (2015). The effect of magnocellular-based visual-motor intervention on Chinese children with developmental dyslexia. *Frontiers in Psychology, 6*, 1529.

Quaglino, V., Bourdin, B., Czternasty, G. et al. (2008). Differences in effective connectivity between dyslexic children and normal readers during a pseudoword reading task: An fMRI study. *Neurophysiologie Clinique/Clinical Neurophysiology, 38*, 73–82.

Schlaggar, B. L., & McCandliss, B. D. (2007). Development of neural systems for reading. *Annual Review Neuroscience, 30*, 475–503.

Shaywitz, B. A., Shaywitz, S. E., Pugh, K. R. et al. (2002). Disruption of posterior brain systems for reading in children with developmental dyslexia. *Biological Psychiatry, 52*, 101–110.

Shaywitz, S. E., Shaywitz, B. A., Pugh, K. R. et al. (1998). Functional disruption in the organization of the brain for reading in dyslexia. *Proceedings of the National Academy of Sciences of the United States of America, 95*, 2636–2641.

Shu, H., McBride-Chang, C., Wu, S., & Liu, H. (2006). Understanding Chinese developmental dyslexia: Morphological awareness as a core cognitive construct. *Journal of Educational Psychology, 98*, 122–133.

Siok, W. T., & Fletcher, P. (2001). The role of phonological awareness and visual-orthographic skills in Chinese reading acquisition. *Developmental Psychology, 37*, 886–899.

Siok, W. T., Niu, Z., Jin, Z., Perfetti, C. A., & Tan, L. H. (2008). A structural-functional basis for dyslexia in the cortex of Chinese readers. *Proceedings of the National Academy of Sciences of the United States of America, 105*, 5561–5566.

Siok, W. T., Perfetti, C. A., Jin, Z., & Tan, L. H. (2004). Biological abnormality of impaired reading is constrained by culture. *Nature, 431*, 71–76.

Siok, W. T., Spinks, J. A., Jin, Z., & Tan, L. H. (2009). Developmental dyslexia is characterized by the co-existence of visuospatial and phonological disorders in Chinese children. *Current Biology, 19*, R890–R892.

Song, S., Su, M., & Kang, C. et al. (2015). Tracing children's vocabulary development from preschool through the school-age years: An 8-year longitudinal study. *Developmental Science, 18*, 119–131.

Spironelli, C., Penolazzi, B., Vio, C., & Angrilli, A. (2010). Cortical reorganization in dyslexic children after phonological training: Evidence from early evoked potentials. *Brain, 133*, 3385–3395.

Stein, J. (2001). The magnocellular theory of developmental dyslexia. *Dyslexia, 7*, 12–36.

Stein, J., & Walsh, V. (1997). To see but not to read; the magnocellular theory of dyslexia. *Trends in Neurosciences, 20*, 147–152.

Stevenson, H. W., Stigler, J. W., Lucker, G. W. et al. (1982). Reading disabilities: The case of Chinese, Japanese, and English. *Child Development*, *53*, 1164–1181.

Su, M., Wang, J., Maurer, U. et al. (2015). Gene–environment interaction on neural mechanisms of orthographic processing in Chinese children. *Journal of Neurolinguistics*, *33*, 172–186.

Sun, Y., Gao, Y., Zhou, Y. et al. (2014). Association study of developmental dyslexia candidate genes DCDC2 and KIAA0319 in Chinese population. *American Journal of Medical Genetics Part B: Neuropsychiatric Genetics*, *165*, 627–634.

Tan, L. H., Laird, A. R., Li, K., & Fox, P. T. (2005). Neuroanatomical correlates of phonological processing of Chinese characters and alphabetic words: A meta-analysis. *Human Brain Mapping*, *25*, 83–91.

Tan, L. H., Liu, H. L., Perfetti, C. A. et al. (2001). The neural system underlying Chinese logograph reading. *NeuroImage*, *13*, 836–846.

Tan, L. H., Spinks, J. A., Eden, G. F., Perfetti, C. A., & Siok, W. T. (2005). Reading depends on writing, in Chinese. *Proceedings of the National Academy of Sciences of the United States of America*, *102*, 8781–8785.

Tan, L. H., Spinks, J. A., Feng, C. M. et al. (2003). Neural systems of second language reading are shaped by native language. *Human Brain Mapping*, *18*, 158–166.

Tan, L. H., Xu, M., Chang, C. Q., & Siok, W. T. (2013). China's language input system in the digital age affects children's reading development. *Proceedings of the National Academy of Sciences of the United States of America*, *110*, 1119–1123.

Taylor, I., & Taylor, M. M. (1995). *Writing and literacy in Chinese, Korean and Japanese*. Philadelphia, PA: John Benjamins Publishing.

Temple, E., Deutsch, G. K., Poldrack, R. A. et al. (2003). Neural deficits in children with dyslexia ameliorated by behavioral remediation: Evidence from functional MRI. *Proceedings of the National Academy of Sciences of the United States of America*, *100*, 2860–2865.

van der Mark, S., Klaver, P., Bucher, K. et al. (2011). The left occipitotemporal system in reading: disruption of focal fMRI connectivity to left inferior frontal and inferior parietal language areas in children with dyslexia. *NeuroImage*, *54*, 2426–2436.

Wagner, R. K., Torgesen, J. K., Rashotte, C. A. et al. (1997). Changing relations between phonological processing abilities and word-level reading as children develop from beginning to skilled readers: A 5-year longitudinal study. *Developmental Psychology*, *33*, 468–479.

Wang, G., Zhou, Y., Gao, Y. et al. (2015). Association of specific language impairment candidate genes CMIP and ATP2C2 with developmental dyslexia in Chinese population. *Journal of Neurolinguistics*, *33*, 163–171.

Wang, J. J., Bi, H. Y., Gao, L. Q., & Wydell, T. N. (2010). The visual magnocellular pathway in Chinese-speaking children with developmental dyslexia. *Neuropsychologia*, *48*, 3627–3633.

Wang, Z., Cheng-Lai, A., Song, Y. et al. (2014). A perceptual learning deficit in Chinese developmental dyslexia as revealed by visual texture discrimination training. *Dyslexia*, *20*, 280–296.

Woo, E. Y., & Hoosain, R. (1984). Visual and auditory functions of Chinese dyslexics. *Psychologia: An International Journal of Psychology in the Orient*, *27*, 164–170.

Xu, M., Yang, J., Siok, W. T., & Tan, L. H. (2015). Atypical lateralization of phonological working memory in developmental dyslexia. *Journal of Neurolinguistics*, *33*, 67–77.

Yan, M., Pan, J., Laubrock, J., Kliegl, R., & Shu, H. (2013). Parafoveal processing efficiency in rapid automatized naming: A comparison between Chinese normal and dyslexic children. *Journal of Experimental Child Psychology, 115*, 579–589.

Yang, Y., Bi, H.-Y., Long, Z.-Y., & Tao, S. (2013). Evidence for cerebellar dysfunction in Chinese children with developmental dyslexia: An fMRI study. *International Journal of Neuroscience, 123*, 300–310.

Yang, Y.-H., Yang, Y., Chen, B.-G., Zhang, Y.-W., & Bi, H.-Y. (2016). Anomalous cerebellar anatomy in Chinese children with dyslexia. *Frontiers in Psychology, 7*, 324.

Zhang, C. F., Zhang, J. H., Yin, R. S., Zhou, J., & Chang, S. M. (1996). Experimental research on the reading disability of Chinese students (in Chinese). *Journal of Psychological Science, 19*, 222–226.

Zhang, Y., Li, J., Tardif, T. et al. (2012). Association of the DYX1C1 dyslexia susceptibility gene with orthography in the Chinese population. *PLoS One, 7*(9), e42969.

Zhao, J., Qian, Y., Bi, H.-Y., & Coltheart, M. (2014). The visual magnocellular-dorsal dysfunction in Chinese children with developmental dyslexia impedes Chinese character recognition. *Scientific Reports, 4*, 7068.

Zhou, Y. (1978). Xian dai han zi zhong sheng pang de biao yin gong neng wen ti [To what degree are the "phonetics" of present-day Chinese characters still phonetic?]. *Zhongguo Yuwen [Chinese Language and Writing], 146*, 172–177.

Zhou, Y., McBride-Chang, C., Law, A. B.-Y. et al. (2014). Development of reading-related skills in Chinese and English among Hong Kong Chinese children with and without dyslexia. *Journal of Experimental Child Psychology, 122*, 75–91.

Ziegler, J. C., & Goswami, U. (2005). Reading acquisition, developmental dyslexia, and skilled reading across languages: A psycholinguistic grain size theory. *Psychological Bulletin, 131*, 3–29.

Part II

Cross-Linguistic Perspectives on Developmental Dyslexia

11 Behavioral Precursors of Developmental Dyslexia

Karin Landerl

11.1 Introduction

Learning to read requires mapping the units of a particular writing system onto its corresponding spoken language units. While such a mapping process is universal to all orthographies, there is considerable variation in (1) the visual characteristics of writing systems (e.g., Chinese, Arabic, Latin-based), (2) the grain size of the spoken language units that are represented by a writing system (e.g., words/morphemes in Chinese vs. phonemes in Western alphabets), and (3) the consistency and regularity of the correspondences between spoken and written language units, which is often called orthographic depth (Katz & Frost, 1992). Shallow orthographies like Finnish represent the sound structure of the spoken language in a highly consistent and transparent way while deep orthographies like English represent deeper linguistic structures (i.e. morphology) rather than the phonological surface structure of words, which makes them rather opaque to the developing reader.

Establishing fast and automatic mappings between written and spoken language during reading development is a complex process that relies on the integration of a range of linguistic skills, and also on certain visual, attentional, and sensory skills which children must have readily available. In dyslexia, a failure in this mapping process induces serious impairments in the development of efficient and automatic word recognition. While there is largely consensus that the explanations for this failure are multifactorial (e.g., Peterson & Pennington, 2012), there are different perspectives as to which deficits are at the core of this developmental disorder. This chapter provides an overview of the dominant perspectives on mechanisms explaining reading failure.

During reading acquisition, individual precursors interact with environmental factors like print exposure (Mol & Bus, 2011), home-literacy environment (Hamilton et al., 2016; Sénéchal & LeFevre, 2002), or type of reading instruction (Ehri et al., 2001). Orthographic structure is one of the environmental factors that will be the focus of the current chapter. Cross-linguistic research designs integrating data from more than one orthography into one and the same study are particularly relevant to determining the impact of orthographic structure on children's reading development. Overall, this evidence suggests that the basic mechanisms of reading are largely similar across languages; nevertheless, there are also a number of fine-grained but critical differences which will be discussed in this chapter. Implications of the current evidence on linguistic, cognitive, and sensory precursors on early identification of dyslexia as well as on approaches of intervention will be presented in Section 11.6.

11.2   Theoretical Background

11.2.1   Role of Linguistic Precursors

The dominant causal theory of dyslexia is that a deficit in phonological processing induces persistent deficits in reading and/or spelling by preventing the individual from fully understanding and systematically exploiting the mappings between graphic symbols and the sound structure of spoken language. Within the domain of phonological processing, research has identified three subcomponents that are typically deficient in dyslexic individuals, namely phonological awareness, phonological working memory, and lexical access (Vellutino et al., 2004).

Phonological awareness refers to the ability to consciously access and manipulate sub-lexical phonological segments such as syllable onsets, rimes, and phonemes. In a typical phonological awareness task, a child might be instructed to delete a certain sound from a word or nonword pronunciation (e.g., "Say/nilt/without the/l/"). The child then has to maintain the sound sequence in phonological working memory, identify the/l/-sound in the phoneme string, delete it from the pronunciation, and blend the remaining sound parts. Thus, although such tasks are taken to measure phonological awareness, they usually also require a certain amount of phonological memory capacity.

Lexical access is usually assessed by rapid automatized naming (RAN) tasks measuring the speed with which an individual can pronounce the names of a sequentially and repeatedly presented limited set of stimuli like letters, Arabic digits, color patches, or pictures of familiar objects. Performing RAN tasks certainly requires phonological skills (accessing the phonological output programs of the required word pronunciations as quickly as possible) and is therefore sometimes seen as a third subcomponent of phonological processing (Torgesen et al., 1997; Vaessen, Gerretsen, & Blomert, 2009). However, there is now ample evidence that "naming speed is phonological, but not only phonological" (Kirby et al., 2010, p. 356) and constitutes a second cognitive mechanism underpinning reading development that is largely independent from phonological awareness, a view that is specified in the double-deficit theory of dyslexia (Wolf & Bowers, 1999).

While behavioral deficits in these domains have been reported for dyslexia in a large range of different orthographies, their impact on the manifestations of dyslexia may well differ, depending on the structure of the particular orthography. The dominantly researched orthography of English is an exceptionally nontransparent alphabetic orthography, making it particularly difficult to understand the complex relationship between spoken and written language. In more transparent orthographies like German or Italian, even dyslexic readers are usually able to work out the reliable correspondences between graphemes and phonemes. As a consequence, dyslexic readers in transparent orthographies are usually able to achieve relatively high reading accuracy for words as well as nonwords (e.g., de Jong & van der Leij, 2002; Landerl, Wimmer, & Frith, 1997; Wimmer, 1993). However, they experience marked and persistent problems with establishing an efficient and automatized reading system, a problem that manifests itself very clearly in seriously impaired reading speed. In terms of cognitive precursors, it has been suggested that deficits in phonological awareness might be less detrimental in transparent orthographies, as milder problems in this domain might still allow a sufficient understanding of the relatively simple and straightforward grapheme–phoneme correspondences. At the same time, the relevance of RAN deficits might increase with orthographic consistency, as RAN is most strongly associated with reading fluency (Kirby et al., 2010; Norton & Wolf, 2012) and reading fluency deficits are the predominant symptoms of dyslexia in transparent orthographies. The empirical evidence associated with these predictions is discussed in the next section.

11.2.2   Role of Non-Linguistic Precursors

While it is generally accepted that phonological processing is strongly associated with reading acquisition and dyslexia, there are different perspectives as to whether such a deficit in the linguistic domain is consequential on more general cognitive or sensory deficits and to what extent reading failure can be caused by other precursors in the domain of visual processing or attention/executive functions. For example, the magnocellular theory of dyslexia (Stein & Walsh, 1997) postulates that phonological deficits result from a domain-general deficit in the perception of quickly changing information. In the auditory domain, such a deficit is assumed to prevent children from forming clear phoneme boundaries (Tallal, 2004). In the visual domain (Stein, 2012), unstable visual images of letter sequences hinder proper word recognition. However, although sensory deficits in the auditory as well as visual domain occur in many dyslexic individuals, their causal status is highly controversial (Ramus, 2003).

Various aspects of visuo-spatial processing have also been causally related to reading acquisition and dyslexia: Valdois and colleagues (Valdois, Bosse, & Tainturier, 2004) argue that children vary in their visual attention span, which limits the number of letters that can be processed in parallel, and that a deficit in visual attention span constitutes a causal factor of dyslexia independent of phonological deficits. Another relevant visual factor is how well children are able to allocate their visuo-spatial attention to the letter sequence (Facoetti, 2012; Hari & Renvall, 2001). Different causal factors would well explain the heterogeneity of symptoms in dyslexia; however, the research evidence on such deficits, which will be discussed in the next section, is less consistent than on linguistic factors.

11.3   Research Evidence

As described in the first part of this book, evidence on behavioral precursors of reading acquisition and dyslexia comes from a range of different languages and orthographies. However, studies vary considerably in the predictive strength of phonological awareness, phonological memory, and rapid-naming tasks. Comparing findings across studies is often difficult because of differences in study design (longitudinal or cross-sectional), selection criteria (random sample vs. dyslexic readers), age and educational background of participants, predictor measures included, dependent measures included (word or nonword reading accuracy or speed, reading comprehension, spelling), and – last but not least – the language and the orthography to be acquired. In order to examine whether the relationship between these behavioral precursors and impairments in reading and spelling are universal or language-specific, cross-linguistic studies are of particular relevance. It should be noted that the cross-linguistic studies which will be presented in the following mostly focused on the relevance of linguistic precursors in different orthographies, while such comparative studies are largely lacking for other, non-linguistic precursors.

11.3.1   Predictors of Learning to Read

Up to date, cross-linguistic research has mostly focused on typical reading development in alphabetic orthographies. A number of cross-sectional studies provided empirical support for the hypothesis that phonological awareness may indeed be less relevant in transparent orthographies: Ziegler et al. (2010) investigated a large sample of 1263 European second graders in five orthographies with increasing degrees of complexity (Finnish, Hungarian, Dutch, Portuguese, and French) and found that the impact of phonological awareness (measured by phoneme deletion) increased systematically with orthographic complexity. Nevertheless, phonological awareness was significantly associated with word and nonword reading accuracy and speed in all orthographies and was the strongest concurrent predictor in all orthographies, except in the most transparent Finnish writing system, where vocabulary was, equally with phoneme deletion, the strongest predictor of word-reading speed and predicted word- and nonword-reading accuracy. RAN was only moderately associated with reading speed, which is surprising given that there is consistent evidence for a strong RAN–reading association (Kirby et al., 2010). It is possible, that this low association is due to the fact that Ziegler et al. (2010) used an object-naming paradigm while other studies indicate that naming of alphanumeric stimuli (letter, digits) is more closely related to reading than naming of such non-alphanumeric stimuli (Bowey, McGuigan, & Ruschena, 2005). Importantly, the RAN–reading association was not modulated by orthographic complexity.

The unusually low RAN–reading speed association in the European comparison by Ziegler et al. (2010) may be due to the fact that relatively young readers were investigated. This was indicated by a study on the concurrent prediction of word and nonword reading fluency in Hungarian, Dutch, and Portuguese, three orthographies with increasing complexity (Vaessen et al., 2010). Findings suggested a shift of cognitive mechanisms underlying reading fluency with increasing age and reading competence. In Grades 1 and 2, the association of phonological awareness and RAN with reading fluency was largely comparable, while in Grades 3 and 4 RAN was clearly more strongly associated with reading fluency than phonological awareness. Importantly, Vaessen et al. (2010) also found that cognitive mechanisms underlying reading were similar across the three alphabetic orthographies that were included, but again, the association of reading with phonological awareness was modulated by orthographic complexity, while this was not the case for RAN or phonological memory.

Can the cross-linguistic findings of these large-scale European studies be extended to English, arguably the most inconsistent among the alphabetic orthographies (Share, 2008)? This was investigated in another European project comparing elementary-school children (Grades 2 to 7) learning to read and spell in English, French, German, Hungarian, or Finnish (Moll et al., 2014). In this sample, phonological skills (awareness and memory) accounted for significant amounts of variance in reading accuracy and spelling in all orthographies, while RAN was the best concurrent predictor of reading fluency. No major language differences were found between patterns of concurrent prediction. However, overall, the regression models accounted for higher amounts of variance in English than in the other orthographies. Interestingly, it was not so much phonological awareness that showed a stronger association to literacy measures in English than in the other orthographies, but RAN that accounted for significantly more variance in English children's reading accuracy.

Only a few cross-linguistic studies have assessed the behavioral precursors of (typical) reading and spelling before the onset of schooling and investigated their impact on later reading and spelling skills in longitudinal designs: Georgiou et al. (2012) compared reading and spelling acquisition in English, Greek and Finnish. In the context of a European network, Caravolas et al. (2012) and Caravolas et al. (2013) followed a cross-linguistic sample including English and two more consistent alphabetic orthographies, Spanish and Czech. In another longitudinal study, Furnes and Samuelsson (2011) contrasted reading acquisition in English with two more consistent Scandinavian alphabetic orthographies, Swedish and Norwegian. Georgiou et al. (2012) identified interesting differences in the predictive patterns of early precursors: Phonological awareness and RAN were significant predictors of nonword reading accuracy in English, but not in Greek and Finnish, whereas RAN was a significant predictor of spelling in English and Greek, but not in Finnish. The authors argued that Greek was more similar to Finnish in the case of nonword reading because letter–sound correspondences are consistent in both orthographies, while Greek was more similar to English in the case of spelling given that sound–letter correspondences are inconsistent in both orthographies. Overall, the behavioral precursors included in this study (phoneme awareness, RAN, and letter–sound knowledge) accounted for more variance when correspondences between written and spoken language were relatively nontransparent (reading and spelling in English and spelling in Greek) than when they were transparent (reading in Greek and reading and spelling in Finnish). However, Caravolas et al. (2012, 2013) and Furnes and Samuelsson (2011) did not find differential predictive patterns between orthographies. They argued that the developmental trajectories would progress faster in consistent orthographies due to the high reliability of their letter–sound correspondences, whereas the underlying mechanisms would remain mostly language-universal, at least for alphabetic orthographies. Finally, two recent large-scale cross-linguistic longitudinal investigations of cross-lagged relations between precursors and reading development demonstrate the important point that the relationship is mostly interactive for phonological awareness (Landerl et al., 2019) and - at least very early on, before naming is automatized, also for RAN (Peterson et al., 2018).

11.3.2   *Predictors of Developmental Dyslexia*

Even though these cognitive precursors may be generally relevant in learning to read, specific evidence for dyslexia is still needed for theoretical as well as for practical reasons. We need to test whether impairments of the cognitive mechanisms specified for successful reading acquisition induce similar patterns of reading failure across orthographies or whether certain deficits (most importantly phonological awareness) constitute a more serious handicap in some orthographies than in others. From a practical point of view, it needs to be established whether the predictive quality of cognitive precursors of dyslexia is similar across orthographies. Again, it is important to note that cross-language studies almost exclusively focused on linguistic predictors of dyslexia, while comparisons across different orthographies for visual and other non-linguistic factors are largely lacking.

To what extent is the impact of phonological awareness, naming speed, and phonological memory modulated by orthographic depth? This was examined in a large European research network, assessing data from about 1,000 dyslexic and 1,000 typically developing children learning to read in English, French, German, Dutch, Hungarian, or Finnish (Landerl et al., 2013). The six orthographies were categorized into three complexity levels based on the consistency of letter–sound relationships in the reading as well as in the spelling direction: English and French were assigned the most complex level, with inconsistent grapheme–phoneme as well as phoneme–grapheme correspondences, German and Dutch were assigned to a medium complexity level, with largely consistent grapheme–phoneme correspondences but inconsistent phoneme–grapheme correspondences, and Hungarian and Finnish constituted the lowest level of complexity, with consistent correspondences between letters and sounds in both directions. A major advantage of this European research initiative was that the same criteria, based on ICD-10 (World Health Organization, 2008), were applied in each national subsample: Children with more general learning, attentional, or neurological problems as well as children whose first language was not the instructional language were not admitted to the study. Reading was assessed by language-specific standardized word-reading tests. Dyslexic readers had to perform more than 1.25 standard deviations below grade level, which was a pragmatic compromise between the standard criteria of -1 and -1.5 standard deviations that are widely applied in research and clinical practice.

As expected, phoneme deletion and RAN were strong concurrent predictors of developmental dyslexia in all orthographies, while phonological memory and general verbal abilities played a comparatively minor role. Importantly, the study nicely demonstrated that orthographic complexity exacerbates the manifestation of dyslexia: As evident from Figure 11.1, overall more participants were classified correctly by the cognitive predictors phonological awareness, RAN, and phonological memory when orthography was more complex. The impact of phoneme deletion was clearly stronger in complex than in less complex orthographies: Figure 11.2 shows that one z-unit in the phoneme deletion measure multiplied the probability of dyslexia by two within low-complexity orthographies, whereas it multiplied it by almost three in the medium- and by more than four in the high-complexity orthographies.

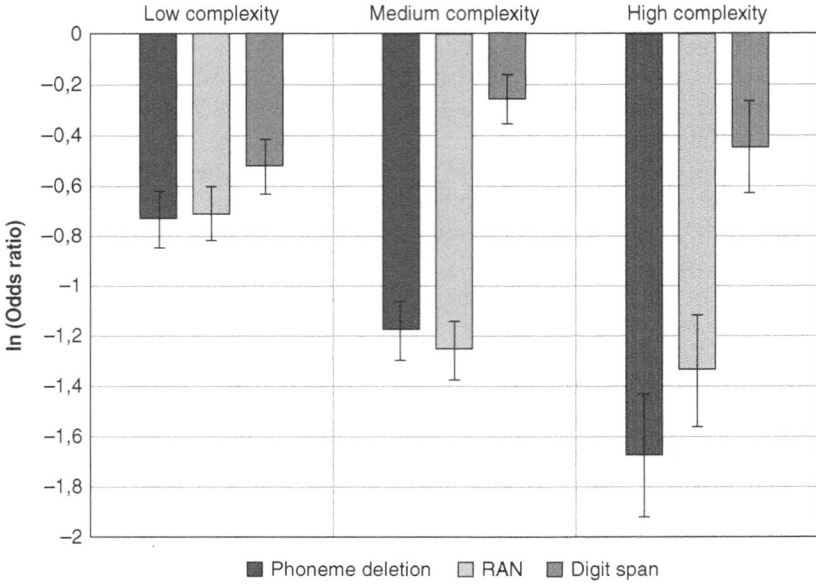

Figure 11.1 Estimates (in OR) and their 95 percent confidence limits per orthographic complexity group for phoneme deletion, RAN, and digit span respectively (data from Landerl et al., 2013)

Heterogeneity between orthographies was also found for the RAN measure. However, findings were not in line with the assumption that RAN might be more relevant in consistent orthographies, where disfluent reading is the central marker of dyslexia: quite the contrary, the orthographic heterogeneity was driven by the low-complexity group, which showed significantly higher odds ratios than both the medium- and the high-complexity group, indicating that its impact was weaker in the low than in the other two complexity groups (see Figure 11.2). Note that in this study findings were very similar for RAN objects and RAN digits, not confirming earlier evidence that alphanumeric RAN is more closely related with reading than non-alphanumeric RAN (Bowey et al., 2005).

A serious methodological limitation was that the age and grade levels of participants in this European sample were diverse, ranging from 8 to almost 13 years of age, with systematically lower grade levels in the low- than in the high-complexity orthographies. However, a second set of analyses restricted to grade levels 2, 3, and 4 fully confirmed the results. Note that the concurrent assessment of

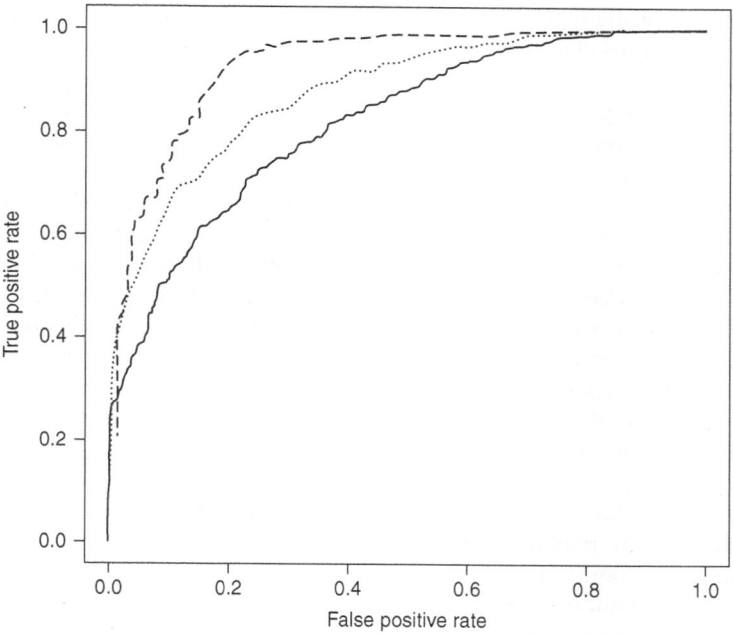

Figure 11.2   ROC-curves (high complexity: dashed, medium complexity: dotted, low complexity: full) (from Landerl et al., 2013)

cognitive and reading measures does not allow a causal interpretation of the findings. However, longitudinal assessments of dyslexia, ideally starting before the onset of reading acquisition, are a challenging enterprise: given a prevalence rate of about 4 to 6 percent for dyslexia, very large sample sizes would be required at the start of such a study in order to include a sufficiently large sample of dyslexic individuals to allow a statistical analysis.

To date, only one longitudinal cross-linguistic analysis on reading and spelling deficits has been carried out in the context of the International Longitudinal Twin Study (ILTS) on early language and literacy development conducted in the USA, Australia, Sweden, and Norway. Furnes and Samuelsson (2010) used logistic regression models to predict poor readers and poor spellers (performing more than 1 SD below age level) in Grades 1 and 2 based on a range of cognitive measures (phonological awareness, RAN, letter knowledge, phonological memory, and broader language measures) assessed at the ages of 5 and about 6½ years. In this study, the overall predictive quality of the logistic regression models was largely comparable for the non-transparent English and the transparent Scandinavian orthographies, but again, the predictive patterns were different depending on the acquired orthography: In English, phonological awareness, RAN and letter knowledge at both early assessment points were consistent predictors of difficulties in reading as well as spelling. In the more consistent Scandinavian orthographies, however, letter knowledge assessed at the age of 5 was not significantly related to later reading and spelling problems, probably because of generally low familiarity with letters in the Scandinavian sample, where early reading preparation has no cultural tradition (see also Mann & Wimmer, 2002, for similar findings in a comparison of English and German). The theoretically more important difference to the English findings was that phonological awareness assessed at age 6½ ceased to predict reading problems in Grade 2 (see also Furnes et al., 2019). This finding is in line with the assumption that in consistent orthographies phonemic decoding skills are pretty much at ceiling, even among poor readers, so that early phonological deficits are less detrimental than in nontransparent writing systems like English, where phonological skills are constantly needed to work out the complex relationships between spoken and written languages. This interpretation is confirmed by the finding that early phonological awareness significantly predicted spelling in the Scandinavian as well as in the English sample, probably because the phoneme–grapheme correspondences in both orthographies are inconsistent and simple phoneme-based procedures are not sufficient to spell words correctly.

Finally, a highly interesting way to investigate early precursors of dyslexia is to follow the early development of preschool children who have an increased familial risk of developing this disorder because they have a dyslexic first-grade relative. Such projects have been carried out in a number of different orthographies ranging from the highly consistent Finnish orthography (e.g., Lyytinen et al., 2004) via the medium consistent orthography of Dutch (Boets et al., 2006; van Bergen et al., 2011) and highly inconsistent orthographies of Danish (Petersen & Elbro, 1999) and English (Moll, Loff, & Snowling, 2013; Nash et al., 2013; Scarborough, 1989; Snowling, Gallagher, & Frith, 2003) to the non-alphabetic Chinese orthography (Ho, Leung, & Cheung, 2011). While all these projects clearly indicated early deficits in speech and language processing among the at-risk samples, it is again difficult to compare findings across projects because of marked differences in research designs (age of assessment, constructs and measures included, criteria for dyslexia diagnosis at school age). Fine-grained differences in the complex interactions between early precursors, orthographic structure, and reading outcome can probably only be detected in cross-linguistic research initiatives.

11.4   Explanatory Mechanisms

11.4.1   Phonological Deficit

In all the orthographies investigated to date, phonological awareness has been found to show close associations with reading acquisition and dyslexia. Especially during the early stages of reading development phonological awareness was consistently found to be a reliable concurrent (Caravolas, Volín, & Hulme, 2005; Georgiou, Parrila, & Papadopoulos, 2008; Vaessen et al., 2010; Ziegler et al., 2010) and longitudinal (Caravolas et al., 2012, 2013; Furnes & Samuelsson, 2011) predictor of reading accuracy as well as speed across different orthographies. However, findings were mixed with respect to the relative importance of phonological awareness as a function of orthographic consistency. While some studies showed that the impact of phonological awareness on reading was stronger in less than in more consistent orthographies (Landerl et al., 2019; Mann & Wimmer; 2002; Vaessen et al., 2010; Ziegler et al., 2010), others reported an equally strong prediction of phonological awareness in English and in more transparent orthographies (Caravolas et al., 2005, 2012, 2013; Peterson et al., 2018).

Differences between orthographies have also been suggested with respect to the impact of phonological awareness on reading over time. It has been argued that in more consistent orthographies the predictive strength of phonological awareness decreases after about one year of reading instruction (Furnes & Samuelsson, 2011; Georgiou et al., 2008; Vaessen et al., 2010), because decoding skills have by then already been sufficiently acquired. In inconsistent orthographies, phonological awareness remains a strong predictor beyond Grade 1, reflecting the fact that the development of decoding skills takes longer in inconsistent compared to consistent orthographies.

While deficits in decoding skills were identified as a specific (Rack, Snowling, & Olson, 1992) and persistent (Bruck, 1992) problem of dyslexia in English, the situation seems to be quite different in phonologically more transparent orthographies. Relatively simple and highly reliable correspondences between written and spoken language, in accordance with reading instruction that is usually phonics-based (as this seems to be the most natural way to teach the alphabetic code), encourage even children with early phonological deficits to apply the limited number of letter–sound correspondences during decoding, which in turn helps them to understand the alphabetic basis of their orthography. What is more, this early focus on decoding skills may even help them to overcome and compensate for their early problems in phonological processing. Indeed, Wimmer, Mayringer, and Landerl (2000) identified a sample of German-speaking children with a marked and specific deficit in phonological awareness at school entry who did not develop any reading problems later on. However, their spelling skills did not develop adequately.

German orthography is quite inconsistent in the spelling direction: there is usually more than one grapheme that corresponds to a certain phoneme (see Landerl, 2017, for a more detailed description of German orthography). In spite of what might be expected, children with early phonological deficits learned to segment spoken words into their constituent sounds and to translate them into adequate letters. Nevertheless, their spellings were mostly orthographically incorrect. This may indicate that the phoneme-based strategies these children applied during reading and spelling were mostly compensatory, but their phonological word representations were still not sufficiently structured to allow orthographic mapping (Ehri, 2014) with the corresponding word spellings. Thus, it seems that the relevance of a well-developed phonological system may decrease with the transparency of the relationships between spoken and written language. Most orthographies are less transparent in the spelling than in the reading direction, which may explain why phonological awareness was found to be a consistent predictor of spelling skills (Caravolas et al., 2012, 2013; Furnes & Samuelsson, 2011; Moll et al., 2014) and spelling deficits (Caravolas et al., 2005; Furnes & Samuelsson, 2010) across orthographies.

The concurrent associations of phonological awareness with reading competence (Moll et al., 2014; Vaessen et al., 2010) and dyslexia (Landerl et al., 2013) in older children may at least partly be explained by the fact that reading and spelling skills are correlated (Moll & Landerl, 2009). At least for German orthography, Moll and Landerl (2009) found a phonological deficit only for children with combined deficits in reading as well as spelling, but not for children with reading problems whose spelling skills were age-adequate. It would be highly interesting to test whether this finding replicates in other orthographies. The finding that orthographic consistency impacts on the phonology-reading association in dyslexic (Landerl et al., 2013) but not in typically developing readers (Moll et al., 2014) may point to the compensatory role of orthography: The more consistent and phonologically transparent the orthography, the more practicing reading and spelling helps to overcome problems in phonological processing in dyslexic individuals. Typically developing children are probably less dependent on such compensation through orthography.

11.4.2   Naming-Speed Deficit

The association of RAN with reading and dyslexia increases during reading development (Vaessen et al., 2010) and has been found to be either comparable across orthographies (Caravolas et al., 2012; Furnes & Samuelsson, 2011; Georgiou et al., 2008; Vaessen et al., 2010; see also a recent metaanalysis by Araújo & Faísca, 2019) or again stronger in inconsistent than in consistent orthographies (Landerl et al., 2013; Moll et al., 2014). Assumptions that RAN might be more relevant in consistent orthographies because of a supposedly higher relevance of reading fluency could not be confirmed. The theoretical explanation for the RAN–reading relationship is under extensive debate (Kirby et al., 2010). The finding that orthographic complexity is associated with the predictive strength of RAN may be explained by the higher variability in all reading measures, including reading fluency, in the complex orthography of English compared to more consistent orthographies like German (Landerl et al., 1997). It is also supportive of explanatory accounts assuming that RAN reflects the complexity of the reading process and represents a "microcosm of the reading system" (Norton & Wolf, 2012) by indexing an individual's ability to integrate multiple neural processes.

11.4.3   Phonological Working Memory Deficit

Learning to read requires the ability to store and manipulate phonological information in working memory. In the context of Baddeley's (1992) working-memory model, both the storage component of the phonological loop and the control component of the central executive constitute relevant precursors to reading, particularly in the early stages of reading acquisition, when letter–sound translation is not yet automatized. Later on, phonological working memory seems to be more relevant for reading-comprehension processes than for word recognition (e.g., Cain, Oakhill, & Bryant, 2004). Deficits in phonological memory are also frequently associated with dyslexia, although they are often less prominent than the deficits in phoneme awareness and rapid naming (see, e.g., Figure 11.2, presenting data from the cross-linguistic study by Landerl et al., 2013).

11.4.4   Other Explanations

Over the last decades, research on linguistic factors has clearly dominated the field while other, non-linguistic factors have been less often investigated and findings are less consistent. Deficits in visual attention span are assumed to limit the amount of visual information that can be processed at a glance (Valdois et al., 2004). Processing of visual input during reading is also assumed to be deficient because of limitations in adequately assigning visuo-spatial attention to graphic symbols (Facoetti, 2012; Hari & Renvall, 2001). Positive evidence for both accounts is currently limited to a few European orthographies. It would be highly interesting to know whether these visual factors have a differential impact depending on the visual complexity of the particular writing system. There is some evidence that dynamic visual processing predicts reading Chinese characters (e.g., Meng et al., 2011), but it is unknown whether the amount of variance explained in visually complex orthographies like Chinese or Korean Hangul is higher than in Latin-script-based orthographies.

An account that attempts to explain the heterogeneity of dyslexia symptoms and the high rates of comorbidity with other developmental disorders is presented by Nicolson and Fawcett (2011), who postulate deficits in procedural learning rooted in cerebellar brain functions as a main causal factor. In this view, cerebellar deficits cause mild motor and articulatory problems which in turn prevent affected children from developing adequate phonological awareness. In addition, the cerebellar deficit induces more general problems in automatizing skill and knowledge that may also impair word-reading fluency and orthographic learning. From a cross-linguistic perspective, it is difficult to see whether this rather broad account can make differential predictions depending on particular characteristics of orthographic systems. Furthermore, while, indeed, many children with dyslexia experience problems in motor skills and other aspects of procedural learning, the causal status of such deficits is under debate. In a neurobiological model proposed by Ramus (2004), focal cortical anomalies in left perisylvian language areas cause deficits in phonological processing which in turn induce problems in reading development. Under certain hormonal conditions during gestation, these cortical anomalies can induce secondary disruption in sensory pathways and may even extend to the cerebellum. In these cases, affected individuals show sensorimotor impairments, which may in some cases aggravate the reading impairment. In this view then, sensorimotor deficits are a marker of problems in early brain development, but are not causal factors of dyslexia.

11.5   Cross-Language Issues

A cross-linguistic approach can certainly not eliminate all methodological problems that are inherent in comparisons across different educational, cultural, and language backgrounds, but findings are still easier to interpret within such designs, which aim to assess the same constructs in similar populations, than between studies that are carried out in different orthographic systems independently. One problem for cross-linguistic studies is the lack of a common metric to describe orthographic and linguistic differences. Writing systems vary widely with respect to their visual structure and complexity. Furthermore, written language units can represent phonemes, syllables, or words, and these units are not always represented linearly (e.g., in the alphabetic writing system of Korean Hangul, character blocks represent syllables; Semitic writing systems have optional diacritics that can represent vowels above or below the letters of the consonant grid). Writing systems also vary widely in their orthographic depth, referring to the reliability of print-to-speech. Although there is notable agreement on where to place particular writing systems on a continuum of orthographic depth (e.g., Borgwaldt, Hellwig, & De Groot, 2005; Seymour, Aro, & Erskine, 2003), the adequate levels of description are still under discussion and their quantification is an ongoing enterprise for psycholinguistic research. Schmalz et al. (2015) recently suggested that the complexity of print-to-speech correspondences and the unpredictability of the derivation of the pronunciations should be differentiated as two separable subcomponents of orthographic depth. French, for instance, has a clearly lower number of irregular words than English, but the consistencies between written and spoken language are often not on the grapheme–phoneme level, but concern more complex multi-letter clusters. Detailed analyses of different writing systems as provided by Perfetti and Verhoeven (2017) will be seminal in order to further develop a unitary system of description.

A major issue in cross-linguistic studies is the extent to which linguistic tasks designed in different languages tap similar cognitive processes and represent similar levels of difficulty. One possibility is to choose languages that are sufficiently close (such as English and German) to match all the material (e.g., Frith, Wimmer, & Landerl, 1998; Landerl et al., 1997; Rau et al., 2016; Rau et al., 2015; Ziegler et al., 2003). When one wants to study a broader range of languages, this is not an option anymore. There is simply no way to design equivalent lists of words or nonwords across languages as different as English and Finnish. Furthermore, even if the material is matched, the difficulty of certain tasks (such as phoneme deletion) might not be, as this is partly dependent on the structure of the particular language (e.g., Caravolas & Landerl, 2010). Thus, it is inevitable that in cross-linguistic studies some tasks tap different levels of performance and thus have different sensitivities in different languages.

To date, cross-linguistic studies have been almost exclusively carried out in the context of Western alphabetic orthographies, which constitutes a major limitation to the generalizability of findings toward a universal model of reading (Perfetti, 2003; Perfetti & Harris, 2013). Even if non-Western writing systems like Arabic or Chinese are the subject of investigation, the research often attempts to confirm the validity of the standard precursors of reading identified for English (phonological processing and RAN) for these orthographies (e.g., Elbeheri & Everatt, 2007; Ho et al., 2004). It will be highly important in the future to identify cognitive mechanisms that may be more relevant in other languages than in English. One reason why research is often limited to phonological awareness and RAN is probably that these tasks are easier to match across orthographies than other constructs like morphological or orthographic processing, which may be realized by distinct parameters in different languages. Thus, research on the world language of English and on its complex orthography has made tremendous contributions to our understanding of reading acquisition and dyslexia, but it has also confined our view to characteristics that may be more relevant in English than in other writing systems (Share, 2008, 2014).

11.6   Clinical Implications

11.6.1   Assessment

The central clinical application of research on precursors of dyslexia is to enable early identification (ideally before reading problems become manifest) and efficient intervention via improvement of the cognitive mechanisms underlying reading failure. However, the cross-linguistic research summarized in this chapter seems to suggest that the precursors identified in the context of reading acquisition in English might be of lower predictive quality in phonologically more transparent writing systems. Some studies suggest that lower amounts of variance of reading skills in the general population are explained in consistent than in inconsistent orthographies. Note that both Moll et al. (2014) and Ziegler et al. (2010) reported that measures of phonological awareness, phonological memory and RAN could only explain between 10 percent and 25 percent of variance in reading and spelling in Finnish. Even more relevant for dyslexia diagnosis is the finding that the predictive quality of these constructs was about twice as high in the high-complexity orthographies of English and French as in the low- complexity orthographies of Finnish and Hungarian (Landerl et al., 2013). So how useful are early screening measures of phonological awareness and RAN in orthographies that are more transparent than English? In a recent review of such preschool screening batteries for dyslexia in German, Marx and Lenhard (2010) have criticized their overall low prognostic validity. This low validity should not at all be interpreted as evidence that these constructs are irrelevant to acquire German orthography. It is more likely to be a consequence of the interactions of phonological processing with a consistent orthographic structure and phonics reading instruction: being taught and encouraged to sound out unfamiliar letter strings and having the positive experience that sounding out is a successful strategy to identify words is probably a very efficient means of remediation for children with poor phonological processing skills. Thus, the presumably most efficient intervention is available to children with early phonological processing deficits, and helps them to overcome their problems so that they never qualify for a dyslexia diagnosis.

11.6.2   Early Intervention

Research has clearly demonstrated that phonology-based interventions help children with dyslexia to improve their reading accuracy (Bus & van IJzendoorn, 1999; Suggate, 2016). Importantly, such training should not only focus on phonological awareness, but should help children to establish links between spoken and written language units (Hatcher, Hulme & Ellis, 1994; Galuschka et al., 2014). A limitation of this research domain is that most of the evidence comes from samples learning to read the complex English orthography. In more consistent orthographies phonics-based intervention is often provided in the context of standard reading instruction and reading accuracy is not considered a primary problem for dyslexic individuals. For the majority of children with dyslexia in a consistent orthography, helping them to crack the alphabetic code is not the central issue. The main task is probably to help them to use this code efficiently and automatically and to integrate their explicit knowledge about letters and sounds with their implicit language competence. However, our knowledge of how to improve the automaticity and fluency of reading is still rather limited. Intervention approaches that aim to improve letter–sound integration (e.g., Breznitz, 1997), automaticity of access to sub-lexical units (Heikkilä et al., 2013), or the lexical quality of single words in order to make them more accessible during the reading process (e.g., Wolf & Katzir-Cohen, 2001) are certainly interesting. Their efficiency in remediating reading problems in different writing systems still needs to be demonstrated in well-controlled intervention studies.

Learning software that fosters reading- and letter–sound-based activities offers promising perspectives as computer technology provides a number of general advantages: Interactive learning software can be very engaging and keep struggling learners motivated, even for tasks that are highly repetitive. A good example is Graphogame, a computer software program that focuses on establishing and automatizing print–speech correspondences, which was originally developed for the transparent Finnish orthography and was then adapted for numerous different languages (Ojanen et al., 2015). In general, it is important that information and communications technology (ICT) training programs are based on current theories of reading acquisition and that their efficacy is tested in high-quality randomized control trials.

11.7   Discussion and Conclusion

Phonological awareness and RAN are cognitive predictors of reading acquisition and dyslexia in all orthographic systems that have been investigated to date. Undoubtedly, the introduction of the concept of phonological processing to reading research in the 1970s (Brady & Shankweiler, 1991) has made a tremendous contribution to our understanding of the reading process as well as to the causes for reading failure. Still, the strong dominance of research on the world language of English with its uncommonly complex orthography may have led us to overestimate the relevance of phonology. All orthographies represent language, and understanding the relationships between spoken and written language is essential in order to learn to read in any language and thus constitutes a universal challenge in learning to read. But orthographies represent spoken language in quite different ways and therefore pose different challenges to the learning child. Orthographies that are phonologically more transparent than English certainly require phonological awareness, but it seems that the acquisition of phonological awareness is less of a stumbling block than in the complex English orthography.

Cross-linguistic research helps to identify fine-grained differences that are induced by differences in orthographic structure. A number of recent international research initiatives have revealed important insights; however, most of them investigated typical reading acquisition in various alphabetic orthographies. It will be important to expand this type of research to dyslexia in different orthographies as it cannot be taken for granted that the impact of early precursors on later reading is constant across the whole range of reading skills.

While associations between reading acquisition and certain linguistic precursors are clearly established, evidence on non-linguistic precursors in the domain of visual or attentional processing is often less clear. Better controlled longitudinal and intervention studies will be necessary in order to specify the exact causal connections between a certain precursor and particular subcomponents of written language processing. The phonological-deficit account makes clear predictions for differences between languages based on the consistency of their orthographic systems, and these predictions have received empirical support. Analogously, it should be possible to make predictions for visual factors based on the visual characteristics and complexity of different writing systems.

It is generally agreed that dyslexia is a multifactorial developmental disorder (e.g., Peterson & Pennington, 2012) and the current chapter has provided an overview of the different factors that can induce problems in children's reading development. However, our understanding of how different precursors interact with each other is still limited. Learning to read universally involves the efficient processing of the visual–verbal correspondences between written and spoken language. Failure to develop such efficient orthographic processing skills depends not only on the linguistic and cognitive profile of the individual child, but also on the linguistic and visual characteristics of the writing system, which may well place differential demands on children's sensory and cognitive processing systems. Thus, continuing research efforts on dyslexia in different orthographies will be seminal in order to further improve our understanding of the cognitive mechanisms underlying reading as well as reading failure.

References

Araújo, S. & Faísca, L. (2919). A meta-analytic review of naming speed deficits in developmental dyslexia. *Scientific Studies of Reading*. doi: https://doi.org/10.1080/10888438.2019.1572758 epub ahead of print.

Baddeley, A. (1992). Working memory. *Science, 255*, 556–559. doi: http://dx.doi.org/10.1126/science.1736359.

Boets, B., Wouters, J., Van Wieringen, A., & Ghesquière, P. (2006). Auditory temporal information processing in preschool children at family risk for dyslexia: Relations with phonological abilities and developing literacy skills. *Brain and Language*, *97*, 64–79. doi: http://dx.doi.org/10.1016/j.bandl.2005.07.026.

Borgwaldt, S. R., Hellwig, F. M., & de Groot, A. M. B. (2005). Onset entropy matters: Letter-to-phoneme mappings in seven languages. *Reading and Writing*, *18*, 211–229. doi: http://dx.doi.org/10.1007/s11145-005-3001-9.

Bowey, J. A., McGuigan, M., & Ruschena, A. (2005). On the association between serial naming speed for letters and digits and word-reading skill: Towards a developmental account. *Journal of Research in Reading*, *28*, 400–422. doi: http://dx.doi.org/10.1111 /j.1467-9817.2005.00278.x.

Brady, S. A., & Shankweiler, D. (1991). *Phonological processes in literacy: A tribute to Isabelle Y. Liberman*. Hillsdale, UK: Lawrence Erlbaum Associates.

Breznitz, Z. (1997). Effects of accelerated reading rate on memory for text among dyslexic readers. *Journal of Educational Psychology*, *89*, 289–297. doi: http://dx .doi.org/10.1037/0022-0663.89.2.289.

Bruck, M. (1992). Persistence of dyslexics' phonological awareness deficits. *Developmental Psychology*, *28*, 874–886. doi: http://dx.doi.org/10.1037/0012-1649 .28.5.874.

Bus, A. G., & van IJzendoorn, M. H. (1999). Phonological awareness and early reading: A meta-analysis of experimental training studies. *Journal of Educational Psychology*, *91*, 403–414. doi: http://dx.doi.org/10.1037/0022-0663.91.3.403.

Cain, K., Oakhill, J., & Bryant, P. (2004). Children's reading comprehension ability: Concurrent prediction by working memory, verbal ability, and component skills. *Journal of Educational Psychology*, *96*, 31–42. doi: http://dx.doi.org/0.1037/0022-0 663.96.1.31.

Caravolas, M., & Landerl, K. (2010). The influences of syllable structure and reading ability on the development of phoneme awareness: A longitudinal, cross-linguistic study. *Scientific Studies of Reading*, *14*, 464–484. doi: http://dx.doi.org/10.1080 /10888430903034804.

Caravolas, M., Lervåg, A., Defior, S., Seidlová Málková, G., & Hulme C. (2013). Different patterns, but equivalent predictors, of growth in reading in consistent and inconsistent orthographies. *Psychological Science*, *24*, 1398–1407. doi: http://dx .doi.org/10.1177/0956797612473122.

Caravolas, M., Lervåg, A., Mousikou, P. et al. (2012). Common patterns of prediction of literacy development in different alphabetic orthographies. *Psychological Science*, *23*, 678–686. doi: http://dx.doi.org/10.1177/0956797611434536.

Caravolas, M., Volín, J., & Hulme, C. (2005). Phoneme awareness is a key component of alphabetic literacy skills in consistent and inconsistent orthographies: Evidence from Czech and English children. *Journal of Experimental Child Psychology*, *92*, 107–139. doi: http://dx.doi.org/10.1016/j.jecp.2005.04.003.

de Jong, P. F., & van der Leij, A. (2002). Effects of phonological abilities and linguistic comprehension on the development of reading. *Scientific Studies of Reading*, *6*, 51–77. doi: http://dx.doi.org/10.1207/S1532799XSSR0601_03.

Ehri, L. C. (2014). Orthographic mapping in the acquisition of sight word reading, spelling memory, and vocabulary learning. *Scientific Studies of Reading*, *18*, 5–21. doi: http://dx.doi.org/10.1080/10888438.2013.819356.

Ehri, L. C., Nunes, S. R., Stahl, S. A., & Willows, D. M. (2001). Systematic phonics instruction helps students learn to read: Evidence from the national reading panel's meta-analysis. *Review of Educational Research, 71*, 393–447. doi: http://dx.doi.org /10.3102/00346543071003393.

Elbeheri, G., & Everatt, J. (2007). Literacy ability and phonological processing skills amongst dyslexic and non-dyslexic speakers of Arabic. *Reading and Writing, 20*, 273–294. doi: http://dx.doi.org/10.1007/s11145-006-9031-0.

Facoetti, A. (2012). Spatial attention disorder in developmental dyslexia: Towards the prevention of reading acquisition deficits. In J. Stein & Z. Kapoula (Eds.), *Visual aspects of dyslexia* (pp. 123–136). Oxford, UK: Oxford University Press. doi: http:// dx.doi.org/10.1093/acprof:oso/9780199589814.003.0008.

Frith, U., Wimmer, H., & Landerl, K. (1998). Differences in phonological recoding in German- and English-speaking children. *Scientific Studies of Reading, 2*, 31–54. doi: http://dx.doi.org/10.1207/s1532799xssr0201_2.

Furnes, B., & Samuelsson, S. (2010). Predicting reading and spelling difficulties in transparent and opaque orthographies: A comparison between Scandinavian and US/Australian children. *Dyslexia, 16*, 119–142. doi: http://dx.doi.org/10 .1002/dys.401.

Furnes, B., Elwèr, A., Samuelsson, S., Olson, R.K., & Byrne, B. (2019). Investigating the double-deficit hypothesis in more and less transparent orthographies: A long-itudinal study from preschool to Grade 2. *Scientific Studies of Reading*, doi: https:// doi.org/10.1080/10888438.2019.1610410 epub ahead of print.

Furnes, B., & Samuelsson, S. (2011). Phonological awareness and rapid automatized naming predicting early development in reading and spelling: Results from a cross-linguistic longitudinal study. *Learning and Individual Differences, 21*, 85–95. doi: http://dx.doi.org/10.1016/j.lindif.2010.10.005.

Galuschka, K., Ise, E., Krick, K., & Schulte-Körne, G. (2014). Effectiveness of treat-ment approaches for children and adolescents with reading disabilities: A meta-analysis of randomized control trials. *PLoS One, 9*(2), e89900. doi: http://dx .doi.org/10.1371/journal.pone.0089900.

Georgiou, G. K., Parrila, R., & Papadopoulos, T. C. (2008). Predictors of word decoding and reading fluency across languages varying in orthographic consistency. *Journal of Educational Psychology, 100*, 566–580. doi: http://dx.doi.org/10.1037/0022-0663 .100.3.566.

Georgiou, G. K., Torppa, M., Manolitsis, G., Lyytinen, H., & Parrila, R. (2012). Longitudinal predictors of reading and spelling across languages varying in ortho-graphic consistency. *Reading and Writing, 25*, 321–346. doi: http://dx.doi.org/10 .1007/s11145-010-9271-x.

Hamilton, L. G., Hayiou-Thomas, M. E., Hulme, C., & Snowling, M. J. (2016). The home literacy environment as a predictor of the early literacy development of children at family-risk of dyslexia. *Scientific Studies of Reading, 20*, 401–419. doi: http://dx .doi.org/10.1080/10888438.2016.1213266.

Hari, R., & Renvall, H. (2001). Impaired processing of rapid stimulus sequences in dyslexia. *Trends in Cognitive Science, 5*, 525–532. doi: http://dx.doi.org/10.1016/S 1364-6613(00)01801-5.

Hatcher, P. J., Hulme, C., & Ellis, A. W. (1994). Ameliorating early reading failure by integrating the teaching of reading and phonological skills: The phonological linkage hypothesis. *Child Development, 65*, 41–57. doi: http://dx.doi.org/10.1111/j.1467-86 24.1994.tb00733.x.

Heikkilä, R., Aro, M., Närhi, V., Westerholm, J., & Ahonen, T. (2013). Does training in syllable recognition improve reading speed? A computer-based trial with poor readers from second and third grade. *Scientific Studies of Reading, 17*, 398–414. doi: htt p://dx.doi.org/10.1080/10888438.2012.753452.

Ho, C. S.-H., Chan, D. W.-O., Lee, S.-H., Tsang, S.-M., & Luan, V. H. (2004). Cognitive profiling and preliminary subtyping in Chinese developmental dyslexia. *Cognition, 91*, 43–75. doi: http://dx.doi.org/10.1016/S0010-0277(03)00163-X.

Ho, C. S.-H., Leung, M.-T., & Cheung, H. (2011). Early difficulties of Chinese preschoolers at familial risk for dyslexia: deficits in oral language, phonological processing skills, and print-related skills. *Dyslexia, 17*, 143–164. doi: http://dx.doi.org/10 .1002/dys.429.

Katz, L., & Frost, R. (1992). The reading process is different for different orthographies: The orthographic depth hypothesis. In R. Frost & L. Katz (Eds.), *Orthography, phonology, morphology, and meaning* (pp. 67–84). Amsterdam: Elsevier Science Publishers.

Kirby, J. R., Georgiou, G. K., Martinussen, R., & Parrila, R. (2010). Naming speed and reading: From prediction to instruction. *Reading Research Quarterly, 45*, 341–362. doi: http://dx.doi.org/10.1598/RRQ.45.3.4.

Landerl, K. (2017). Reading acquisition in German language. In C. Perfetti & L, Verhoeven (Eds.), *Learning to read across languages and writing systems* (pp. 299–323). Cambridge, UK: Cambridge University Press.

Landerl, K., Freudenthaler, H.H., Heene, M., et al. (2019). Phonological awareness and rapid automatized naming as longitudinal predictors of reading in five alphabetic orthographies with varying degrees of consistency. *Scientific Studies of Reading, 23*, 220–234. doi: https://doi.org/10.1080/10888438.2018.1510936.

Landerl, K., Ramus, F., Moll, K. et al. (2013). Predictors of developmental dyslexia in European orthographies with varying complexity. *Journal of Child Psychology and Psychiatry, 54*, 686–694. doi: http://dx.doi.org/10.1111/jcpp.12029.

Landerl, K., Wimmer, H., & Frith, U. (1997). The impact of orthographic consistency on dyslexia: A German-English comparison. *Cognition, 63*, 315–334. doi: http://dx .doi.org/10.1016/S0010-0277(97)00005-X.

Lyytinen, H., Aro, M., Eklund, K. et al. (2004). The development of children at familial risk for dyslexia: Birth to early school age. *Annals of Dyslexia, 54*, 184–220. doi: ht tp://dx.doi.org/10.1007/s11881-004-0010-3.

Mann, V., & Wimmer, H. (2002). Phoneme awareness and pathways into literacy: A comparison of German and American children. *Reading and Writing, 15*, 653–682. doi: http://dx.doi.org/10.1023/A:1020984704781.

Marx, P., & Lenhard, W. (2010). Diagnostische Merkmale von Screeningverfahren. In M. Hasselhorn & W. Schneider (Eds.), *Frühprognose schulischer Kompetenzen*. Göttingen, Germany: Hogrefe.

Meng, X., Cheng-Lai, A., Zeng, B., Stein, J. F., Zhou, X. (2011). Dynamic visual perception and reading development in Chinese school children. *Annals of Dyslexia, 61*, 161–176. doi: http://dx.doi.org/10.1007/s11881-010-0049-2

Mol, S. E., & Bus, A. G. (2011). To read or not to read. A meta-analysis of print exposure from infancy to early adulthood. *Psychological Bulletin, 137*, 267–296. doi: http://dx.doi.org/10.1037/a0021890.

Moll, K., & Landerl, K. (2009). Double dissociation between reading and spelling deficits. *Scientific Studies of Reading, 13,* 359–382. doi: http://dx.doi.org/10.1080/10888430903162878.

Moll, K., Loff, A., & Snowling, M. J. (2013). Cognitive endophenotypes of dyslexia. *Scientific Studies of Reading, 17,* 385–397. doi: http://dx.doi.org/10.1080/10888438.2012.736439.

Moll, K., Ramus, F., Bartling, J. et al. (2014). Cognitive mechanisms underlying reading and spelling development in five European orthographies: Is English an outlier orthography? *Learning and Instruction, 29,* 65–77. doi: http://dx.doi.org/10.1016/j.learninstruc.2013.09.003.

Nash, H. M., Hulme, C., Gooch, D., & Snowling, M. J. (2013). Preschool language profiles of children at family risk of dyslexia: Continuities with specific language impairment. *Journal of Child Psychology and Psychiatry, 54,* 958–968. doi: http://dx.doi.org/10.1111/jcpp.12091.

Nicolson, R. I., & Fawcett, A. J. (2011). Dyslexia, dysgraphia, procedural learning and the cerebellum. *Cortex, 47,* 117–127. doi: http://dx.doi.org/10.1016/j.cortex.2009.08.016.

Norton, E. S., & Wolf, M. (2012). Rapid Automatized Naming (RAN) and reading fluency: Implications for understanding and treatment of reading disabilities. *Annual Review of Psychology, 63,* 427–452. doi: http://dx.doi.org/10.1146/annurev-psych-120710-100431.

Ojanen, E., Ronimus, M., Ahonen, T. et al. (2015). GraphoGame – a catalyst for multi-level promotion of literacy in diverse contexts. *Frontiers in Psychology, 6,* e671. doi: http://dx.doi.org/10.3389/fpsyg.2015.00671.

Perfetti, C. A. (2003). The universal grammar of reading. *Scientific Studies of Reading, 7,* 3–24. doi: http://dx.doi.org/10.1207/S1532799XSSR0701_02.

Perfetti, C. A. & Harris, L. N. (2013). Universal reading processes are modulated by language and writing system. *Language Learning and Development, 9,* 296–316. doi: http://dx.doi.org/10.1080/15475441.2013.813828.

Perfetti, C. A., & Verhoeven, L. (2017). *Learning to read across languages and writing systems.* Cambridge, UK: Cambridge University Press.

Petersen, D. K. & Elbro, C. (1999). Pre-school prediction and prevention of dyslexia: A longitudinal study with children of dyslexic parents. In T. Nunes (Ed.), *Learning to read: An integrated view from research and practice* (pp. 133–154). Dordrecht: Kluwer.

Peterson, R. L., Arnett, A. B., Pennington, B. F., et al. (2018). Literacy acquisition influences children's rapid automatized naming. *Developmental Science, 21,* e12589. doi: https://doi.org/10.1111/desc.12589.

Peterson, R. L., & Pennington, B. F. (2012). Developmental dyslexia. *Lancet, 379,* 1997–2007. doi: http://dx.doi.org/10.1016/S0140-6736(12)60198-6.

Rack, J. P., Snowling, M. J., & Olson, R. K. (1992). The nonword reading deficit in developmental dyslexia: A review. *Reading Research Quarterly, 27,* 28–53. doi: http://dx.doi.org/10.2307/747832.

Ramus, F. (2003). Developmental dyslexia: specific phonological deficit or general sensorimotor dysfunction? *Current Opinion in Neurobiology, 13,* 212–218. doi: http://dx.doi.org/10.1016/S0959-4388(03)00035-7.

Ramus, F. (2004). Neurobiology of dyslexia: A reinterpretation of the data. *Trends in Neurosciences, 27,* 720–726. doi: http://dx.doi.org/10.1016/j.tins.2004.10.004.

Rau, A. K., Moll, K., Moeller, K. et al. (2016). Same same, but different: Word and sentence reading in German and English. *Scientific Studies of Reading, 20*, 203–219. doi: http://dx.doi.org/10.1080/10888438.2015.1136913.

Rau, A. K., Moll, K., Snowling, M. J., & Landerl, K. (2015). Effects of orthographic consistency on eye movement behavior: German and English children and adults process the same words differently. *Journal of Experimental Child Psychology, 130*, 92–105. doi: http://dx.doi.org/10.1016/j.jecp.2014.09.012.

Scarborough, H. S. (1989). Prediction of reading disability from familial and individual differences. *Journal of Educational Psychology, 81*, 101–108. doi: http://dx.doi.org /10.1037//0022-0663.81.1.101.

Schmalz, X., Marinus, E., Coltheart, M., & Castles, A. (2015). Getting to the bottom of orthographic depth. *Psychonomic Bulletin & Review, 22*, 1614–1629. doi: http://dx .doi.org/10.3758/s13423-015-0835-2.

Sénéchal, M., & LeFevre, J.-A. (2002). Parental involvement in the development of children's reading skill: A five-year longitudinal study. *Child Development, 73*, 445–460. doi: http://dx.doi.org/10.1111/1467-8624.00417.

Seymour, P. H. K., Aro, M., & Erskine, J. M. (2003). Foundation literacy acquisition in European orthographies. *British Journal of Psychology, 94*, 143–174. doi: http://dx .doi.org/10.1348/000712603321661859.

Share, D. L. (2008). On the Anglocentricities of current reading research and practice: the perils of over-reliance on an "outlier" orthography. *Psychological Bulletin, 134*, 584–615. doi: http://dx.doi.org/10.1037/0033-2909.134.4.584.

Share, D. L. (2014). Alphabetism in reading science. *Frontiers in Psychology, 5*, e752. doi: http://dx.doi.org/10.3389/fpsyg.2014.00752.

Snowling, M. J., Gallagher, A., & Frith, U. (2003). Family risk of dyslexia is continuous: Individual differences in the precursors of reading skill. *Child Development, 74*, 358–373. doi: http://dx.doi.org/10.1111/1467-8624.7402003.

Stein, J. (2012). Visual contributions to reading difficulties: The magnocellular theory. In J. Stein & Z. Kapoula (Eds.), *Visual aspects of dyslexia* (pp. 171–197). Oxford, UK: Oxford University Press.

Stein, J., & Walsh, V. (1997). To see but not to read: The magnocellular theory of dyslexia. *Trends in Neuroscience, 20*, 147–152. doi: http://dx.doi.org/10.1016/S016 6-2236(96)01005-3.

Suggate, S. P. (2016). A meta-analysis of the long-term effects of phonemic awareness, phonics, fluency, and reading comprehension interventions. *Journal of Learning Disabilities, 49*, 77–96. doi: http://dx.doi.org/10.1177/0022219414528540.

Tallal, P. (2004). Improving language and literacy is a matter of time. *Nature Reviews Neuroscience, 5*, 721–728. doi: http://dx.doi.org/10.1038/nrn1499.

Torgesen, J. K., Wagner, R. K., Rashotte, C. A., Burgess, S., & Hecht, S. (1997). Contributions of phonological awareness and rapid automatized naming ability to growth of word-reading skills in second- to fifth-grade children. *Scientific Studies of Reading, 1*, 161–185. doi: http://dx.doi.org/10.1207/s1532799xssr0102_4.

Vaessen, A., Bertrand, D., Tóth, D. et al. (2010). Cognitive development of fluent word reading does not qualitatively differ between transparent and opaque orthographies. *Journal of Educational Psychology, 102*, 827–842. doi: http://dx.doi.org/10.1037 /a0019465.

Vaessen, A., Gerretsen, P., & Blomert, L. (2009). Naming problems do not reflect a second independent core deficit in dyslexia: Double deficits explored. *Journal of Experimental Child Psychology*, *103*, 202–221. doi: http://dx.doi.org/10.1016/j.jecp.2008.12.004.

Valdois, S., Bosse, M.-L., & Tainturier, M.-J. (2004). The cognitive deficits responsible for developmental dyslexia: Review of evidence for a selective visual attentional disorder. *Dyslexia*, *10*, 339–363. doi: http://dx.doi.org/10.1002/dys.284.

van Bergen, E., de Jong, P. F., Regtvoort, A. et al. (2011). Dutch children at family risk of dyslexia: precursors, reading development, and parental effects. *Dyslexia*, *17*, 2–18. doi: http://dx.doi.org/10.1002/dys.423.

Vellutino, F. R., Fletcher, J. M., Snowling, M. J., & Scanlon, D. M. (2004). Specific reading disability (dyslexia): What have we learned in the past four decades? *Journal of Child Psychology and Psychiatry*, *45*, 2–40. doi: http://dx.doi.org/10.1046/j.0021-9630.2003.00305.x.

Wimmer, H. (1993). Characteristics of developmental dyslexia in a regular writing system. *Applied Psycholinguistics*, *14*, 1–33. doi: http://dx.doi.org/10.1017/S0142716400010122.

Wimmer, H., Mayringer, H., & Landerl, K. (2000). The double-deficit hypothesis and difficulties in learning to read a regular orthography. *Journal of Educational Psychology*, *92*, 668–680. doi: http://dx.doi.org/10.1037/0022-0663.92.4.668.

Wolf, M., & Bowers, P. G. (1999). The double-deficit hypothesis for the developmental dyslexias. *Journal of Educational Psychology*, *91*, 415-438. doi: http://dx.doi.org/10.1037/0022-0663.91.3.415.

Wolf, M., & Katzir-Cohen, T. (2001). Reading fluency and its intervention. *Scientific Studies of Reading*, *5*, 211–239. doi: http://dx.doi.org/10.1207/S1532799XSSR0503_2.

World Health Organization. (2008). *International statistical classification of diseases and related health problems - Tenth revision* (2nd ed.). Geneva, Switzerland: World Health Organization.

Ziegler, J. C., Bertrand, D., Tóth, D. et al. (2010). Orthographic depth and its impact on universal predictors of reading: A cross-language investigation. *Psychological Science*, *21*, 551–559. doi: http://dx.doi.org/10.1177/0956797610363406.

Ziegler, J. C., Perry, C., Ma-Wyatt, A., Ladner, D., & Schulte-Körne, G. (2003). Developmental dyslexia in different languages: Language-specific or universal? *Journal of Experimental Child Psychology*, *86*, 169–193. doi: http://dx.doi.org/10.1016/S0022-0965(03)00139-5.

12 Neural Predictors of Developmental Dyslexia

Elizabeth S. Norton, John D. E. Gabrieli,
and Nadine Gaab

12.1 Introduction

Dyslexia, or difficulty in learning to read that is not caused by a sensory deficit or lack of effort or education, affects readers of all languages (Caravolas, 2005). Based on this definition, dyslexia cannot be diagnosed until children have demonstrated trouble with reading acquisition. However, it would be ideal to identify which children will go on develop reading problems before they struggle or fail to learn to read. Children who are identified early and who receive early intervention are likely to have better reading outcomes (Bowyer-Crane et al., 2008; Torgesen, 2004; Schatschneider & Torgesen, 2004; Vellutino, Scanlon, & Tanzman, 1998) and may suffer fewer of the negative consequences associated with poor reading. Further, an understanding of which children are at greatest risk for reading difficulties would allow educators and clinicians to allocate limited intervention resources to students who need them most. Extensive behavioral research has sought to answer this question and yet models predicting reading are rarely employed in practice. In order to potentially improve accuracy of these models in predicting later reading ability, researchers have investigated the role of neural measures in such predictions. In this chapter, we review how neural measures have contributed to our evolving understanding of early precursors of reading ability and dyslexia.

Dyslexia is caused by neurobiological differences thought to be present from birth (Langer et al., 2017; Leppänen et al., 1999; Leppänen et al., 2010, 2012; Norton, Beach, & Gabrieli, 2015; Peterson & Pennington, 2015), and thus markers of dyslexia are likely to exist before children learn to read. Dyslexia is moderately heritable, but the genetic basis of reading ability is not so strong that we can use familial history alone as a method of early identification. Among children who have a parent or sibling with dyslexia, approximately one third to one half develop dyslexia (Hensler et al., 2010; McBride-Chang et al., 2011; Pennington & Lefly, 2001), whereas the prevalence of dyslexia in the general population is approximately 7–10 percent (Peterson & Pennington, 2015; Snowling, 2013; Snowling & Melby-Lervåg, 2016). Thus, a family history of dyslexia is a risk indicator, but not a perfect predictor of future reading ability. Note that because of the heterogeneity in diagnostic and inclusion/exclusion criteria across studies, we here use the term dyslexia to refer to a difficulty with accurate and/or fluent word reading (e.g., Lyon, Shaywitz, & Shaywitz, 2003); particular criteria vary from study to study.

Reading depends on several language and cognitive abilities that can be assessed before children learn to read. Oral language is a foundation of reading, and children with deficits in areas such as vocabulary or oral comprehension struggle when learning to read (Snowling & Melby-Lervåg, 2016). Additional key reading-related abilities include phonological processing and phonological awareness (PA; the ability to identify and manipulate the sound units of language), rapid automatized naming (RAN; the speed with which one can name an array of familiar items), and letter-name and -sound knowledge (Elbro, Borstrom, & Petersen, 1998; Landerl & Wimmer, 2008; McBride-Chang et al., 2011; Schatschneider et al., 2004; see also Landerl, Chapter 11 in this volume). Measures of these abilities in pre-reading children tend to correlate with later reading scores in most alphabetic languages, with relatively minor variations depending on the characteristics of the particular language and reading system (Caravolas et al., 2013; Moll et al., 2014). Predictive models derived from research studies that combine these behavioral measures to identify risk for dyslexia achieve varying levels of success (discussed below in Section 12.2.1), and are not widely employed in educational practice (Catts et al., 2001; Ozernov-Palchik & Gaab, 2016).

Across studies of many different conditions, adding brain measures to behavioral measures improves prediction of which individuals will develop a disorder or respond to a particular intervention (Gabrieli, Ghosh, & Whitfield-Gabrieli, 2015). Thus, researchers have turned to safe and child-friendly brain-imaging measures to examine the development of reading skills, investigate the etiology of dyslexia, and evaluate potential neural predictors of later reading ability. We first discuss the methods and challenges of assessing possible neural predictors of reading ability in infants and young children. We then review studies that have examined the neural predictors of later reading across languages using electrophysiology, and structural and functional magnetic resonance imaging (MRI). Finally, we discuss the clinical implications of our current knowledge in this area, and the state of our understanding of neural predictors and how they might be employed to help the many children around the world who struggle to learn to read.

12.2   Theoretical Background

12.2.1   Predictive Models of Reading

Research studies that classify children as at risk of dyslexia are usually based on a statistical regression model that incorporates the different predictor measures (e.g., Catts et al., 2001). The model assigns weights to each of the different predictor variables (e.g., test scores, demographics) and produces a probability value of risk for each individual. Then, a cutoff score must be set at a certain probability value, separating the continuum of risk scores into two distinct groups, those at risk and those not at risk. Choosing the cutoff criterion comes with a trade-off between specificity (the ability to detect true negatives) and sensitivity (the ability to detect true positives) (O'Connor & Jenkins, 1999). One approach is to set a criterion designed to maximize *specificity* of prediction. With this approach, a smaller number of children, those with the highest probabilities, are identified as at risk. This way, children who are unlikely to need early intervention will not be flagged as at risk. In this case, though, it is likely that a number of additional children who will develop dyslexia will be missed (false negatives). On the other hand, the criterion can be set to maximize *sensitivity*, with the goal of ensuring that all children who are truly at risk are identified. In this case, the number of false positives will likely increase. Even though additional reading intervention is not harmful for typically developing children, there are downsides to over-identification. On a practical basis, schools rarely have the resources to provide time and cost-intensive interventions to children who may not benefit from them. Further, being labeled as at risk of dyslexia may have negative psychosocial effects and may affect a child's self-concept (Humphrey & Mullins, 2002).

12.2.2   In Search of Neural Predictors of Dyslexia

There are several challenges associated with conducting studies to determine whether there are neural predictors that can aid in prediction of future reading ability before children learn to read. First, in order to prospectively study a sufficiently large sample of children who have a diagnosis of dyslexia, studies need to recruit and follow very large groups of children from birth or an early age through to school age. Thus, many studies have enrolled infants and children with, versus those without, a family history of dyslexia. As noted above, children who have a first-degree family member with dyslexia are three to five times more likely to have dyslexia than children with no family history (Pennington & Lefly, 2001; Puolakanaho et al., 2007). Children in these two groups differ based on their family history of dyslexia, but not necessarily the state of having dyslexia themselves; approximately half of the children with family history of dyslexia (FHD+) will become typical readers, and a small proportion of children with no family history (FHD–) will have dyslexia. Beginning these studies in infancy is difficult, but offers the advantage that any brain differences between FHD+ children and FHD– controls present very early in life are more likely to reflect genetic/biological differences associated with dyslexia rather than factors related to experience and environment. On the other hand, studies that begin with infant participants must follow them until they can be evaluated for reading ability, meaning that they take at least 6 years to complete.

Second, conducting brain-imaging studies with infants and children is challenging (Perlman, 2012; Raschle et al., 2009, 2012), especially because head movements of just a few millimeters can introduce artifact and noise into both structural and functional MRI images (e.g., Reuter et al., 2015). Head or body motion, as well as eye blinks, create artifacts in electroencephalography (EEG) recordings (Luck, 2014). Experiments must be designed to obtain sufficient artifact-free data in a reasonable amount of time. Experimental paradigms must also be engaging, and not too easy or too difficult, in order to obtain good data from young children.

Third, many brain measures are also expensive and are likely not feasible for the clinic or classroom. MRI scanners cost millions of dollars to purchase and require consistent upkeep and maintenance. EEG can be measured with systems that cost in the thousands rather than millions of dollars. Collecting and interpreting data from these types of equipment also requires substantial training. Thus, an important practical concern is whether any potential predictive brain measure will be feasible to acquire in a large sample. Additional research is also needed to determine the reliability and validity of these measures if they are to be used clinically (Bishop, 2007; Poldrack et al., 2017).

Finally, finding brain measures that predict dyslexia is made difficult by the heterogeneity of the disorder and a lack of consensus on its causes. In the literature, objective physical correlates of a condition are often referred to as "biomarkers" (e.g., Kraemer, Schultz, & Arndt, 2002). Here, we use the term "predictors," because this heterogeneity means that there is unlikely to be a single biomarker that underlies all cases of dyslexia. Different theories of the cause of dyslexia posit different underlying core deficits. Some consider core deficits in phonological processing (Boada & Pennington, 2006; Boets et al., 2013; Ramus & Szenkovits, 2008). Others suggest a multiple-deficit view of dyslexia, in which deficits in any one or more different reading-related skills can cause dyslexia (Wolf & Bowers, 1999; Pennington et al., 2012). Whereas the underlying cause of dyslexia has not been fully established, the discovery of potential biomarkers that predict dyslexia could offer insight into its etiology and assist in the development of remediation strategies.

12.3   Research Evidence of Auditory and Language Processing Differences from Event-Related Potentials (ERPs)

Electroencephalography measures the brain's function by recording electrical activity from electrodes in a fabric cap or net fitted over the scalp. The EEG signal reflects the electrical activity of many neurons in similar alignment firing at the same time. EEG can be used to measure responses to particular stimuli; these time-locked EEG responses are called event-related potentials (ERPs). EEG/ERP measures provide temporal resolution on the order of milliseconds, but less precise information about the brain regions generating the observed signals. Thus, studies tend to use ERPs to look at the timing or magnitude of neural responses to particular stimuli rather than to determine the source of neural responses.

12.3.1   ERP Measures of Speech Processing Predicting Dyslexia

ERP responses to auditory stimuli are often measured during passive listening, and thus do not require explicit attention to the stimuli or any responses from participants. Thus, these paradigms are relatively unaffected by effort or task-performance differences between groups. Further, passive auditory EEG recording is ideal for studying infants and children because stimuli can be played over earphones or speakers while participants are sleeping or watching a soundless movie. Studies of infants also take advantage of the fact that the human auditory system is relatively well developed at birth (Moore & Linthicum, 2009), whereas the development of other systems depends more heavily on postnatal experience. Several studies have used a simple paradigm, recording the brain's responses to speech syllables, to investigate whether these differences may be associated with dyslexia or future reading ability.

12.3.1.1 Speech Processing in Infants at Risk of Dyslexia   As discussed above, one of the most widely used methods for understanding early brain differences associated with reading ability is to study infants with a family history of dyslexia (FHD). These studies can be conducted very early in life, thus any differences between the groups are more likely to be related to genetic/ biological causes rather than environmental influences. A drawback of these types of studies is that because dyslexia is only moderately heritable, not all of the infants in the at-risk group will go on to evince dyslexia. Nonetheless, studies of infants with a family history of dyslexia have provided important insights into the early auditory and language processes that may be implicated in dyslexia.

A series of studies from the Jyväskylä research group in Finland examined forty-nine infants within seven days of birth and compared those with versus without FHD (Guttorm et al., 2001; Guttorm et al., 2003). While infants slept, their automatic ERP responses to syllables /ba/, /ga/, and /da/ were measured. The amplitude of ERP responses to the syllables differed significantly between the two groups. The authors used a discriminant function analysis to determine if membership in the FHD+ versus FHD– group could be predicted from ERP measures alone; the model correctly classified 69 percent of the infants (Guttorm et al., 2001), with 73 percent sensitivity and 65 percent specificity. This means that ERP patterns were somewhat, but not completely, distinct between the two groups of infants. In a follow-up study, the same syllables plus a second set, /paa/, /taa/, and /kaa/, were tested (Guttorm et al., 2003). Differences were again found in the groups' ERPs among the first set of syllables, but there was no difference in the two groups' ERPs to the second set of syllables.

Differences in language sound processing were also associated with FHD among a group of 17-month-old Dutch infants (van Herten et al., 2008). FHD+ versus FHD– groups differed in their neural processing of language, both in the latency of early and mid-latency ERP components, and in the laterality of neural processing of speech. Taken together, these results indicate that magnitude and laterality of ERP responses may differ in very young children with family history of dyslexia. Because these three studies used different sounds and paradigms, and because differences were not seen in all conditions, it is difficult to draw conclusions across studies.

12.3.1.2 Speech Processing in Children with Dyslexia   Longitudinal studies indeed provide valuable information that informs our understanding of how family risk and brain measures relate to later pre-reading and reading skills. The Jyväskylä Longitudinal Study examined correlations between newborn ERPs and later language and pre-reading abilities through age 5 in children with and without FHD. The authors examined infants with FHD (n=26) and controls (n=23). In the combined sample of children, ERP responses were significantly correlated with scores on receptive language at age 2.5 years and verbal memory at age 5 years (Guttorm et al., 2005). However, no correlations were seen with language or memory abilities at age 3.5 years. In a subsequent follow-up at age 6.5 with a smaller subsample from the same group, the children who displayed the "at-risk" pattern of brain response in infancy (n=11) had significantly lower phonological awareness, rapid naming, and letter knowledge than did controls (n=10) (Guttorm et al., 2010). Children with vs. without family history did not differ significantly in these three behavioral markers of pre-reading ability; however, the group of children with family history who showed the at-risk pattern of ERP responses scored significantly lower on the phonology, RAN, and letter-naming measures than children with no family history and a "typical" pattern of ERP responses to speech in infancy. Similar results, in which only the group who developed dyslexia showed a difference, were seen from pre-readers at age 6 (Hämäläinen et al., 2013).

Another set of studies followed babies in the United States from birth to age 8. Here, researchers measured ERPs to syllables /bi/ and /gi/ in forty-eight infants within thirty-six hours of birth (Molfese, 2000). At age 8, children were classified into three groups: typical readers, "dyslexics" (poor reading with higher IQ), and "poor readers" (poor reading and lower IQ). Curiously, the amplitude of the ERP response in the control group fell in between the group who developed dyslexia and the group who were poor readers with lower IQ. A discriminant function analysis based on the ERP measures classified thirty-nine of the forty-eight children (81.3 percent) into the correct group. In an extension of the study with a larger sample of ninety-six children, the influence of home literacy environment, socioeconomic status (SES), and early language and perceptual skills were considered as additional predictors of reading outcome (Molfese, Molfese, & Modgline, 2001). In several competing regression models predicting reading ability at age 8, the ERP measures were always significant predictors. Regressions revealed that behavioral and ERP measures accounted for approximately equal proportions of the variance in age-8 reading scores; however, the models accounted at most 19 percent of overall variance in reading.

The results from these studies indicate that considering family history, behavioral measures, and brain responses together predicts future reading and reading-related abilities more accurately than either factor alone. Further, because such differences are present very early and persist to school age, they may be potentially useful markers of later reading ability. However, further studies are needed with large samples to determine whether these measures have sufficient sensitivity and specificity to be used in early identification of dyslexia.

12.3.2   ERP Measures of Auditory Change Detection Predicting Dyslexia

One widely used approach for studying auditory ERPs is to present stimuli in an oddball paradigm, in which a standard stimulus is presented repeatedly and a different stimulus (called the oddball or deviant) is presented infrequently among the standards. The difference in ERP brain responses between the standard and deviant stimuli is called the mismatch negativity (MMN; Näätänen, 2001; Näätänen et al., 2012), as it is a negative-going wave in typical adults. Among infants, the mismatch is sometimes a positive rather than a negative deflection, and thus is sometimes called a mismatch response (MMR) or mismatch positivity (MMP). Depending on the stimulus type and age, the mismatch stimulus sometimes elicits two separate negative peaks, the first usually called the MMN and the second called the late MMN or late discriminative negativity (LDN); these may reflect different stages of stimulus processing (Halliday et al., 2014).

In many studies of older children and adults with dyslexia, the MMN response is reduced in amplitude, later in latency, or differently lateralized or located in the brain (see Bishop, 2007, for a review). The standard and deviant stimuli for MMN studies are usually very similar, thus detecting the difference depends on auditory perception, but the fact that the MMN is fast and pre-attentive means that the MMN may also reflect the automaticity of brain processes. The robust association between RAN and reading across languages may be because RAN taps the same processes of automaticity that support accurate and fluent reading.

12.3.2.1 Auditory Change Detection in Children at Risk of Dyslexia   As with simple auditory ERP studies, much of the research on MMN and genetic risk for reading disorders comes from longitudinal studies of children with family history of dyslexia. Researchers from the Jyväskylä Longitudinal Study examined the mismatch response to two syllables in seventy-three Finnish infants with vs. without FHD within seven days of birth and again at age 6 months (Pihko et al., 1999). As newborns, only the at-risk FHD+ infants showed an MMR (i.e., a significant difference in the ERPs to the standard versus deviant stimuli). The FHD− newborns did not show any difference between the standard and deviant stimuli. At age 6 months, both groups showed a mismatch response, left-lateralized in the FHD− children and right-lateralized in the FHD+ children. Another mismatch study with two pseudo-words as stimuli was carried out with 6-month-old infants in the Jyväskylä study (Leppänen et al., 2002). The FHD+ and FHD− groups showed similar amplitude responses across most of the scalp, but a significant MMR was observed in the FHD− group, whereas no significant MMR was observed in the FHD+ group. These results again reveal a potential difference associated with genetic risk for dyslexia but some inconsistency across studies.

The Dutch Dyslexia Program has also included studies examining MMN responses and family history of dyslexia. In these studies, the word /bAk/ was the standard and /dAk/ was the deviant stimulus. Two-month-old FHD− infants had a significant MMR, whereas the FHD+ infants had no observable MMR (van Leeuwen et al., 2006, and extended in van Leeuwen et al., 2008). The authors report that the source of the MMR was traceable to the superior temporal auditory cortices in FHD− infants, but not in FHD+ infants. In a follow-up study that examined ERPs to different stimuli on the continuum from /bAk/ to /dAk/, FHD− children showed significantly different amplitude responses for the stimuli on opposite sides of the phoneme category boundary, whereas FHD+ children showed a similar response to all of the stimuli (van

Leeuwen et al., 2007). This finding is consistent with the notion that individuals with dyslexia may be more generally sensitive to discriminating sounds regardless of whether the sounds make a linguistically meaningful phoneme change, whereas individuals with typical language and reading are more attuned to the phoneme boundaries (Noordenbos et al., 2012; Serniclaes et al., 2004).

Several studies have also examined the MMN in pre-reading children at early school age. In such studies, it is important to control for other factors that may differ between groups, such as language abilities, which may account for differences in the MMN. One study examined MMN responses in Finnish children ages 5–6 using tone stimuli that included frequency, intensity, and duration deviants relative to a standard tone (Hämäläinen et al.,2015). The FHD+ group scored significantly lower on language measures, but did not differ in age, phonological processing, or RAN from the FHD– group. There were no significant group differences in the tone duration or intensity comparisons, despite previous findings of speech-sound duration MMR differences in Finnish infants related to FHD (Leppänen et al., 1999, 2002). The FHD+ children did show significantly larger MMN responses to the tone frequency deviant than did FHD– children. Amplitude of the MMN response to frequency change was correlated with better scores on RAN and sentence repetition. This correlation with behavior provides a clue that in addition to phonological processes, automaticity and language processes may play a role in the relation between MMN and reading ability. However, others found that tone and speech-stimuli MMNs may have differential relations to risk for dyslexia (Lovio, Näätänen, & Kujala, 2010).

MMN paradigms with both tone and phoneme conditions were directly compared in German-speaking children. Responses to syllables (/ba/, /da/, /ta/), as well as tones differing in frequency (pitch), were compared among sixty 6- to 7-year-olds with and without FHD who were matched on age, gender, and handedness (Maurer et al., 2003). The FHD+ children scored lower in phonological awareness than the FHD– group. Only the late MMN response differed between the groups, with the FHD+ showing a more right-lateralized response in the tone condition and reduced amplitude and lateralization in the phoneme condition. Given that the phoneme condition overall showed a more pronounced difference between groups, this suggests that language stimuli may elicit responses that are more closely related to dyslexia or risk for dyslexia.

Taken together, a common theme across many, but not all, of the MMR studies is that FHD– groups are more likely to evince a significant MMR, indicating detection of the sound change. Often, the MMR is more right-lateralized in the infants and children with FHD and left-lateralized in the children without FHD. We also see that the stimuli and experimental parameters used can substantially affect findings. Another substantial challenge in interpreting the results of studies that among the FHD+ children, only some will evince dyslexia. Thus, FHD+ groups could be considered to be more heterogeneous than FHD– groups, which again could affect results, biasing this group toward a lower response amplitude because of the greater variability between individuals.

12.3.2.2 Auditory Change Detection in Children with Dyslexia   Longitudinal follow-up studies of infants can help clarify whether the MMR differences are predictive of dyslexia, and not just family history. In the Jyväskylä study, children who completed an MMN paradigm with tones within 7 days of birth were assessed in Grade 2 and classified as typical or poor readers (Leppänen et al., 2010). FHD– children who became typical readers showed an MMR to the tone stimuli as infants, but FHD+ children did not, regardless of whether they became typical or poor readers. Thus, it seems that at the group level, MMR was related to genetic risk rather than overall reading ability. Early and late MMRs were significantly correlated with several language and pre-reading skills, as well as with children's reading speed and accuracy in Grade 2. MMR responses accounted for significant variance in reading speed and accuracy. The correlations between MMRs and reading speed were strongest in the FHD– children, suggesting that these measures may not be as useful for differentiating which at-risk children will have dyslexia.

Children from the Dutch Dyslexia Program who completed the /bAk/ vs. /dAk/ paradigm at 2 months were followed to Grade 2 and classified as controls (no FHD, fluent reader) or children at risk who became fluent or non-fluent readers (n=10–16 per group) (van Zuijen et al., 2013). The FHD+ children who became non-fluent readers did not show an MMR. Typical readers, regardless of their FHD status, had significant MMRs as infants (i.e., significant differences between standard and deviant stimuli), but these differed in location on the scalp. Thus, the MMR responses tracked with both reading outcome and family risk, providing support for the notion that neural data could help predict later reading ability among children at risk of dyslexia.

An additional Dutch Dyslexia Program study examined MMN responses to a different auditory feature: amplitude rise time (ART), which has been suggested as a potential core deficit in dyslexia (Goswami et al., 2002). ERPs were measured to tones with ART deviants and frequency deviants in 3-year-old children with (n=25) and without FHD (n=13) (Plakas et al., 2013). The MMN responses to a frequency deviant at age 3.5 were significantly greater in controls than in FHD+ children who had dyslexia in second grade. When the FHD+ children were pooled into one group regardless of their reading outcome, that group's MMN to both the frequency deviant and the ART deviant was reduced as compared to controls. Despite the lack of clear separation between risk groups who had typical reading versus dyslexia, significant small-to-medium size correlations were observed between greater MMN amplitudes in both deviant conditions and better word-reading fluency.

Another study explicitly tested whether ERP measures add to prediction beyond the power of behavioral measures from kindergarten to Grade 2 and Grade 5. Swiss-German children with and without FHD completed MMN paradigms with tone and with phoneme stimuli in kindergarten (Maurer et al., 2009). The centroid of the response (a way of measuring degree of lateralization) was significantly more leftward in children who became typical readers versus those who developed dyslexia. Models including behavior and ERP measures accounted for 39–45 percent of variance in reading outcomes. This study also used logistic regression to predict group membership; the best model including the phoneme MMN measure correctly classified 66 percent of children as below the 10th percentile in reading (sensitivity 21 percent, specificity 87 percent) and 75 percent of children as below the 20th percentile (sensitivity 68 percent, specificity 80 percent). These values are generally lower than those reported for behavioral prediction in English-speaking kindergartners (reviewed in Ozernov-Palchik & Gaab, 2016).

Considering how MMN responses relate to reading ability, it may be that MMN responses and behavioral characteristics, such as family history of dyslexia and language abilities, could be combined to yield more accurate prediction of dyslexia. The fact that relations with reading are stronger and more consistent when speech stimuli are used is consistent with the idea that deficits observed in dyslexia are at the level of speech sounds and not the purely acoustic level. Greater predictive power in large samples would need to be demonstrated before these measures are used in practice.

12.3.3   ERP Measures in Other Domains Predicting Dyslexia

Beyond auditory and phonological skills, a variety of other skills relate to later reading, including knowledge of letters, and automaticity of language processing. Thus, researchers have also examined ERPs during processing of letters and words. Though these measures probably cannot be extended to very young children the way that passive auditory paradigms can, they may provide different types of information that relate to reading.

One such study examined whether differences in the ERP component associated with orthographic processing in mature readers, called the N170, was altered in kindergarten children who would later be poor readers (Bach et al., 2013). These children were drawn from a more general population not selected for family history of dyslexia. During EEG recording, children (n=19) were presented with auditory words, altered speech, printed words, or false fonts; children were asked to simply respond as to whether each stimulus was presented in the visual or auditory modality. Beyond behavioral measures of RAN and IQ, adding the ERP N170 response magnitude to words versus false fonts significantly improved prediction of Grade 2 reading speed. Together, behavioral and ERP measures accounted for approximately 67 percent of variance in Grade 2 scores. This value is somewhat higher than what has been seen in other auditory ERP studies. This could be because visual measures are a better predictor, or could reflect a regression model that may be overfit in a small sample.

Researchers in Norway examined lexical and semantic priming in 20- to 24-month-old children, nine with FHD and seventeen without FHD (Torkildsen et al., 2007). The children with FHD had smaller vocabularies on average. The N400 ERP component, which is sensitive to semantic effects, was the focus of analysis in a semantic categorization experiment. FHD– children showed an early response and FHD+ children showed a later response. The FHD– group also had a more bilateral pattern of activation for the N400 response, whereas the FHD+ group showed a left-lateralized pattern of activation. This study provides interesting evidence that semantic knowledge may differ in children with versus without FHD, however the differences in children's vocabularies associated with their FHD status make the results more challenging to interpret.

Whereas theories of dyslexia increasingly espouse a multiple-deficit view, future studies should examine factors such as orthographic and semantic processing alongside phonological and automaticity measures in the same children. Ideally, such work would also account for different patterns of single or multiple deficits across individuals in order to better reveal patterns associated with these heterogeneous profiles (e.g., Norton, Black et al. 2014; Ozernov-Palchik et al., 2017; Pennington et al., 2012).

12.4   Research Evidence of Brain Structure and Function Differences from MRI

12.4.1   *Structural Gray-Matter Predictors of Dyslexia*

Magnetic resonance imaging (MRI) measures differences in the magnetic properties of various tissues, and thus can be used to image both the structure and function of the brain (Huettel, Song, & McCarthy, 2009). Structural MRI images are used to examine the detailed anatomical structure of the brain, with spatial resolution as fine as a few millimeters. From structural scans, the gray-matter volume of a region or the thickness of cortex can be determined, as can the size or morphology of brain structures.

In children and adults with dyslexia, gray-matter volume and cortical thickness are altered throughout the reading network (Richlan, Kronbichler & Wimmer, 2013). A meta-analysis of eleven MRI studies of pre-readers found differences associated with risk for dyslexia in the left fusiform gyrus, temporo-parietal region, and cerebellum, as well as a right parietal area (Vandermosten, Hoeft, & Norton, 2016). Researchers have also begun to examine sulcal patterns, meaning the global pattern of arrangement, number and size of brain folds, which are set very early in development; atypical sulcal patterns have been reported in children with developmental dyslexia and pre-readers with FHD (Im et al., 2015; Williams et al., 2018). Though several studies have used MRI to study pre-readers, fewer have followed children longitudinally to determine whether MRI measures can help predict future reading ability.

The first study to examine structural differences associated with family history of dyslexia in pre-reading children with and without FHD (n=10 per group) used voxel-based morphometry, a measure of regional gray-matter volume, and was performed within the Boston Longitudinal Dyslexia Study (Raschle, Chang, & Gaab, 2011). The FHD+ children had less gray matter in the bilateral temporal-parietal cortex and ventral occipitotemporal cortex, despite no differences in gray matter or brain size overall. The authors concluded that the differences seen in older readers with dyslexia in previous studies could be related to the etiology of dyslexia, rather than differences in reading experience or expertise.

The Bergen Longitudinal Dyslexia Study in Norway examined children's behavioral profiles beginning in kindergarten and their brain structure with MRI in the spring of Grade 1 (before reading instruction began), as well as in Grades 3 and 6 (Clark et al., 2014). Children were classified as having dyslexia or not in sixth grade. Significant brain differences were found among the brains of the typical and dyslexic groups in Grade 1. The group with dyslexia had significantly thinner cortex in left-hemisphere language regions including Heschl's gyrus, lingual gyrus, and medial frontal gyrus, as well as the right orbitofrontal cortex. Despite the small sample size (n=17) the individuals in each group had distinct scores with very little overlap on these measures.

German children completed a structural MRI scan at age 5–6 and then were classified at age 7–8 as having typical reading or dyslexia (n=10 per group) (Skeide et al., 2016). Researchers first identified regions of interest by mapping associations between candidate dyslexia genes and regional gray-matter and white-matter volume of the brains of these children and older children. Then, a pattern-classification algorithm was used to determine whether these measures could classify which children were in the typical readers versus dyslexia group. Classification based on gray-matter volume in the left fusiform gyrus, which houses the visual word form area, led to 75 percent accuracy; sensitivity and specificity were approximately 70–80 percent. Classification based on gray matter in the left parieto-occipital cortex led to 80 percent accuracy.

There are some similarities in the regions identified as candidate predictors in these three studies, despite the fact that structural measures and approaches were somewhat different. The major regions identified are consistent with structural and functional differences in dyslexia (e.g., Richlan et al., 2013). Though each study found significant results, larger studies with greater statistical power should be run (Kraft et al., 2015).

12.4.2   Structural White-Matter Predictors of Dyslexia

White-matter tracts are bundles of myelinated neurons, akin to highways connecting different brain regions. Regions that must communicate with one another often and efficiently tend to be connected by strong white-matter tracts. Diffusion-weighted MRI scans are designed to allow visualization and measurement of white-matter tracts in the brain, often via the diffusion-tensor imaging (DTI) technique (Soares et al., 2013). From diffusion MRI scans, researchers can measure how large and how well organized these tracts are. Fractional anisotropy (FA) is often used as a proxy for microstructural organization of the tract.

As with structural and functional MRI, there are alterations in white-matter tracts in dyslexia throughout the reading network. Both the size and organization of the left arcuate fasciculus and the corona radiata tracts have been reported to be reduced in individuals with dyslexia (Odegard et al., 2009). Among kindergartners and pre-readers, phonological awareness ability is correlated with the volume and FA of the left arcuate fasciculus in English-speaking (Saygin et al., 2013) and Dutch-speaking children (Vandermosten et al., 2015). Ventral tracts, primarily the left inferior fronto-occipital fasciculus, also show lower FA values in children with family history of dyslexia (Vandermosten et al., 2015).

Several studies have examined how white-matter structure relates to future reading ability. In one study that predicted later reading outcomes, English-speaking children of a variety of reading abilities in the United States were scanned in kindergarten (Myers et al., 2014). Reading in Grade 3 was correlated with increases in volume of the left hemisphere arcuate and corona radiata between kindergarten and Grade 3, once other cognitive and pre-reading skills were accounted for. In a regression model, adding the white-matter measures in these two areas significantly improved prediction over pre-reading measures. Together, the behavior and brain measures accounted for 59 percent of variance in Grade 3 reading scores. A region of the left arcuate fasciculus showed lower FA and different development in FHD+ children than FHD− children (Wang et al., 2016). Interestingly, the rate of FA development did not differ between the FHD groups, but did differ by reading outcome: Eventual good readers showed faster rates of FA increases than eventual poor readers. Rate of left AF development was correlated with increases in word-reading ability. Brain and behavior measures together accounted for 56–62 percent of variance in reading outcomes.

Similarly, a study of Dutch-speaking children with and without FHD found that from kindergarten to second grade, FA of the arcuate and inferior frontal-occipital tracts increased overall (Vanderauwera et al., 2017). Children with dyslexia in second grade had lower FA in the left arcuate at both kindergarten and second grade. In a regression model predicting which children had dyslexia, behavioral measures correctly classified 80 percent of cases, whereas adding the FA of left arcuate increased the model accuracy significantly to 84 percent of cases. Though the sample in the regression with dyslexia was small (n=11 with dyslexia and 34 without dyslexia), the left arcuate measure was stronger than behavioral measures and improved classification primarily among children with dyslexia. A similar study of German children found an important role for left-hemisphere white matter that correlated with family risk and predicted reading outcome (Kraft et al., 2016). Among fifty-three children who had an MRI scan at kindergarten age, thirty-five were assessed at the end of Grade 1 or 2. Left arcuate fasciculus intensity (an indicator of reduced myelination) was greater in the FHD+ children than the FHD− children. After adding IQ, phonological processing, and working-memory measures into a logistic regression predicting reading outcome, the only significant predictor was the left arcuate fasciculus measure, which improved prediction by 17 percent over behavioral measures. The overall model accounted for 47 percent of variance in reading, and classification accuracy was 80 percent (90 percent sensitivity, 64 percent specificity). However, this model did not include FHD status, which makes understanding whether brain measures truly improve prediction beyond that factor difficult to discern. Further, the sample size for the group with dyslexia was relatively small (n=12).

These studies highlight the potential important role of structural connections among brain areas as a potential deficit in dyslexia. There is promising convergence among these studies in their common finding that integrity of the left arcuate fasciculus is related to reading ability, even in different samples and languages. In each case, adding white-matter measures to a regression model improved prediction over behavioral measure alone. Though white-matter measures and behavior together accounted for substantial variance in later reading, the contribution of MRI measures was often small relative to behavioral scores. Further, these studies show that considering developmental trajectory of brain or behavioral measures may be important, rather than their assessment at a single time point.

12.4.3   Functional MRI Differences Associated with Risk for Dyslexia

Functional MRI, or fMRI, measures what is called the blood-oxygen-level-dependent (BOLD) signal, which is a correlate of local neuronal activity (Huettel, Song, & McCarthy, 2009). As neurons fire, their oxygen and energy are replenished through increased flow of oxygenated blood, which has different magnetic properties than deoxygenated blood. The BOLD signal reflects this contrast between oxygenated and deoxygenated blood, which peaks several seconds after an area has become activated. Thus, fMRI is most often used to look at differences in magnitude and location of activation, rather than differences in timing of brain processes.

A study of correlates of FHD in pre-readers was carried out in the Boston cohort (Raschle, Zuk, & Gaab, 2012). In the MRI scanner, children completed two tasks with auditory word stimuli, a first-sound-matching task (requiring phonological awareness) and a control voice-matching task. By subtracting the control task from the first-sound-matching task, the researchers were able to isolate the regions of the brain that support phonological awareness. Reduced activation in the FHD+ children was found in the left occipito-temporal region, left temporo-parietal region, and bilateral cerebellum. These areas of difference are consistent with those seen in older readers with dyslexia, suggesting that they might be related to the etiology of dyslexia rather than differences in reading ability or experience. However, the single time-point measurement reported in that study does not provide information about how these regions relate to reading outcomes.

Another study compared functional brain activation in children who were at risk of dyslexia because of poor performance on early reading measures. Groups of seven children were studied who were either "on track" or "at risk" (<35th percentile) in terms of their letter-naming and phonological skills at the beginning of kindergarten (Yamada et al., 2011). In the MRI scanner, children performed a one-back task (detecting a repeated stimulus) with letter and with false-font stimuli. Children completed the scan twice, with the at-risk group completing an intervention between scans. At time 1, the on-track readers engaged several bilateral regions more for letters than for false fonts including the reading network: inferior frontal, temporal, lateral and medial parietal regions. At time 2, activation was more similar between groups and the at-risk group showed greater activation in many of these same areas. These findings highlight the plasticity of the reading network. The authors also note another source that may help us understand early risk for reading problems: The children in the at-risk group moved significantly more in the scanner, which may indicate less developed self-regulation and attention skills.

One study obtained fMRI in addition to ERP measures in the same Swiss-German children in kindergarten and then followed them to Grade 2 to determine whether brain measures improved prediction of dyslexia over behavioral measures (Bach et al., 2013). During EEG and MRI, children completed a word and false-font reading/judgment task. In multiple regression analyses, pre-reading behavioral measures accounted for 51 percent of variance in Grade 2 reading scores. Adding a measure of ERP N170 response to words/false fonts significantly improved prediction, reaching 67 percent of variance. Further, adding MRI measures of word/false-font processing in the left fusiform gyrus/ visual word form region improved prediction still more, reaching 84 percent of variance explained.

Together, these studies point to differences in a variety of regions that are involved in reading that are already present before children learn to read, and which may predict later reading. Most of these studies have relatively small participant samples, and larger samples might allow more precise analyses to determine which measures best differentiate between children who will develop dyslexia versus typical reading skills. Furthermore, developmental trajectories are rarely examined, despite the value of such trajectories in providing insights into the etiology of dyslexia and its neural correlates over time. Continuing advances in technology that make MRI scanning more child-friendly, such as shorter acquisition time and better methods to prevent and correct for motion artifacts (e.g., Tisdall et al., 2012) will also make this process easier.

12.5   Discussion and Conclusion

12.5.1   Neural Predictors of Dyslexia Revisited

Though there has been much progress in finding measures that relate to later reading, the differences in neural predictors of dyslexia reported across studies are perhaps greater than the similarities. Even within languages and experimental methods, differences at infancy between groups with family history of dyslexia vary substantially. There are several factors that may explain these differences. One source of variance is differences in diagnosis across studies. There are no universal standard criteria for dyslexia, and identification of individuals as having dyslexia or not (whether parents of infants being studied, or children being studied once they enter school) varies within and between languages. It is also difficult to estimate the effects of differences in other behavioral pre-reading abilities (e.g., phonological awareness, RAN) that exist between many of the groups compared in these studies. Because reading is a complex behavior, it is also unlikely that a single biomarker or predictor would account for all the proposed deficits in dyslexia.

We also know very little about children without family history of dyslexia who go on to develop dyslexia, because in most longitudinal studies focused on family history of dyslexia, there are usually too few of these children to study. Furthermore, children who have a strong genetic risk but subsequently develop average or above-average reading skills are often ignored, but data on these children may be able to provide important insights into protective or compensatory mechanisms in the brain.

Another reason that studies may not find the same reliable predictors is a lack of statistical power. Most studies have somewhat small sample sizes; none of the studies reported here include more than 200 children, and most are closer to 40 total children. Small sample sizes can lead to overfitting of models, such that they are not generalizable to other groups. Neuroimaging data is very rich, with data from many sites (EEG or MEG sensors or MRI voxels) over many time points, and some findings may be spurious due to a failure to control for multiple statistical comparisons (Button et al., 2013).

To date, most imaging studies have examined averages for a group of individuals because there is so much individual variation and noise in the data. If we are to be able to use imaging to aid in diagnosis or classification of individuals as at risk of dyslexia, it is crucial that we find measures that are robust (not sensitive to noise or variance within the individual) (Poldrack et al., 2017) and that are strongly related to our constructs of interest, dyslexia and reading outcomes. Further, the hardware, software, and procedures used to acquire and analyze data vary widely and can strongly impact results.

12.5.2   Clinical Implications

Predicting which children will develop dyslexia before they have learned to read is still a challenge in all languages. Despite the current lack of well-validated early predictors, it is possible to consider how a brain-based reading screening would be implemented. Giving every infant or child an MRI scan seems impractical and cost-prohibitive (several hundred dollars per child, plus time for travel and scanning). However, if reliable markers are identified, a potential solution would be to employ a more intensive screening strategy for children who have other risk factors, such as a family history of dyslexia. Behavioral studies find that this type of "tiered" approach is effective in identifying and providing intervention earlier (e.g., Catts et al., 2015).

Whereas brain measures seem to be inconsistent in their accuracy for predicting future reading level among children at risk of dyslexia, this may be because there is no single universal predictor across individuals or languages. Both from the research presented here and other literature, the heterogeneity in dyslexia and its brain basis is evident. Even individuals who have the same diagnosis of dyslexia based on the same criteria can have very different patterns of abilities. Thus, it seems unlikely that all individuals with dyslexia share a single core deficit. Understanding what abilities and measures predict dyslexia will go hand in hand with a more nuanced understanding of the etiology (or etiologies) of dyslexia. Multiple-deficit models that allow for different core deficits may lead to more nuanced understanding of dyslexia and prediction of later reading abilities.

12.6   Conclusion

A major hurdle in our ability to diagnose and intervene early and effectively is that the core etiologies of dyslexia, and whether they differ across languages, have not yet been determined. As we come to determine how behavioral and neural predictors relate to dyslexia within orthographies, we can begin to learn more about how predictors differ across orthographies. The goal of understanding the neurobiological cause(s) of dyslexia will be mutually informative with the search for methods to identify children with dyslexia earlier and provide effective intervention in direct response to early identification.

Acknowledgments

This work was supported by National Institutes of Health–National Institute of Child Health and Human Development (Grant #R01 HD067312) to NG and JG. We thank Sean McWeeny for assistance with manuscript preparation.

References

Bach, S., Richardson, U., Brandeis, D., Martin, E., & Brem, S. (2013). Print-specific multimodal brain activation in kindergarten improves prediction of reading skills in second grade. *Neuroimage*, *82*, 605–615.

Bishop, D. V. M. (2007). Using mismatch negativity to study central auditory processing in developmental language and literacy impairments: Where are we, and where should we be going? *Psychological Bulletin*, *133*(4), 651–672.

Boada, R., & Pennington, B. F. (2006). Deficient implicit phonological representations in children with dyslexia. *Journal of Experimental Child Psychology*, *95*(3), 153–193.

Boets, B., Op de Beeck, H. P., Vandermosten, M., et al. (2013). Intact but less accessible phonetic representations in adults with dyslexia. *Science*, *342*, 1251–1254.

Bowyer-Crane, C., Snowling, M. J., Duff, F. J. et al. (2008). Improving early language and literacy skills: Differential effects of an oral language versus a phonology with reading intervention. *Journal of Child Psychology and Psychiatry*, *49*(4), 422–432.

Button, K. S., Ioannidis, J. P., Mokrysz, C. et al. (2013). Power failure: Why small sample size undermines the reliability of neuroscience. *Nature Reviews Neuroscience*, *14*(5), 365–376.

Caravolas, M. (2005). The nature and causes of dyslexia in different languages. In M. J. Snowling & C. Hulme (Eds.), *The science of reading: A handbook* (pp. 336–355). Malden, MA: Blackwell Publishing.

Caravolas, M., Lervåg, A., Defior, S., Málková, G. S., & Hulme, C. (2013). Different patterns, but equivalent predictors, of growth in reading in consistent and inconsistent orthographies. *Psychological Science*, *24*(8), 1398–1407.

Catts, H. W., Fey, M. E., Zhang, X., & Tomblin, J. B. (2001). Estimating the risk of future reading difficulties in kindergarten children: a research-based model and its clinical implementation. *Language, Speech, and Hearing Services in Schools*, *32*(1), 38–50.

Catts, H. W., Nielsen, D. C., Bridges, M. S., Liu, Y. S., & Bontempo, D. E. (2015). Early identification of reading disabilities within an RTI framework. *Journal of Learning Disabilities*, *48*(3), 281–297.

Clark, K. A., Helland, T., Specht, K. et al. (2014). Neuroanatomical precursors of dyslexia identified from pre-reading through to age 11. *Brain*, *137*(12), 3136–3141.

Elbro, C., Borstrom, I., & Petersen, D. K. (1998). Predicting dyslexia from kindergarten: The importance of distinctness of phonological representations of lexical items. *Reading Research Quarterly*, *33*, 36–60.

Gabrieli, J. D., Ghosh, S. S., & Whitfield-Gabrieli, S. (2015). Prediction as a humanitarian and pragmatic contribution from human cognitive neuroscience. *Neuron*, *85*(1), 11–26.

Goswami, U., Thomson, J., Richardson, U. et al. (2002). Amplitude envelope onsets and developmental dyslexia: A new hypothesis. *Proceedings of the National Academy of Sciences*, *99*(16), 10911–10916.

Guttorm, T. K., Leppänen, P. H., Hämäläinen, J. A., Eklund, K. M., & Lyytinen, H. J. (2010). Newborn event-related potentials predict poorer pre-reading skills in children at risk for dyslexia. *Journal of Learning Disabilities*, *43*(5), 391–401.

Guttorm, T. K., Leppänen, P. H., Poikkeus, A. M. et al. (2005). Brain event-related potentials (ERPs) measured at birth predict later language development in children with and without familial risk for dyslexia. *Cortex*, *41*(3), 291–303.

Guttorm, T. K., Leppänen, P. H., Richardson, U., & Lyytinen, H. (2001). Event-related potentials and consonant differentiation in newborns with familial risk for dyslexia. *Journal of Learning Disabilities*, *34*(6), 534–544.

Guttorm, T. K., Leppänen, P. H. T., Tolvanen, A., & Lyytinen, H. (2003). Event-related potentials in newborns with and without familial risk for dyslexia: Principal component analysis reveals differences between the groups. *Journal of Neural Transmission*, *110*, 1059–1074.

Hämäläinen, J. A., Guttorm, T. K., Richardson, U. et al. (2013). Auditory event-related potentials measured in kindergarten predict later reading problems at school age. *Developmental Neuropsychology*, *38*(8), 550–566.

Hämäläinen, J. A., Lohvansuu, K., Ervast, L., & Leppänen, P. H. (2015). Event-related potentials to tones show differences between children with multiple risk factors for dyslexia and control children before the onset of formal reading instruction. *International Journal of Psychophysiology*, *95*(2), 101–112.

Halliday, L. F., Barry, J. G., Hardiman, M. J., & Bishop, D. V. (2014). Late, not early mismatch responses to changes in frequency are reduced or deviant in children with dyslexia: an event-related potential study. *Journal of Neurodevelopmental Disorders*, *6*(21).

Hensler, B. S., Schatschneider, C., Taylor, J., & Wagner, R. K. (2010). Behavioral genetic approach to the study of dyslexia. *Journal of Developmental and Behavioral Pediatrics*, *31*(7), 525–32.

Huettel, S. A., Song, A. W., & McCarthy, G. (2009). *Functional magnetic resonance imaging*. Sunderland, MA: Sinauer Associates.

Humphrey, N., & Mullins, P. M. (2002). Self-concept and self-esteem in developmental dyslexia. *Journal of Research in Special Educational Needs*, *2*, 1–13.

Im, K., Raschle, N. M., Smith, S. A., Grant, P. E., & Gaab, N. (2015). Atypical sulcal pattern in children with developmental dyslexia and at-risk kindergarteners. *Cerebral Cortex*, *26*(3), 1138–1148.

Kraemer, H. C., Schultz, S. K., & Arndt, S. (2002). Biomarkers in psychiatry: methodological issues. *The American Journal of Geriatric Psychiatry*, *10*(6), 653–659.

Kraft, I., Cafiero, R., Schaadt, G. et al. (2015). Cortical differences in preliterate children at familiar risk of dyslexia are similar to those observed in dyslexic readers. *Brain*, *138*(9), e378-e378.

Kraft, I., Schreiber, J., Cafiero, R. et al. (2016). Predicting early signs of dyslexia at a preliterate age by combining behavioral assessment with structural MRI. *NeuroImage, 143*, 378–386.

Landerl, K., & Wimmer, H. (2008). Development of word reading fluency and spelling in a consistent orthography: An 8-year follow-up. *Journal of Educational Psychology, 100*(1), 150–161.

Langer, N., Peysakhovich, B., Zuk, J. et al. (2017). White matter alterations in infants at risk for developmental dyslexia. *Cerebral Cortex, 27*(2), 1027–1036.

Leppänen, P. H. T., Hämäläinen, J. A., & Guttorm, T. K. et al. (2012). Infant brain responses associated with reading-related skills before school and at school age. *Clinical Neurophysiology, 42*, 35–41.

Leppänen, P. H., Hämäläinen, J. A., & Salminen, H. K. et al. (2010). Newborn brain event-related potentials revealing atypical processing of sound frequency and the subsequent association with later literacy skills in children with familial dyslexia. *Cortex, 46*(10), 1362–1376.

Leppänen, P. H., Pihko, E., Eklund, K. M., & Lyytinen, H. (1999). Cortical responses of infants with and without a genetic risk for dyslexia: II. Group effects. *NeuroReport, 10*(5), 969–973.

Leppänen, P. H. T., Richardson, U., & Pihko, E. (2002). Brain responses to changes in speech sound durations differ between infants with and without familial risk for dyslexia. *Developmental Neuropsychology, 22*(1), 407–422.

Lovio, B. R., Näätänen, R., & Kujala, T. (2010). Abnormal pattern of cortical speech feature discrimination in 6-year-old children at risk for dyslexia. *Brain Research, 1335*, 53–62.

Luck, S. J. (2014). *An introduction to the event-related potential technique* (2nd ed.). Cambridge, MA: MIT Press.

Lyon, G. R., Shaywitz, S. E., & Shaywitz, B. A. (2003). A definition of dyslexia. *Annals of Dyslexia, 53*(1), 1–14.

Maurer, U., Bucher, K., & Brem, S. et al. (2009). Neurophysiology in preschool improves behavioral prediction of reading ability throughout primary school. *Biological Psychiatry, 66*, 341–348.

Maurer, U., Bucher, K., Brem, S., & Brandeis, D. (2003). Altered responses to tone and phoneme mismatch in kindergartners at familial dyslexia risk. *Neuroreport, 14*(17), 2245–2250.

McBride-Chang, C., Lam, F., & Lam, C. et al. (2011). Early predictors of dyslexia in Chinese children: Familial history of dyslexia, language delay, and cognitive profiles. *Journal of Child Psychology and Psychiatry, 52*(2), 204–211.

Molfese, D. (2000). Predicting dyslexia at 8 years of age using neonatal brain responses. *Brain and Language, 72*, 238–245.

Molfese, V. J., Molfese, D. L., & Modgline, A. A. (2001). Newborn and preschool predictors of second-grade reading scores: An evaluation of categorical and continuous scores. *Journal of Learning Disabilities, 34*(6), 545–554.

Moll, K., Ramus, F., & Bartling, J. et al. (2014). Cognitive mechanisms underlying reading and spelling development in five European orthographies. *Learning and Instruction, 29*, 65–77.

Moore, J. K., & Linthicum, F. H. (2009). The human auditory system: A timeline of development. *International Journal of Audiology, 46*(9), 460–478.

Myers, C. A., Vandermosten, M., Farris, E. A. et al. (2014). Structural changes in white matter are uniquely related to children's reading development. *Psychological Science, 25*(10), 1870–1883.

Näätänen, R. (2001). The perception of speech sounds by the human brain as reflected by the mismatch negativity (MMN) and its magnetic equivalent (MMNm). *Psychophysiology, 38*(1), 1–21.

Näätänen, R., Kujala, T., & Escera, C. et al. (2012). The mismatch negativity (MMN): A unique window to disturbed central auditory processing in ageing and different clinical conditions. *Clinical Neurophysiology, 123*(3), 424–458.

Noordenbos, M. W., Segers, E., Serniclaes, W., Mitterer, H., & Verhoeven, L. (2012). Neural evidence of allophonic perception in children at risk for dyslexia. *Neuropsychologia, 50*(8), 2010–2017.

Norton, E. S., Beach, S. D., & Gabrieli, J. D. E. (2015). Neurobiology of dyslexia. *Current Opinion in Neurobiology, 30*, 73–78.

Norton, E. S., Black, J. M., Stanley, L. M., Tanaka, H., Gabrieli, J. D. E., Sawyer, C., & Hoeft, F. (2014). Functional neuroanatomical evidence for the double-deficit hypothesis of developmental dyslexia. *Neuropsychologia, 61*, 235–246.

O'Connor, R. E., & Jenkins, J. R. (1999). Prediction of reading disabilities in kindergarten and first grade. *Scientific Studies of Reading, 3*, 159–197.

Odegard, T. N., Farris, E. A., Ring, J., McColl, R., & Black, J. (2009). Brain connectivity in non-reading impaired children and children diagnosed with developmental dyslexia. *Neuropsychologia, 47*(8), 1972–1977.

Ozernov-Palchik, O., & Gaab, N. (2016). Tackling the 'dyslexia paradox': reading brain and behavior for early markers of developmental dyslexia. *WIREs Cognitive Science, 7*: 156–176.

Ozernov-Palchik, O., Norton, E. S., Sideridis, G., Beach, S. D., Gabrieli, J. D. E., & Gaab, N. (2017). Early-reading profiles of children at kindergarten and longitudinally: Implications for early screening and theories of reading. *Developmental Science, 20*(5).

Pennington, B. F., & Lefly, D. L. (2001). Early reading development in children at family risk for dyslexia. *Child Development, 72*(3), 816–833.

Pennington, B. F., Santerre-Lemmon, L., Rosenberg, J. et al. (2012). Individual prediction of dyslexia by single vs. multiple deficit models. *Journal of Abnormal Psychology, 121*(1), 212–224.

Perlman, S. B. (2012). Neuroimaging in child clinical populations: Considerations for a successful research program. *Journal of the American Academy of Child & Adolescent Psychiatry, 51*(12), 1232–1235.

Peterson, R. L., & Pennington, B. F. (2015). Developmental dyslexia. *Annual Review of Clinical Psychology, 11*, 283–307.

Pihko, E., Leppänen, P. H., Eklund, K. M. et al. (1999). Cortical responses of infants with and without a genetic risk for dyslexia: I. Age effects. *Neuroreport, 10*(5), 901–5.

Plakas, A., van Zuijen, T., van Leeuwen, T., Thomson, J. M., & van der Leij, A. (2013). Impaired non-speech auditory processing at a pre-reading age is a risk-factor for dyslexia but not a predictor: an ERP study. *Cortex, 49*(4), 1034–1045.

Poldrack, R. A., Baker, C. I., Durnez, J. et al. (2017). Scanning the horizon: towards transparent and reproducible neuroimaging research. *Nature Reviews Neuroscience, 18*(2), 115–126.

Puolakanaho, A., Ahonen, T., Aro, M. et al. (2007). Very early phonological and language skills: Estimating individual risk of reading disability. *Journal of Child Psychology and Psychiatry, and Allied Disciplines*, *48*(9), 923–931.

Ramus, F., & Szenkovits, G. (2008). What phonological deficit? *Quarterly Journal of Experimental Psychology*, *61*(1), 129–141.

Raschle, N. M., Chang, M., & Gaab, N. (2011). Structural brain alterations associated with dyslexia predate reading onset. *NeuroImage*, *57*, 742–749.

Raschle, N., Lee, M., Buechler, R. et al. (2009). Making MR imaging child's play: Pediatric neuroimaging protocol, guidelines, and procedure. *Journal of Visualized Experiments*, *29*. www.jove.com/index/Details.stp?ID=1309

Raschle, N. M., Zuk, J.,& Gaab, N. (2012). Functional characteristics of developmental dyslexia in left-hemispheric posterior brain regions predate reading onset. *Proceedings of the National Academy of Sciences of the United States of America*, *109*, 2156–2161.

Raschle, N., Zuk, J., Ortiz-Manilla, S. et al. (2012). Pediatric neuroimaging in early childhood and infancy: Challenges and practical guidelines. *Annals of the New York Academy of Sciences*, *1252*, 43–50.

Reuter, M., Tisdall, D., Qureshi, A. et al. (2015). Head motion during MRI acquisition reduces gray matter volume and thickness estimates. *NeuroImage*, *107*, 107–115.

Richlan, F., Kronbichler, M., & Wimmer, H. (2013). Structural abnormalities in the dyslexic brain: A meta-analysis of voxel-based morphometry studies. *Human Brain Mapping*, *34*(11), 3055–3065.

Saygin, Z. M., Norton, E. S., Osher, D. et al. (2013). Tracking the roots of reading ability: White matter volume and integrity correlate with phonological awareness in pre- and early-reading kindergarten children. *The Journal of Neuroscience*, *33*(33), 13251–13258.

Schatschneider, C., Fletcher, J. M., Francis, D. J., Carlson, C. D., & Foorman, B. R. (2004). Kindergarten prediction of reading skills: A longitudinal comparative analysis. *Journal of Educational Psychology*, *96*(2), 265–282.

Schatschneider, C., & Torgesen, J. (2004). Using our current understanding of dyslexia to support early identification and intervention. *Journal of Child Neurology*, *19*(10), 759–765.

Serniclaes, W., van Heghe, S., Mousty, P., Carre, R. & Sprenger-Charolles, L. (2004). Allophonic mode of speech perception in dyslexia. *Journal of Experimental Child Psychology*, *87*, 336–361.

Skeide, M. A., Kraft, I., Müller, B. et al. (2016). NRSN1 associated grey matter volume of the visual word form area reveals dyslexia before school. *Brain*, *139*(10), 2792–2803.

Snowling, M. J. (2013). Early identification and interventions for dyslexia: A contemporary view. *Journal of Research in Special Educational Needs*, *13* (1), 7–14.

Snowling, M. J., & Melby-Lervåg, M. (2016). Oral language deficits in familial dyslexia: A meta-analysis and review. *Psychological Bulletin*, *142*(5), 498–545.

Soares, J. M., Marques, P., Alves, V., & Sousa, N. (2013). A hitchhiker's guide to diffusion tensor imaging. *Frontiers in Neuroscience*, *7*, 31.

Tisdall, M. D., Hess, A. T., Reuter, M., et al. (2012). Volumetric navigators for prospective motion correction and selective reacquisition in neuroanatomical MRI. *Magnetic Resonance in Medicine*, *68*(2), 389–399.

Torgesen, J. K. (2004). Avoiding the devastating downward spiral: the evidence that early intervention prevents reading failure. *American Educator, 28,* 6–19.

Torkildsen, J.von K., Syversen, G., Simonsen, H. et al. (2007). Brain responses to lexical-semantic priming in children at-risk for dyslexia. *Brain and Language, 102,* 243–261.

Vanderauwera, J., Wouters, J., Vandermosten, M., & Ghesquière, P. (2017). Early dynamics of white matter deficits in children developing dyslexia. *Developmental Cognitive Neuroscience, 27,* 69–77.

Vandermosten, M., Hoeft, F., & Norton, E. S. (2016). Integrating MRI brain imaging studies of pre-reading children with current theories of developmental dyslexia: A review and quantitative meta-analysis. *Current Opinion in Behavioral Science, 10,* 155–161.

Vandermosten, M., Vanderauwera, J., Theys, C. et al. (2015). A DTI tractography study in pre-readers at risk for dyslexia. *Developmental Cognitive Neuroscience, 14,* 8–15.

van Herten, M., Pasman, J., van Leeuwen, T. H. et al. (2008). Differences in AERP responses and atypical hemispheric specialization in 17-month-old children at risk of dyslexia. *Brain Research, 1201,* 100–105.

van Leeuwen, T., Been, P., & Kuijpers, C. et al. (2006). Mismatch response is absent in 2-month-old infants at risk for dyslexia. *Neuroreport, 17*(4), 351–355.

van Leeuwen, T., Been, P., van Herten, M. et al. (2007). Cortical categorization failure in 2-month-old infants at risk for dyslexia. *Neuroreport, 18*(9), 857–861.

van Leeuwen, T., Been, P., van Herten, M. et al. (2008). Two-month-old infants at risk for dyslexia do not discriminate/bAk/from/dAk: A brain-mapping study. *Journal of Neurolinguistics, 21*(4), 333–348.

van Zuijen, T. L., Plakas, A., Maassen, B. A. M., Maurits, N. M., & van der Leij, A. (2013). Infant ERPs separate children at risk of dyslexia who become good readers from those who become poor readers. *Developmental Science, 16,* 554–563.

Vellutino, F. R., Scanlon, D. M., & Tanzman, M. S. (1998). The case for early intervention in diagnosing specific reading disability. *Journal of School Psychology, 36*(4), 367–397.

Wang, Y., Mauer, M. V., & Raney, T. et al. (2017). Development of tract-specific white matter pathways during early reading development in at-risk children and typical controls. *Cerebral Cortex., 27*(4), 2469–2485.

Williams, V. J., Juranek, J., Cirino, P., & Fletcher, J. M. (2018). Cortical thickness and local gyrification in children with developmental dyslexia. *Cerebral Cortex., 28*(3), 963–973

Wolf, M., & Bowers, P. G. (1999). The double-deficit hypothesis for the developmental dyslexias. *Journal of Educational Psychology, 91*(3), 415.

Yamada, Y., Stevens, C., Dow, M. et al. (2011). Emergence of the neural network for reading in five-year-old beginning readers of different levels of pre-literacy abilities: an fMRI study. *Neuroimage, 57*(3), 704–713.

13 Neurocognitive Markers of Developmental Dyslexia

Lan Shuai, Stephen J. Frost, Nicole Landi, W. Einar Mencl, and Kenneth Pugh

13.1 Introduction

In the history of human evolution, reading and writing skills were developed about 5,400 years ago (Dehaene, 2009), which is fairly late in the context of the 350,000–150,000 years of history of human speech (Perreault & Mathew, 2012). In terms of ontogeny, the acquisition of reading also follows that of speech over the course of the child's early years. Nonetheless, reading has become one of the most important cognitive functions for daily life and reading difficulties can severely limit an individual's ability to thrive in the modern world (Calfee, 1982; Rawson, 1978). Across languages and cultures, approximately 5–20 percent of the population (depending on definitional criteria) is affected by developmental dyslexia (DD), a specific reading impairment presents in the absence of other cognitive impairments (S. E. Shaywitz & Shaywitz, 2003). Neuroimaging studies from the past two decades have shown that DD is a brain-based disorder, usually associated with phonological processing deficits and corresponding anomalies in phonological circuits in the brain, which give rise to difficulties in decoding. Given that basic speech and visual processing appear essentially normal for most dyslexics, it is of interest to explore how this anomaly (at the level of brain and behavior) develops. In this chapter, we discuss recent neurocognitive findings concerning typical and atypical reading development that help to shed light on this condition, and we do so, wherever possible, with a cross-language focus to address the question of whether the mechanisms involved in DD are language-universal.

In the past decades, there have been significant advances in reading research and theory, mostly with alphabetic languages. Existing cognitive and neural models are largely based on data from English-speaking populations and cross-linguistic differences are largely interpreted as reflecting the transparency in the mappings between written and spoken forms (typically referred to as orthographic depth; R. Frost, Katz, & Bentin, 1987). How these differences might impact typical and atypical reading development has only recently becoming a prominent research topic (Landerl et al., 2013; Moll, 2014; Ziegler et al., 2010). However, across cultures and continents, there exists many languages and types of writing systems, including alphabets, syllabaries, and logographic systems, all of which vary in the level and systematicity of the mappings between orthography and phonology, as well as the mappings between orthography and meaning. Within these writing systems, the first two types can be viewed as coding systems of sounds at either phoneme or syllable level, whereas logographic writing systems may provide a greater weighting toward the mapping from orthography to whole-word phonology and semantics. For this reason, studying logographic languages such as Chinese as well as alphabetic languages that differ in orthographic depth (R. Frost, 2012) may provide a more comprehensive picture on how we process written language in general and allow us to address the questions of whether there are universals in learning to become a fluent reader and whether the neurocognitive foundation of dyslexia is similar or different across vastly different writing systems (W. S. Wang & Tsai, 2011).

At the time of writing, there is increasing support for a language-universal cognitive model (and underlying neural mechanisms) of skilled reading (R. Frost, 2012), with minor differences depending on whether the spelling-to-sound mappings are transparent or opaque (Richlan, 2014), but this model is certainly not accepted by all researchers (Siok et al., 2008; Siok et al., 2004). Moreover, there remains a rather contentious debate on whether reading mechanisms in logographic languages such as Chinese deviate from the general models developed for alphabetic languages, and all of this has an impact on how we think about the neural basis of DD (Hu et al., 2010; Nakamura et al., 2012). In this chapter, we will review cognitive and neuroimaging studies of alphabetic languages and will also address the controversial issues regarding Chinese. In the following sections, Section 13.2 will discuss the cognitive accounts of reading and reading difficulties by summarizing the multifaceted cognitive functions and predictors of reading abilities across languages. Starting from a general neural model of reading and reading difficulties (Pugh, Mencl, Jenner et al., 2000) in Section 13.3 we will discuss the related brain regions in detail, by comparing studies of opaque and transparent alphabetic orthographies, as well as logographic languages such as Chinese. Section 13.4 will provide an update on recent developments that utilize new techniques for studying skilled and impaired reading, and some of the remaining issues in the field. Finally, Section 13.5 will summarize our views on the mechanisms of reading difficulty across languages and point out future directions for research.

13.2   Theoretical Background

Behavioral studies have characterized the cognitive processes necessary to acquire skilled reading, and how these processes are usually compromised in DD individuals (Fletcher et al., 1994). For most struggling readers, a core difficulty manifests itself as a deficiency within the language system, specifically at the level of phonological processing. To learn to read in alphabetic orthographies, a child must develop an understanding of the segmental nature of speech and come to realize that spoken words are composed of the smallest of these segments, phonemes. This appreciation of the segmental nature of speech is termed *phonemic awareness*. It is phonemic awareness and the metalinguistic understanding that the constituents of a printed word – its letters – bear a relationship to phonemes that allows the beginning reader to connect printed words to the corresponding words in his/her speech lexicon (Griffith & Olson, 1992; Kamii & Manning, 2002).

There is strong evidence that phonemic awareness is a source of difficulty in emergent DD readers, who will have difficulty developing efficient routines for mapping alphabetic characters onto the phonetic constituents they represent (Brady & Shankweiler, 1991; Bruck, 1992; Fletcher et al., 1994; Rieben & Perfetti, 1991; Shankweiler et al., 1995). Although the underlying neurocognitive causes of these deficits are not fully understood (Pugh et al., 2013; Scarborough, 1998), there is some support for the notion that at least part of the difficulty resides in the phonological component of a larger specialization for spoken language (A. M. Liberman, 1996; I. Y. Liberman, Shankweiler, & Liberman, 1989). If that component is fuzzy or less then ideally specified the perception of phonemes may be less than ideally distinctive (Ziegler & Goswami, 2005). For children with adequate phonological processing and representations, word identification in reading quickly becomes fluent and automated; skilled readers can access the lexicon for printed words exceedingly fast. Although the struggle with various aspects of phonological processing (including phonemic awareness, phonological working memory, and rapid naming) appears to be common for DD children across alphabetic languages (Caravolas et al., 2012; Caravolas, Volín, & Hulme, 2005), there is debate on the specific role of phonemic awareness and whether it is more essential for opaque orthographies like English, than for more transparent orthographies such as German or Finnish where speed of retrieval measured by rapid naming tasks appears to be more predictive (Lyytinen et al., 2004; Wimmer, Mayringer, & Landerl, 2000). However, this issue remains unresolved, and one recent large-scale study of emergent readers in regular (Spanish, Czech) vs. irregular (English) orthographies has argued that phonological awareness contributes similarly to outcomes across these contrastive languages (Caravolas et al., 2013). In any event, the notion that phonological processing is affected in DD is not controversial (Ramus, 2003).

Research on non-alphabetic languages like Chinese suggests that phonological deficits also appear to play a significant role in DD in these languages (e.g., Shu et al., 2005) but there are contrasting views (see Ho et al., 2007). Some findings in Chinese suggest a heightened role of *morphological* awareness in learning to read Chinese (McBride-Chang et al., 2005; McBride-Chang et al., 2003; Shu et al., 2006), and although this still reflects phonological competence to a large extent in our view, the findings may also reflect a heightened importance of semantic organization as a constraint on efficient lexical access in this writing system (Verhoeven & Perfetti, 2003). Moving toward causal accounts of DD, we must systematically examine the role of phonological processing skills and how deficits therein modulate reading similarly or differently in contrastive languages. As discussed below, neurobiological evidence is relevant to this issue.

Beyond the role of phonological deficits in the initial stages of learning to read, in all languages learning to read words fluently and automatically requires that orthographic, phonological, and semantic component processes become well integrated. Current theories differ mainly in how these components are organized, both within languages (in good and poor readers) and across languages that vary in orthographic depth. According to the orthographic-depth hypothesis (Katz & Frost, 1992), word reading in a transparent orthography should differ from an opaque orthography in the relative weighting of different component processes. Thus, in transparent languages (e.g., Spanish) the orthography-to-phonology mapping provides reliable information about word pronunciations; thus, the O–P pathway should play a heightened role, in comparison to irregular/opaque orthographies (e.g., English), in which readers should tend to rely more on direct mapping from orthography to semantics and then obtain word pronunciations via a lexical lookup procedure. Another hypothesis, predicated on the orthographic depth framework that also addresses variation in the weighting of component process across languages, is the psycholinguistic grain-size theory (Ziegler & Goswami, 2005). This hypothesis emphasizes variation in the consistency with which phonology is represented at the phoneme, body, syllable level, the grain size at which there is a match between orthographic and phonological units, and their impact on developmental differences in the grain size of lexical representations. This theory not only summarizes the phenomenon in skilled readers (readers of more opaque orthographies will rely on larger units) but also yields predictions concerning behavioral performance of DD across languages. For example, Ziegler and colleagues point out that there should be common indices for dyslexia across languages with different manifestations caused by varieties of orthographic depth, but that dyslexia would not become less prominent even in languages relying on larger units. Although the grain size is emphasized here, the sound–print correspondence is still the most important factor in comparing different orthographies, no matter whether the correspondence is at the phoneme or syllable level. For example, phonological deficits are hypothesized to present similarly in developmental dyslexics regardless of whether individuals are readers of Japanese Kana or an alphabetic orthography such as Spanish, even though Kana is a syllabary writing system (Ziegler & Goswami, 2005).

Both the orthographic-depth hypothesis and the psycholinguistic grain-size theory mainly discuss how differences in the regularity of spelling-to-sound mappings impact reading in contrastive alphabetic orthographies, ranging from transparent ones like Spanish to opaque ones like English. However, a full account also requires that we understand cross-language differences in mechanisms associated with semantic access from print as we move toward non-alphabetic reading systems. Thus, neither hypothesis provides clear guidance in how to consider the role of the semantic radicals in reading Chinese; some of these radicals actually have no corresponding pronunciation in this opaque writing system and yet they are functional in word reading. As recently pointed out by R. Frost (2012), "the actual computation of an orthographic code in a given language is determined online by the transparency of mapping of graphemes into phonemes, on the one hand, and by morphological and semantic considerations on the other hand, given the language properties in which reading occurs" (p. 277).

In summary, individual differences in both phonological awareness and naming speed (rapid naming) are predictive of reading outcomes in emergent learners (Caravolas, 2005; Goswami, Ziegler, & Richardson, 2005; Landerl et al., 2013; Mann & Wimmer, 2002; Moll et al., 2014; Ziegler et al., 2010). As noted above, in Chinese, although phonological awareness and naming speed are also important predictors (Newman et al., 2011; Shu, Anderson, & Wu, 2000; Shu, Peng, & McBride-Chang, 2008; Tan, Hoosain, & Peng, 1995; N. N. Wu, Zhou, & Shu, 1999; Zhou & Marslen-Wilson, 1999, 2000), some research suggests a heightened role of morphological awareness as an important factor in learning to read Chinese (McBride-Chang et al., 2005; McBride-Chang et al., 2003; Shu et al., 2006). Ongoing debates in all orthographies continue the focus on developing better accounts of how phonological processing and speed of processing influence reading, and whether additional deficits in sensory-motor processing, temporal processing, or visual attention underpin higher-order phonological deficits in some or most DD children (Bosse, Tainturier, & Valdois, 2007; Goswami et al., 2002; Goswami et al., 2011; Lallier et al., 2009; Tallal, 1984; Viana et al., 2013; Jing Zhao et al., 2014). A great challenge for theory is to develop accounts that identify both invariance in the biology and how variance in writing systems moderates and shapes reading circuits (R. Frost, 2012). New research on the neural bases of reading are relevant here, and we consider this topic next.

13.3   Research Evidence from Neuroimaging Studies

Neuroimaging provides useful tools with which to further explore the extent to which deficits in DD are universal. Multimodal imaging techniques can help to reveal the brain circuits that are more involved in language and reading tasks. Techniques such as functional magnetic resonance imaging (fMRI) provide evidence about regional activation and measures of functional connections between regions, whereas structural MRI provides information about pathways connecting different brain regions (white-matter tracts) using diffusion tensor imaging (DTI), and both cortical thickness and gray-matter volume using voxel-based morphometry (VBM). Additional techniques provide information regarding the temporal dynamics of concurrent neural firing using electroencephalography (EEG) and event-related potential (ERP). Another recent advance in this field is the use of magnetic resonance spectroscopy (MRS) to trace neurochemical alterations that are associated with reading difficulties (Pugh et al., 2014). These techniques address not only cortical structural and functional abnormalities, but also subcortical contributions.

13.3.1   Neural Models of Reading and Reading Disability

One early brain-based model of reading development and reading difficulties was proposed by our group (Pugh, Mencl, Jenner et al., 2000). The model, grounded by extant research on the functional organization of typically developing (TD) vs. DD readers, posits three neural circuits in the left hemisphere that are important for reading. The ventral circuit includes both the middle/inferior temporal gyrus (MTG/ITG) and the posterior fusiform gyrus (FFG) where the putative visual word form area (VWFA; Cohen et al., 2002; Dehaene & Cohen, 2011) is located. The specificity of this posterior FFG or occipito-temporal (OT) region in its response to printed language is late developing in emergent readers and supports fluent-word recognition (B. A. Shaywitz et al., 2004). Greater activation within this region is associated with higher reading skills; activation increases with age and experience (B. A. Shaywitz et al., 2002). The dorsal circuit includes the temporo-parietal (TP) cortex, involving angular and supramarginal gyri (AG and SMG) in the inferior parietal lobule (IPL), and the Wernicke's area in the posterior superior temporal gyrus (pSTG). In contrast to the ventral circuit, activation within the dorsal region increases with complexity of phonological analysis (Pugh et al., 1996) and dorsal regions, particularly the AG, are critical for binding orthographic, phonologic, and lexical semantic information. The anterior circuit sits in and around Broca's area in the left inferior frontal gyrus (LIFG). Posterior aspects of this network are thought to play a role in sequencing of speech articulatory output for reading (Wheat et al., 2010), and activation in this region is sensitive to the spelling-to-sound consistency of word mappings, suggesting a role in phonologically analytic processing (Lee et al., 2004). We proposed that this region works in concert with the dorsal system in shaping reading acquisition and in training up fluent pattern recognition in the posterior OT (Pugh et al., 2013).

With respect to DD, initial studies suggest reduced activation and functional connectivity in DD in both TP and OT systems with somewhat heightened engagement of RH homologues and IFG (Pugh, Mencl, Shaywitz et al., 2000; S. E. Shaywitz et al., 1998), and the model reflects this.

Certain details of the initial model proposed by Pugh, Mencl, Jenner et al. (2000) have been challenged, most recently by Richlan (2012) based on a meta-analysis of TD/DD studies; Richlan stated that the deficit phonological decoding in reading disability is not general in left hemisphere dorsal systems (not seen in pSTG in particular), but at more specific components of left IPL. Following a more detailed segregation based on the meta-analysis of TD/DD differences, Richlan (2014) proposed a new account, which separates the left posterior dorsal TP region into IPL and STG, and the left anterior region into IFG and dorsal precentral gyrus (PreG). In this more fine-grained demarcation, there are five regions with functions distinct from the basic model: the left posterior OT cortex processes both visual-orthographic whole-word and serial grapheme–phoneme conversion; the left IPL is in charge of serial decoding related to attention control; the left STG is only concerned with fine-grained phonological analysis or audiovisual integration; the left IFG accesses phonological output representations, and under-activates in DD; and the left dorsal PreG supports a compensation function relying on articulatory processing in the sublexical phonological decoding route, and over-activates in DD. The more fine-grained taxonomy has potential for disentangling detailed partitions of altered neural regions in DD readers, yet it needs to be tested with more neuroimaging data across languages and compared to other studies aimed at developing more fine-grained accounts (Church et al., 2011). In the following section, we first summarize neuroimaging research pointing to the dependence of reading on reorganization of spoken-language networks (Dehaene et al., 2015), and then discuss the functions of individual brain regions in DD within the framework of our basic model.

13.3.2 Reading and Its Relation to Spoken Language Processing

Generally speaking, the reading network is not a stand-alone system dissociated from speech; instead, it must become well integrated into extant language processing networks in the human brain in order for reading to become fluent (S. J. Frost et al., 2009; Preston et al., 2016; Shankweiler et al., 2008). Print and speech processing share in common a large number of brain regions (Binder, 2009; Binder & Price, 2001; Démonet, Thierry, & Cardebat, 2005; S. J. Frost et al., 2009; Price, 2000; Shankweiler et al., 2008) in a widespread network in the left temporal and frontal lobes (Braze et al., 2011; Shankweiler et al., 2008; Spitsyna et al., 2006), with frequently reported overlap of modalities in STG respectively (mainly Wernicke's area, although studies have also shown overlap in the superior temporal sulcus [STS] and ventral STG; see Cohen et al., 2002; DeWitt & Rauschecker, 2013; IFG, Shankweiler et al., 2008), and with a wider network for print–speech co-activation extending to IPL and OT (Démonet, Taylor, & Chaix, 2004; Yoncheva et al., 2010).

Importantly, several studies from our lab have recently reported that individual differences in reading skill (in English) are directly associated with degree of print–speech convergence; we observed this in both emergent readers (S. J. Frost et al., 2009; Preston et al., 2016) and in older readers with varying degrees of reading comprehension skills (Shankweiler et al., 2008). In S. J. Frost et al. (2009), individual differences in phonological awareness were positively correlated with the relative degree of print–speech overlap/convergence in the left STG and OT regions in beginning readers at age 7; thus, the better the phonological skills and reading readiness the more print and speech tokens activated common tissue in the LH cortex. In a recent follow-up outcome study at age 9 (Preston et al., 2016) we found that print–speech convergence across all major components of the LH reading circuit predicted reading outcomes two years later (indeed, convergence at age 7, and not overall activation levels for print or speech, was the significant predictor). In a similar study by another lab, McNorgan, Randazzo-Wagner, and Booth (2013) also found a strong correlation between phonological awareness and activation in posterior STS and FFG during a visual-auditory cross-modal task, but only in TD children. No correlation in a unimodal task was found in TD children, and no significant brain–behavior correlation was obtained in either a unimodal or cross-modal task in DD children. The cross-modal integration effect found in TD children and the absence of such an effect in DD children are consistent with the findings of S. J. Frost et al. (2009), while the failure to show a correlation between the auditory unimodal phonological task and the brain activation confirms the requirement of reading experience for phonological skill development (Mann & Wimmer, 2002; Newman et al., 2011). The importance of convergence at the level of print and speech networks can be seen even in adults at the level of reading comprehension. Thus, in another study from our team (Shankweiler et al., 2008) we focused on individual differences in reading comprehension in relation to brain activation for spoken vs. written sentences in young adults with varied comprehension abilities. The key finding was that in LH IFG, a region sensitive to sentential complexity for print and speech, the greater the convergence (integration) in an individual's activation patterns for print and speech the higher their reading comprehension scores.

In general, all these studies reveal that fluent reading depends upon leveraging speech and language tissue in processing written forms. Thus, it is unsurprising that early phonological skills create the necessary conditions for this major reorganization of language cortex for print, and together these studies reinforce the notion that skilled reading, in English at least, is parasitic on speech (see Dehaene et al., 2015, for similar arguments). Proficient reading depends on the ability to, at the neural level, process print and speech tokens in common networks that in preliterate individuals serve only speech (Castro-Caldas et al., 1999). Given this, we must ask whether print–speech convergence would be expected to vary in any important ways across orthographies depending on factors like orthographic depth. An initial study from our group examined print-speech convergence in English, Spanish, Hebrew, and Chinese skilled adult readers and found that convergence across the LH reading circuitry was remarkably similar across all four contrastive languages (Rueckl et al., 2015). Clearly, ongoing work on the interdependence of literate language and spoken language (Dehaene et al., 2015) suggests important ways in which early phonological abilities would support the development of fluent reading (S. J. Frost et al., 2009), and further work on developmental aspects of this convergence across languages will be important going forward.

13.3.3   Neural Markers of Developmental Dyslexia

The symptoms of reading difficulties in the DD population emerge early on when children learn to read, and research suggests that some aspects of the functional neuroanatomy of reading disability may change across development. Here, we highlight some neuroimaging studies that map the neural alterations during development, from young readers through adolescence and into early adulthood.

In general, for both children and adults with a reading disability, there are marked functional differences, relative to TD readers, with regard to activity generated in the TP, OT, and IFG systems during reading (Brunswick et al., 1999; Helenius, Uutela, & Hari, 1999; Paulesu et al., 2001; Pugh, Mencl, Shaywitz et al., 2000; Richlan, Kronbichler, & Wimmer, 2009, 2011; Rumsey et al., 1992; Salmelin et al., 1996; B. A. Shaywitz et al., 2002; S. E. Shaywitz et al., 1998; Temple et al., 2003). Specifically, DD readers tend to underactivate the TP and OT systems used by TD readers; and this disruption is also evident as reduced functional connectivity among these regions during reading (Hampson et al., 2006; Horwitz, Rumsey, & Donohue, 1998; Pugh, Mencl, Shaywitz et al., 2000). Instead, DD readers often show evidence of two, apparently compensatory, responses to their LH posterior dysfunction: an increased functional role for RH posterior sites (Pugh et al., 2006; Sarkari et al., 2002; S. E. Shaywitz et al., 1998) and increased bi-hemispheric IFG activation (Brunswick et al., 1999; B. A. Shaywitz et al., 2002; S. E. Shaywitz et al., 1998). The neurophenotype of reduced LH posterior activation and connectivity in DD appears to be stable across a large number of studies to date (see Gabrieli, 2009, for a review). The next major focus must be developmental; when and why do these differences in neural organization emerge in children learning to read and what are the underlying gene-brain-cognitive mechanisms that cause them?

Developmental imaging studies allow us to measure those systems that support reading acquisition and the development of fluent decoding over time. In one developmental fMRI study using a cross-sectional design, we examined changes in the functional organization for reading in large TD and DD cohorts ranging in age from 7 through 17 (B. A. Shaywitz et al., 2002). The primary finding was that as TD readers mature, there is a shift in weighting of the functional neuroanatomy for reading toward a more consolidated "expert" response in the LH OT ventral system. Indeed, when multiple regression analyses examined both age and reading skill (measured by performance on standardized measures of reading skill) the critical predictor was reading-skill level: the higher the reading skill, the stronger the response in the LH OT cortex (with several other areas showing both age- and skill-related reductions). Thus, a beginning reader on a successful trajectory employs a widely distributed cortical system for print processing including TP, frontal, and RH posterior areas. As reading skill increases, LH OT subregions become more critical in fluent recognition of printed (word) stimuli (see Booth et al., 2001; Church et al., 2008; Turkeltaub et al., 2003, for similar arguments).

As we dig more deeply into the earliest stages of learning to read we can gain insights on the neural circuits that support literacy acquisition and how they differ in DD. In one recent study by our team (Pugh et al., 2013) with beginning readers (age 7) we found that behavioral measures of phonological awareness, pseudo-word decoding, and rapid auditory processing jointly reveal a strong positive correlation between neural responses in left TP, OT, IFG, visual cortex, and thalamus in print tasks, with a similar pattern for IFG in speech tasks, together with several other loci in the left and right hemispheres for print or speech tasks respectively. This study indicated that the *learning circuit* for emergent readers reflects tight coupling of LH language with visual regions, but also implicates a strong role for frontal lobe systems, cortical (cingulate; precuneus), and subcortical (pulvinar) attentional control systems in learning to read. At-risk learners showed reduced activation across this entire network.

In another recent study comparing both reading- and age-matched children around 9 and 11 years old respectively, Hoeft et al. (2006) found under-activation in the left TP region, bilateral frontal cortices, and right OT and TP regions in DD children. The separation of phonological and orthographic tasks denotes disrupted left TP region for rhyming task and disrupted occipito-parietal region in the extrastriate cortex for a letter-matching task in DD (Temple et al., 2001). Cao et al. (2006) compared DD children compared to age-matched controls on a rhyme task with similarly spelled (MINT-HINT) and dissimilarly spelled (JAZZ-HAS) pairs. Similar to the results of Hoeft et al. (2006), DD children showed less activation in left IFG,

IPL, and MTG in the TP region, and ITG and FFG in the OT region, but only for dissimilarly spelled rhyme pairs. Reading-group differences were also obtained when comparing activation for similarly and dissimilarly spelled rhyme pairs, with less activation in the left IFG and MFG for DD children. The under-activation of the left IFG for DD children, especially in resolving the mapping between orthographic and phonological forms, is explained as a lack of top-down modulation during reading. The work done by Hoeft et al. (2007), however, found over-activation in the left IFG and MFG, caudate, and thalamus in contrasting DD children with age-matched controls around 14.5 years old, and no over-activation in these regions when comparing DD children with reading-matched controls around 10 years old. In addition, activation in the left parietal and bilateral fusiform cortices was weaker for DD children relative to both reading- and age-matched controls. The dissociation between the consistent hypo-activation in comparison to both control groups and the hyper-activation obtained only when compared to age-matched controls reveals a dyslexic related neural circuit of hypo-activation and a developmental-related neural circuit of hyper-activation. This study found an over-activation in frontal regions when comparing DD and age-matched groups, consistent with the basic model; however, the absence of over-activation in comparison to the reading-matched group provides an alternative explanation to the conventional compensatory hypothesis. The inconsistent patterns of altered neural circuits in Hoeft et al. (2006) and Hoeft et al. (2007) may well represent developmental-related changes, which may also explain the discrepancies between our initial model and Richlan's model given that the data may come from different age groups. More imaging studies on the acquisition of literacy across languages will help address issues of language universals and specificities going forward.

13.3.4   Cross-Language Neuroimaging Studies in Skilled Readers

Next, we consider the status of cross-language neuroimaging studies on skilled reading and reading difficulties. Most of the aforementioned neuroimaging studies were conducted with alphabetic languages, especially English. For the past ten years, findings have been accumulating in Chinese and other non-alphabetic languages. We start with a direct comparison within alphabetic writing systems and between alphabetic and logographic writing systems, and then discuss studies on non-alphabetic languages.

For the comparison of transparent and opaque orthographies in alphabetic writing systems, the classic study from Paulesu and colleagues (2000) compared Italian and English TD speakers' brain activations using positron emission tomography (PET), and discovered largely a similar reading network in the left IFG, PreG, STG, MTG, ITG, FFG, and right STG in the two groups, with greater left posterior Inferior Temporal Gyrus (pITG) and anterior Inferior Frontal Gyrus (aIFG) activation in English speakers during pseudo-word reading and greater left STG activation in Italian speakers during both word and pseudo-word reading. Recent work contrasting alphabetic and non-alphabetic orthographies in skilled readers also suggests a high degree of overlap with some regions playing an enhanced role in Chinese reading and in discriminating DD and TD readers in Chinese, including LH MFG, RH OT, and superior parietal lobule (SPL) (Siok et al., 2008; Siok et al., 2004; Siok et al. 2009). In a comparison between skilled readers of Chinese and French, Nakamura et al. (2012) found the same brain activation patterns for word-shape recognition in the LH OT and writing-sequence recognition in the left dorsal PreG in the two groups in a repetition priming design. There were cross-language-specific activations induced by repetition reduction in priming: French readers showed significant priming effects in the left posterior inferior prefrontal cortex and bilateral posterior parietal cortex, and Chinese readers showed significant priming effects in the bilateral anterior MFG, in addition to common activations in the left posterior IFG and VWFA in both groups. However, no significant cross-language differences were obtained when contrasting the two groups, probably not seen because of the small effective size by repetition priming in general. This work clearly shows the common core brain regions in Chinese and French readers, especially in word shape and gesture-related recognition, but the most important properties of Chinese-character reading, regarding its opaque print–sound matching as well as the transparency of semantic access in comparison to alphabetic languages, still need to be addressed.

The behavioral studies of Chinese have already shown that word morphology is crucial in addition to phonology, which points to a more balanced weighting between semantics and phonology in Chinese reading. Such balanced labor division between semantic and phonological processing in Chinese is shown in Jingjing Zhao et al. (2014) in comparison to the case in English (Sandak et al., 2004). Most strikingly, using similar phonological or semantic training paradigms, English readers show distinctive neural circuits between the two types of training, whereas Chinese readers have largely the same neural network in the FFG, IPL, MTG, IFG, and MFG for both types of training, and all these areas are generally in common with alphabetic languages. This work not only shows common neural circuits in reading Chinese compared to alphabetic languages, but also highlights two of the most important characteristics of logographic writing systems compared to alphabetic writing systems, namely the opaque orthography-to-phonology matching and the heavy reliance on direct orthography to semantic mapping.

Meanwhile, the largely shared network for semantic and phonological processing in Jingjing Zhao et al. (2014) does not mean that there are no differences between the two types of processing. A small number of brain regions such as the left IFG and STG as well as right hemisphere and subcortical regions are sensitive to the modulation of semantic or phonological training (Jingjing Zhao et al., 2014). Tasks of semantic association and phonological matching without training in Dong et al. (2005) show a greater semantic processing in the left ventral IFG compared to phonological processing, together with robust common posterior inferior temporal cortex activation in both tasks in Chinese readers. Consistently, Booth et al. (2006) has found the left anterior ventral IFG/MFG and STG/MTG are more engaged for semantic association, and the left dorsal IFG/MFG and IPL are more engaged in phonological rhyming, in addition to a common activation in left IFG/MFG, bilateral MFG, FFG, and the cerebellum in both tasks. Yang et al. (2011) also pinpointed a sublexical spelling-to-sound matching area in the left TP region. This separation of semantic or phonological systems is also consistent with findings from alphabetic languages. As for orthographic in contrast to phonological processing, Kuo et al. (2004) found greater activation in the left OT, IPL, and right MFG for physical orthographic-form judgments relative to homophone judgments. They also discovered that the left PreG, MFG/IFG, SMA, and TP regions respond to the homophone-judgment task greater than orthographic-form tasks. In addition, they also pointed out that the set of concomitantly activated brain regions in their study support a distributed parallel processing of orthography and phonology. Importantly, X. Wang et al. (2015) found that such language-specific effects are task dependent, showing MFG and right FFG were more active for Chinese than for English speakers during a lexical-decision task, whereas no difference between the two groups was obtained during naturalistic text-reading tasks.

The similar brain regions involved in reading Chinese and alphabetic languages and the distributed parallel processing also manifest when examining the orthography–phonology conversion by manipulating character frequency and consistency (Lee et al., 2004). In this study, bilateral IFG and insula, the left TP (SMG and SPL), and left OT regions show greater activation in naming inconsistent characters than consistent ones, especially in low character frequency cases. The low-frequency characters are expressed in the left PreG/IFG, SMA, anterior insula, pITG, SPL and lingual gyrus more than high-frequency characters, while high-frequency activate the left SMG/AG and precuneus more than low-frequency characters (Kuo et al., 2003). Apart from the frequency and consistency effects shown in relatively distinguished neural regions that largely overlap with alphabetic languages, Liu et al. (2008) pinpointed the two most robust areas in reading Chinese characters: the VWFA and left MFG. The focus on these two regions is in line with findings from Nakamura et al. (2012), which further clarified the shape and gesture properties for the VWFA and left MFG respectively in Chinese reading.

As for developmental studies, Cao et al. (2010) investigated developmental differences in phonological and orthographic processing in Chinese children of 9 and 11 years old as well as adults. They found greater activations in the right SPL and ITG in responding to spelling tasks than rhyming tasks, together with activation in the bilateral occipital cortex that increased with age. The rhyming task showed greater activation than the spelling task in the left STG, with its strength decreasing with age, which has been interpreted as either reflecting reduced phonological processing or more mature phonological representations developing with reading acquisition. There were also age-related increases in left IPL activation, a region involved in orthography–phonology mapping, and age-related increases in left anterior IFG and posterior MFG activations; these latter regions are thought to be involved in lexical retrieval and selection. They pointed out that there is a continuous development of bilateral visuo-orthography regions in occipital regions for developing skilled Chinese read-ing, in addition to other similar brain-region development as in alphabetic languages. Meanwhile, a greater reliance on Pinyin (a phonetic transcription of the Mandarin pronunciation of Chinese characters in Latin letters) in begin-ner Chinese readers and less dependence on Pinyin in adults may contribute to the decrease of activation in the STG (Snowling & Hulme, 2008).

More convergences and differences observed when comparing the neural regions used in reading Chinese and those used in reading alphabetic languages are discussed in the meta-analysis work on Chinese (C.-Y. Wu, Ho, & Chen, 2012). There are three left hemisphere regions that are consistently activated in Chinese reading: the OT, MFG, and IPL. The modulation of task demands reveals greater involvement of left IPL and right STG for phonological processing, and left MTG for semantic processing, with bilateral ventral OT regions recruited in both semantic and phonological processing. These regions are largely consistent with findings in alphabetic languages, such as the inferior OT region for word-form processing, MTG/ITG regions for semantic processing, and the IFG for phonological and semantic processing. However, in Chinese reading, there is an absence of activation in the posterior TP region for grapheme–phoneme conver-sion, and the activation in the left MFG and right FFG seems to be more prevalent in Chinese-character reading (C.-Y. Wu et al., 2012).

13.4   Cross-Language Issues

13.4.1   *Role of Orthographic Depth*

For skilled readers of opaque and transparent orthographies (e.g., English and Italian), there is evidence that the set of brain regions involved in reading is largely identical, with small language-specific differences (Paulesu et al., 2000). Along similar lines, for the DD population, comparisons between Italian, French, and English groups show commonly impaired regions in the left MTG, ITG, STG, and middle occipital gyrus, despite better behavioral reading performance in DD readers of transparent Italian relative to the more opaque French and English (Paulesu et al., 2001). These results can be taken as support for a universal neural basis for dyslexia across alphabetic languages; namely, a core phonological deficit among DD readers in all.

13.4.2 Dyslexia in Chinese

For Chinese skilled readers, almost the same set of brain regions is involved as that of alphabetic language users but some regions, including the MFG, appear to be more engaged in Chinese than in alphabetic languages. The left MFG region has also been argued to be anomalous in Chinese DD readers both functionally (Siok et al., 2004) and structurally (Siok et al., 2008), together with under-activation in the right MFG, left OT, and bilateral posterior IFG in a lexical-decision task, and over-activation in the left anterior IFG in a rhyming task. Although Siok argued that the LH regions typically implicated in DD in alphabetic languages – such as STG and IPL – are not implicated in Chinese, that view has been challenged recently by Hu et al. (2010) who reported under-activation in the left AG, MFG, posterior temporal and OT regions for both Chinese and English DD relative to TD readers in a semantic-decision task, despite the fact that there were language-specific effects in TD readers (i.e., TD Chinese yielded greater activation in the left inferior frontal sulcus [IFS], whereas greater activation was observed in the left posterior STS for English TD readers). It needs to be noted that the activation in the left MFG among the four groups shows the greatest response in the Chinese TD group, whereas the responses from both Chinese and English DD groups are compatible. Such a pattern would not appear to support the explanation that Chinese dyslexia has an entirely distinct impaired neural circuit in MFG compared to that of dyslexia in alphabetic languages; instead, the degraded neural networks are universal across languages, and it is the greater activation in MFG in adaptation to Chinese reading in skilled readers that enhances the contrast between DD and TD groups in this brain region (Hu et al., 2010). In addition, left OT (VWFA) impairment in Chinese DD readers is shown in semantic and lexical-decision tasks but not in phonological tasks. Thus in simple word recognition, deficits in VWFA are seen in both Hu et al. (2010) and and Siok et al. (2004), and appear to be uni versal (Paulesu et al., 2001). In general, research on dyslexia across languages supports a universally altered neural network for reading disability, with equivocal evidence for the cross-language differences more commonly observed in TD readers.

13.4.3   Dyslexia in Other Non-Alphabetic Languages

Abugida writing systems like Hindi denote both consonants and vowels, as in alphabetic languages. Hence, mechanisms of Hindi reading should appear similar to those of alphabetic languages, but there might be a greater visual complexity in reading Hindi because vowel notations are affixed to consonant notations, occupy smaller spaces, and appear at various positions surrounding consonants. It is found that the visuospatial complexity of Hindi writing increases brain responses in the OT and decreases those in the left posterior temporal cortex, which is consistent with the OT's having an orthographic role and the posterior STG and MTG having phonological and semantic roles, as has been proposed by some for alphabetic languages (Rao & Singh, 2015). Rao and Singh also found that word frequency modulates the left IFG, IPL, SPL, OT, and bilateral occipital and putamen areas, which indicates that effortful phonological processing is integrated with visuospatial processing.

In Korean and Japanese, a Chinese character system coexists with a phonologically transparent writing system. When users of these languages read Chinese characters, highly proficient Chinese readers activate the anterior cingulate cortex (ACC), MFG, and FFG, which has been interpreted as a greater dependency on rapid and direct orthographic–semantic mapping, whereas less proficient Chinese readers activate the IPL and IFG, denoting a dependency on a sublexical orthographic–phonological mapping (Jeon, 2012). As for phonological processing in reading Japanese Kana, Kita et al. (2013) found that the left IFG, MFG, STG, and bilateral basal ganglia respond to phonological manipulations, and that the subtype of phonological dyslexic children have under-activation in the left STG and over-activation in the basal ganglia, both of which reflect impaired phonological processing.

13.5   **Explanatory Mechanisms**

Most of the above studies are based on fMRI, a measurement of the brain's hemodynamic responses. However, there is also a rich body of information provided by the analysis of electrophysiological data, neurochemistry, morphostructure of the cerebral cortex, and structural connectivity when examining brain-behavior functions, that we have not reviewed and will briefly describe here.

In a recent study, we used MRS to explore the neurochemistry of typically and atypically developing beginning readers in a longitudinal tracking study (Pugh et al., 2014); the first MRS study in dyslexic children. We found that the concentrations of glutamate (Glu) and choline (Cho) measured in the visual cortex were negatively correlated with reading performance at age 7, and Glu predicted reading outcomes two years later at age 9. Although the visual cortex is not usually the focus of dyslexic research, there are studies reporting dysfunction, mainly over-activation, in the occipital lobe in both DD children and adults (Schlaggar et al., 2002; Temple et al., 2001; Wimmer et al., 2010). Given that Glu and gamma-aminobutyric acid (GABA) are major excitatory and inhibitory neurotransmitters in the brain, too much Glu may cause an imbalanced status in neural excitation and inhibition (Petroff, 2002). Imbalance in Glu/GABA has also been shown to contribute to neuroinflammation and synaptic disorder associated with autism spectrum disorders (El-Ansary & Al-Ayadhi, 2014). Such imbalance not only causes neural firing disorders, but also affects neuronal migration during brain maturation (Manent & Represa, 2007), thus resulting in disrupted cortical architecture in dyslexic individuals (Giraud & Ramus, 2013). This research into the neurochemistry of learning and plasticity holds promise for gaining insights into potential mechanisms underlying differences in language and reading organization in TD and DD readers. Moreover, we suggest that research into differences in neurochemistry provides closer links to genetics and the promise of gene-brain-behavior accounts of reading (dis)ability.

Structural studies of both gray-matter volume and white-matter connectivity have also helped to refine our understanding of reading skill and disability. For example, Blackmon et al. (2010) found gray-matter-thickness differences between adult DD and TD readers such that better reading performance was associated with thicker cortex in the bilateral anterior STG, AG/pSTG, and left intraparietal sulcus. In contrast, better reading performance was associated with thinner cortex in the left posterior FFG and central sulcus, bilateral IFG, and right lingual gyrus and SMG. Klingberg et al. (2000) also found a strong correlation between white-matter connectivity in the left TP region and reading scores both in DD and TD groups. Moreover, white-matter connectivity from AG to pSTG correlates positively with semantic processing efficiency in reading in nonimpaired adult readers (Graves et al., 2014). Boets et al. (2013) found impaired functional and structural connectivity between the auditory cortex and left IFG, which has been interpreted as revealing deficient phonological access with intact phonetic representation in the primary and secondary auditory cortices in DD readers. Such functional and structural connectivity deficiencies can be better described by systematic graph theory analysis in the whole brain. The structural connectivity analysis indicates differences in left posterior cingulate, hippocampus, and left PreG between children at risk and controls (Hosseini et al., 2013), whereas functional connectivity analysis reveals divergent connectivities within the visual pathway and between visual areas and prefrontal attention areas, with an increased right hemisphere connectivity, a reduced connectivity in the VWFA, and persistent connectivities to anterior language areas including and around left IFG in DD (Finn et al., 2014).

Findings from Finn et al. (2014) indicate degraded visual integration and impaired visual-attention modulation that hamper the orthographic processing in DD, and reveal an altered and laborious articulation system in DD compensating for the non-automated visual-based reading, all of which support the basic model (Pugh, Mencl, Jenner et al., 2000).

A functional disconnection between posterior and anterior language regions in dyslexia was actually proposed almost twenty years ago (Paulesu et al., 1996). Throughout the years, various findings have reported connectivity disruptions in DD, such as between the AG and occipital and temporal regions (Horwitz et al., 1998; Pugh, Mencl, Shaywitz et al., 2000), between the left TP area and ventral visual association cortex (Simos et al., 2000), and between the left IFG and left posterior temporal areas including FFG, ITG, MTG, and STG (Schurz et al., 2014). Studies examining functional connectivity with the IFG have yielded mixed results, indicating a compromised information transfer between extrastriate visual cortex and the IFG via the OT in DD readers, whereas the connectivity between the IFG and left anterior language regions including medial prefrontal cortex, anterior cingulate, and left caudate is greater in DD than in TD readers (Finn et al., 2014). The strengthened prefrontal cortex connectivity seems consistent with the proposed compensatory over-activation of frontal region in the general model (Pugh, Mencl, Jenner et al., 2000) while the reduced connectivity between the IFG and VWFA might result from reduced activation in tasks that access to speech gestural coding (Richlan, 2014). Connectivity results, while less stable at present than activation findings promise to generate important systems-level mechanistic models and, ass pointed out by Price (2012), brain connectivity research will become more and more essential in studying reading and language functions going forward.

Most of the studies described above focus on findings within cortical regions; however, an increasing body of literature indicates that subcortical regions such as the thalamus (Díaz et al., 2012; Hoeft et al., 2007; Maisog et al., 2008; Pugh et al., 2008; Pugh et al., 2013) and the cerebellar cortex (Baillieux et al., 2009) also show anomalous patterns of activation in DD readers. In addition to the fMRI findings on subcortical regions, auditory brainstem response (ABR) abnormalities in responding to speech sounds are also found in DD readers (Banai et al., 2009; Hornickel et al., 2012; Hornickel et al., 2009). Evidence supporting differences in subcortical regions between DD and TD readers adds important information to the neural models of dyslexia, yet the functions of subcortical regions in reading are not well understood. More investigations of the subcortical correlates of reading ability are also needed. This will help reconcile cerebellar, magnocellular, auditory temporal theories of reading disability with the more prevalent phonological-deficit and naming-speed hypotheses of dyslexia, thus revealing the underlying sensory-motor deficit during phoneme acquisition and development of automated grapheme–phoneme processing.

In addition, the relation of visual and attentional processes to reading disabilities and phonological deficits is not well explored in neuroimaging studies. Only recent neuroimaging studies have started to explore neural correlates with visuospatial (Diehl, Frost, & Sherman, 2014) and attention span (Lobier et al., 2014) deficits. Recent work by our group (Diehl et al., 2014) provides support for an advantage in certain types of visuospatial processing in DD adolescents, consistent with previous behavioral findings (Von Karolyi et al., 2003), as well as identifying multiple cortical and sub-cortical regions showing a reversed activation pattern in responding to print and figures compared to a TD comparison group. These results support a possible trade-off between visuospatial and reading functions. Lobier et al. (2014) also revealed that SPL coactivates with OT in a DD group with attention span deficits and the activations in both SPL and OT regions are reduced in a DD compared to a TD group, which indicates an attentional network deficit in DD. Another recent study by Paulesu, Danelli, & Berlingeri (2014) indicates that altered functionality of the dorsal left fronto-parietal cortex may be associated with motor and attentional deficits in DD readers. These findings suggest that more neuroimaging studies, focused on general cognitive correlates in DD readers in relation to orthographic, semantic, and phonological processing, are needed to provide a more comprehensive understanding of the mechanisms concerning dyslexia.

Although the basic functional neuroanatomy of reading skill and disability is fairly well established, the incorporation of findings from the temporal domain into brain models of reading is still an underdeveloped area. Although several ERP components, such as visual P100 (Dujardin et al., 2011), N170 (Bar-Kochva & Breznitz, 2014; Dujardin et al., 2011; Kast et al., 2010), visual MMN (J.-J. Wang et al., 2010), P3 (Bar-Kochva & Breznitz, 2014), and N400 under a homophonic condition (Meng et al., 2007), have been found compromised in DD groups, there is no neural model that incorporates this temporal information. It is worth investigating the sources of these ERP components in dyslexia studies and incorporating them into the general neural model of reading. Moreover, evidence suggests there may be abnormalities in the EEG oscillation in DD readers, such as less phase coherence in delta and theta bands relative to TD readers (Klimesch, Doppelmayr, Wimmer, Schwaiger et al., 2001; Power et al., 2013; Soltész et al., 2013) and greater power in alpha, theta, and beta bands (Ackerman et al., 1994; Klimesch, Doppelmayr, Wimmer, Gruber et al., 2001), less left lateralized gamma band oscillation (Lehongre et al., 2013; Lehongre et al., 2011), and reduced interhemispheric coherence of alpha-band oscillation in central-parietal electrodes (Dhar et al., 2010). These spectral analyses need further systematic investigations together with time-frequency information.

13.6   Discussion and Conclusion

The current review covers cognitive models and behavioral and neuroimaging studies of reading and dyslexia. With regard to the neural model, the general division of (1) ventral, (2) dorsal, and (3) anterior brain subcircuits with differential involvement in semantic orthographic, and phonological coding. In addition, developmental changes across these systems seem to be a succinct and reasonable way to summarize the neural mechanisms of reading and reading difficulties in the cerebral cortex. As discussed in the previous sections, a detailed functional segregation of brain regions, especially Broca's area, is necessary in resolving the inconclusive activation pattern in DD. In addition, state-of-the-art multivariate analytical tools (e.g., graph theory) applied to structural and functional analysis will become crucial in understanding the neural mechanisms of dyslexia at a systems level. Such a system-level account must also take subcortical regions into consideration and address the developmental changes. Only with a more comprehensive evaluation of the whole-brain dynamics in not only semantics, phonology, and orthography, but also general cognitive functions such as attention and sensory related issues, can we better understand the underlying reasons behind phonological, naming-speed, and other cognition-related reading problems, and predict or intervene in the development of high-risk children even before reading acquisition. In this regard, neurochemistry study and neural oscillatory analysis can provide useful tools.

A comparison of cross-language readers with and without reading difficulties shows both a general picture and a common core of the problem from the behavioral and neuroimaging results. Phonological processing and naming-speed deficit are universal across languages in DD readers; however, these factors are not as prominent as morphological awareness in Chinese reading, as shown in behavioral studies. For neural mechanisms, TD readers across languages share a similar neural network supporting reading with minor differences in different writing systems, such as extra STG activation for transparent orthographies, posterior Inferior Temporal Gyrus (pITG) and anterior Inferior Frontal Gyrus (aIFG) or opaque orthographies, and MFG for opaque and logographic orthographies, whereas DD readers across languages have a common dysfunction of the neural systems. Moreover, we should not ignore subtypes of dyslexia and possible proportional differences in each subtype across languages. Perhaps further study of languages with multiple writing systems, such as Japanese, and research on bilingual and multilingual DD populations can provide more information regarding dyslexia subtypes and writing-system interactions.

Finally, reading is a cognitive function built upon speech, both in evolution and development. Research from Haskins Laboratories shows that the degree of recruitment of speech regions predicts the level of reading in emergent readers (S. J. Frost et al. 2009; Preston et al., 2016), and forthcoming data from several languages, including English, Hebrew, Spanish, and Chinese, indicate that overlap in regional activation for print and speech is associated with skilled reading in each of these languages (Rueckl et al., 2015). Research in this line will help us better understand the cognitive and neural mechanisms of reading and reading difficulty.

References

Ackerman, P. T., Dykman, R. A., Oglesby, D. M., & Newton, J. E. (1994). EEG power spectra of children with dyslexia, slow learners, and normally reading children with ADD during verbal processing. *Journal of Learning Disabilities, 27,* 619–630.

Baillieux, H., Vandervliet, E. J., Manto, M. et al. (2009). Developmental dyslexia and widespread activation across the cerebellar hemispheres. *Brain and Language, 108,* 122–132.

Banai, K., Hornickel, J., Skoe, E. et al. (2009). Reading and subcortical auditory function. *Cerebral Cortex, 19,* 2699–2707.

Bar-Kochva, I., & Breznitz, Z. (2014). Reading proficiency and adaptability in orthographic processing: An examination of the effect of type of orthography read on brain activity in regular and dyslexic readers. *PLoS One, 9,* e86016. doi: http://dx.doi.org /10.1371/journal.pone.0086016.

Binder, J. (2009). fMRI of language systems. In M. Filippi (Ed.), *fMRI techniques and protocols* (Vol. 41, pp. 323–351). Totowa, NJ: Humana Press.

Binder, J., & Price, C. J. (2001). Functional neuroimaging of language. In R. Cabeza & A. Kingstone (Eds.), *Handbook of functional neuroimaging of cognition* (pp. 187–251). Cambridge, MA: MIT press.

Blackmon, K., Barr, W. B., Kuzniecky, R. et al. (2010). Phonetically irregular word pronunciation and cortical thickness in the adult brain. *Neuroimage, 51,* 1453–1458.

Boets, B., Op de Beeck, H. P., Vandermosten, M. et al. (2013). Intact but less accessible phonetic representations in adults with dyslexia. *Science, 342,* 1251–1254.

Booth, J. R., Burman, D. D., Van Santen, F. W. et al. (2001). The development of specialized brain systems in reading and oral-language. *Child Neuropsychology, 7,* 119–141.

Booth, J. R., Lu, D., Burman, D. D. et al. (2006). Specialization of phonological and semantic processing in Chinese word reading. *Brain Research, 1071,* 197–207.

Bosse, M.-L., Tainturier, M. J., & Valdois, S. (2007). Developmental dyslexia: The visual attention span deficit hypothesis. *Cognition, 104,* 198–230.

Brady, S. A., & Shankweiler, D. P. (1991). *Phonological processes in literacy: A tribute to Isabelle Y. Liberman.* Hillsdale, NJ: Lawrence Erlbaum.

Braze, D., Mencl, W. E., & Tabor, W. et al. (2011). Unification of sentence processing via ear and eye: An fMRI study. *Cortex, 47,* 416–431.

Bruck, M. (1992). Persistence of dyslexics' phonological awareness deficits. *Developmental Psychology, 28,* 874–886.

Brunswick, N., McCrory, E., Price, C., Frith, C., & Frith, U. (1999). Explicit and implicit processing of words and pseudowords by adult developmental dyslexics. *Brain, 122,* 1901–1917.

Calfee, R. (1982). Literacy and illiteracy: Teaching the nonreader to survive in the modern world. *Annals of Dyslexia, 32*, 71–91. doi: http://dx.doi.org/ 10.1007/BF02647954.

Cao, F., Bitan, T., Chou, T. L., Burman, D. D., & Booth, J. R. (2006). Deficient orthographic and phonological representations in children with dyslexia revealed by brain activation patterns. *Journal of Child Psychology and Psychiatry, 47*, 1041–1050.

Cao, F., Lee, R., Shu, H. et al. (2010). Cultural constraints on brain development: Evidence from a developmental study of visual word processing in Mandarin Chinese. *Cerebral Cortex, 20*, 1223–1233.

Caravolas, M. (2005). The nature and causes of dyslexia in different languages. In M. Snowling & & C. Hulme (Eds.), *The science of reading: A handbook* (pp. 336–355). Oxford, UK: Blackwell.

Caravolas, M., Lervåg, A., Defior, S., Málková, G. S., & Hulme, C. (2013). Different patterns, but equivalent predictors, of growth in reading in consistent and inconsistent orthographies. *Psychological Science, 24*, 1398–1407.

Caravolas, M., Lervåg, A., Mousikou, P. et al. (2012). Common patterns of prediction of literacy development in different alphabetic orthographies. *Psychological Science, 23*, 678–686.

Caravolas, M., Volín, J., & Hulme, C. (2005). Phoneme awareness is a key component of alphabetic literacy skills in consistent and inconsistent orthographies: Evidence from Czech and English children. *Journal of Experimental Child Psychology, 92*, 107–139.

Castro-Caldas, A., Miranda, P. C., Carmo, I. et al. (1999). Influence of learning to read and write on the morphology of the corpus callosum. *European Journal of Neurology, 6*, 23–28.

Church, J. A., Balota, D. A., Petersen, S. E., & Schlaggar, B. L. (2011). Manipulation of length and lexicality localizes the functional neuroanatomy of phonological processing in adult readers. *Journal of Cognitive Neuroscience, 23*, 1475–1493.

Church, J. A., Coalson, R. S., Lugar, H. M., Petersen, S. E., & Schlaggar, B. L. (2008). A developmental fMRI study of reading and repetition reveals changes in phonological and visual mechanisms over age. *Cerebral Cortex, 18*, 2054–2065.

Cohen, L., Lehéricy, S., Chochon, F. et al. (2002). Language-specific tuning of visual cortex? Functional properties of the Visual Word Form Area. *Brain, 125*, 1054–1069.

Dehaene, S. (2009). *Reading in the brain: The new science of how we read*. London: Penguin Publishing Group.

Dehaene, S., & Cohen, L. (2011). The unique role of the visual word form area in reading. *Trends in Cognitive Sciences, 15*, 254–262.

Dehaene, S., Cohen, L., Morais, J., & Kolinsky, R. (2015). Illiterate to literate: Behavioural and cerebral changes induced by reading acquisition. *Nature Reviews Neuroscience, 16*, 234–244.

Démonet, J.-F., Taylor, M. J., & Chaix, Y. (2004). Developmental dyslexia. *The Lancet, 363*, 1451–1460.

Démonet, J.-F., Thierry, G., & Cardebat, D. (2005). Renewal of the neurophysiology of language: Functional neuroimaging. *Physiological Reviews, 85*, 49–95.

DeWitt, I., & Rauschecker, J. P. (2013). Wernicke's area revisited: Parallel streams and word processing. *Brain and Language, 127*, 181–191.

Dhar, M., Been, P. H., Minderaa, R. B., & Althaus, M. (2010). Reduced interhemispheric coherence in dyslexic adults. *Cortex, 46*, 794–798.

Díaz, B., Hintz, F., Kiebel, S. J., & von Kriegstein, K. (2012). Dysfunction of the auditory thalamus in developmental dyslexia. *Proceedings of the National Academy of Sciences of the United States of America, 109*, 13841–13846.

Diehl, J. J., Frost, S. J., & Sherman, G. (2014). Neural correlates of language and non-language visuospatial processing in adolescents with reading disability. *Neuroimage, 101*, 653–666.

Dong, Y., Nakamura, K., & Okada, T. (2005). Neural mechanisms underlying the processing of Chinese words: An fMRI study. *Neuroscience Research, 52*, 139–145.

Dujardin, T., Etienne, Y., Contentin, C. et al. (2011). Behavioral performances in participants with phonological dyslexia and different patterns on the N170 component. *Brain and Cognition, 75*, 91–100.

El-Ansary, A., & Al-Ayadhi, L. (2014). GABAergic/glutamatergic imbalance relative to excessive neuroinflammation in autism spectrum disorders. *Journal Neuroinflammation, 11*, 189. doi: http://dx.doi.org/10.1186/s12974-014-0189-0.

Finn, E. S., Shen, X., & Holahan, J. M. (2014). Disruption of functional networks in dyslexia: A whole-brain, data-driven analysis of connectivity. *Biological Psychiatry, 76*, 397–404.

Fletcher, J. M., Shaywitz, S. E., Shankweiler, D. P. et al. (1994). Cognitive profiles of reading disability: Comparisons of discrepancy and low achievement definitions. *Journal of Educational Psychology, 86*, 6–23.

Frost, R. (2012). Towards a universal model of reading. *Behavioral and Brain Sciences, 35*, 263–279.

Frost, R., Katz, L., & Bentin, S. (1987). Strategies for visual word recognition and orthographical depth: A multilingual comparison. *Journal of Experimental Psychology: Human Perception and Performance, 13*, 104–115. doi: http://dx .doi.org/10.1037/0096-1523.13.1.104.

Frost, S. J., Landi, N., & Mencl, W. E. et al. (2009). Phonological awareness predicts activation patterns for print and speech. *Annals of Dyslexia, 59*, 78–97.

Gabrieli, J. D. (2009). Dyslexia: A new synergy between education and cognitive neuroscience. *Science, 325*, 280–283.

Giraud, A.-L., & Ramus, F. (2013). Neurogenetics and auditory processing in developmental dyslexia. *Current Opinion in Neurobiology, 23*, 37–42.

Goswami, U., Thomson, J., Richardson, U. et al. (2002). Amplitude envelope onsets and developmental dyslexia: A new hypothesis. *Proceedings of the National Academy of Sciences of the United States of America, 99*, 10911–10916.

Goswami, U., Wang, H.-L. S., Cruz, A. et al. (2011). Language-universal sensory deficits in developmental dyslexia: English, Spanish, and Chinese. *Journal of Cognitive Neuroscience, 23*, 325–337.

Goswami, U., Ziegler, J. C., & Richardson, U. (2005). The effects of spelling consistency on phonological awareness: A comparison of English and German. *Journal of Experimental Child Psychology, 92*, 345–365.

Graves, W. W., Binder, J. R., Desai, R. H. et al. (2014). Anatomy is strategy: Skilled reading differences associated with structural connectivity differences in the reading network. *Brain and Language, 133*, 1–13.

Griffith, P. L., & Olson, M. W. (1992). Phonemic awareness helps beginning readers break the code. *The Reading Teacher, 45*, 516–523.

Hampson, M., Tokoglu, F., Sun, Z. et al. (2006). Connectivity–behavior analysis reveals that functional connectivity between left BA39 and Broca's area varies with reading ability. *Neuroimage*, *31*, 513–519.

Helenius, P., Uutela, K., & Hari, R. (1999). Auditory stream segregation in dyslexic adults. *Brain*, *122*, 907–913.

Ho, C. S.-H., Chan, D. W., Chung, K. K., Lee, S.-H., & Tsang, S.-M. (2007). In search of subtypes of Chinese developmental dyslexia. *Journal of Experimental Child Psychology*, *97*, 61–83.

Hoeft, F., Hernandez, A., McMillon, G. et al. (2006). Neural basis of dyslexia: A comparison between dyslexic and nondyslexic children equated for reading ability. *The Journal of Neuroscience*, *26*, 10700–10708.

Hoeft, F., Meyler, A., Hernandez, A. et al. (2007). Functional and morphometric brain dissociation between dyslexia and reading ability. *Proceedings of the National Academy of Sciences of the United States of America*, *104*, 4234–4239.

Hornickel, J., Anderson, S., Skoe, E., Yi, H.-G., & Kraus, N. (2012). Subcortical representation of speech fine structure relates to reading ability. *Neuroreport*, *23*, 6–9.

Hornickel, J., Skoe, E., Nicol, T., Zecker, S., & Kraus, N. (2009). Subcortical differentiation of stop consonants relates to reading and speech-in-noise perception. *Proceedings of the National Academy of Sciences of the United States of America*, *106*, 13022–13027.

Horwitz, B., Rumsey, J. M., & Donohue, B. C. (1998). Functional connectivity of the angular gyrus in normal reading and dyslexia. *Proceedings of the National Academy of Sciences of the United States of America*, *95*, 8939–8944.

Hosseini, S. H., Black, J. M., Soriano, T. et al. (2013). Topological properties of large-scale structural brain networks in children with familial risk for reading difficulties. *Neuroimage*, *71*, 260–274.

Hu, W., Lee, H. L., & Zhang, Q. (2010). Developmental dyslexia in Chinese and English populations: Dissociating the effect of dyslexia from language differences. *Brain*, *133*, 1694–1706.

Jeon, H.-A. (2012). Effect of lexical proficiency on reading strategies used for shallow and deep orthographies. *Neuroreport*, *23*, 979–983.

Kamii, C., & Manning, M. (2002). Phonemic awareness and beginning reading and writing. *Journal of Research in Childhood Education*, *17*, 38–46.

Kast, M., Elmer, S., Jancke, L., & Meyer, M. (2010). ERP differences of pre-lexical processing between dyslexic and non-dyslexic children. *International Journal of Psychophysiology*, *77*, 59–69.

Katz, L., & Frost, R. (1992). The reading process is different for different orthographies: The orthographic depth hypothesis. *Advances in Psychology*, *94*, 67–84.

Kita, Y., Yamamoto, H., Oba, K. et al. (2013). Altered brain activity for phonological manipulation in dyslexic Japanese children. *Brain*, *136*, 3696–3708.

Klimesch, W., Doppelmayr, M., Wimmer, H., Gruber, W. et al. (2001). Alpha and beta band power changes in normal and dyslexic children. *Clinical Neurophysiology*, *112*, 1186–1195.

Klimesch, W., Doppelmayr, M., Wimmer, H. E. A., Schwaiger, J. et al. (2001). Theta band power changes in normal and dyslexic children. *Clinical Neurophysiology*, *112*, 1174–1185.

Klingberg, T., Hedehus, M., & Temple, E. (2000). Microstructure of temporo-parietal white matter as a basis for reading ability: evidence from diffusion tensor magnetic resonance imaging. *Neuron, 25,* 493–500.

Kuo, W.-J., Yeh, T.-C., Lee, C.-Y. et al. (2003). Frequency effects of Chinese character processing in the brain: An event-related fMRI study. *Neuroimage, 18,* 720–730.

Kuo, W.-J., Yeh, T.-C., Lee, J.-R. et al. (2004). Orthographic and phonological processing of Chinese characters: An fMRI study. *Neuroimage, 21,* 1721–1731.

Lallier, M., Thierry, G., Tainturier, M.-J. et al. (2009). Auditory and visual stream segregation in children and adults: An assessment of the amodality assumption of the "sluggish attentional shifting" theory of dyslexia. *Brain Research, 1302,* 132–147.

Landerl, K., Ramus, F., Moll, K. et al. (2013). Predictors of developmental dyslexia in European orthographies with varying complexity. *Journal of Child Psychology and Psychiatry, 54,* 686–694. http://dx.doi.org/10.1111/jcpp.12029.

Lee, C.-Y., Tsai, J.-L., Kuo, W.-J. et al. (2004). Neuronal correlates of consistency and frequency effects on Chinese character naming: An event-related fMRI study. *Neuroimage, 23,* 1235–1245.

Lehongre, K., Morillon, B., Giraud, A.-L., & Ramus, F. (2013). Impaired auditory sampling in dyslexia: Further evidence from combined fMRI and EEG. *Frontiers in Human Neuroscience, 7,* 454.

Lehongre, K., Ramus, F., Villiermet, N., Schwartz, D., & Giraud, A.-L. (2011). Altered low-gamma sampling in auditory cortex accounts for the three main facets of dyslexia. *Neuron, 72,* 1080–1090.

Liberman, A. M. (1996). *Speech: A special code.* London: MIT press.

Liberman, I. Y., Shankweiler, D., & Liberman, A. M. (1989). The alphabetic principle and learning to read. In D. Shankweiler & I. Y. Liberman (Eds.), *International academy for research in learning disabilities monograph series, no. 6. Phonology and reading disability: Solving the reading puzzle* (pp. 1–33). Ann Arbor, MI: The University of Michigan Press.

Liu, C., Zhang, W.-T., Tang, Y.-Y. et al. (2008). The visual word form area: Evidence from an fMRI study of implicit processing of Chinese characters. *Neuroimage, 40,* 1350–1361.

Lobier, M. A., Peyrin, C., Pichat, C., Le Bas, J.-F., & Valdois, S. (2014). Visual processing of multiple elements in the dyslexic brain: Evidence for a superior parietal dysfunction. *Frontiers in Human Neuroscience, 8,* 479.

Lyytinen, H., Aro, M., Eklund, K. et al. (2004). The development of children at familial risk for dyslexia: Birth to early school age. *Annals of Dyslexia, 54,* 184–220.

Maisog, J. M., Einbinder, E. R., Flowers, D. L., Turkeltaub, P. E., & Eden, G. F. (2008). A Meta-analysis of functional neuroimaging studies of dyslexia. *Annals of the New York Academy of Sciences, 1145,* 237–259.

Manent, J.-B., & Represa, A. (2007). Neurotransmitters and brain maturation: Early paracrine actions of GABA and glutamate modulate neuronal migration. *The Neuroscientist, 13,* 268–279.

Mann, V., & Wimmer, H. (2002). Phoneme awareness and pathways into literacy: A comparison of German and American children. *Reading and Writing, 15,* 653–682. doi: http://dx.doi.org/10.1023/A:1020984704781.

McBride-Chang, C., Cho, J.-R., Liu, H. et al. (2005). Changing models across cultures: Associations of phonological awareness and morphological structure awareness with vocabulary and word recognition in second graders from Beijing, Hong Kong, Korea, and the United States. *Journal of Experimental Child Psychology, 92*, 140–160.

McBride-Chang, C., Shu, H., Zhou, A. et al. (2003). Morphological awareness uniquely predicts young children's Chinese character recognition. *Journal of Educational Psychology, 95*, 743–751.

McNorgan, C., Randazzo-Wagner, M., & Booth, J. R. (2013). Cross-modal integration in the brain is related to phonological awareness only in typical readers, not in those with reading difficulty. *Frontiers in Human Neuroscience, 7*, 388. http://dx.doi.org/10.3389/fnhum.2013.00388.

Meng, X., Tian, X., Jian, J., & Zhou, X. (2007). Orthographic and phonological processing in Chinese dyslexic children: An ERP study on sentence reading. *Brain Research, 1179*, 119–130.

Moll, K., Ramus, F., Bartling, J. et al. (2014). Cognitive mechanisms underlying reading and spelling development in five European orthographies. *Learning and Instruction, 29*, 65–77.

Nakamura, K., Kuo, W.-J., Pegado, F. et al. (2012). Universal brain systems for recognizing word shapes and handwriting gestures during reading. *Proceedings of the National Academy of Sciences of the United States of America, 109*, 20762–20767. doi: http://dx.doi.org/10.1073/pnas.1217749109.

Newman, E. H., Tardif, T., Huang, J. Y., & Shu, H. (2011). Phonemes matter: The role of phoneme-level awareness in emergent Chinese readers. *Journal of Experimental Child Psychology, 108*, 242–259.

Paulesu, E., Danelli, L., & Berlingeri, M. (2014). Reading the dyslexic brain: Multiple dysfunctional routes revealed by a new meta-analysis of PET and fMRI activation studies. *Frontiers in Human Neuroscience, 8*, 830. doi: http://dx.doi.org/10.3389/fnhum.2014.00830.

Paulesu, E., Démonet, J.-F., Fazio, F. et al. (2001). Dyslexia: Cultural diversity and biological unity. *Science, 291*, 2165–2167.

Paulesu, E., Frith, U., Snowling, M. et al. (1996). Is developmental dyslexia a disconnection syndrome. *Brain, 119*, 143–157.

Paulesu, E., McCrory, E., Fazio, F. et al. (2000). A cultural effect on brain function. *Nature Neuroscience, 3*, 91–96.

Perreault, C., & Mathew, S. (2012). Dating the origin of language using phonemic diversity. *PLoS One, 7*, e35289. doi: http://dx.doi.org/10.1371/journal.pone.0035289.

Petroff, O. A. (2002). Book review: GABA and glutamate in the human brain. *The Neuroscientist, 8*, 562–573.

Power, A. J., Mead, N., Barnes, L., & Goswami, U. (2013). Neural entrainment to rhythmic speech in children with developmental dyslexia. *Frontiers in Human Neuroscience, 7*, 777.

Preston, J. L., Molfese, P. J., Frost, S. J. et al. (2016). Print-speech convergence predicts future reading outcomes in early readers. *Psychological Science, 27*, 75–84.

Price, C. J. (2000). The anatomy of language: Contributions from functional neuroimaging. *Journal of Anatomy, 197*, 335–359.

Price, C. J. (2012). A review and synthesis of the first 20 years of PET and fMRI studies of heard speech, spoken language and reading. *Neuroimage, 62*, 816–847.

Pugh, K. R., Frost, S. J., Rothman, D. L. et al. (2014). Glutamate and choline levels predict individual differences in reading ability in emergent readers. *The Journal of Neuroscience, 34*, 4082–4089.

Pugh, K. R., Frost, S. J., Sandak, R. et al. (2008). Effects of stimulus difficulty and repetition on printed word identification: An fMRI comparison of nonimpaired and reading-disabled adolescent cohorts. *Journal of Cognitive Neuroscience, 20,* 1146–1160.

Pugh, K. R., Landi, N., Preston, J. L. et al. (2013). The relationship between phonological and auditory processing and brain organization in beginning readers. *Brain and Language, 125,* 173–183. doi: http://dx.doi.org/10.1016/j.bandl.2012.04.004.

Pugh, K. R., Mencl, W. E., Jenner, A. R. et al. (2000). Functional neuroimaging studies of reading and reading disability (developmental dyslexia). *Mental Retardation & Developmental Disabilities Research Reviews, 6,* 207–213.

Pugh, K. R., Mencl, W. E., Shaywitz, B. A. et al. (2000). The angular gyrus in developmental dyslexia: Task-specific differences in functional connectivity within posterior cortex. *Psychological Science, 11,* 51–56.

Pugh, K. R., Sandak, R., Frost, S. J., Moore, D. L., & Mencl, W. E. (2006). Neurobiological investigations of skilled and impaired reading. In D. K. Dickinson & S. B. Neuman (Eds.), *Handbook of early literacy research* (Vol. 2, pp. 64–74). New York, NY: Guilford Publications.

Pugh, K. R., Shaywitz, B. A., Shaywitz, S. E. et al. (1996). Cerebral organization of component processes in reading. *Brain, 119,* 1221–1238.

Ramus, F. (2003). Developmental dyslexia: Specific phonological deficit or general sensorimotor dysfunction? *Current Opinion in Neurobiology, 13,* 212–218.

Rao, C., & Singh, N. C. (2015). Visuospatial complexity modulates reading in the brain. *Brain and Language, 141,* 50–61.

Rawson, M. (1978). Dyslexia and learning disabilities: Their relationship. *Bulletin of the Orton Society, 28,* 43–61. doi: http://dx.doi.org/10.1007/BF02653425.

Richlan, F. (2012). Developmental dyslexia: Dysfunction of a left hemisphere reading network. *Frontiers in Human Neuroscience, 6,* 120.

Richlan, F. (2014). Functional neuroanatomy of developmental dyslexia: The role of orthographic depth. *Frontiers in Human Neuroscience, 8,* 347. doi: http://dx.doi.org /10.3389/fnhum.2014.00347.

Richlan, F., Kronbichler, M., & Wimmer, H. (2009). Functional abnormalities in the dyslexic brain: A quantitative meta-analysis of neuroimaging studies. *Human Brain Mapping, 30,* 3299–3308.

Richlan, F., Kronbichler, M., & Wimmer, H. (2011). Meta-analyzing brain dysfunctions in dyslexic children and adults. *Neuroimage, 56,* 1735–1742.

Rieben, L., & Perfetti, C. A. (1991). *Learning to read: Basic research and its implications.* Hillsdale, NJ: Lawrence Erlbaum Associates.

Rueckl, J. G., Paz-Alonso, P. M., & Molfese, P. J. et al. (2015). Universal brain signature of proficient reading: Evidence from four contrasting languages. *Proceedings of the National Academy of Sciences, 112,* 15510–15515.

Rumsey, J. M., Andreason, P., & Zametkin, A. J. (1992). Failure to activate the left temporoparietal cortex in dyslexia: An oxygen 15 positron emission tomographic study. *Archives of Neurology, 49,* 527–534. doi: http://dx.doi.org/10.1001/archneur .1992.00530290115020.

Salmelin, R., Kiesilä, P., Uutela, K., Service, E., & Salonen, O. (1996). Impaired visual word processing in dyslexia revealed with magnetoencephalography. *Annals of Neurology, 40,* 157–162.

Sandak, R., Mencl, W. E., Frost, S. J. et al. (2004). The neurobiology of adaptive learning in reading: A contrast of different training conditions. *Cognitive, Affective, & Behavioral Neuroscience, 4,* 67–88.

Sarkari, S., Simos, P., Fletcher, J. et al. (2002). The emergence and treatment of developmental reading disability: Contributions of functional brain imaging. *Seminars in Pediatric Neurology, 9,* 227–236.

Scarborough, H. S. (1998). Early identification of children at risk for reading disabilities: Phonological awareness and some other promising predictors. In B. K. Shapiro, P. J. Accardo, & A. J. Capute (Eds.), *Specific reading disability: A view of the spectrum* (pp. 75–119). Timonium, MD: York Press.

Schlaggar, B. L., Brown, T. T., Lugar, H. M. et al. (2002). Functional neuroanatomical differences between adults and school-age children in the processing of single words. *Science, 296,* 1476–1479.

Schurz, M., Wimmer, H., Richlan, F. et al. (2014). Resting-state and task-based functional brain connectivity in developmental dyslexia. *Cerebral Cortex, 25,* 3502–3514. doi: http://dx.doi.org/10.1093/cercor/bhu184.

Shankweiler, D., Crain, S., Katz, L. et al. (1995). Cognitive profiles of reading-disabled children: Comparison of language skills in phonology, morphology, and syntax. *Psychological Science, 6,* 149–156.

Shankweiler, D., Mencl, W. E., Braze, D. et al. (2008). Reading differences and brain: Cortical integration of speech and print in sentence processing varies with reader skill. *Developmental Neuropsychology, 33,* 745–775.

Shaywitz, S. E., & Shaywitz, B. A. (2003). The science of reading and dyslexia. *Journal of American Association for Pediatric Ophthalmology and Strabismus, 7,* 158–166. doi: http://dx.doi.org/10.1016/s1091-8531(03)00002-8.

Shaywitz, B. A., Shaywitz, S. E., Blachman, B. A. et al. (2004). Development of left occipitotemporal systems for skilled reading in children after a phonologically-based intervention. *Biological Psychiatry, 55,* 926–933.

Shaywitz, S. E., Shaywitz, B. A., & Pugh, K. R. et al. (1998). Functional disruption in the organization of the brain for reading in dyslexia. *Proceedings of the National Academy of Sciences of the United States of America, 95,* 2636–2641.

Shaywitz, B. A., Shaywitz, S. E., Pugh, K. R. et al. (2002). Disruption of posterior brain systems for reading in children with developmental dyslexia. *Biological Psychiatry, 52,* 101–110.

Shu, H., Anderson, R. C., & Wu, N. N. (2000). Phonetic awareness: Knowledge of orthography-phonology relationships in the character acquisition of Chinese children. *Journal of Educational Psychology, 92,* 56–62.

Shu, H., McBride-Chang, C., Wu, S., & Liu, H. Y. (2006). Understanding Chinese developmental dyslexia: Morphological awareness as a core cognitive construct. *Journal of Educational Psychology, 98,* 122–133.

Shu, H., Meng, X., Chen, X., Luan, H., & Cao, F. (2005). The subtypes of developmental dyslexia in Chinese: Evidence from three cases. *Dyslexia, 11,* 311–329.

Shu, H., Peng, H., & McBride-Chang, C. (2008). Phonological awareness in young Chinese children. *Developmental Science, 11,* 171–181. doi: http://dx.doi.org/10.1111/j.1467-7687.2007.00654.x.

Simos, P. G., Breier, J., Fletcher, J., Bergman, E., & Papanicolaou, A. (2000). Cerebral mechanisms involved in word reading in dyslexic children: A magnetic source imaging approach. *Cerebral Cortex, 10,* 809–816.

Siok, W. T., Niu, Z., Jin, Z., Perfetti, C. A., & Tan, L. H. (2008). A structural–functional basis for dyslexia in the cortex of Chinese readers. *Proceedings of the National Academy of Sciences of the United States of America*, *105*, 5561–5566. doi: http://dx.doi.org/10.1073/pnas.0801750105.

Siok, W. T., Perfetti, C. A., Jin, Z., & Tan, L. H. (2004). Biological abnormality of impaired reading is constrained by culture. *Nature*, *431*, 71–76.

Siok, W. T., Spinks, J. A., Jin, Z., & Tan, L. H. (2009). Developmental dyslexia is characterized by the co-existence of visuospatial and phonological disorders in Chinese children. *Current Biology*, *19*, R890–R892.

Snowling, M. J., & Hulme, C. (2008). *The science of reading: A handbook* (Vol. 9). Malden, MA: Blackwell Publishing. doi: http://dx.doi.org/10.1002/9780470757642.

Soltész, F., Szűcs, D., Leong, V., White, S., & Goswami, U. (2013). Differential entrainment of neuroelectric delta oscillations in developmental dyslexia. *PLoS One*, *8*, e76608. doi: http://dx.doi.org/10.1371/journal.pone.0076608.

Spitsyna, G., Warren, J. E., Scott, S. K., Turkheimer, F. E., & Wise, R. J. (2006). Converging language streams in the human temporal lobe. *The Journal of Neuroscience*, *26*, 7328–7336.

Tallal, P. (1984). Temporal or phonetic processing deficit in dyslexia? That is the question. *Applied Psycholinguistics*, *5*, 167–169.

Tan, L. H., Hoosain, R., & Peng, D.-L. (1995). Role of early presemantic phonological code in Chinese character identification. *Journal of Experimental Psychology: Learning, Memory, and Cognition*, *21*, 43–54.

Temple, E., Deutsch, G. K., Poldrack, R. A. et al. (2003). Neural deficits in children with dyslexia ameliorated by behavioral remediation: Evidence from functional MRI. *Proceedings of the National Academy of Sciences of the United States of America*, *100*, 2860–2865.

Temple, E., Poldrack, R. A., Salidis, J. et al. (2001). Disrupted neural responses to phonological and orthographic processing in dyslexic children: An fMRI study. *Neuroreport*, *12*, 299–307.

Turkeltaub, P. E., Gareau, L., Flowers, D. L., Zeffiro, T. A., & Eden, G. F. (2003). Development of neural mechanisms for reading. *Nature Neuroscience*, *6*, 767–773.

Verhoeven, L., & Perfetti, C. (2003). Introduction to this special issue: The role of morphology in learning to read. *Scientific Studies of Reading*, *7*, 209–217.

Viana, A. R., Razuk, M., de Freitas, P. B., & Barela, J. A. (2013). Sensorimotor integration in dyslexic children under different sensory stimulations. *PLoS One*, *8*, e72719. doi: http://dx.doi.org/10.1371/journal.pone.0072719.

Von Karolyi, C., Winner, E., Gray, W., & Sherman, G. F. (2003). Dyslexia linked to talent: Global visual-spatial ability. *Brain and Language*, *85*, 427–431.

Wang, J.-J., Bi, H.-Y., Gao, L.-Q., & Wydell, T. N. (2010). The visual magnocellular pathway in Chinese-speaking children with developmental dyslexia. *Neuropsychologia*, *48*, 3627–3633.

Wang, W. S., & Tsai, Y. (2011). The alphabet and the sinogram. *Dyslexia across cultures*. Baltimore, MD: Brookes Publishing.

Wang, X., Yang, J., Yang, J. et al. (2015). Language differences in the brain network for reading in naturalistic story reading and lexical decision. *PLoS One*, *10*, e0124388. doi: http://dx.doi.org/10.1371/journal.pone.0124388.

Wheat, K. L., Cornelissen, P. L., Frost, S. J., & Hansen, P. C. (2010). During visual word recognition, phonology is accessed within 100 ms and may be mediated by a speech production code: Evidence from magnetoencephalography. *The Journal of Neuroscience, 30*, 5229–5233.

Wimmer, H., Mayringer, H., & Landerl, K. (2000). The double-deficit hypothesis and difficulties in learning to read a regular orthography. *Journal of Educational Psychology, 92*, 668–680. doi: http://dx.doi.org/10.1037/0022-0663.92.4.668.

Wimmer, H., Schurz, M., Sturm, D. et al. (2010). A dual-route perspective on poor reading in a regular orthography: An fMRI study. *Cortex, 46*, 1284–1298.

Wu, C.-Y., Ho, M.-H. R., & Chen, S.-H. A. (2012). A meta-analysis of fMRI studies on Chinese orthographic, phonological, and semantic processing. *Neuroimage, 63*, 381–391.

Wu, N. N., Zhou, X. L., & Shu, H. (1999). Sublexical processing in reading Chinese: A development study. *Language and Cognitive Processes, 14*, 503–524.

Yang, J., Wang, X., Shu, H., & Zevin, J. D. (2011). Brain networks associated with sublexical properties of Chinese characters. *Brain and Language, 119*, 68–79.

Yoncheva, Y. N., Zevin, J. D., Maurer, U., & McCandliss, B. D. (2010). Auditory selective attention to speech modulates activity in the visual word form area. *Cerebral Cortex, 20*, 622–632.

Zhao, J. [Jing], Qian, Y., Bi, H.-Y., & Coltheart, M. (2014). The visual magnocellular-dorsal dysfunction in Chinese children with developmental dyslexia impedes Chinese character recognition. *Scientific Reports, 4*, 7068. doi: http://dx.doi.org/10.1038/srep07068.

Zhao, J. [Jingjing], Wang, X., Frost, S. J. et al. (2014). Neural division of labor in reading is constrained by culture: A training study of reading Chinese characters. *Cortex, 53*, 90–106.

Zhou, X., & Marslen-Wilson, W. (1999). Phonology, orthography, and semantic activation in reading Chinese. *Journal of Memory and Language, 41*, 579–606.

Zhou, X., & Marslen-Wilson, W. (2000). The relative time course of semantic and phonological activation in reading Chinese. *Journal of Experimental Psychology: Learning, Memory, and Cognition, 26*, 1245–1265.

Ziegler, J. C., Bertrand, D., Tóth, D. et al. (2010). Orthographic depth and its impact on universal predictors of reading: A cross-language investigation. *Psychological Science, 21*, 551–559. doi: http://dx.doi.org/10.1177/0956797610363406.

Ziegler, J. C., & Goswami, U. (2005). Reading acquisition, developmental dyslexia, and skilled reading across languages: A psycholinguistic grain size theory. *Psychological Bulletin, 131*, 3–29.

14 Role of Visual Attention in Developmental Dyslexia

Andrea Facoetti, Sandro Franceschini, and Simone Gori

14.1 Introduction

Attention is a neurocognitive process composed by subprocesses located in several brain areas and controlled by specific neurotransmitters (Petersen & Posner, 2012). This process aims to select relevant information and modulates sensory processing, perception, memory, and learning. This selection of information processing – based on the combination of perceptual noise exclusion and signal enhancement – is fundamental in developing fine object representations in the brain (see Corbetta & Shulman, 2011; Petersen & Posner, 2012; Roelfsema, van Ooyen, & Watanabe, 2010, for reviews).

Alerting and orienting are the two main processes involved in reading acquisition. Alerting is defined as the multisensory attentional process that increases performance during tasks (Petersen & Posner, 2012), producing a phasic change in alertness (e.g., Ronconi et al., 2016). The alerting system can already be measured in the infant brain (e.g., Ronconi, Facoetti et al., 2014). Attention orienting is the ability to select a spatial location (Petersen & Posner, 2012) or time event (Battelli, Pascual-Leone, & Cavanagh, 2007, for a review) inside the sensory field. Attention orienting is described as a spotlight that moves to the attended area (Carrasco, 2011). The attention spotlight is not only oriented in a specific spatiotemporal location, but can also be adjusted in its size (i.e., zoom-in and zoom-out of focusing attention, e.g., Facoetti et al., 2000, 2003; Facoetti & Molteni, 2000; Ronconi, Facoetti et al., 2014; Ronconi et al., 2013, 2016). Frontal and parietal areas are the neural substrate of the orienting and focusing of attention (Battelli et al., 2007; Corbetta & Shulman, 2002; Ronconi, Basso et al., 2014). The subcortical lateral geniculate nucleus (LGN) and the pulvinar, both in the thalamus, have also been shown to participate in attentional orienting (Schneider & Kastner, 2009).

In this chapter, we will start out by providing a theoretical background on how visual attention may be involved in reading and developmental dyslexia. In addition, the research evidence that is predominantly cited in the literature on the occurrence of a visual deficit independently from a phonological deficit will be summarized; see Chapter 12). Explanatory mechanisms for such a visual deficit in dyslexia will also be discussed. Finally, clinical implications will be provided along with a final conclusion.

14.2   Theoretical Background

Individuals with developmental dyslexia (DD) present difficulties with accurate and fluent word recognition and spelling despite adequate instruction, intelligence, and sensory abilities. DD is characterized by difficulties with decoding, while comprehension is more intact (Peterson & Pennington, 2015).

DD is often associated with an impaired phonological awareness, which refers to the ability to perceive and manipulate the sounds of spoken words (Castles & Coltheart, 2004). A phonological awareness deficit could impair the ability to map speech sounds onto their homologous visual letters (see Vellutino et al., 2004). Impaired phonological awareness is largely assumed to be the core deficit in DD (see Gabrieli, 2009; Peterson & Pennington, 2015). However, reading acquisition can profoundly refine the neurocognitive organization of the auditory-phonological reading network (see Dehaene et al., 2015). In particular, previous research has established that learning to read improves children's performance on reading-related phonological tasks, including phoneme awareness (PA), and nonword repetition as well as rapid automatized naming (Peterson et al., 2017). These findings imply that the association between literacy and phonological skills is moderated by development. Consequently, also the findings of structurally (e.g., less gray-matter volume) and functionally (e.g., less activated cortical and subcortical areas) different reading circuits in DD may represent the consequence of a reduced reading development (e.g., Krafnick et al., 2014).

Longitudinal studies have suggested a causal link between impaired phonological awareness and reading difficulties (see Peterson & Pennington, 2015, for a review). However, there is a lack of longitudinal studies investigating phonological skills in DD that have controlled for existing literacy skills and grapheme-to-phoneme mapping in their participants (Castles & Coltheart, 2004). Moreover, it has been shown that specific phonological awareness training does not always automatically transfer to better reading skills (e.g., Galuschka et al., 2014; but see Ball & Blachman, 1988; Bradley & Bryant, 1983; Moats, 1994, for positive effects of phonological awareness training on reading remediation in children with DD). It is important to note that recent studies suggest that also other neurocognitive deficits might cause

DD (Valdois, Bosse, & Tainturier, 2004; e.g., Boets et al., 2011; Franceschini, Bertoni et al., 2017; Franceschini et al., 2012, 2013, 2015; Franceschini, Trevisan et al., 2017; Gori, Bertoni et al., 2016; Gori et al., 2015, 2016; Gori, Molteni, & Facoetti, 2016; Kevan & Pammer, 2009).

Indeed, it can be assumed that DD is a multi-componential and probabilistic, rather than uni-causal and deterministic, neurodevelopmental disorder of learning to read (e.g., Carroll, Solity, & Shapiro, 2016; Franceschini et al., 2012). As a case in point, a longitudinal study by Clark and colleagues (2014) showed that the primary neuroanatomical abnormalities that precede DD are in lower-level areas responsible for visual and auditory processing, and frontal-attentional functions. These findings suggest that dysfunctions in the reading network (e.g., Pugh et al., 2000) may be also a consequence of different reading experiences and deficits. Although Langer and colleagues (2017) showed abnormalities in the white matter in the areas related to speech in children at risk for DD, explaining DD with a single cause seems to be an unsuccessful approach. It will be argued that at least one cause of DD should be sought in the area of visual perceptual and attentional deficits.

14.3   Research Evidence

It is now considered that one cause of DD is a visual attention deficit, independent of the subject's auditory-phonological abilities (e.g., Franceschini et al., 2012, 2013, 2015; Gabrieli & Norton, 2012; Gori, Seitz et al., 2016). The visual-orthographic system receives an attention-orienting influence that modulates all visual processing levels (for reviews see Corbetta & Shulman, 2002, 2011; Facoetti, 2012; Vidyasagar & Pammer, 2010) from the primary visual cortex (V1) to the visual word form area. This specific region of the fusiform gyrus is involved in identifying words and letters from the visual input, preceding the association with phonology or semantics (Dehaene et al., 2015). During word decoding, attentional orienting is considered the resultant of the engagement mechanism onto a letter or grapheme – which has to be mapped to its corresponding speech sound – and the subsequent disengagement mechanism (see Vidyasagar & Pammer, 2010, for a review). It is important to note that engagement and disengagement of visuo-attention orienting occur before linguistic sublexical and lexical mapping, making the efficient functioning of these mechanisms crucial for reading acquisition in writing systems, irrespective of the varying degrees of consistency in letter-to-speech-sound relationships of those systems.

A visual attentional orienting deficit has been systematically found in DD, irrespective of the transparency of the alphabetic writing system (for reviews see Facoetti, 2004, 2012; Franceschini, Trevisan et al., 2017; Gori & Facoetti, 2014, 2015; Gori et al., 2016; Hari & Renvall, 2001; Stein, 2014; Valdois et al.,

2004; Vidyasagar & Pammer, 2010), and more specifically in individuals with DD characterized by poor phonological decoding skills (e.g., Cestnick & Coltheart, 1999; Facoetti, Trussardi et al., 2010; Facoetti et al., 2006; Roach & Hogben, 2007; Ruffino et al., 2010, 2014). Interestingly, Liu, Chen, and Chung (2015) found that attentional abilities – independently from phonology and orthography – predict reading skills also in morpheme-based orthographies, such as Chinese.

Evidence on the role of visual attention in decoding also comes from a training study by Franceschini et al. (2013). They showed the effects of an action video-game (AVG) training session on the spotlight of attention in children with DD in the visual attention span task (Bosse, Tainturier, & Valdois, 2007), whereby participants had to identify one of six visual stimuli. Training with AVG, compared to non-action video-game (NAVG) training, led children with DD to improve their abilities in stimulus discrimination both in a condition of zoom-out (large) and zoom-in (small) attention spotlight (Franceschini et al., 2013). It could be argued that the zoom-in attention spotlight is crucial in shallow languages (e.g., Italian) because the reading unit is primarily composed of one or two letters, while the zoom-out attention spotlight is necessary to read larger group of letters that are at the basis of reading in opaque languages (e.g., English; Franceschini, Trevisan et al., 2017). Consequently, regardless of the consistency between orthography and phonology, training with AVG could make the weaker attention spotlight of individuals with DD more efficient (e.g., Moores, Tsouknida, & Romani, 2015).

It is important to note that word reading in individuals with DD may be slowed down because of greater crowding effects, which is in agreement with the peculiar spatial distribution of attention that is also found in these individuals (Martelli et al., 2009; Zorzi et al., 2012; see Gori & Facoetti, 2015 for a review). Visual crowding occurs when an object becomes harder to identify when surrounded by other objects than when it is in isolation (see Whitney & Levi, 2011 for a review). Recognition is impaired when objects are closer to each other than a critical degree of spacing (e.g., Yu et al., 2007), which is the distance between objects at which target recognition is restored (Martelli et al., 2009). Crowding might thus be the result of a limit in the resolution of spatial attention (e.g., He, Cavanagh, & Intriligator, 1996; Petrov & Meleshkevich, 2011; see Gori & Facoetti, 2015 for a review).

Extra-large spacing between letters and words can reduce crowding. Zorzi et al. (2012) showed that a simple manipulation of letter spacing improved text-reading performance in online reading without any training in a large, unselected sample of Italian and French children with DD. Written French is much more opaque than Italian. In contrast, younger controls matched on reading level (RL) did not show any improvement with extra-large spacing. This result is congruent with a previous study of Italian children by Spinelli et al. (2002) in which a moderate increase in spacing between letters improved reading only in individuals with DD. Perea et al. (2012) demonstrated that slight increases in inter-letter spacing improved the readability of texts aimed at Spanish children, especially those with DD. Recently, Schneps and colleagues (Schneps, Thomson, Chen et al., 2013; Schneps, Thomson, Sonnert et al., 2013) showed that reducing crowding by presenting fewer words in a line on a small screen improved reading abilities in English-speaking individuals with DD. This reading improvement is interpreted as a consequence of the reduced amount of attention necessary to perform tasks (Schneps, Thomson, Chen et al., 2013; Schneps, Thomson, Sonnert et al., 2013; Zorzi et al., 2012). Difficulties with both, words and symbols, indicate that the crowding effect takes place before the process of letter-to-speech sound integration (Moores et al., 2015; Spinelli et al., 2002).

Importantly, there is also evidence that temporal orienting of attention in the so-called attentional blink task may result in impairments for individuals with DD (Stein, 2014). The attentional blink task (Raymond, Shapiro, & Arnell, 1992) consists of two targets shown in rapid sequence among distractors. This task evaluates the subject's temporal attention disengagement abilities. Longer recovery times in individuals with DD and in children with a specific language impairment (SLI) was found relative to controls in disengaging attention from the first target (Facoetti et al., 2008; Hari, Renvall, & Tanskanen, 2001; Laasonen et al., 2012; Lum, Conti-Ramsden, & Lindell, 2007; see Badcock & Kidd, 2015 for a recent review). Individuals with DD and SLI also show poorer performance in temporal attention engagement on the target when it is rapidly followed by a second object (i.e., backward masking; Di Lollo, Hanson, & McIntyre, 1983; Dispaldro et al., 2013; Facoetti et al., 2008; Ruffino et al., 2010, 2014). This temporal attention engagement deficit was recently demonstrated to be causally linked to DD by the use of perceptual-learning training (Gori, Seitz et al., 2016) that improved reading abilities alongside temporal attention performance.

Individuals with DD suffer from a deficit of rapid attentional orienting, affecting not only single-sensory but also cross-sensory attention (e.g., Virsu, Lahti-Nuuttila, & Laasonen, 2003). Auditory processing deficits are characteristic of DD (Tallal, 2004). Children with SLI and DD show difficulties in perceiving speech–sound when it is presented with background noise (e.g., Boets et al., 2011; Geiger et al., 2008; Ziegler et al., 2005). Rapid auditory processing in infants and toddlers can predict their future language acquisition skills (Benasich & Tallal, 2002). These disorders in auditory perceptual noise exclusion could be caused by an attentional deficit (Facoetti et al., 2005, 2003, Facoetti, Trussardi et al., 2010; Renvall & Hari, 2002). The temporo-parietal phonological system is influenced by auditory attention, which modulates the primary auditory cortex up to the left perisylvian language network (Boets et al., 2013; Dehaene et al., 2015).

Although some researchers have argued that there is a lack of evidence on causal links between visual attentional deficit and DD (Goswami, 2015), long-itudinal studies and studies with pre-reading children at risk for DD have shown that visual attention orienting is one of the most important predictors of early reading abilities (e.g., Carroll et al., 2016; Facoetti, Corradi et al., 2010; Franceschini et al., 2012). In addition, the relationship between attentional skills in pre-reading children and their future reading abilities has been found to be fully independent of phonological processing (Franceschini et al., 2012; Gori, Seitz et al., 2016). These results clearly rule out the possible explanation suggested by Goswami (2015) according to which the reading experience is supposed to play a major role in explaining the attentional deficit found in children with DD. It is important to remember that these studies involved samples that were composed of children with DD but without ADHD. In conclusion, it is proposed that one of the core cognitive deficits underlying DD is that of the fundamental multimodal spatial and temporal attention-orienting mechanisms (which affect both visual and auditory perception) that mediate efficient orthographic–phonological binding (Gori & Facoetti, 2014, 2015; Hari & Renvall, 2001); this suggests that attention could also influence the typical auditory-phonological deficits associated with DD (e.g., Facoetti, Trussardi et al., 2010; Franceschini, Trevisan et al., 2017).

14.4   Explanatory Mechanisms

A possible neurobiological substrate of temporal and spatial-attention-orienting deficits in DD could be a weakened magnocellular–dorsal (M–D) stream, and a consequent dysfunction of the main fronto-parietal attentional network (Facoetti, 2012; Livingstone et al., 1991; Stein & Walsh, 1997). Although Wright, Conlon, and Dyck (2012) suggested that in DD the weaker M sensitivity and visual spatial attention deficits may be independent, an impaired attentional orienting system (Boden & Giaschi, 2007; Hari & Renvall, 2001; Vidyasagar & Pammer, 2010) is anatomically contained in the M–D stream. Accordingly, several neurophysiological and neuroimaging studies of both typical and atypical reading development (e.g., Cao et al., 2013; Takashima et al., 2014; Turkeltaub et al., 2003; see for review Richlan, 2012) have consistently implicated M–D areas that are known to be part of the visual attention-orienting system (Corbetta & Shulman, 2011). The visual word form area is functionally connected with the dorsal fronto-parietal attention network in the inferior parietal lobule (Vogel et al., 2012). Vidyasagar (1999) proposed that an attentional deficit – strongly related to an M–D deficit – could be the main cause of DD (Vidyasagar & Pammer, 2010).

The theory of a mild M–D deficit as the basis of DD stemmed from the observation that the majority of reading-disabled children are impaired specifically in the visual M–D pathway (Boden & Giaschi, 2007; Gori & Facoetti, 2014, 2015; Stein, 2014; Stein & Walsh, 1997; Vidyasagar & Pammer, 2010). The M–D deficit theory is a dominant, albeit controversial, account (e.g., Olulade, Napoliello, & Eden, 2013). The M–D pathway originates in the ganglion cells of the retina, passes through the M layer of the LGN, and finally reaches the occipital and parietal cortices (Maunsell & Newsome, 1987). This pathway consists of large, heavily myelinated neurons with high conduction velocity (Pammer, 2014). The M–D stream is blind to colors and responds optimally to contrast differences, low spatial frequencies, high temporal frequencies, and both real and illusory motion (e.g., Agrillo, Gori, & Beran, 2015; Gori, Agrillo et al., 2014; Gori, Giora, & Stubbs, 2010; Gori et al., 2011; Gori & Hamburger, 2006; Gori & Yazdanbakhsh 2008; Livingstone & Hubel, 1987; Morrone et al., 2000; Ruzzoli et al., 2011; Yazdanbakhsh & Gori, 2011). Much of the evidence supporting the M–D deficit theory of DD is related to research on perception of coherent dot motion (CDM; e.g., Boets et al., 2011; Cornelissen et al., 1995), which heavily relies upon processing within the M–D pathway (Newsome & Pare, 1998).

Consistent with the M–D deficit theory of DD, individuals with DD and prereaders at risk of DD show poor performance on CDM tasks compared to typical reading controls (Boets et al., 2011; Eden, VanMeter, & Rumsey, 1996; Gori, Seitz et al., 2016; Kevan & Pammer, 2008), while performing similarly to the controls on tasks mainly associated with the parvocellular-ventral pathway (Gori, Cecchini et al., 2014, Gori et al., 2015; Kevan & Pammer, 2009). It has been reported that up to 75 percent of dyslexic individuals show visual M–D processing deficits (Lovegrove, Martin, & Slaghuis, 1986). Moreover, a postmortem study showed that M-neurons of the LGN were significantly smaller in individuals with DD than those of normal readers. On the contrary, the parvocellular neurons did not vary between the two groups (Livingstone et al., 1991). These findings were confirmed by an in vivo MRI study (Giraldo-Chica, Hegarty, & Schneider, 2015). Recently, Gori et al. (2015) demonstrated that children with DD showed lower performance in tasks related to visual illusions that rely upon the M–D pathway (i.e., the spatial frequency doubling illusion, Kelly, 1966; the rotating tilted lines illusion and the accordion grating illusion, Gori et al., 2010, 2011, 2013; Gori & Hamburger 2006; Gori & Yazdanbakhsh, 2008; Yazdanbakhsh & Gori, 2011) in comparison with both age-matched and RL controls. Gori et al. (2015) also reported the first association between a genetic variance (the DCDC2-Intron 2 deletion) and M–D deficits in both individuals with DD and typical readers. Interestingly the M–D deficit in individuals with DD was found also in logographic languages such as Chinese (e.g., Zhao et al., 2014).

While a substantial body of evidence suggests a relationship between M–D processing and DD (Stein, 2014), the main criticism of this theory has been that M–D deficits may not be causal to DD and, instead, could be a consequence of lack of reading experience (Goswami, 2015; Olulade et al., 2013) since children with DD read far less than their peers (e.g., Cunningham & Stanovich, 1997). Recently, Gori, Seitz, and colleagues (2016) showed that: (i) motion perception was impaired in children with DD in comparison both to age-matched and to RL controls; (ii) pre-reading visual motion perception – independent of auditory-phonological skill – predicted future reading development; (iii) targeted M–D training sessions – not involving any phonological stimulation – led to improved reading skill in children and adults with DD; and (iv) in a parvocellular-ventral task involving noise exclusion, no difference in the DD group was found. These findings demonstrate, for the first time, a causal relationship between M–D deficits and DD, although it should be noted that this study was conducted on unselected samples. However, notwithstanding the heterogenic nature of the cognitive profiles on DD, the M–D deficit seems to be so basic that it may have a cascade effect on the other cognitive functions.

14.5   Clinical Implications

Evidence shows that there is no word identification without spatial attention orienting (e.g., Robidoux, Rauwerda, & Besner, 2014). Specific intervention studies led to improvements in both auditory and visual orienting of attention children with DD (e.g., Facoetti et al., 2003; Franceschini, Trevisan et al., 2017; Franceschini et al., 2013; Geiger, Lettvin, & Fahle, 1994). These studies demonstrated that the inhibitory mechanism of attentional orienting – which is crucial for perceptual noise exclusion – can be remediated with appropriate rehabilitation programs. Computer games have proven to be efficient in improving auditory temporal processing and spatial attention in children with SLI (Stevens et al., 2008; see Tallal, 2004; Tallal et al., 1996, for a review).

There is evidence that playing action video games also significantly improves visual and auditory attentional orienting (Green & Bavelier, 2003; Green, Pouget, & Bavelier, 2010). AVG training generalizes to various tasks beyond game situations, allowing gamers to better allocate their attention across both space and time. AVGs share an extraordinary speed in terms of transient events and moving objects, a high degree of perceptual and motor load, and an emphasis on peripheral processing. All these visual characteristics are processed by the M–D stream; consequently the AVG treatment could be mainly tapping into the M–D pathway (Franceschini et al., 2013; Gori & Facoetti, 2014; Gori, Seitz et al., 2016). In a study by Franceschini et al. (2013), it was demonstrated, for the first time, that AVG training makes children with DD read better. These authors measured the phonological decoding of pseudowords and words and text-reading skills in children with DD before and after two video-game training sessions (AVG or NAVG). After twelve hours of treatment (nine days in total) the AVG training players improved in basic phonological decoding and in lexical recognition as measured by reading words in a text. Results, in syllables per second, showed that children treated with AVG training showed a level of improvement higher than that which would be expected in a child with DD after one year of schooling, and greater than or equal to those obtained by the highly demanding traditional DD training (Franceschini et al., 2013). Individual analysis showed that 80 percent of AVG players differed statistically from the NAVG group. After AVG training, attentional and reading improvements were highly correlated even after controlling for phonological-training-induced changes, suggesting that such gains cannot be explained by phonological factors as argued by Goswami (2015). These results have been confirmed in a second study (Gori, Seitz et al., 2016), in which a group of children with DD were trained, using NAVG before and AVG after, in a within-subject design. The NAVG training led to no significant effects. On the contrary, training with AVG showed significant improvements in word and pseudoword text reading, which stresses the importance of using AVG as a possible training method in DD. These results were further confirmed when children with DD were in comorbidity with dyscalculia (Gori, Tait et al., 2014). In these AVG training studies (Franceschini et al., 2013; Gori, Seitz et al., 2016; Gori, Tait et al., 2014) no drop-out was observed.

Although the association between a mild M–D deficit and DD has been consistently observed (see Boden & Giaschi, 2007; Gori & Facoetti, 2014, 2015; Hari & Renvall, 2001; Laycock & Crewther, 2008; Schulte-Körne & Bruder, 2010; Stein, 2012, 2014; Stein & Walsh, 1997; Vidyasagar, 1999; Vidyasagar & Pammer, 2010; Walsh, 1995, for reviews), the lack of studies employing training designs has led to debate regarding the relationship between M–D pathway deficits and reading disorders (Goswami, 2015). Interestingly, Gori, Seitz, and colleagues (2016) showed that not only reading skills, but also M–D pathway functionality were specifically improved after AVG training in children with DD, whereas parvocellular-ventral performances were unaffected. The specific effect of AVG training on the M–D pathway is confirmed also by improved illusory motion perception; this is an accepted proxy of M–D functionality that is not related to perceptual noise exclusion (Gori, Seitz et al., 2016). These results not only expand on previous findings, but also indicate that the underlying neural substrate of the AVG training appears to be the M–D pathway.

AVG training presents important advantages to the development of specific training modules for DD, because it features an appealing task that encourages compliance. However, the complex tasks involved in commercial video games make it difficult to isolate the core mechanisms of how this type of training impacts DD. Consequently, a form of training that is specifically based on the M–D pathway is necessary to further establish the causal role of the M–D deficit in DD. In the same study, Gori, Seitz, and colleagues (2016) showed that direct training of the M–D pathway based on a *CDM* perceptual-learning procedure drastically improved the reading skills of adults with DD. Improvements in the M–D pathway functioning directly translated to better reading skills. Specific M–D pathway training also increased both peripheral visual perception and the temporal mechanism of visual attention orienting, confirming the suggested link between M–D pathway functioning and attentional mechanisms. Moreover, the training-induced perceptual and attentional changes explained a large proportion of variance in the reading performance gain of the individuals with DD, which demonstrates the causal link between M–D pathway and reading skills (see also Lawton, 2016).

Furthermore, Gori, Seitz, and colleagues (2016) found significant improvement in auditory-phonological abilities after AVG treatment, showing that M–D functioning and attentional training can also affect phonological skills (see also Lawton, 2016). These findings confirm the cross- and multisensory effects of the AVG training (e.g., Franceschini, Trevisan et al., 2017; Franceschini et al., 2013; Green et al., 2010). Indeed, Green et al. (2010) demonstrated that AVG can improve a range of spatial and temporal aspects of visual and auditory attention, not strictly connected to those directly trained by the video-game use per se. The authors also showed that a better use of sensory evidence (or target filtering) could be obtained by AVG players in tasks that involved not only visual, but also auditory stimuli (see Bavelier et al., 2012; Dye, Green, & Bavelier, 2009; Green & Bavelier, 2012, for reviews of the "learn-to-learn" effects of AVGs). There is consistent evidence in support of the M–D temporal hypothesis that explicitly claims that phonological decoding deficits in individuals with DD could arise from impairments in sensory processing of visual and auditory dynamic stimuli (e.g., Facoetti, Trussardi et al., 2010; Lallier, Tainturier et al., 2010; Vidyasagar, 2013; Witton et al., 1998).

It is important to note that the studies by Franceschini et al. (2013), Gori, Cecchini et al. (2014), and Gori, Seitz et al. (2016) were based on Italian, a relatively transparent orthography in comparison to other languages, such as English. One may argue that these results could not be easily generalized to opaque orthographies, such as English, because of the high level of transparency characterizing Italian. In transparent orthographies it is possible that phonological deficits may be less relevant for DD than in more opaque ones. However, difference in orthographic transparency does not seem to be crucial. Indeed, there is evidence that both word recognition and phonological decoding have also been significantly and clinically improved in English-speaking children with DD thus confirming the pattern even in this language

(Franceschini, Trevisan et al., 2017). In this recent study, auditory-phonological working memory, as well as visual-to-auditory attention orienting, were significantly improved, confirming that the direct role of multisensory and cross-modal attention-orienting mechanisms in reading remediation is also present in more opaque orthographies. It could be supposed that the perceptual and the attentional mechanisms controlled by the M–D pathway precede the orthographic-to-phonological mapping (e.g., Pammer et al., 2006; Zorzi et al., 2012). Attentional and M–D deficits are peripheral by definition. The DD characterized by peripheral deficits is often found irrespective of varying degrees of orthographic transparency (Zorzi et al., 2012). Thus, it is likely that attentional and M–D training will be beneficial to individuals with DD regardless of the DD subtype and the depth of the language.

To date, DD prevention is only a dream, far from being realized (Gabrieli, 2009). However, Gori, Bertoni and colleagues (2016) showed that only twenty hours of playing AVG – which did not involve any direct phonological or orthographic training – improved early visual and auditory predictors of future reading abilities in pre-reading children at risk of DD. Gori, Bertoni, and colleagues (2016) tested rapid naming, letter knowledge, auditory-phonological skills and visuo-attentional spotlight efficiency (i.e., earliest predictors of reading acquisition) in three matched groups of pre-reading children at cognitive risk of DD before and after they played AVG or NAVG, as well as a no-treatment group, for twenty sessions of sixty minutes per day. It was found that only playing AVG improved the visual and phonological predictors of future reading abilities in pre-reading children. These results show that attention-orienting improvements can directly translate into better language abilities in pre-reading children at risk of DD, providing a new, fast, and fun training method for the prevention of DD.

14.6   Discussion and Conclusion

In summary, several findings, which are consistent across methods and languages, demonstrate the causal role of visual attention and M–D pathway deficits in DD. It can thus be assumed that the unsuccessful search for a single cause of DD makes the identification of causes other than phonological awareness of utmost importance. Attentional and M–D pathway training were found to remediate DD independently of auditory-phonological approaches. Inside a multifactorial and probabilistic hypothesis for DD (Menghini et al., 2010), attentional and M–D pathway training seems to be a very promising future practice that should be added to the more traditional approaches for DD remediation. The most intriguing aspect of these types of visual training is the possibility to obtain generalization of the visual aspect of reading by using visual stimuli that are far from strings of letters, often on the basis of more traditional language and phonological decoding training modules. A combination of these kinds of treatment may further reduce drop-out rate improve reading remediation for children with DD. The fact that both visual attentional and M–D pathway deficits can be tested and trained during infancy paves the way for more effective DD remediation and prevention programs.

References

Agrillo, C., Gori, S., & Beran, M. J. (2015). Do rhesus monkeys (Macacamulatta) perceive illusory motion? *Animal Cognition*, *18*, 895–910. doi: http://dx.doi.org/10 .1007/s10071-015-0860-6.

Badcock, N. A., & Kidd, J. C. (2015). Temporal variability predicts the magnitude of between-group attentional blink differences in developmental dyslexia: A meta-analysis. *PeerJ*, *3*(e746), 1–18. doi: http://dx.doi.org/10.7717/peerj.746.

Ball, E. W., & Blachman, B. A. (1988). Phoneme segmentation training: Effect on reading readiness. *Annals of Dyslexia*, *38*, 208–225.

Battelli, L., Pascual-Leone, A., & Cavanagh, P. (2007). The "when" pathway of the right parietal lobe. *Trends in Cognitive Sciences*, *11*, 204–210. doi: http://dx.doi.org/10 .1016/j.tics.2007.03.001.

Bavelier, D., Green, C. S., Pouget, A., & Schrater, P. (2012). Brain plasticity through the life span: Learning to learn and action video games. *Annual Review of Neurosciences*, *35*, 391–416.

Benasich, A. A., & Tallal, P. (2002). Infant discrimination of rapid auditory cues predicts later language impairment. *Behavioural Brain Research*, *136*, 31–49.

Boden, C., & Giaschi, D. (2007). M-stream deficits and reading-related visual processes in developmental dyslexia. *Psychological Bulletin*, *133*, 346–366. doi: http://dx .doi.org/10.1037/0033-2909.133.2.346.

Boets, B., de Beeck, H. P. O., Vandermosten, M. et al. (2013). Intact but less accessible phonetic representations in adults with dyslexia. *Science*, *342*(6163), 1251–1254.

Boets, B., Vandermosten, M., Cornelissen, P., Wouters, J., & Ghesquière, P. (2011). Coherent motion sensitivity and reading development in the transition from pre-reading to reading stage. *Child Development*, *82*, 854–869. doi: http://dx .doi.org/10.1111/j.1467-8624.2010.01527.x.

Bosse, M. L., Tainturier, M. J., & Valdois, S. (2007). Developmental dyslexia: The visual attention span deficit hypothesis. *Cognition*, *104*, 198–230. doi: http://dx .doi.org/10.1016/j.cognition.2006.05.009.

Bradley, L., & Bryant, P. E. (1983). Categorizing sounds and learning to read – A causal connection. *Nature*, *301*, 419–421.

Cao, F., Rickles, B., Vu, M. et al. (2013). Early stage visual-orthographic processes predict long-term retention of word form and meaning: A visual encoding training study. *Journal of Neurolinguistics*, *26*, 440–461.

Carrasco, M. (2011). Visual attention: The past 25 years. *Vision Research*, *51*, 1484–1525. doi: http://dx.doi.org/10.1016/j.visres.2011.04.012.

Carroll, J. M., Solity, J., & Shapiro, L. R. (2016). Predicting dyslexia using pre-reading skills: The role of sensorimotor and cognitive abilities. *Journal of Child Psychology and Psychiatry*, *57*, 750–758.

Castles, A., & Coltheart, M. (2004). Is there a causal link from phonological awareness to success in learning to read? *Cognition, 91,* 77–111. doi: http://dx.doi.org/10.1016/S0010-0277(03)00164-1.

Cestnick, L., & Coltheart, M. (1999). The relationship between language-processing and visual-processing deficits in developmental dyslexia. *Cognition, 71,* 231–255. doi: http://dx.doi.org/10.1016/S0010-0277(99)00023-2.

Clark, K. A., Helland, T., Specht, K. et al. (2014). Neuroanatomical precursors of dyslexia identified from pre-reading through to age 11. *Brain, 137,* 3136–3141. doi: http://dx.doi.org/10.1093/brain/awu229.

Corbetta, M., & Shulman, G. L. (2002). Control of goal-directed and stimulus-driven attention in the brain. *Nature Review Neuroscience, 3,* 201–215. doi: http://dx.doi.org/10.1038/nrn755.

Corbetta, M., & Shulman, G. L. (2011). Spatial neglect and attention networks. *Annual Review of Neuroscience, 34,* 569–599. doi: http://dx.doi.org/10.1146/annurev-neuro-061010-113731.

Cornelissen, P., Richardson, A., Mason, A., Fowler, S., & Stein, J. (1995). Contrast sensitivity and coherent motion detection measured at photopic luminance levels in dyslexics and controls. *Vision Research, 35,* 1483–1494.

Cunningham, A. E., & Stanovich, K. E. (1997). Early reading acquisition and its relation to reading experience and ability 10 years later. *Developmental Psychology, 33,* 934–945.

Dehaene, S., Cohen, L., Morais, J., & Kolinsky, R. (2015). Illiterate to literate: Behavioural and cerebral changes induced by reading acquisition. *Nature Review Neuroscience, 16,* 234–244. doi: http://dx.doi.org/10.1038/nrn3924.

Di Lollo, V., Hanson, D., & McIntyre, J. S. (1983). Initial stages of visual information processing in dyslexia. *Journal of Experimental Psychology: Human Perception & Performance, 9,* 923–935. doi: http://dx.doi.org/10.1037/0096-1523.9.6.923.

Dispaldro, M., Leonard, L. B., Corradi, N. et al. (2013). Visual attentional engagement deficits in children with Specific Language Impairment and their role in real-time language processing. *Cortex, 49,* 2126–2139. doi: http://dx.doi.org/10.1016/j.cortex.2012.09.012.

Dye, M. W., Green, C. S., & Bavelier, D. (2009). Increasing speed of processing with action video games. *Current Direction in Psychology Science, 18,* 321–326.

Eden, G. F., VanMeter, J. W., & Rumsey, J. M. (1996). Abnormal processing of visual motion in dyslexia revealed by functional brain imaging. *Nature, 382,* 66–69. doi:10.1038/382066a0.

Facoetti, A. (2004). Reading and selective spatial attention: Evidence from behavioral studies in dyslexic children. In H. D. Tobias (Ed.), *Trends in dyslexia research* (pp. 35–71). New York, NY: Nova Biomedical Books.

Facoetti, A. (2012). Spatial attention disorders in developmental dyslexia: Towards the prevention of reading acquisition deficits. In J. Stein & Z. Kapoula (Eds.), *Visual aspects of dyslexia* (pp. 123–136). Oxford: Oxford University Press. doi: http://dx.doi.org/10.1093/acprof:oso/9780199589814.003.0008.

Facoetti, A., Corradi, N., Ruffino, M., Gori, S., & Zorzi, M. (2010). Visual spatial attention and speech segmentation are both impaired in preschoolers at familial risk for developmental dyslexia. *Dyslexia, 16,* 226–239. doi: http://dx.doi.org/10.1002/dys.413.

Facoetti, A., Lorusso, M. L., Cattaneo, C., Galli, R., & Molteni, M. (2005). Visual and auditory attentional capture are both sluggish in children with developmental dyslexia. *Acta NeurobiologiaeExperimentalis, 65*, 61–72.

Facoetti, A., Lorusso, M. L., Paganoni, P., Umiltà, C., & Mascetti, G. G. (2003). The role of visuospatial attention in developmental dyslexia: Evidence from a rehabilitation study. *Cognitive Brain Research, 15*, 154–164. doi: http://dx.doi.org /10.1016/S0926-6410(02)00148-9.

Facoetti, A., & Molteni, M. (2000). Is attentional focusing an inhibitory process at distractor location? *Cognitive Brain Research, 10*, 185–188. doi: http://dx.doi.org/10 .1016/S0926-6410(00)00031-8.

Facoetti, A., Paganoni, P., Turatto, M., Marzola, V., & Mascetti, G. G. (2000). Visual-spatial attention in developmental dyslexia. *Cortex, 36*, 109–123.

Facoetti, A., Ruffino, M., Peru, A., Paganoni, P., & Chelazzi, L. (2008). Sluggish engagement and disengagement of non-spatial attention in dyslexic children. *Cortex, 44*, 1221–1233. doi: http://dx.doi.org/10.1016/j.cortex.2007.10.007.

Facoetti, A., Trussardi, A. N., Ruffino, M. et al. (2010). Multisensory spatial attention deficits are predictive of phonological decoding skills in developmental dyslexia. *Journal of Cognitive Neuroscience, 22*, 1011–1025. doi: http://dx.doi.org/10.1162/j ocn.2009.21232.

Facoetti, A., Zorzi, M., Cestnick, L. et al. (2006). The relationship between visuo-spatial attention and nonword reading in developmental dyslexia. *Cognitive Neuropsychology, 23*, 841–855. doi: http://dx.doi.org/10.1080/02643290500483090.

Franceschini, S., Bertoni, S., Gianesini, T., Gori, S., & Facoetti, A. (2017). A different vision of dyslexia: Local precedence on global perception. *Scientific Reports, 7*, 17462. doi: http://dx.doi.org/10.1038/s41598-017-17626-1.

Franceschini, S., Bertoni, S., Ronconi, L. et al. (2015). "Shall we play a game?": Improving reading through action video games in developmental dyslexia. *Current Developmental Disorders Reports, 2*, 318–329. doi: http://dx.doi.org/10.1007/s404 74-015-0064-4.

Franceschini, S., Gori, S., Ruffino, M., Pedrolli, K., & Facoetti, A. (2012). A causal link between visual spatial attention and reading acquisition. *Current Biology, 22*, 814–819. doi: http://dx.doi.org/10.1016/j.cub.2012.03.013.

Franceschini, S., Gori, S., Ruffino, M. et al. (2013). Action video games make dyslexic children read better. *Current Biology, 23*, 462–466. doi: http://dx.doi.org/10.1016/j .cub.2013.01.044.

Franceschini, S., Trevisan, P., Ronconi, L. et al. (2017). Action video games improve reading abilities and visual-to-auditory attentional shifting in English-speaking children with dyslexia. *Scientific Reports, 7*, 5863.

Gabrieli, J. D. (2009). Dyslexia: A new synergy between education and cognitive neuroscience. *Science, 325*, 280–283. doi: http://dx.doi.org/10.1126/science .1171999.

Gabrieli, J. D., & Norton, E. S. (2012). Reading abilities: Importance of visual-spatial attention. *Current Biology, 22*, R298–R299. doi: http://dx.doi.org/10.1016/j .cub.2012.03.041.

Galuschka, K., Ise, E., Krick, K., & Schulte-Körne, G. (2014). Effectiveness of treatment approaches for children and adolescents with reading disabilities: A meta-analysis of randomized controlled trials. *PLoS One, 9*(2), e89900. doi: http://dx .doi.org/10.1371/journal.pone.0089900.

Geiger, G., Cattaneo, C., Galli, R. et al. (2008). Wide and diffuse perceptual modes characterize dyslexics in vision and audition. *Perception, 37*, 1745–1764.

Geiger, G., Lettvin, J. Y., & Fahle, M. (1994). Dyslexic children learn a new visual strategy for reading: A controlled experiment. *Vision Research, 34*, 1223–1233. doi:10.1016/0042-6989(94)90303-4.

Giraldo-Chica, M., Hegarty, J. P., & Schneider, K. A. (2015). Morphological differences in the lateral geniculate nucleus associated with dyslexia. *Neuroimage Clinical, 7*, 830–836. doi:10.1016/j.nicl.2015.03.011.

Gori, S., Agrillo, A., Dadda, M., & Bisazza,A. (2014). Do fish perceive illusory motion? *Scientific Reports, 4*, 6443. doi: http://dx.doi.org/10.1038/srep06443.

Gori, S., Bertoni, S., Sali, M. E. et al. (2016). Dyslexia prevention by action video game training: Behavioural and neurophysiological evidence. *Journal of Vision, 16*, 489. doi: http://dx.doi.org/10.1167/16.12.489.

Gori, S., Cecchini, P., Bigoni, A., Molteni, M., & Facoetti, A. (2014). Magnocellular-dorsal pathway and sub-lexical route in developmental dyslexia. *Frontiers in Human Neuroscience, 8*, 460. doi: http://dx.doi.org/10.3389/fnhum.2014.00460.

Gori, S., & Facoetti, A. (2014). Perceptual learning as a possible new approach for remediation and prevention of developmental dyslexia. *Vision Research, 99*, 78–87. doi: http://dx.doi.org/10.1016/j.visres.2013.11.011.

Gori, S., & Facoetti, A. (2015). How the visual aspects can be crucial in reading acquisition? The intriguing case of crowding and developmental dyslexia. *Journal of Vision, 15*, 8. doi: http://dx.doi.org/10.1167/15.1.8.

Gori, S., Giora, E., & Stubbs, D. A. (2010). Perceptual compromise between apparent and veridical motion indices: The Unchained-Dots illusion. *Perception, 39*, 863–866. doi: http://dx.doi.org/10.1068/p6678.

Gori, S., Giora, E., Yazdanbakhsh, A., & Mingolla, E. (2011). A new motion illusion based on competition between two kinds of motion processing units: The Accordion Grating. *Neural Networks, 24*, 1082–1092. doi: http://dx.doi.org/10.1016/j.neunet.2011.06.017.

Gori, S., Giora, E., Yazdanbakhsh, A., & Mingolla, E. (2013). The novelty of the "Accordion Grating Illusion." *Neural Network, 39*, 52. doi: http://dx.doi.org/10.1016/j.neunet.2012.07.008.

Gori, S., & Hamburger, K. (2006). A new motion illusion: The Rotating-Tilted-Lines illusion. *Perception, 35*, 853–857. doi: http://dx.doi.org/10.1068/p5531.

Gori, S., Mascheretti, S., Giora, E. et al. (2015). The *DCDC2* intron 2 deletion impairs illusory motion perception unveiling the selective role of magnocellular-dorsal stream in reading (dis)ability. *Cerebral Cortex, 25*, 1685–1695. doi: http://dx.doi.org/10.1093/cercor/bhu234.

Gori, S., Molteni, M., & Facoetti, A. (2016). Visual illusions: An interesting tool to investigate developmental dyslexia and autism spectrum disorder. *Frontiers in Human Neuroscience, 10*, 175. doi: http://dx.doi.org/10.3389/fnhum.2016.00175.

Gori, S., Seitz, A. R., Ronconi, L., Franceschini, S., & Facoetti, A. (2016). Multiple causal links between magnocellular–dorsal pathway deficit and developmental dyslexia. *Cerebral Cortex, 26*, 4356–4369.

Gori, S., Tait, M., Franceschini, S. et al. (2014, July). *Dyscalculia remediation by action video games*. Abstract Number: FENS-3332. Poster session presented at Forum of Neuroscience (FENS), Milan, Italy.

Gori, S., & Yazdanbakhsh, A. (2008). The riddle of the Rotating-Tilted-Lines illusion. *Perception, 37,* 631–635. doi: http://dx.doi.org/10.1068/p5770.

Goswami, U. (2015). Sensory theories of developmental dyslexia: Three challenges for research. *Nature Reviews Neuroscience, 16,* 43–54. doi: http://dx.doi.org/10.1038/nrn3836.

Green, C. S., & Bavelier, D. (2003). Action video game modifies visual selective attention. *Nature, 423,* 534–537.

Green, C. S., & Bavelier, D. (2012). Learning, attentional control and action video games. *Current Biology, 22,* R197–R206. doi: http://dx.doi.org/10.1016/j.cub.2012.02.012.

Green, C. S., Pouget, A., & Bavelier, D. (2010). Improved probabilistic inference as a general learning mechanism with action video games. *Current Biology, 20,* 1573–1579. doi: http://dx.doi.org/10.1016/j.cub.2010.07.040.

Hari, R., & Renvall, H. (2001). Impaired processing of rapid stimulus sequences in dyslexia. *Trends in Cognitive Sciences, 5,* 525–532. doi: http://dx.doi.org/10.1016/S1364-6613(00)01801-5.

Hari, R., Renvall, H., & Tanskanen, T. (2001). Left minineglect in dyslexic adults. *Brain, 124,* 1373–1380.

He, S., Cavanagh, P., & Intriligator, J. (1996). Attentional resolution and the locus of visual awareness. *Nature, 383,* 334–337. doi: http://dx.doi.org/10.1038/383334a0.

Kelly, D. (1966). Frequency doubling in visual responses. *Journal of the Optical Society of America, 56,* 1628–1633. doi: http://dx.doi.org/10.1364/JOSA.56.001628.

Kevan, A., & Pammer, K. (2008). Visual deficits in pre-readers at familial risk for dyslexia. *Vision Research, 48,* 2835–2839. doi: http://dx.doi.org/10.1016/j.visres.2008.09.022.

Kevan, A., & Pammer, K. (2009). Predicting early reading skills from pre-reading measures of dorsal stream functioning. *Neuropsychologia, 47,* 3174–3181. doi: http://dx.doi.org/10.1016/j.neuropsychologia.2009.07.016.

Krafnick, A. J., Flowers, D. L., Luetje, M. M., Napoliello, E. M., & Eden, G. F. (2014). An investigation into the origin of anatomical differences in dyslexia. *Journal of Neuroscience, 34,* 901–908. doi: http://dx.doi.org/10.1523/JNEUROSCI.2092-13.2013.

Laasonen, M., Salomaa, J., Cousineau, D. et al. (2012). Project DyAdd: Visual attention in adult dyslexia and ADHD. *Brain and Cognition, 80,* 311–327.

Lallier, M., Tainturier, M. J., Dering, B. et al. (2010). Behavioral and ERP evidence for amodal sluggish attentional shifting in developmental dyslexia. *Neuropsychologia, 48,* 4125–4135.

Langer, N., Peysakhovich, B., Zuk, J. et al. (2017). White matter alterations in infants at risk for developmental dyslexia. *Cerebral Cortex, 27,* 1027–1036.

Lawton, T. (2016). Improving dorsal stream function in dyslexics by training figure/ground motion discrimination improves attention, reading fluency, and working memory. *Frontiers Human Neuroscience, 10,* 397.

Laycock, R., & Crewther, S. G. (2008). Towards an understanding of the role of the "magnocellular advantage" in fluent reading. *Neuroscience & Biobehavioral Review, 32,* 1494–1506. doi: http://dx.doi.org/10.1016/j.neubiorev.2008.06.002.

Liu, D., Chen, X., & Chung, K. K. H. (2015). Performance in a visual search task uniquely predicts reading abilities in third-grade Hong Kong Chinese children. *Scientific Studies of Reading, 19,* 307–324.

Livingstone, M. S., & Hubel, D. H. (1987). Psychophysical evidence for separate channels for the perception of form, color, movement, and depth. *Journal of Neuroscience, 7,* 3416–3468.

Livingstone, M. S., Rosen, G. D., Drislane, F. W., & Galaburda, A. M. (1991). Physiological and anatomical evidence for a magnocellular defect in developmental dyslexia. *Proceedings of the National Academy of Sciences of the United States of America, 88,* 7943–7947. doi: http://dx.doi.org/10.1073/pnas.88.18.7943.

Lovegrove, W., Martin, F., & Slaghuis, W. A. (1986). A theoretical and experimental case for visual deficit in specific reading disability. *Cognitive Neuropsychology, 3,* 225–267.

Lum, J. A., Conti-Ramsden, G., & Lindell, A. K. (2007). The attentional blink reveals sluggish attentional shifting in adolescents with specific language impairment. *Brain and Cognition, 63,* 287–295.

Martelli, M., Di Filippo, G., Spinelli, D., & Zoccolotti, P. (2009). Crowding, reading, and developmental dyslexia. *Journal of Vision, 9,* 14. doi: http://dx.doi.org/10.1167/9.4.14.

Maunsell, J. H., & Newsome, W. T. (1987). Visual processing in monkey extrastriate cortex. *Annual review of Neuroscience, 10,* 363–401.

Menghini, D., Finzi, A., Benassi, M. et al. (2010). Different underlying neurocognitive deficits in developmental dyslexia: A comparative study. *Neuropsychologia, 48,* 863–872. doi: http://dx.doi.org/10.1016/j.neuropsychologia.2009.11.003.

Moats, L. C. (1994). The missing foundation in teacher education: Knowledge of the structure of spoken and written language. *Annals of Dyslexia, 44,* 81–102.

Moores, E., Tsouknida, E., & Romani, C. (2015). Adults with dyslexia can use cues to orient and constrain attention but have a smaller and weaker attention spotlight. *Vision Research, 111,* 55–65.

Morrone, M. C., Tosetti, M., Montanaro, D. et al. (2000). A cortical area that responds specifically to optic flow, revealed by fMRI. *Nature Neuroscience, 3,* 1322–1328. doi: http://dx.doi.org/10.1038/81860.

Newsome, W. T., & Pare, E. B. (1998). A selective impairment of motion perception following lesions of the middle temporal visual area (MT). *Journal of Neuroscience, 8,* 2201–2211.

Olulade, O. A., Napoliello, E. M., & Eden, G. F. (2013). Abnormal visual motion processing is not a cause of dyslexia. *Neuron, 79,* 180–190. doi: http://dx.doi.org/10.1016/j.neuron.2013.05.002.

Pammer, K. (2014). Temporal sampling in vision and the implications for dyslexia. *Frontiers in Human Neuroscience, 7,* 933. doi: http://dx.doi.org/10.3389/fnhum.2013.00933.

Pammer, K., Hansen, P., Holliday, I., & Cornelissen, P. (2006). Attentional shifting and the role of the dorsal pathway in visual word recognition. *Neuropsychologia, 44,* 2926–2936.

Perea, M., Panaderó, V., Moret-Tatay, C., & Góméz, P. (2012). The effects of inter-letter spacing in visual-word recognition: Evidence with young normal readers and developmental dyslexics. *Learning and Instruction, 22,* 420–430.

Petersen, S. E., & Posner, M. I. (2012). The attention system of the human brain: 20 years after. *Annual Review of Neuroscience, 35,* 73–89. doi: http://dx.doi.org/10.1146/annurev-neuro-062111-150525.

Peterson, R. L., Arnett, A. B., Pennington, B. F. et al. (2017). Literacy acquisition influences children's rapid automatized naming. *Developmental Science.* Advance online publication doi: http://dx.doi.org/10.1111/desc.12589.

Peterson, R. L., & Pennington, B. F. (2015). Developmental dyslexia. *Annual Review of Clinical Psychology, 11*, 283–307. doi: http://dx.doi.org/10.1146/annurev-clinpsy-0 32814-112842.

Petrov, Y., & Meleshkevich, O. (2011). Locus of spatial attention determines inward–outward anisotropy in crowding. *Journal of Vision, 11*, 1. doi: http://dx.doi.org/10 .1167/11.4.1.

Pugh, K. R., Mencl, W. E., Shaywitz, B. A. et al. (2000). The angular gyrus in developmental dyslexia: Task-specific differences in functional connectivity within posterior cortex. *Psychological Science, 11*, 51–56. doi: http://dx.doi.org/10.1111/1 467-9280.00214.

Raymond, J. E., Shapiro, K. L., & Arnell, K. M. (1992). Temporary suppression of visual processing in an RSVP task: An attentional blink? *Journal of Experimental Psychology: Human Perception and Performance, 18*, 849–860.

Renvall, H., & Hari, R. (2002). Auditory cortical responses to speech-like stimuli in dyslexic adults. *Journal of Cognitive Neuroscience, 14*, 757–768.

Richlan, F. (2012). Developmental dyslexia: Dysfunction of a left hemisphere reading network. *Frontiersin Human Neuroscience, 6*, 120. doi: http://dx.doi.org/10.3389/f nhum.2012.00120.

Roach, N. V., & Hogben, J. H. (2007). Impaired filtering of behaviourally irrelevant visual information in dyslexia. *Brain, 130*, 771–785. doi: http://dx.doi.org/10.1093 /brain/awl353.

Robidoux, S., Rauwerda, D., & Besner, D. (2014). Basic processes in reading aloud and colour naming: Towards a better understanding of the role of spatial attention. *The Quarterly Journal of Experimental Psychology, 67*, 979–990. doi: http://dx.doi.org /10.1080/17470218.2013.838686.

Roelfsema, P. R., van Ooyen, A., & Watanabe, T. (2010). Perceptual learning rules based on reinforcers and attention. *Trends in Cognitive Sciences, 14*, 64–71. doi: http://dx .doi.org/10.1016/j.tics.2009.11.005.

Ronconi, L., Basso, D., Gori, S., & Facoetti, A. (2014). TMS on right frontal eye fields induces an inflexible focus of attention. *Cerebral Cortex, 24*, 396–402. doi: http://dx .doi.org/10.1093/cercor/bhs319.

Ronconi, L., Facoetti, A., Bulf, H. et al. (2014). Paternal autistic traits are predictive of infants visual attention. *Journal of Autism and Developmental Disorders, 44*, 1556–1564. doi: http://dx.doi.org/10.1007/s10803-013-2018-1.

Ronconi, L., Gori, S., Ruffino, M., Molteni, M., & Facoetti, A. (2013). Zoom-out attentional impairment in children with autism spectrum disorder. *Cortex, 49*(4), 1025–1033.

Ronconi, L., Pincham, H. L., Szűcs, D., & Facoetti, A. (2016). Inducing attention not to blink: Auditory entrainment improves conscious visual processing. *Psychological Research, 80*, 774–784. doi: http://dx.doi.org/10.1007/s00426-015-0691-8.

Ruffino, M., Gori, S., Boccardi, D., Molteni, M., & Facoetti, A. (2014). Spatial and temporal attention in developmental dyslexia. *Frontiers in Human Neuroscience, 8*, 331. doi: http://dx.doi.org/10.3389/fnhum.2014.00331.

Ruffino, M., Trussardi, A. N., Gori, S. et al. (2010). Attentional engagement deficits in dyslexic children. *Neuropsychologia, 48*, 3793–3801. doi: http://dx.doi.org/10.1016/j .neuropsychologia.2010.09.002.

Ruzzoli, M., Gori, S., Pavan, A. et al. (2011). The neural basis of the Enigma illusion: A transcranial magnetic stimulation study. *Neuropsychologia, 49*, 3648–3655. doi: http://dx.doi.org/10.1016/j.neuropsychologia.2011.09.020.

Schneider, K. A., & Kastner, S. (2009). Effects of sustained spatial attention in the human lateral geniculate nucleus and superior colliculus. *Journal of Neuroscience*, *29*, 1784–1795. doi: http://dx.doi.org/10.1523/JNEUROSCI.4452-08.2009.

Schneps, M. H., Thomson, J. M., Chen, C., Sonnert, G., & Pomplun, M. (2013). E-readers are more effective than paper for some with dyslexia. *PLoS One, 8*(9), e75634. doi: http://dx.doi.org/10.1371/journal.pone.0075634.

Schneps, M. H., Thomson, J. M., Sonnert, G. et al. (2013). Shorter lines facilitate reading in those who struggle. *PLoS One, 8*(8), e71161. doi: http://dx.doi.org/10.1371/journal.pone.0071161.

Schulte-Körne, G., & Bruder, J. (2010). Clinical neurophysiology of visual and auditory processing in dyslexia: A review. *Clinical Neurophysiology, 121*, 1794–1809. doi: http://dx.doi.org/10.1016/j.clinph.2010.04.028.

Spinelli, D., De Luca, M., Judica, A., & Zoccolotti, P. (2002). Crowding effects on word identification in developmental dyslexia. *Cortex, 38*, 179–200.

Stein, J. (2012). Visual contributions to reading difficulties: The magnocellular theory. In J. Stein & Z. Kapoula (Eds.), *Visual aspect of dyslexia* (pp. 171–197). Oxford, UK: Oxford University Press.

Stein, J. (2014). Dyslexia: The role of vision and visual attention. *Current Developmental Disorders Reports, 1*, 267–280.

Stein, J., & Walsh, V. (1997). To see but not to read: The magnocellular theory of dyslexia. *Trends in Neurosciences, 20*, 147–152.

Stevens, C., Fanning, J., Donna, C., Sanders, L., & Neville, H. (2008). Neural mechanisms of selective auditory attention are enhanced by computerized training: Electrophysiological evidence from language-impaired and typically developing children. *Brain Research, 1205*, 55–69. doi: http://dx.doi.org/10.1016/j.brainres.2007.10.108.

Takashima, A., Wagensveld, B., van Turennout, M. et al. (2014). Training-induced neural plasticity in visual-word decoding and the role of syllables. *Neuropsychologia, 61*, 299–314. doi: http://dx.doi.org/10.1016/j.neuropsychologia.2014.06.017.

Tallal, P. (2004). Improving language and literacy is a matter of time. *Nature Reviews Neuroscience, 5*, 721–728.

Tallal, P., Miller, S. L., Bedi, G. et al. (1996). Language comprehension in language-learning impaired children improved with acoustically modified speech. *Science, 271*, 81–84.

Turkeltaub, P. E., Gareau, L., Flowers, D. L., Zeffiro, T. A., & Eden, G. F. (2003). Development of neural mechanisms for reading. *Nature Neuroscience, 6*, 767–773. doi: http://dx.doi.org/10.1038/nn1065.

Valdois, S., Bosse, M. L., & Tainturier, M. J. (2004). The cognitive deficits responsible for developmental dyslexia: Review of evidence for a selective visual attentional disorder. *Dyslexia, 10*, 339–363. doi: http://dx.doi.org/10.1002/dys.284.

Vellutino, F. R., Fletcher, J. M., Snowling, M. J., & Scanlon, D. M. (2004). Specific reading disability (dyslexia): What have we learned in the past four decades? *Journal of Child Psychology and Psychiatry, 45*, 2–40. doi: http://dx.doi.org/10.1046/j.0021-9630.2003.00305.x.

Vidyasagar, T. R. (1999). A neuronal model of attentional spotlight: Parietal guiding the temporal. *Brain Research Reviews, 30*, 66–76. doi: http://dx.doi.org/10.1016/S0165-0173(99)00005-3.

Vidyasagar, T. R. (2013). Reading into neuronal oscillations in the visual system: Implications for developmental dyslexia. *Frontiers in Human Neuroscience, 7*, 811. doi: http://dx.doi.org/10.3389/fnhum.2013.00811.

Vidyasagar, T. R., & Pammer, K. (2010). Dyslexia: A deficit in visuo-spatial attention, not in phonological processing. *Trends in Cognitive Sciences, 14*, 57–63. doi: http://dx.doi.org/10.1016/j.tics.2009.12.003.

Virsu, V., Lahti-Nuuttila, P., & Laasonen, M. (2003). Crossmodal temporal processing acuity impairment aggravates with age in developmental dyslexia. *Neuroscience Letters, 336*, 151–154. doi: http://dx.doi.org/10.1016/S0304-3940(02)01253-3.

Vogel, A. C., Miezin, F.M., Petersen, S. E., & Schlaggar, B. L. (2012). The putative visual word form area is functionally connected to the dorsal attention network. *Cerebral Cortex, 22*, 537–549. doi: http://dx.doi.org/10.1093/cercor/bhr100.

Walsh, V. (1995). Dyslexia: Reading between the laminae. *Current Biology, 5*, 1216–1217.

Whitney, D., & Levi, D.M. (2011). Visual crowding: A fundamental limit on conscious perception and object recognition. *Trends in Cognitive Sciences, 15*, 160–168.

Wright, C. M., Conlon, E. G., & Dyck, M. (2012). Visual search deficits are independent of magnocellular deficits in dyslexia. *Annals of Dyslexia, 62*, 53–69.

Witton, C., Talcott, J. B., Hansen, P. C. et al. (1998). Sensitivity to dynamic auditory and visual stimuli predicts nonword reading ability in both dyslexic and normal readers. *Current Biology, 8*, 791–797.

Yazdanbakhsh, A., & Gori, S. (2011). Mathematical analysis of the accordion grating illusion: A differential geometry approach to introduce the 3D aperture problem. *Neural Networks, 24*, 1093–1101. doi: http://dx.doi.org/10.1016/j.neunet.2011.06.016.

Yu, D., Cheung, S. H., Legge, G. E., & Chung, S. T. L. (2007). Effect of letter spacing on visual span and reading speed. *Journal of Vision, 7*(2), 1–10. doi: http://dx.doi.org/10.1167/7.2.2.

Zhao, J., Qian, Y., Bi, H. Y., & Coltheart, M. (2014). The visual magnocellular-dorsal dysfunction in Chinese children with developmental dyslexia impedes Chinese character recognition. *Scientific Reports, 4*, 7068, 1–7. doi: http://dx.doi.org/10.1038/srep07068

Zorzi, M., Barbiero, C., Facoetti, A. et al. (2012). Extra-large letter spacing improves reading in dyslexia. *Proceedings of the National Academy of Sciences of the United States of America, 109*, 11455–11459. doi: http://dx.doi.org/10.1073/pnas.1205566109.

Ziegler, J. C., Pech-Georgel, C., George, F., Alario, F. X., & Lorenzi, C. (2005). Deficits in speech perception predict language learning impairment. *Proceedings of the National Academy of Sciences of the United States of America, 102*, 14110–14115.

15 Morphological and Semantic Processing in Developmental Dyslexia

S. Hélène Deacon, Xiuli Tong, and Catherine Mimeau

15.1 Introduction

This chapter examines the theoretical and empirical foundations of the roles of morphological and semantic skills in developmental dyslexia. Morphemes are the minimal units of meaning by which we create new words in any given language (e.g., "magic"+"ian" = "magician"). Semantics is the study of meaning, broadly speaking. In this chapter, we review data on children's access to meaning at the word and sentence level in tasks, primarily in the oral modality. This review is important because of two common assumptions. The first is of the dominant role of phonological skills in dyslexia, an assumption that has limited the scope of empirical exploration into other potentially implicated factors. The second is that people with dyslexia have a strength in morphology and semantics, a speculation with surprisingly little empirical foundation. We first review the theoretical background for these speculations. We then present the available research evidence, focusing specifically on children with dyslexia, for alphabetic, morphosyllabic, and abjad writing systems. We then review explanatory mechanisms, before turning to cross-linguistic dimensions. We conclude with a broad discussion of these theories and findings, including clinical implications.

15.2 Theoretical Background

15.2.1 Morphological Awareness and Semantic Deficits

Phonological awareness and decoding are viewed as foundational to reading acquisition. In sharp contrast, morphemes play a minimal role in most models of reading. When morphological awareness is included, it is typically described as late emerging and closely connected to orthographic skills (e.g., Ehri, 2005; Seymour, 1999). For instance, according to Ehri's phase model (1995), children first learn to read through phonological decoding. On this foundation, children's reading strategies later extend beyond strict adherence to letter–sound correspondences to the use of rimes, syllables, and morphemes. According to this model, children experience difficulty in acquiring skill because of challenges with phonological awareness and phonological decoding, which in turn, cause difficulties in morphological awareness.

Semantics is also considered to be relatively neglected (Keenan & Betjemann, 2008) in models of reading. For instance, while Goodman (1967) postulated that semantic cues from the sentence are helpful in reading, others have suspected that this attention to semantics is to the detriment of that which should be paid to orthography (Ehri, 2005). At the word level, connectionist models of reading also state that semantic processing is involved in word reading (Plaut et al., 1996) and reading comprehension (Perfetti & Hart, 2002). Despite its inclusion in some prominent models, semantics has received limited empirical attention. As a striking example, Seidenberg and McClelland (1989) entirely omitted the semantic component from their original simulations in their triangle model of word reading (though see Harm & Seidenberg, 2004).

Following on the centrality of phonological awareness and phonological decoding in theoretical models of dyslexia (see, e.g., Vellutino & Fletcher, 2005, for a review), morphological awareness and semantic deficits in dyslexia are widely viewed as a consequence of more fundamental phonological deficits.

15.2.2   A Compensatory Perspective

Established phonological deficits in dyslexia have led to an alternative hypothesis: Morphological and semantic processing might in fact be a strength in dyslexia (Catts, Adlof, & Weismer, 2006; Elbro & Arnbak, 1996). In Stanovich's (1980) interactive-compensatory model, smaller units of words (e.g., letters) are processed to attain higher levels of information (such as meaning; e.g., LaBerge & Samuels, 1974), and higher levels of information support the processing of smaller units (e.g., Goodman, 1967). This simultaneous processing means that "a deficit in any particular process will result in a greater reliance on other knowledge sources, regardless of their level in the processing hierarchy" (Stanovich, 1980, p. 32). In relation to dyslexia, this model would thus predict that poor phonological skills could result in a greater reliance on semantic and morphological skills, thereby reducing cognitive resources available for reading comprehension (see also Perfetti, 1985).

Dual-route models of reading traditionally encompass a lexical and a non-lexical route for accessing pronunciation from print (Coltheart et al., 1993, 2001; Ellis & Young, 1988; from Grainger & Ziegler, 2011 article). These provide a framework for compensation. The lexical route involves direct access to whole-word orthographic representations in the lexicon. The non-lexical route applies letter–sound correspondences prior to accessing phonological and semantic representations. According to this theoretical approach, dyslexics' impairments in phonological decoding lead to reliance on the lexical route. More recent conceptualizations of dual-route models suggest that the use of morphological information speeds lexical access, with both direct and indirect lexical access via letter co-occurrences, such as complex graphemes and morphemes (e.g., TH, CH and RE, ED, respectively; Grainger & Ziegler, 2011). This provides a theoretical context for the speculation that dyslexics might rely on a lexical route that includes morphemes.

Nonetheless, Betjemann and Keenan (2008) argued against the notion that semantic processing is a strength in dyslexia, an idea that can be applied equally to morphological processing. The authors explained that dyslexic children rely on semantic cues more than typical readers because they need to compensate for their poor phonological skills when trying to read, rather than because they have particularly strong semantic skills. Like Stanovich's (1980) interactive-compensatory model, Betjemann and Keenan (2008) incorporate the paradoxical hypotheses that dyslexics have impaired morphological and semantic processing, and yet rely greatly on these while reading. Together, these approaches provide theoretical justification for the possibility that dyslexics' established phonological deficits might be associated with relative strengths in morphological and/or semantic processing.

15.2.3 Insights from Chinese

These aforementioned models suggest that dyslexics may show a strength in morphological and/or semantic processing, but remain limited because these models focus almost exclusively on studies of alphabetic writing systems. Chinese provides a fascinating window into the role of morphological and semantic skills in dyslexia because of its unique morphosyllabic writing system, which emphasizes the role of semantics instead of phonology in word-recognition systems.

Unlike English and other alphabetic orthographies that emphasize letter–phoneme mappings, the Chinese character, the basic unit of Chinese writing, maps onto a syllable or a morpheme (DeFrancis, 1989). The majority of Chinese characters are semantic-phonetic compounds containing a semantic radical (a clue to meaning) and a phonetic radical (a clue to sound). As an example, the character 清/tsʰɪŋ1/ (clean) consists of a semantic radical inline indicating a water-related concept and a phonetic radical 青 with the pronunciation /tsʰɪŋ1/. Notably, the phonetic radical maps onto a whole syllable instead of the phoneme. Of the two radicals, the semantic radical is far more predictive; for semantic-phonetic compound characters, roughly 26 percent share the same sounds with their phonetic radicals, while more than 80 percent are semantically related to their semantic radicals (Shu et al., 2003, 2006). As such, the Chinese writing system itself is more reliable in terms of its orthography–semantic links than its orthography–phonology links (Seidenberg, 2011). The centrality of the direct orthography–semantic links (i.e., semantic radicals) encourages the examination of the possibility that a semantic-related construct, such as morphological awareness but not phonological awareness, is a key construct of understanding Chinese developmental dyslexia (McBride-Chang et al., 2008; Shu et al., 2006; Tong & McBride-Chang, 2010).

Furthermore, Chinese has unique morphological properties, strikingly different from the derivational and inflectional morphology used in alphabetic orthographies, whose presence further supports the possibility that morphological awareness is key to understanding developmental dyslexia in Chinese. First, lexical compounding is the main vehicle of word formation in Chinese, with the majority of compound words semantically transparent (e.g., 電動車 / tin6 tʊŋ6 tsʰɛ1/ (*electric vehicle*) = 電 /tin6/ (*electric*) + 動 /tʊŋ6/ (*motor*) + 車 / tsʰɛ1/ (*vehicle*)). The transparent nature of the component units of meaning may make Chinese readers attend more to semantics rather than phonology (Shu et al., 2003). Second, there are a large number of homophones in Chinese for which meaning is clarified in their writing or word context. For example, the tonal syllable /si6/ has at least six visually distinctive characters, 視 "see," 士 "solider," 示 "show," 是 "is," 事 "work," 侍 "serve," indicating six meanings, respectively. This large number of homophones, each with distinctive characters, makes sound information less reliable in reading Chinese words. This may promote access of exact meaning of each individual morpheme, strengthening the semantic representations of the individual words (Tong, McBride-Chang, & Wong, 2011).

Collectively, the unique characteristics of Chinese orthography, specifically, the predictability of the semantic radical, lexical-compounding morphology and the large number of homophones, are likely to make morphological awareness deficits much more evident than those in phonological awareness in Chinese developmental dyslexia.

15.2.4   Insights from Abjad Languages

Languages represented with abjads, such as Hebrew and other Semitic languages, are of interest in part because they have morphology at the core of their orthographic representation, albeit in a different manner than Chinese writing systems. As an example, in Hebrew each individual word is constructed from two basic morphemes: the root and word pattern (Berman, 1987; Ravid, 1996; Schiff & Ravid, 2007). The root contains the core meaning of all morphologically related forms and is represented in print by three or four consonants. The word pattern is a set of vowels intermingled between the consonants. For example, the root *g-d-l* means grow, and it is contained within the set related words of *gadal* "grew," *gidel* "raised," and *gudal* "was raised" (examples from Schiff & Ravid, 2007). The centrality of morphology in the writing system and the rich and complex morphology might make it particularly difficult to learn to use morphological analysis in reading, and all the more so for students with dyslexia (Schiff & Ravid, 2007). In terms of models of word reading, these features of the orthography might cause morphological, rather than phonological awareness to be foundational in word-reading development. As such, a morphological deficit might underlie the emergence of reading difficulties in Arabic and Hebrew.

15.3   Research Evidence

We review here studies of the morphological and semantic skills of dyslexic children learning to read across a range of orthographies. We first do so for morphological awareness, the ability to manipulate morphemes in the oral language. We then turn to the role of morphemes in reading and in lexical organization, given the theoretical predictions on morphology as a compensatory reading strategy. We prioritize studies with a reading-level match design, contrasting performance of children with dyslexia to that of younger children with reading skill. If dyslexics perform poorer than reading-ability-matched controls, then the difference cannot be explained by reading skill (or experience with print). We think that this design is vital in evaluating evidence on morphological and semantic skills in dyslexics because of the clear evidence that children learn about both skills during their reading (e.g., Cunningham, 2005; Deacon, Benere, & Pasquarella, 2013; Kruk & Bergman, 2013). Uncovered differences can then be considered a potential causal factor in poor reading (e.g., Goswami & Bryant, 1989) or a consequence of a more primary deficit, such as phonological awareness (see, e.g., Casalis, Colé, & Sopo, 2004). In this design, we need to be wary of factors that are not matched, such as explicit instruction in the classroom, which could provide an alternative explanation of differences.

15.3.1   Morphological Awareness in Dyslexics

Alphabetic Orthographies. Across several studies, French and English children with dyslexia have been shown to perform similarly to or better than younger children of similar reading skill on a range of measures of morphological awareness (Egan & Pring, 2004; Egan & Tainturier, 2011; Robertson et al., 2013; Tsesmeli & Seymour, 2006). As an example, Egan and Tainturier contrasted 9-year-old children with two or more years of reading delay with 7-year-old children matched on reading level. Children judged whether there was a smaller word within a larger word that was related to the larger word (e.g., *farmer*, which contains the related word *farm* versus *corner*, which contains the unrelated word *corn*). Children also completed morphological sentence analogies, and inflected nonsense words presented within sentence context. Across these diverse measures of morphological awareness, dyslexics performed similarly to reading-level-match controls. That said, we need to be aware that, in studies of English, French, and Bosnian, children with dyslexia have been shown to underperform their chronological-age-matched peers on morphological awareness (Berthiaume & Daigle, 2014; Carlisle, 1987; Duranovic, Tinjak, & Turbic-Hadzagic, 2014; Egan & Pring, 2004; Egan & Tainturier, 2011; Joanisse et al., 2000; Leong, 1999; Siegel, 2008; Tsesmeli & Seymour, 2006; Vogel, 1977; but see Robertson et al., 2013). As such, dyslexics may have a deficit in morphological awareness relative to their typically developing peers, but this level may be commensurate with their reading skill. One common interpretation of such findings is that parity in performance by dyslexics relative to reading-level matches suggests that morphological awareness is not a deficit causing the dyslexics' reading difficulties.

The use of morphemes in reading is a key test of whether dyslexics might use morphemes as a compensatory avenue to reading. A single study shows greater use of a morphemic strategy in word reading than reading-level controls. Elbro and Arnbak (1996) found that Danish dyslexic adolescents were significantly better in reading text parsed into morphemes than into syllables. In another paradigm, 15-year-old dyslexic Danish students were faster in reading words with than without a semantically transparent morphological structure (e.g., *sunburn* versus *window* as an example in English). Two other studies show use of a morphemic strategy across more word types by dyslexics than reading-level-matched controls. Burani et al. (2008) found that 11-year-old Italian dyslexics were faster in reading morphologically complex over simple words (e.g., *cassiere* versus *cammello*, translates as "cashier" versus "camel") for both real and nonwords. A similar pattern emerged for reading-level-matched controls for nonwords, but not for real words, with no differences between any word types for chronological-age controls (see also Suárez-Coalla & Cuetos, 2013; but see Deacon, Parrila, & Kirby, 2006; Lázaro, Camacho, & Burani, 2013). Burani et al. (2008) argued that children might rely on morphemes in their reading of words not yet automatized at the whole-word level; certainly, there might be more such words for dyslexics. Intriguingly, in Elbro and Arnbak's original study, the size of the difference in performance between the words with and without morphological structure was correlated with better reading comprehension, offering support for the possibility that use of morphemes in reading is a compensatory mechanism to support dyslexics' reading. Comparable studies clearly need to be conducted in more opaque languages, such as English and French, and in languages that do not use letter–sound mapping, such as Chinese.

Chinese. There is empirical evidence that Chinese developmental dyslexics have challenges in morphological awareness, at least in comparison to their peers of the same age (e.g., McBride-Chang et al., 2008, 2012; Shu et al., 2006). For example, Shu and colleagues (2006) found that Grade 5 and 6 Mandarin-speaking Chinese dyslexic children had poorer performance in both a morpheme production and a morpheme judgment tasks than their chronological-age controls. Moreover, the dyslexics and chronological-age control groups were most accurately separated by the morpheme production task. McBride-Chang and colleagues (2008) also showed that Cantonese-speaking preschool children at risk for dyslexia underperformed their chronological-age-matched peers in a lexical-compounding morphological awareness task. They therefore provided evidence that morphological awareness is a hallmark of reading disorders and identifies children at risk of dyslexia in Chinese.

To date, two studies compared the morphological awareness of a group of dyslexics with both a reading-level and chronological-age control group. In one study, Chung, Ho, Chan, Tsang, and Lee (2011) compared a group of Cantonese-speaking dyslexic middle-school students with these two normally achieving control groups in a morpheme discrimination task and a morpheme production task. In both tasks, the dyslexic group underperformed the chronological-age-matched group, but performed similarly to the reading-level-matched group. In a second study, Zhou and colleagues (2014) compared a group of 6-year-old Cantonese-speaking dyslexics with two control groups. In a morphological construction task tapping Chinese lexical compounding, the authors found that the dyslexic group outperformed their reading-level-matched peers, but had indistinguishable performance with their chronological-age-matched peers at the end of the two years.

Collectively, one convergent finding emerges from these studies with Chinese dyslexics. Across multiple morphological tasks, morphological awareness is a key factor distinguishing children with dyslexia from their chronological-age-matched normally achieving readers. However, there is lack of convincing evidence supporting that Chinese children with dyslexia underperformed reading-level-matched normal readers. This is especially critical given that many morphological awareness tasks in Chinese involve print (e.g., Chung et al., 2011). As such, it seems that the difficulties experienced by dyslexics with morphological awareness tasks is as one would expect based on their reading level and there is little evidence to date to support the conclusion that morphological awareness is a causal factor leading to developmental dyslexia for Chinese readers. Further, we were not able to identify any studies of the use of morphemes in reading by dyslexic child readers of Chinese. Thus, future longitudinal research with reading-level control groups is needed to examine the role that morphological awareness and morphological reading strategies play in dyslexia. Additionally, future research might set out to provide a more comprehensive understanding of Chinese dyslexic children's deficits in the use of phonetic and semantic radicals by assessing Chinese dyslexic children's sensitivity to both phonetic and semantic radicals. Previous research with typically developing Chinese children has shown that school-aged Chinese readers are sensitive to the sound cuing function of phonetic radicals by showing the use of full or partial information of phonetic radicals in Chinese character recognition (Anderson et al., 2003; Ho & Bryant, 1997). However, no study to date has systematically evaluated Chinese dyslexic children's use of phonetic and semantic information of radicals in character reading. It would be worthwhile to examine this issue in future research.

Abjads. A very small set of studies of Hebrew- or Arabic-learning children with dyslexia attempted to include reading-level-matched controls; we focus first on data from these studies to provide the most stringent evaluation. A single study was able to include comparison groups that were well matched on the basis of reading level. Schiff, Schwartz-Nahshon, and Nagar (2011) contrasted the performance of 12-year-old children with dyslexia to reading-level-matched peers in Grade 3. Dyslexics performed similarly to these reading-level-matched children on a word-analogy task, and better than reading-level-matched peers on a sentence-completion task. Several other studies attempted to find reading-level matches to younger dyslexics, but did not succeed, with large remaining differences in word-level reading. These studies, in general showed poorer performance by dyslexics than younger children on several morphological tasks, including the ability to judge morphological relationships between written words (Abu-Rabia, Share, & Mansour, 2003; Ben-Dror, Bentin, & Frost, 1995; see also Leikin, 2002) and skill in generating morphologically related words (Abu-Rabia et al., 2003, but see Ben-Dror et al., 1995). As we noted at the outset, however, only one of these included a true reading-level match (Schiff et al., 2011) and this showed that dyslexics performed similarly to or better than reading-level matched controls. This evidence can be paired with findings that dyslexic Hebrew children underperformed their chronological-age peers on a wide range of tests of morphological awareness (Abu-Rabia, 2007; Abu-Rabia et al., 2003; Ben-Dror et al., 1995; Schiff & Ravid, 2004; references from Schiff et al., 2011, see Leikin & Zur Hagit, 2006; Schiff & Ravid, 2013, for similar patterns with adults with dyslexia). As such, it seems that dyslexics have difficulties in morphological awareness relative to typically developing children of the same age, but these difficulties appear to be as expected on the basis of their reading skill. Similarity in performance by dyslexics on morphological awareness tasks to reading-level matches suggests that morphological awareness is not a deficit causing the dyslexics' reading difficulties for readers of Hebrew and Arabic.

Unfortunately, to our knowledge, there are no studies on the use of morphemes in reading by dyslexic child readers of Hebrew and Arabic; as such, we cannot evaluate whether they have a strength in reading strategies based on morphemes, as is suggested by evidence with dyslexic readers of alphabets (e.g., Elbro & Arnbak, 1996). Given this paucity of evidence with children, we expand our purview to a handful of studies of university students with dyslexia.

One study suggests potentially greater reliance on morphemes by dyslexics in reading, as revealed by a masked priming paradigm prior to lexical decision. There was greater priming following a morphologically than orthographically related prime for university students with than without dyslexia (e.g., 200 ms versus 30 ms priming effect); they also showed poorer performance on morphological awareness tasks (Leikin & Zur Hagit, 2006). Of course, as with any written task, it is not clear what effect dyslexics' slower reading time had on results. That said, these findings support the possibility of increased reliance on morphemes in reading, despite non-exceptional morphological awareness skills.

In contrast, university students with dyslexia showed marked insensitivity to either morphological or repetition priming in another study that contrasted visual and auditory prime presentation. In a long-term unmasked priming paradigm, adults with dyslexia showed no priming when the prime was visual, either repetition or morphological; there was both types of priming for the adults without dyslexia as well as for the reading-level matches. In sharp contrast, when the prime was presented in the auditory domain, adults with dyslexia showed similar morphological priming to chronological-age-matched peers (Raveh & Schiff, 2008). These results are compelling in that they reveal a pattern of stability in morphological representations in the auditory lexicon, with impairments in orthographic representations in general in dyslexics, not just specific to morphology (see Schiff & Raveh, 2007, for similar results in a fragment completion paradigm).

To date, the findings then are conflicting as to whether Hebrew and Arabic university students with dyslexia, who have likely compensated to some extent for their reading difficulties, use morphemes in their word recognition. Further studies need to be done specifically with children with dyslexia.

15.3.2   Semantic Skills in Dyslexics

Although research on semantic skills in dyslexics is far more limited than that on morphology, a range of studies in speakers of various languages suggest that dyslexic children also suffer from semantic impairment. Indeed, some studies comparing dyslexic children with same-age typical readers have found evidence of deficits in early semantic skills (Liu et al., 2010; Lyytinen et al., 2001; Torppa et al., 2010). For instance, a comprehensive study examined the early language skills of Finnish-speaking children identified as dyslexic at 9 years of age. At 2, 3, and 5 years of age, the children who went on to become dyslexic recognized and produced fewer words in vocabulary and naming tasks (Torppa et al., 2010). Furthermore, dyslexic children's semantic skills seem to remain impaired through the elementary school years, at least in comparison with age-matched controls (Ben-Dror et al., 1995; Chik et al., 2012; Schulz et al., 2008; Vellutino, Scanlon, & Spearing, 1995). As an example, Ben-Dror et al. (1995) showed that 10- to 12-year-old Hebrew-speaking dyslexics performed worse than age-matched controls in producing and classifying words from different semantic categories. These semantic impairments could have a neural basis. Indeed, studies conducted in Polish (Jednoróg et al., 2010), Finnish (Helenius et al., 1999), and German (Schulz et al., 2008) have consistently indicated that dyslexics, in comparison with normal readers, showed delayed and weaker cerebral activations during the completion of tasks assessing semantic skills.

However, it remains unclear whether the behavioral and neural deficits in semantics observed in dyslexics (e.g., Ben-Dror et al., 1995; Jednoróg et al., 2010) are an underlying cause of their reading difficulties because the empirical evidence to date is contradictory. Whereas some studies have shown that dyslexic children had poorer semantic skills than reading-level-matched controls, others have shown no differences between the two groups. For instance, in a masked priming study, Betjemann and Keenan (2008) compared 11- to 13-year-old English-speaking dyslexic children with a reading-level-matched control group. The authors asked the children to indicate whether written stimuli were words. Both groups showed facilitation effects when the stimuli were preceded by a semantically related prime, but the size of the priming effect was significantly smaller for the dyslexic group compared with the control group. These findings suggest that dyslexics' processing of semantic information was poorer than that of typical readers of the same level of reading ability. Likewise, when 7- to 11-year-old Chinese-speaking children were asked to complete a synonym judgment task, the dyslexic group underperformed the reading-level-matched control group (Xiao & Ho, 2014). In contrast, Tsesmeli and Seymour (2006) showed that English-speaking 13- to 15-old dyslexics were better than their reading-level-matched controls at formulating definitions of words. Similarly, in a study conducted with 9-year-old Chinese-speaking children, the dyslexics were found to be as accurate as their reading-level-matched controls at using target words in sentences and at identifying synonyms (Chik et al., 2012). This mixed evidence from studies on both English and Chinese makes it difficult to postulate whether semantics has a causal role to play in dyslexia.

Regarding the use of semantic information while reading, dyslexics were found to rely more on semantic context than typical readers, as seems to be the case for morphemes (Burani et al., 2008; Elbro & Arnbak, 1996; Suárez-Coalla & Cuetos, 2013). As an example, in a study conducted in English, Nation and Snowling (1998) asked a group of dyslexic 11-year-olds and a group of reading-level-matched 8-year-olds to read words either presented in isolation or preceded by a sentence. The authors observed a contextual facilitation effect that was greater for the dyslexics than for the typical readers. Likewise, in a study of English-speaking adults diagnosed with dyslexia in childhood (Bruck, 1990), the participants read words embedded in either sentences providing no clue to meaning or in a meaningful passage. The dyslexics showed a greater contextual facilitation effect than reading-level-matched sixth graders. Notably, however, the author did not take into account baseline differences in word reading between the groups, as did Nation and Snowling (1998).

In sum, studies on dyslexics' semantic skills suggest that this population is impaired in comparison with age-matched controls, but it remains very much unclear whether these semantic deficits are the basis for their reading difficulties (e.g., Chik et al., 2012; Xiao & Ho, 2014). Further, there is reasonably consistent evidence that, despite impaired semantic skills, dyslexics tend to rely on semantic context more than typical readers of the same level of reading ability to help them read words (e.g., Nation & Snowling, 1998).

15.4   Explanatory Mechanisms

Our review of empirical evidence to date highlights findings that need to be explained within any theoretical paradigm. To summarize, there is a pattern in which dyslexic readers in a wide range of writing systems have levels of morphological awareness that are concomitant with their reading level. Second, at least for dyslexic readers of alphabets, the use of morphemes in reading might be better than expected on the basis of their reading level. Finally, the evidence to date does not allow the identification of a straightforward pattern for semantics. In this section, we review mechanisms that might explain these general findings.

15.4.1   Morphological Awareness Equals with Reading-Level Matches

Turning to the first pattern, there is abundant evidence that children with dyslexia, regardless of the language in which they are learning to read, perform similarly to reading-level match controls on morphological awareness (e.g., Egan & Pring, 2004; Schiff et al., 2011; Zhou et al., 2014). This general pattern emerges across all the languages in which it has been tested, although notably few studies in Chinese have included this control group. This pattern suggests that morphological awareness is unlikely to be a causal factor leading to these children's reading difficulties; instead, it is likely that some third factor, such as phonological awareness, leads to their challenges both in morphological awareness and word reading.

One explanation of this set of findings is based on the idea, articulated in multiple models of reading (e.g., Ehri, 2005), that phonological awareness is the primary cause of dyslexic children's reading difficulties. Weaknesses in phonological awareness, in turn, cause both morphological and reading problems (e.g., Shankweiler et al., 1995). Several researchers have noted that the phonological quality of morphemes likely makes them more difficult to access and manipulate in oral language tasks (e.g., Egan & Pring, 2004; Joanisse et al., 2000). This explanation is further supported by the abundant evidence of the role of phonological skill in typical reading development (e.g., Bradley & Bryant, 1983; National Reading Panel, 2000). This mechanistic interpretation gained plausibility from a comprehensive evaluation of the morphological awareness skills of French dyslexics. Casalis and her colleagues (2004) found that French children with dyslexia performed similarly to reading-level-matched controls on two tasks evaluating the ability to produce real derived forms, one after having been provided with a sentence context and another following a definition. In contrast, dyslexic children performed more poorly than reading-level-matched peers on two morphological awareness tasks resembling a standard phonological awareness task: blending together or removing a base and suffix (see Berthiaume & Daigle, 2014, for a similar pattern of results, and see also Bryant, Nunes, & Bindman, 1998). Overall, the pattern of results provides support for the possibility that deficits in phonological awareness underlie dyslexics' poorer performance on morphological awareness tasks in comparison to reading-level matches.

It is noteworthy that, even in Hebrew, a language in which morphemes are argued to be a primary means of lexical access, Abu-Rabia et al. (2003) noted that the dyslexic children were "virtually at floor" (p. 434) on the phonological awareness task, while the reading-level controls were virtually at ceiling. As such, even in Hebrew, there is evidence that phonological awareness plays a substantive role in reading difficulties.

The language for which this conclusion is perhaps most contentious is Chinese, for which it has been argued that morphological awareness is a central factor in dyslexia; that said, our review revealed a lack of conclusive empirical evidence to support this. We concur that there is evidence that morphological awareness tasks are able to distinguish dyslexic from non-dyslexic children (McBride-Chang et al., 2012). However, many of the morphological awareness tasks in research to date involve access to the written form of Chinese characters, such as homograph identification (McBride-Chang et al., 2012) and morpheme discrimination (Chung et al., 2011). This raises the question of whether Chinese dyslexic children's deficits in morphological awareness are partly a consequence of their poor orthographic representation.

Further, one of the most commonly used Chinese morphological awareness tasks, morphological construction, may highly depend on children's analogical reasoning abilities. As such, there are confounds with both reading and other cognitive skills. Studies with oral morphological awareness tasks that include reading-level controls are critical in Chinese. Also, as noted earlier, the Chinese reading system itself emphasizes an orthography–semantics connection. It is highly likely that morphological awareness deficits observed in Chinese dyslexics are the consequence of a weak ability to establish orthography–semantic links rather than the cause. Thus, it would be worthwhile to consider separating orthographic knowledge (the written form of words) from the assessment of morphological awareness in Chinese dyslexics.

An alternative explanation is that children develop difficulties with both reading and morphology due to an underlying language deficit, at least for some children with dyslexia. Some support for this possibility came from a study by Joanisse et al. (2000) of third-grade children with poor reading skills. Children with both poor reading and language skills performed significantly worse on a morphological awareness task that involved producing novel inflected forms (e.g., Berko, 1958) than did reading-level controls; no such difference emerged for poor readers as a group. These findings suggest that children with only reading difficulties do not have challenges in morphological awareness beyond what one would expect based on their reading skill, and that deficits in morphological awareness might reflect underlying language impairments for a subset of children. This explanation is supported by the fact that morphology is considered to be a sensitive indicator of language ability (see, e.g., Leonard et al., 1997). This finding demonstrates the need, beyond this single study, to consider morphological awareness along with broader oral language skills in order to pinpoint the sources of deficits.

To summarize the mechanistic interpretation of findings on morphological awareness, the vast majority of current positions regard weaknesses in morphological awareness, as demonstrated in comparison to chronological-age controls, as secondary to primary deficits in some other domain (e.g., general language skills or phonological processing).

15.4.2   More Reliance on Morpho-Semantics in Alphabetic Languages

The second pattern is that dyslexic children learning to read in alphabetic languages demonstrate greater reliance on morphemes and semantic context in reading than one would expect based on their reading level (e.g., Burani et al., 2008; Nation & Snowling, 1998). The use of morphemes and context in reading has not, to our knowledge, been tested for dyslexic children learning to read in either Chinese or abjads, with limited and conflicting evidence from adult Hebrew dyslexics.

There are two postulated mechanisms for findings of greater reliance on morphemes in dyslexics' reading (Quémart & Casalis, 2013; Suárez-Coalla & Cuetos, 2013). Burani et al. (2008; see also Marcolini et al., 2011; Traficante et al., 2011) suggest that children rely on morphemic units when reading long and infrequent words because morphemes are often large phonological units represented with multiple letters. In contrast, Elbro and Arnbak (1996; see also Casalis et al., 2004) argue that it is the semantic quality of morphemes that makes them more accessible units, rather than their phonological and orthographic qualities. To our knowledge, only one study has evaluated these mechanisms.

In a masked priming paradigm administered to French dyslexics, Quémart and Casalis (2013) found that dyslexics showed significant priming in morphological conditions (e.g., *tablette–TABLE*, "little table–TABLE"), and not in the orthographic conditions, regardless of whether this had the appearance of morphological structure or not (e.g., pseudo-derived, e.g., *baguette–BAGUE*, "French stick–ring" and orthographic control *abricot–ABRI*, "apricot–shelter"). In contrast, the reading-level and chronological-age-matched children showed significant priming in both the morphological and pseudo-derived conditions, suggesting a role for orthographic overlap with the appearance of morphological structure. A similar pattern of results emerged in a second experiment that varied the degree of orthographic overlap. These results support the possibility that dyslexics' reliance on morphemes in their processing of written words is due to the semantic rather than orthographic features of morphemes, consistent with their greater use of semantic context during reading (e.g., Nation & Snowling, 1998). However, this pattern needs to be replicated, particularly in dyslexic readers of other orthographies.

15.4.3   *Disparate Findings on Semantics in Dyslexics*

The third broad set of findings that we need to consider comes from evidence on dyslexics' semantics skills; we need to exert caution in doing so as the pattern of results to date remains unclear regarding the question of causality. Whereas some studies suggest that poor semantic skills are partly responsible for dyslexics' reading difficulty (Betjemann & Keenan, 2008; Xiao & Ho, 2014), others have failed to make that demonstration (Chik et al., 2012; Tsesmeli & Seymour, 2006). The disparate findings on dyslexics' impairment at the semantic level are hard to interpret given the limited number of studies. On the one hand, as vocabulary is gained partly through reading (Cunningham, 2005), dyslexics' semantic deficits might result from their reading difficulty rather than the opposite. On the other hand, in two studies (Betjemann & Keenan, 2008; Xiao & Ho, 2014) dyslexic children do not perform as well as their reading-level-matched controls on some semantic tasks; impaired semantic skills could cause reading difficulty, as suggested in some models (e.g., Goodman, 1967; Perfetti & Hart, 2002; Plaut et al., 1996). As meaning is automatically activated when reading a word (Forster & Hector, 2002), semantic information might be helpful to typical readers in word recognition. Given that dyslexics have difficulty retrieving the meaning of words, their word recognition might be diminished partly by this factor. Clearly we need studies designed to elucidate both the general pattern of results and its mechanistic interpretation.

15.5   Cross-Language Issues

We begin by highlighting possible universals across languages, reminding ourselves that not all of these have been demonstrated empirically to date. The overarching empirical pattern to date lies in dyslexics' comparability to reading-level matches on morphological awareness tasks; multiple theoretical positions would argue that the origins of their reading lie in other domains. The other pattern lies in dyslexics' greater use of morphemes in reading in comparison to reading-level matches, possibly originating in a relative semantic strength. These two patterns may be universals, with more empirical evidence on the former. It seems that morphological awareness may not be a source of dyslexics' reading difficulties, even for those learning to read in orthographies relying heavily on morphological principles. Moving forward, we note that these overarching patterns in the data to date exist alongside very clear gaps in the empirical tests of these patterns in specific orthographies. We highlight these here, with the intention of demonstrating the importance of providing empirical tests.

First, we note that rigorous reading-level match controls were included in studies of dyslexics' morphological awareness most prominently in studies of children learning alphabets. It has proven difficult in studies of children learning to read in Arabic or Hebrew, with large remaining differences in reading skill for groups attempted to be matched on reading level (e.g., Abu-Rabia et al., 2003). As such, a stringent reading-level control group has only been included in a single study in Hebrew (Schiff et al., 2011) and a single study in Chinese (Zhou et al., 2014). As such, we have little basis for confidence that the pattern that emerged from studies of children learning to read alphabets is the same or different for children learning to read other orthographies. From a theoretical and linguistic point of view, it is vital that we empirically test morphological awareness of dyslexic children.

As for semantics, two studies in English (Betjemann & Keenan, 2008; Tsesmeli & Seymour, 2006) and two studies in Chinese (Chik et al., 2012; Xiao & Ho, 2014) included reading-level-matched control groups. However, for these languages, the studies obtained opposite patterns. Along with the lack of studies on other languages such as Hebrew and Arabic, these conflicting findings highlight the importance of studying dyslexics' semantic skills in both alphabetic and non-alphabetic languages.

Similarly, from a mechanistic point of view, these studies need to contrast the performance of children with deficits in either or both phonological awareness and oral language (following on Casalis et al., 2004; Joanisse et al., 2000). Such fine-grained investigations will determine the underlying factors influencing morphological awareness and semantic processing.

Finally, all of the evidence that morphemes and semantics might offer a compensatory route to reading for dyslexics comes from studies of alphabetic scripts. Even within alphabets, there is no evidence on use of morphemes in word reading by children learning to read in the most phonologically opaque languages of English and French. Most critically, use of morphemes in reading has not, to our knowledge, been tested for dyslexic children learning to read in either Chinese or abjads. These gaps limit the generalizability of any conclusions.

15.6   Discussion and Conclusion

To summarize, we found, overall, that morphological awareness levels of children with dyslexia are as one would expect on the basis of their reading level. This pattern has been taken to suggest that the cause of dyslexics' reading difficulties lies in domains other than morphology, most likely in phonology, especially for alphabetic orthographies. Intriguingly, we also found that dyslexics appear to rely on morphemes and semantic context in their reading to a greater extent than their reading-level-matched peers. This second set of results provides some support for the captivating possibility that morphology offers a compensatory mechanism. We encourage some remaining skepticism: this pattern is discrepant with performance on morphological awareness tasks, has not been assessed in the majority of the world's orthographies, and exists despite the fact that dyslexics in these studies have ongoing struggles with reading. Also, due to the diversities and complexities of morphology in different writing systems, there is a great variation in the use of different types of morphological awareness tasks to assess different aspects of morphological awareness. This leaves us with a fundamental question about whether the nature of morphological awareness is the same across different writing system. Furthermore, the relative strength of the connection between morphology and phonology, and between morphology and orthography also varies across different orthographies, making it operationally difficult to separately evaluate the contribution of morphological awareness to reading difficulties. Thus, it seems that morphology may not be a silver bullet with which to solve engrained reading difficulties.

This review has clinical implications. First, the absence of clear evidence of morphological awareness and semantic processing as specific deficits, beyond prediction by reading level, suggests that these skills might not be useful to include in a diagnostic toolkit for dyslexia. Certainly, the evidence that many children who struggle with reading also struggle with language (e.g., Joanisse et al., 2000; McArthur et al., 2000) suggests the importance of evaluating both language and reading skill in accurately diagnosing children with either dyslexia or a specific language impairment. Second, and in contrast, there is growing evidence that dyslexics can be skilled in using morphemes and semantic context in their reading (e.g., Bruck, 1990; Elbro & Arnbak, 1996). This latter finding is bolstered by the evidence that instruction in morphological awareness is more effective for poorer readers than for typically developing readers (Bowers, Kirby, & Deacon, 2010). Contrasting the effectiveness of morphological and phonological awareness training is a key next step. As we await data from randomized control trials, we advise treatments of dyslexia focused on morphology only for children who have not responded to intensive phonological awareness intervention.

References

Abu-Rabia, S. (2007). The role of morphology and short vowelization in reading Arabic among normal and dyslexic readers in grades 3, 6, 9, and 12. *Journal of Psycholinguistic Research*, *36*, 89–106. doi: http://dx.doi.org/10.1007/s10936-006-9035-6.

Abu-Rabia, S., Share, D., & Mansour, M. S. (2003). Word recognition and basic cognitive processes among reading-disabled and normal readers in Arabic. *Reading and Writing*, *16*, 423–442. doi: http://dx.doi.org/10.1023/a:1024237415143.

Anderson, R., Li, W., Ku, Y-M., Shu, H., & Wu, N. (2003). Use of partial information in learning to read Chinese characters. *Journal of Educational Psychology*, *95*(1), 52–57.

Ben-Dror, I., Bentin, S., & Frost, R. (1995). Semantic, phonologic, and morphologic skills in reading disabled and normal children: Evidence from perception and production of spoken Hebrew. *Reading Research Quarterly*, *30*, 876–893. doi: http://dx.doi.org/10.1111/j.1467-9280.1995.tb00328.x.

Berko, J. (1958). The child's learning of English morphology. *Word*, *14*, 150–177. doi: http://dx.doi.org/10.1080/00437956.1958.11659661.

Berman, R. A. (1987). Productivity in the lexicon: New-word formation in modern Hebrew. *Folia Linguistica*, *21*, 425–461.

Berthiaume, R., & Daigle, D. (2014). Are dyslexic children sensitive to the morphological structure of words when they read? The case of dyslexic readers of French. *Dyslexia*, *20*, 241–260. doi: http://dx.doi.org/10.1002/dys.1476.

Betjemann, R. S., & Keenan, J. M. (2008). Phonological and semantic priming in children with reading disability. *Child Development*, *79*, 1086–1102. doi: http://dx.doi.org/10.1111/j.1467-8624.2008.01177.x.

Bowers, P. N., Kirby, J. R., & Deacon, S. H. (2010). The effects of morphological instruction on literacy skills: A systematic review of the literature. *Review of Educational Research, 80,* 144–179. doi: http://dx.doi.org/10.3102/0034654309359353.

Bradley, L., & Bryant, P. E. (1983). Categorizing sounds and learning to read: A causal connection. *Nature, 301,* 419–421. doi: http://dx.doi.org/10.1038/301419a0.

Bruck, M. (1990). Word-recognition skills of adults with childhood diagnoses of dyslexia. *Developmental Psychology, 26,* 439–454. doi: http://dx.doi.org/10.1037/0 012-1649.26.3.439.

Bryant, P., Nunes, T., & Bindman, M. (1998). Awareness of language in children who have reading difficulties: Historical comparisons in a longitudinal study. *Journal of Child Psychology and Psychiatry, 39,* 501–510. doi: http://dx.doi.org/10.1111/1469-7610.00346.

Burani, C., Marcolini, S., De Luca, M., & Zoccolotti, P. (2008). Morpheme-based reading aloud: Evidence from dyslexic and skilled Italian readers. *Cognition, 108,* 243–262. doi: http://dx.doi.org/10.1016/j.cognition.2007.12.010.

Carlisle, J. F. (1987). The use of morphological knowledge in spelling derived forms by learning-disabled and normal students. *Annals of Dyslexia, 37,* 90–108. doi: http://dx .doi.org/10.1007/bf02648061.

Casalis, S., Colé, P., & Sopo, D. (2004). Morphological awareness in developmental dyslexia. *Annals of Dyslexia, 54,* 114–138. doi: http://dx.doi.org/10.1007/s11881-0 04-0006-z.

Catts, H. W., Adlof, S. M., & Weismer, S. E. (2006). Language deficits in poor comprehenders: A case for the simple view of reading. *Journal of Speech, Language, and Hearing Research, 49,* 278–293. doi: http://dx.doi.org/10.1044/1092-4388(2006/023).

Chik, P. P. M., Ho, C. S. H., Yeung, P. S. et al. (2012). Contribution of discourse and morphosyntax skills to reading comprehension in Chinese dyslexic and typically developing children. *Annals of Dyslexia, 62,* 1–18. doi: http://dx.doi.org/10.1007/s1 1881-010-0045-6.

Chung, K. K. H., Ho, C. S.-H., Chan, D. W. et al. (2011). Cognitive skills and literacy performance of Chinese adolescents with and without dyslexia. *Reading and Writing, 24,* 835–859. doi: http://dx.doi.org/10.1007/s11145-010-9227-1.

Coltheart, M., Curtis, B., Atkins, P., & Haller, M. (1993). Models of reading aloud: Dual-route and parallel-distributed-processing approaches. *Psychological Review, 100,* 589–608. doi: http://dx.doi.org/10.1037/0033-295x.100.4.589.

Coltheart, M., Rastle, K., Perry, C., Langdon, R., & Ziegler, J. (2001). DRC: A dual route cascaded model of visual word recognition and reading aloud. *Psychological Review, 108,* 204–256. doi: http://dx.doi.org/10.1037/0033-295x.108.1.204.

Cunningham, A. E. (2005). Vocabulary growth through independent reading and reading aloud to children. In E. H. Hiebert & M. L. Kamil (Eds.), *Teaching and learning vocabulary: Bringing research to practice* (pp. 45–68). Mahwah, NJ: Lawrence Erlbaum Associates Publishers.

Deacon, S. H., Benere, J., & Pasquarella, A. (2013). Reciprocal relationship: Children's morphological awareness and their reading accuracy across grades 2 to 3. *Developmental Psychology, 49,* 1113–1126. doi: http://dx.doi.org/10.1037/a0029474.

Deacon, S. H., Parrila, R., & Kirby, J. R. (2006). Processing of derived forms in high functioning dyslexics. *Annals of Dyslexia, 56,* 103–128. doi: http://dx.doi.org/10 .1007/s11881-006-0005-3.

DeFrancis, J. (1989). *Visible speech: The diverse oneness of writing systems*. Honolulu, HI: University of Hawaii Press.

Duranovic, M., Tinjak, S., & Turbic-Hadzagic, A. (2014). Morphological knowledge in children with dyslexia. *Journal of Psycholinguistic Research, 43*, 699–713. doi: http://dx.doi.org/10.1007/s10936-013-9274-2.

Egan, J., & Pring, L. (2004). The processing of inflectional morphology: A comparison of children with and without dyslexia. *Reading and Writing, 17*, 567–591. doi: http://dx.doi.org/10.1023/B:READ.0000044433.30864.23.

Egan, J., & Tainturier, M. J. (2011). Inflectional spelling deficits in developmental dyslexia. *Cortex, 47*, 1179–1196. doi: http://dx.doi.org/10.1016/j.cortex.2011.05.013.

Ehri, L. C. (1995). Phases of development in learning to read words by sight. *Journal of Research in Reading, 18*, 116–125. doi: http://dx.doi.org/10.1111/j.1467-9817.1995.tb00077.x.

Ehri, L. C. (2005). Learning to read words: Theory, findings, and issues. *Scientific Studies of Reading, 9*, 167–188. doi: http://dx.doi.org/10.1207/s1532799xssr0902_4.

Elbro, C., & Arnbak, E. (1996). The role of morpheme recognition and morphological awareness in dyslexia. *Annals of Dyslexia, 46*, 209–240. doi: http://dx.doi.org/10.1007/BF02648177.

Ellis, A. W., & Young, A. W. (1988). Reading: And a composite model for word recognition and production. In A. W. Ellis & A. W. Young (Eds.), *Human cognitive neuropsychology: A textbook with readings* (Augmented ed., pp. 191–238). Hove, UK: Psychology Press.

Forster, K. I., & Hector, J. (2002). Cascaded versus noncascaded models of lexical and semantic processing: The *turple* effect. *Memory & Cognition, 30*, 1106–1117. doi: http://dx.doi.org/10.3758/BF03194328.

Goodman, K. S. (1967). Reading: A psycholinguistic guessing game. *Journal of the Reading Specialist, 6*, 126–135. doi: http://dx.doi.org/10.1080/19388076709556976.

Goswami, U., & Bryant, P. (1989). The interpretation of studies using the reading level design. *Journal of Literacy Research, 21*, 413–424. doi: http://dx.doi.org/10.1080/10862968909547687.

Grainger, J., & Ziegler, J. C. (2011). A dual-route approach to orthographic processing. *Frontiers in Psychology, 2*(54), 1–13. doi: http://dx.doi.org/10.3389/fpsyg.2011.00054.

Harm, M. W., & Seidenberg, M. S. (2004). Computing the meanings of words in reading: Cooperative division of labor between visual and phonological processes. *Psychological Review, 111*, 662–720.

Helenius, P., Salmelin, R., Service, E., & Connolly, J. F. (1999). Semantic cortical activation in dyslexic readers. *Journal of Cognitive Neuroscience, 11*, 535–550. doi: http://dx.doi.org/10.1162/089892999563599.

Ho, C. S.-H., & Bryant, P. (1997). Learning to read Chinese beyond the logographic phase. *Reading Research Quarterly, 32*, 276–289.

Jednoróg, K., Marchewka, A., Tacikowski, P., & Grabowska, A. (2010). Implicit phonological and semantic processing in children with developmental dyslexia: Evidence from event-related potentials. *Neuropsychologia, 48*, 2447–2457. doi: http://dx.doi.org/10.1016/j.neuropsychologia.2010.04.017.

Joanisse, M. F., Manis, F. R., Keating, P., & Seidenberg, M. S. (2000). Language deficits in dyslexic children: Speech perception, phonology, and morphology. *Journal of*

Experimental Child Psychology, *77*, 30–60. doi: http://dx.doi.org/10.1006/jecp .1999.2553.

Keenan, J. M., & Betjemann, R. S. (2008). Comprehension of single words: The role of semantics in word identification and reading disability. In E. L. Grigorenko & A. J. Naples (Eds.), *Single-word reading: Behavioral and biological perspectives* (pp. 191–209). Mahwah, NJ: Lawrence Erlbaum Associates Publishers.

Kruk, R. S., & Bergman, K. (2013). The reciprocal relations between morphological processes and reading. *Journal of Experimental Child Psychology*, *114*, 10–34. doi: http://dx.doi.org/10.1016/j.jecp.2012.09.014.

LaBerge, D., & Samuels, S. J. (1974). Toward a theory of automatic information processing in reading. *Cognitive Psychology*, *6*, 293–323. doi: http://dx.doi.org/10 .1016/0010-0285(74)90015-2.

Lázaro, M., Camacho, L., & Burani, C. (2013). Morphological processing in reading disabled and skilled Spanish children. *Dyslexia*, *19*, 178–188. doi: http://dx.doi.org /10.1002/dys.1458.

Leikin, M. (2002). Processing syntactic functions of words in normal and dyslexic readers. *Journal of Psycholinguistic Research*, *31*, 145–163. doi: http://dx.doi.org/10 .1023/A:1014926900931.

Leikin, M., & Zur Hagit, E. (2006). Morphological processing in adult dyslexia. *Journal of Psycholinguistic Research*, *35*, 471–490. doi: http://dx.doi.org/10.1007/s10936-0 06-9025-8.

Leonard, L. B., Eyer, J. A., Bedore, L. M., & Grela, B. G. (1997). Three accounts of the grammatical morpheme difficulties of English-speaking children with specific language impairment. *Journal of Speech, Language, and Hearing Research*, *40*, 741–753. doi: http://dx.doi.org/10.1044/jslhr.4004.741.

Leong, C. K. (1999). Phonological and morphological processing in adult students with learning/reading disabilities. *Journal of Learning Disabilities*, *32*, 224–238. doi: http:// dx.doi.org/10.1177/002221949903200304.

Liu, P. D., McBride-Chang, C., Wong, A. M.-Y. et al. (2010). Early oral language markers of poor reading performance in Hong Kong Chinese children. *Journal of Learning Disabilities*, *43*, 322–331. doi: http://dx.doi.org/10.1177/0022219410369084.

Lyytinen, H., Ahonen, T., & Eklund, K. et al. (2001). Developmental pathways of children with and without familial risk for dyslexia during the first years of life. *Developmental Neuropsychology*, *20*, 535–554. doi: http://dx.doi.org/10.1207 /S15326942DN2002_5.

Marcolini, S., Traficante, D., Zoccolotti, P., & Burani, C. (2011). Word frequency modulates morpheme-based reading in poor and skilled Italian readers. *Applied Psycholinguistics*, *32*, 513–532. doi: http://dx.doi.org/10.1017/S0142716411000191.

McArthur, G. M., Hogben, J. H., Edwards, V. T., Heath, S. M., & Mengler, E. D. (2000). On the "specifics" of specific reading disability and specific language impairment. *Journal of Child Psychology and Psychiatry*, *41*, 869–874. doi: http://dx.doi.org/10 .1111/1469-7610.00674.

McBride-Chang, C., Lam, F., Lam, C. et al. (2008). Word recognition and cognitive profiles of Chinese pre-school children at risk for dyslexia through language delay or familial history of dyslexia. *Journal of Child Psychology and Psychiatry*, *49*, 211–218. doi: http://dx.doi.org/10.1111/j.1469-7610.2007.01837.x.

McBride-Chang, C., Liu, P. D., Wong, T., Wong, A., & Shu, H. (2012). Specific reading difficulties in Chinese, English, or both: Longitudinal markers of phonological awareness, morphological awareness, and RAN in Hong Kong Chinese children. *Journal of Learning Disabilities, 45,* 503–514. doi: http://dx.doi.org/10.1177 /0022219411400748.

Nation, K., & Snowling, M. J. (1998). Semantic processing and the development of word-recognition skills: Evidence from children with reading comprehension difficulties. *Journal of Memory and Language, 39,* 85–101. doi: http://dx.doi.org/10 .1006/jmla.1998.2564.

National Reading Panel. (2000). *Teaching children to read: An evidence-based assessment of the scientific research literature on reading and its implications for reading instruction: Reports of the subgroups.* Bethesda, MD: National Institute of Child Health and Human Development.

Perfetti, C. A. (1985). *Reading ability.* New York, NY: Oxford University Press.

Perfetti, C. A., & Hart, L. (2002). The lexical quality hypothesis. In L. Verhoeven, C. Elbro, & P. Reitsma (Eds.), *Precursors of functional literacy* (pp. 189–213). Philadelphia, PA: John Benjamins Publishing Company.

Plaut, D. C., McClelland, J. L., Seidenberg, M. S., & Patterson, K. (1996). Understanding normal and impaired word reading: Computational principles in quasi-regular domains. *Psychological Review, 103,* 56–115. doi: http://dx.doi.org/10 .1037/0033-295X.103.1.56.

Quémart, P., & Casalis, S. (2013). Visual processing of derivational morphology in children with developmental dyslexia: Insights from masked priming. *Applied Psycholinguistics, 36,* 1–32. doi: http://dx.doi.org/10.1017/S0142716 41300026X.

Raveh, M., & Schiff, R. (2008). Visual and auditory morphological priming in adults with developmental dyslexia. *Scientific Studies of Reading, 12,* 221–252. doi: http:// dx.doi.org/10.1080/10888430801917068.

Ravid, D. (1996). Cost in language acquisition, language processing and language change. In E. H. Casad (Ed.), *Cognitive linguistics in the redwoods: The expansion of a new paradigm in linguistics* (pp. 117–146). Berlin, Germany: De Gruyter Mouton. doi: http://dx.doi.org/10.1515/9783110811421.117.

Robertson, E. K., Joanisse, M. F., Desroches, A. S., & Terry, A. (2013). Past-tense morphology and phonological deficits in children with dyslexia and children with language impairment. *Journal of Learning Disabilities, 46,* 230–240. doi: http://dx .doi.org/10.1177/0022219412449430.

Schiff, R., & Raveh, M. (2007). Deficient morphological processing in adults with developmental dyslexia: Another barrier to efficient word recognition? *Dyslexia, 13,* 110–129. doi: http://dx.doi.org/10.1002/dys.322.

Schiff, R., & Ravid, D. (2004). Representing written vowels in university students with dyslexia compared with normal Hebrew readers. *Annals of Dyslexia, 54,* 39–64. doi: http://dx.doi.org/10.1007/s11881-004-0003-2.

Schiff, R., & Ravid, D. (2007). Morphological analogies in Hebrew-speaking university students with dyslexia compared with typically developing gradeschoolers. *Journal of Psycholinguistic Research, 36,* 237–253. doi: http://dx.doi.org/10.1007/s10936-0 06-9043-6.

Schiff, R., & Ravid, D. (2013). Morphological processing in Hebrew-speaking students with reading disabilities. *Journal of Learning Disabilities, 46,* 220–229. doi: http://dx .doi.org/10.1177/0022219412449425.

Schiff, R., Schwartz-Nahshon, S., & Nagar, R. (2011). Effect of phonological and morphological awareness on reading comprehension in Hebrew-speaking adolescents with reading disabilities. *Annals of Dyslexia, 61,* 44–63. doi: http://dx.doi.org /10.1007/s11881-010-0046-5.

Schulz, E., Maurer, U., van der Mark, S. et al. (2008). Impaired semantic processing during sentence reading in children with dyslexia: Combined fMRI and ERP evidence. *Neuroimage, 41,* 153–168. doi: http://dx.doi.org/10.1016/j.neuroimage .2008.02.012.

Seidenberg, M. S. (2011). Reading in different writing systems: One architecture, multiple solutions. In P. McCardle, B. Miller, J. R. Lee, & O. L. Tzeng (Eds.), *Dyslexia across languages: Orthography and the brain–gene–behavior link* (pp. 146–168). Baltimore, MD: Paul H. Brookes.

Seidenberg, M. S., & McClelland, J. L. (1989). A distributed, developmental model of word recognition and naming. *Psychological Review, 96,* 523–568. doi: http://dx .doi.org/10.1037/0033-295X.96.4.523.

Seymour, P. H. (1999). Cognitive architecture of early reading. In I. Lindberg, F. E. Tønnessen, & I. Austad (Eds.), *Dyslexia: Advances in theory and practice* (pp. 59–73). Dordrecht, the Netherlands: Springer. doi: http://dx.doi.org/10.1007/97 8-94-011-4667-8_5.

Shankweiler, D., Crain, S., Katz, L. et al. (1995). Cognitive profiles of reading-disabled children: Comparison of language skills in phonology, morphology, and syntax. *Psychological Science, 6,* 149–156. doi: http://dx.doi.org/10.1111/j.1467-9280 .1995.tb00324.x.

Shu, H., Chen, X., Anderson, R. C., Wu, N., & Xuan, Y. (2003). Properties of school Chinese: Implications for learning to read. *Child Development, 74,* 27–47. doi: http:// dx.doi.org/10.1111/1467-8624.00519.

Shu, H., McBride-Chang, C., Wu, S., & Liu, H. (2006). Understanding Chinese developmental dyslexia: Morphological awareness as a core cognitive construct. *Journal of Educational Psychology, 98,* 122–133. doi: http://dx.doi.org/10.1037/0022-0663 .98.1.122.

Siegel, L. S. (2008). Morphological awareness skills of English language learners and children with dyslexia. *Topics in Language Disorders, 28,* 15–27. doi: http://dx .doi.org/10.1097/01.adt.0000311413.75804.60.

Stanovich, K. E. (1980). Toward an interactive-compensatory model of individual differences in the development of reading fluency. *Reading Research Quarterly, 16,* 32–71. doi: http://dx.doi.org/10.2307/747348.

Suárez-Coalla, P., & Cuetos, F. (2013). The role of morphology in reading in Spanish-speaking children with dyslexia. *The Spanish Journal of Psychology, 16,* E51, doi: http://dx.doi.org/ 10.1017/sjp.2013.58.

Tong, X., & McBride-Chang, C. (2010). Developmental models of learning to read Chinese words. *Developmental Psychology, 46,* 1662–1676. doi: http://dx.doi.org/10 .1037/a0020611.

Tong, X., McBride-Chang, C., Wong, A. M.-Y. et al. (2011). Longitudinal predictors of very early Chinese literacy acquisition. *Journal of Research in Reading, 34,* 315–332. doi: http://dx.doi.org/10.1111/j.1467-9817.2009.01426.x.

Torppa, M., Lyytinen, P., Erskine, J., Eklund, K., & Lyytinen, H. (2010). Language development, literacy skills, and predictive connections to reading in Finnish children with and without familial risk for dyslexia. *Journal of Learning Disabilities*, *43*, 308–321. doi: http://dx.doi.org/10.1177/0022219410369096.

Traficante, D., Marcolini, S., Luci, A., Zoccolotti, P., & Burani, C. (2011). How do roots and suffixes influence reading of pseudowords: A study of young Italian readers with and without dyslexia. *Language and Cognitive Processes*, *26*, 777–793. doi: http://dx .doi.org/10.1080/01690965.2010.496553.

Tsesmeli, S. N., & Seymour, P. K. (2006). Derivational morphology and spelling in dyslexia. *Reading and Writing*, *19*, 587–625. doi: http://dx.doi.org/10.1007/s11145-006-9011-4.

Vellutino, F. R., & Fletcher, J. M. (2005). Developmental dyslexia. In M. J. Snowling & C. Hulme (Eds.), *The science of reading: A handbook* (pp. 362–378). Malden, MA: Blackwell Publishing. doi: http://dx.doi.org/10.1002/9780470757642.ch19.

Vellutino, F. R., Scanlon, D. M., & Spearing, D. (1995). Semantic and phonological coding in poor and normal readers. *Journal of Experimental Child Psychology*, *59*, 76–123. doi: http://dx.doi.org/10.1006/jecp.1995.1004.

Vogel, S. A. (1977). Morphological ability in normal and dyslexic children. *Journal of Learning Disabilities*, *10*, 35–43. doi: http://dx.doi.org/10.1177/002221947701000109.

Xiao, X. Y., & Ho, C. S. H. (2014). Weaknesses in semantic, syntactic and oral language expression contribute to reading difficulties in Chinese dyslexic children. *Dyslexia*, *20*, 74–98. doi: http://dx.doi.org/10.1002/dys.1460.

Zhou, Y., McBride-Chang, C., Law, A. B. Y. et al. (2014). Development of reading-related skills in Chinese and English among Hong Kong Chinese children with and without dyslexia. *Journal of Experimental Child Psychology*, *122*, 75–91. doi: http://dx.doi.org/10.1016/j.jecp.2013.12.003.

16 Modeling the Variability of Developmental Dyslexia

Johannes C. Ziegler, Conrad Perry, and Marco Zorzi

16.1 Introduction

Reading is a highly complex task that relies on the integration of visual, orthographic, phonological and semantic information. This complexity is clearly reflected in current computational models of reading (Coltheart et al., 2001; Harm & Seidenberg, 1999, 2004; Perry, Ziegler, & Zorzi, 2007, 2010; Plaut et al., 1996). These models specify the "ingredients" of the reading process in a precise and detailed fashion as they implement the units and computations that are necessary to go from the visual information to word recognition and word production. Such models make it possible to simulate real reading performance in terms of reading latencies (how long it takes to compute the pronunciation of a word or pseudoword) and reading accuracy (whether the output of the model is correct). Computational models are particularly well suited to helping us understand reading impairments, such as developmental or acquired dyslexia. This is because model components can be "impaired" in very specific and focal ways and the consequences of these impairments can be analyzed through simulations (Harm & Seidenberg, 1999; Woollams, 2014; Ziegler et al., 2008). This allows one to understand the *causal* relation between deficits in components of the reading network and performance.

In the present chapter, this approach is applied to the study of developmental dyslexia. Developmental dyslexia is characterized by extremely slow and laborious reading and a failure to automatize parallel visual word recognition that cannot be accounted for by low IQ, poor educational opportunities, or obvious sensory or neurological damage (World Health Organization, 2011). Over the past two decades, it has become increasingly clear that dyslexia is probabilistic and multifactorial rather than deterministic and focused on single causes (Pennington, 2006). Indeed, there seems to be as much variability in the nature of the reading deficits as there is in the underlying cognitive profiles (for a review see Ramus & Ahissar, 2012). Again, computational models are well suited to this domain as they enable us to test to what extent the variability of dyslexia can be accounted for by single- or multi-deficit theories. In the present chapter, we first review the main single- and multiple-deficit theories. We then present the main computational models of skilled reading and how they were used to simulate dyslexia and dyslexia subtypes. Finally, we will describe a developmentally plausible model of learning to read, and show that such a model can be used to understand how deficits that are present at the outset of reading development can affect that learning process.

16.2   Theoretical Background

16.2.1   Single-Deficit Theories of Dyslexia

Single-deficit theories have a long history in the field of dyslexia. The most prominent single-deficit theory is the rapid temporal processing deficit theory (Tallal & Piercy, 1973), which claims that children with dyslexia have difficulties in perceiving auditory stimuli that have short duration and occur in rapid succession. Such a deficit at the basic auditory level would lead to an inability to integrate sensory information delivered in rapid succession and thus prevent a correct temporal analysis of speech at the phoneme level, which consequently results in abnormal phonological development. A more recent theory, the temporal sampling theory of dyslexia, assumes that deficits in temporal sampling and inefficient phase locking at one or more temporal rates could explain abnormal phonological development in children with dyslexia across languages (Goswami, 2011; Goswami et al., 2002).

The most prominent single-deficit theory in the visual domain is the magnocellular-dorsal deficit theory (Stein & Walsh, 1997). The magnocellular pathway is sensitive to low contrast, low spatial frequency, and high temporal frequency. Deficits in the visual magnocellular system would result in impoverished visual guidance of attention and poor letter-position coding, both of which are important abilities for reading development. The magnocellular deficit theory has been supported in studies that reported difficulties in discriminating global motion, spatial frequency grids, or attention shifting (for a review, see Stein, 2014).

Another single-deficit theory in the visual domain is the visual span deficit theory (Bosse, Tainturier, & Valdois, 2007), which assumes that dyslexics show deficits in processing multi-element strings in parallel, such as when they are asked to report a letter in a consonant string (RWXST). This deficit has been attributed to reduced visual attention span or abnormal allocation of attentional resources (but see Ziegler et al., 2010). Although the claim that this deficit is independent from the classic phonological deficits has been recently challenged (Saksida et al., 2016), there are a number of similar theories, which claim that "sluggish attention shifting" (Facoetti et al., 2008) or impoverished allocation of spatial attention (Facoetti et al., 2006, 2009) are associated with dyslexia.

There are a number of single-deficit theories, which have focused on rather general mechanisms. For example, the noise exclusion deficit theory argues that children with dyslexia have deficits in optimizing perceptual filters so that the signals are processed while noise is being excluded (Sperling et al., 2005, 2006). The authors argued that deficits in noise exclusion, not magnocellular or temporal processing, cause dyslexia. The perceptual anchor deficit theory is another general theory, which argues that dyslexics fail to form perceptual anchors in psychophysical tasks that require encoding and matching, such as when deciding whether a tone is lower or higher than a reference (Ahissar, 2007; Ahissar et al., 2006). The important finding was that children with dyslexia do not seem to benefit from the repetition of a reference, which seems to suggest an inability to detect and use stimulus or task regularities (but see Di Filippo, Zoccolotti, & Ziegler, 2008; Ziegler, 2008).

The present list of single-deficit theories is far from being exhaustive. We have simply chosen some of the most prominent or influential single-deficit theories to illustrate an important point for our modeling work. First, at present, there is no single sensory or cognitive deficit that seems to explain all behavioral symptoms of all children with dyslexia (for a review see Ramus & Ahissar, 2012). For example, not all children with dyslexia show a visual span disorder (Saksida et al., 2016) and not all children with dyslexia show auditory deficits (White et al., 2006) or magnocellular-dorsal deficits (Menghini et al., 2010). Second, single-deficit theories run into trouble when it comes to explaining comorbidity, because each single-deficit model would require a distinct account for each comorbidity (for discussion see van Bergen, van der Leij, & de Jong, 2014). Thus, there seems to be some emerging consensus that single-deficit models must give way to multiple-deficit models in understanding developmental disorders.

16.2.2   *Multiple-Deficit Theories of Dyslexia*

Multiple-deficit theories of dyslexia assumes that no single deficit is necessary or sufficient to explain all behavioral symptoms or all reading profiles of children with dyslexia. Instead, a number of sensory or cognitive processes or representations can be impaired to varying degrees, with some being more important or fragile, and some being more easily compensated, than others. In the area of genetics of dyslexia, the multifactorial nature of the disorder has been acknowledged for quite some time (Pennington, 2006). Dyslexia is not caused by a single gene; rather, multiple genetic and environmental risk factors operate probabilistically to cause the disorder.

Cognitive multiple-deficit theories have been supported over the past years by a number of studies, which compared competing accounts of dyslexia within the same study, so-called multiple single-case studies of dyslexia (Ramus et al., 2003). In their study, Ramus et al. administered a full battery of psychometric, phonological, auditory, visual, and cerebellar tests to sixteen dyslexic and sixteen control university students. The results showed that all dyslexics suffered from phonological deficits, whereas only ten showed an auditory deficit, four a motor deficit, and two a visual magnocellular deficit. Importantly, there was quite some overlap between deficits. For example, all children with visual deficits also had auditory deficits. Indeed, only five dyslexics seemed to be entirely unaffected by any sensory or motor/cerebellar disorder. All others had multiple deficits.

In a similar study, Menghini et al. (2010) tested sixty Italian dyslexic children and age-matched normally reading children on tests of phonological abilities, visual processing, selective and sustained attention, implicit learning, and executive functions. While most of the dyslexics had phonological deficits (85 percent had deficits in phonological awareness and 75 percent had deficits in nonword repetition), 16 percent of the dyslexics had deficits in visual-spatial attention, 30 percent in executive functions, 43 percent in sustained attention, 20 percent in visual-spatial perception, and only 10 percent in motion perception, and no significant deficits were found for implicit memory learning tasks. Interestingly, most of the dyslexic children with phonological deficits also showed deficits in other domains, supporting the multiple-deficit model of developmental dyslexia.

In one of our studies (Ziegler et al., 2008), which is summarized in somewhat greater detail here, we designed tasks that tapped the core processing components involved in skilled reading and reading development: sustained attention, letter processing, lexical processing of orthography and phonology, and grapheme–phoneme mapping. The tasks were administered to twenty-four French-speaking children with dyslexia aged between 8 and 11 years and twenty-four age-matched controls. Figure 16.1 presents the performance of each child in each of the component tasks. In order to compare the size of the deficits across the tasks, the performance was standardized by computing z-scores with respect to the mean and standard deviation of the control sample.

The results can be summarized as follows. No deficits were obtained for the sustained attention task (for which only three children were below the 1 SD cutoff). A significant deficit was obtained for letter-in-string perception (e.g., Bosse et al., 2007; Ziegler, Pech-Georgel et al., 2010), which affected about 40 percent of the dyslexic children. No significant deficit

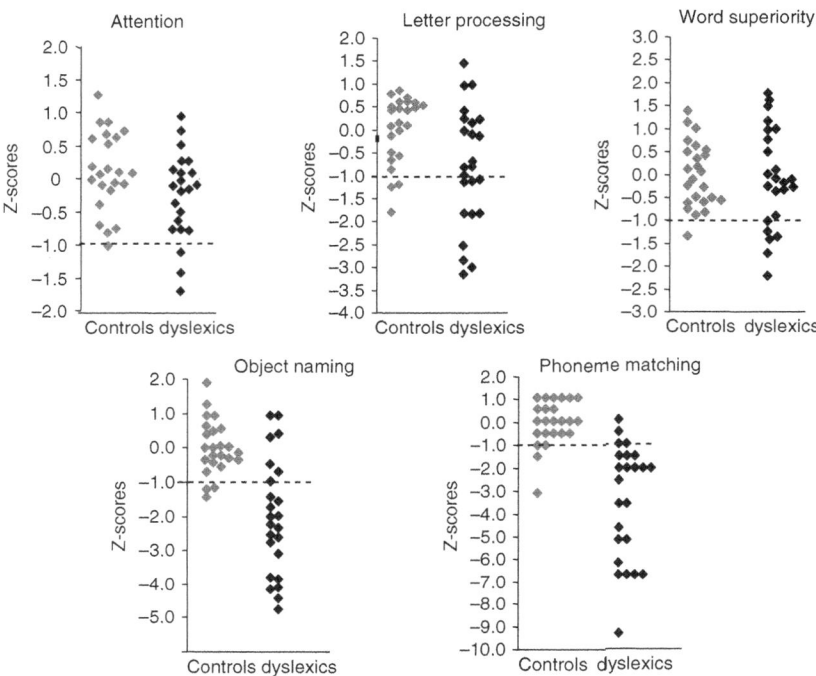

Figure 16.1 Individual patterns of performance of dyslexics (black) and controls (gray) in the five component tasks of reading: sustained attention, letter-in-string perception, word superiority effect, rapid object naming, and phoneme matching

was obtained for the word superiority effect, which was thought to reflect access to and feedback from the orthographic lexicon (only five children showed reduced word superiority effects). A robust deficit was obtained for rapid object naming, which was taken as a proxy for access to the phonological lexicon (70 percent of the dyslexic children exhibited deficits in this task). Finally, over 80 percent of the dyslexic children showed deficits in the phoneme matching task, which was designed to tap grapheme-to-phoneme conversion.

Together, these studies conducted in English, Italian, and French converge to suggest that although most dyslexics exhibited phonological deficits (object naming, phoneme matching), many were deficient in more than one domain or component task. In the study by Ziegler et al. (2008), nine children had a triple deficit, seven had a double deficit, and eight had a single deficit, and the size of the deficits varied substantially between children.

16.3   Modeling Developmental Dyslexia

16.3.1   Models of Reading Processes

A number of computational reading models that have been developed to account for skilled reading have been applied to simulate dyslexia. Broadly speaking, there are two classes. The first are models from the Parallel Distributed Processing (PDP) or triangle family (Plaut et al., 1996; Seidenberg & McClelland, 1989). These models implement a single pathway that is trained with error backpropagation to map orthography onto phonology. Because this mapping is not fully regular/consistent, a hidden layer is needed to learn irregular/inconsistent mappings. This model was able to account for various facts about the reading performance of normal participants (e.g., Plaut et al., 1996). In particular, it showed the classic interaction between word frequency and spelling–sound regularity, which had previously been taken as unequivocal support for dual-route models of reading.

The second class are dual-route models (Coltheart et al., 2001; Perry et al., 2007, 2010; for review see Zorzi, 2010; Zorzi, Houghton, & Butterworth, 1998b). Dual-route models implement two pathways for reading aloud, a lexical (mediated) pathway and a sublexical (direct) pathway. The direct pathway maps letters directly onto orthographic representations in a parallel fashion using the interactive activation model (McClelland & Rumelhart, 1981). The sublexical pathway maps graphemes onto phonemes in a serial manner. In the original dual-route connectionist model (DRC), the sublexical pathway contained a set of hard-wired rules that allowed the model to convert graphemes into phonemes (Coltheart et al., 2001). In the more recent connectionist dual-process model (CDP), the rule system was replaced by a two-layer associative network that was trained to map graphemes onto phonemes (Perry et al., 2007, 2010; Zorzi et al., 1998b). Because it has no hidden layer, unlike PDP models, the associative network uses a simpler learning algorithm (i.e., the delta rule) and it can only learn consistent mappings (for a developmental study of the network's decoding abilities, see Zorzi, Houghton, & Butterworth, 1998a). Thus, the lexical route is needed to read aloud irregular/inconsistent words.

16.3.2   Simulating Dyslexia

Both classes of model have been used to simulate developmental dyslexia. In the important work by Harm and Seidenberg (1999), developmental dyslexia was simulated by impairing the representation of phonological information before training the model to read. That is, prior to reading, an attractor network was implemented that learned phonological structure from phonetic input, a process that was thought to approximate the child's acquisition of phonological knowledge prior to learning to read. Three types of phonological impairments were implemented. In the mild deficit condition, some weight decay was imposed on the weights in the phonological attractor. In the moderate deficit condition, the phonological cleanup units were removed and 50 percent of the connections between the phonological units were lesioned. Finally, in the severe deficit condition, noise was added to each connection weight in the phonological attractor network. The reading model then learned to map orthography onto mildly-to-severely-impaired phonological units. The results showed that a mild phonological impairment resulted in impaired nonword reading but normal exception-word reading. A moderate impairment resulted in a mixed pattern, with strong deficits in nonword reading but smaller deficits in exception-word reading. Finally, a severe deficit resulted in very strong deficits in both nonword and irregular-word reading. These simulations provide proof of the concept that PDP models can simulate developmental dyslexia in a plausible way, but the model was not used to simulate actual data. In the model, the heterogeneity in hypothetical reading patterns is a consequence of the quality of the phonological attractor network prior to reading.

In dual-route models, dyslexia has been simulated either by lesioning the lexical or sublexical routes (Coltheart et al., 2001) or by impairing relevant model components (Ziegler et al., 2008). The latter approach is particularly relevant for simulating inter-individual differences and the multifactorial nature of dyslexia. The basic idea was that one could estimate the efficiency of each model component by using data from so-called component tasks and then set up individual dyslexia models, in which the components were impaired proportionally to the underlying deficit of a given child (see Perry, Zorzi & Ziegler, 2019). For example, if a child had a deficit in phoneme processing, lexical phonology, and letter processing, impaired reading was simulated by simply adding noise to the respective components of the DRC model proportional to the underlying deficit. The actual amount of noise was found by taking the child that was worst at a task and setting the level of noise based on that child (e.g., .1), and then linearly interpolating the level of noise based on the value of the child's z-score. No noise was entered if the z-score of a given child on a given task was positive. For example, if the worst child had a z-score of –4 SDs in phoneme processing, then it would mean that the child with a –2 SD deficit would have the level of noise set to half of that of the worst child (e.g., .05) and a child with a –1 SD deficit would have the level of noise set to one quarter of that of the worst child (e.g., .025). This procedure was applied for each of the twenty-four dyslexic children (for details see Ziegler et al., 2008). One simulation was performed with the normal parameter set (control model). The "normal" and "impaired" models were then presented with a list of regular and irregular words and nonwords, which was the same as the one read by the participants. The results of the

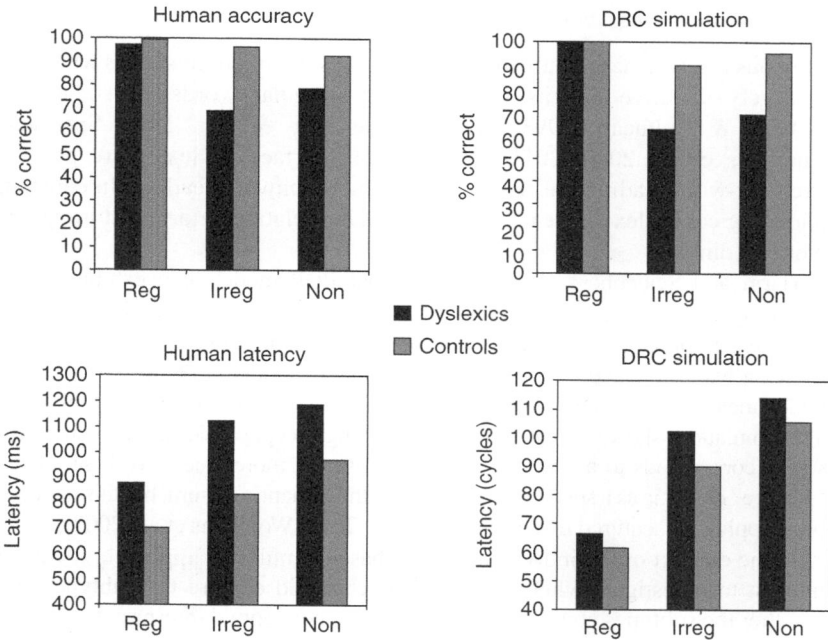

Figure 16.2 Simulations of normal and impaired reading accuracy and reading speed with the DRC model. Impaired reading was simulated by using the individual deficits to determine the noise levels of each of the DRC model's component processes

participants and the model (averaged across the twenty-four participants and the twenty-four simulations) are presented in Figure 16.2.

As expected, children with dyslexia exhibited major deficits in reading aloud. They made significantly more errors than controls when reading irregular words and nonwords and it took them significantly longer to read the three classes of stimuli. Interestingly, accuracy was at ceiling for regular word reading, but the children with dyslexia still showed a robust speed deficit for regular words. As can be seen in Figure 16.2, the impaired model (average of the twenty-four deficit-based simulations) mirrored the impaired reading data almost perfectly. In terms of accuracy, the model showed a ceiling effect for regular words and significantly higher error rates for the dyslexic model than the normal model for irregular words and nonwords (all $ps < .05$). In terms of reading speed, the model showed significant speed deficits for the three classes of stimuli (all $ps < .05$), just like the human data. In sum, the models that were impaired on the basis of the deficits in the component tasks exhibited the same reading deficits as did the children with dyslexia.

16.3.3   Simulating Subtypes of Dyslexia

Previous research has identified two prominent subtypes of dyslexics who have relatively selective deficits when reading irregular words and nonwords (Castles & Coltheart, 1993; Manis, Seidenberg, & Doi, 1999; Sprenger-Charolles et al., 2000, 2011). In particular, surface dyslexics are poor at irregular-word reading but relatively normal at nonword reading. In contrast, phonological dyslexics are poor at nonword but relatively normal at irregular-word reading.

Harm and Seidenberg (1999) showed that PDP models can exhibit "pure" phonological dyslexia when phonological representations are mildly impaired. More severe phonological impairments tend to result in "mixed" profiles. Surface dyslexia was simulated by reducing the number of hidden units from 100 to 20, which meant that the network was no longer able to learn the complete training set. The simulations showed greater impact on reading exception words than nonwords, which corresponds to a "surface" profile. However, more recent work simulated "surface" dyslexia as a specific impairment to the semantic system, but this has only been applied to acquired dyslexia (Woollams, 2014; Woollams et al., 2007).

In the context of the individual-deficit-based simulation approach, it was of interest to investigate whether this approach could capture the subtypes and whether the subtypes could be given a coherent conceptual interpretation based on the ancillary component tasks (for a similar approach, see Griffiths & Snowling, 2002). According to classic dual-route hypotheses, surface dyslexics should show larger deficits on the lexical route (access to the orthographic and phonological lexicons), whereas phonological dyslexics should show larger deficits on the non-lexical route.

The twenty-four dyslexics from the study described above were classified using Castles and Coltheart's (1993) regression procedure, where pseudoword performance was plotted against irregular-word performance (and vice versa). A child was considered a phonological dyslexic if he/she was below the 90 percent confidence interval when pseudowords were plotted against irregular words but within the 90 percent confidence interval when irregular words were plotted against pseudowords. Surface dyslexics were defined conversely. Note that the classification was based on accuracy data only (for a discussion of the limitations of classifications based on accuracy data alone, see Sprenger-Charolles et al., 2011). According to this procedure, 29 percent of the sample were surface dyslexics (seven out of twenty-four) and 19 percent were phonological dyslexics (four out of twenty-four).

We then simulated the reading performance of these surface and phonological dyslexics using the deficit-based simulation approach described above. The performance of the impaired model and the average underlying deficits in the subcomponent tasks are presented in Figure 16.3.

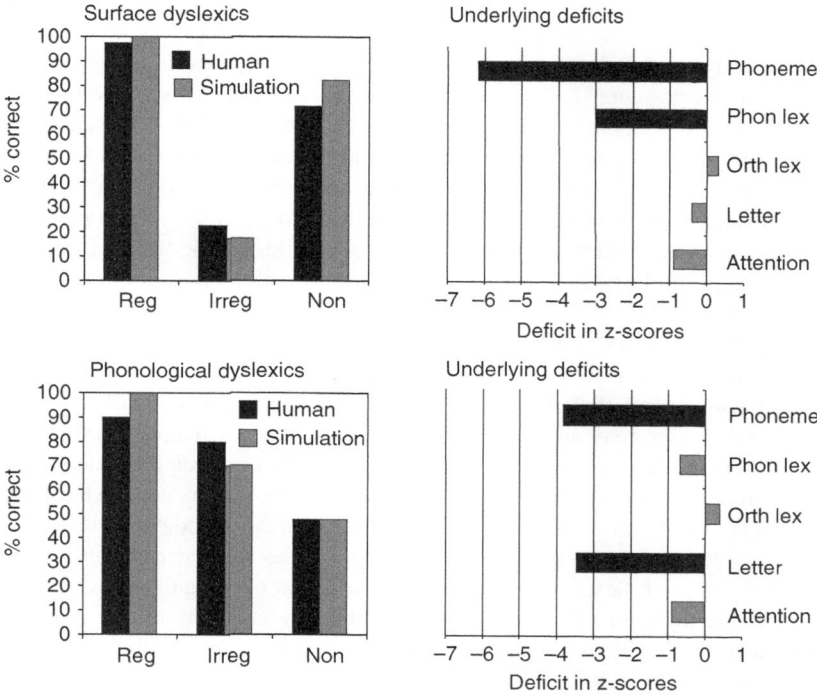

Figure 16.3 Simulations of individuals with surface and phonological dyslexia (left panel) and underlying deficits associated with the dissociated profiles (right panel)

As can be seen in Figure 16.3, the model captured the dissociation between surface and phonological dyslexia surprisingly well. For the surface dyslexics, the model only read 20 percent of the irregular words correctly, even though it read 80 percent of the nonwords correctly. For the phonological dyslexics, the model only read 50 percent of the nonwords correctly even though it read 70 percent of the irregular words correctly. The "simulated" double dissociation is very close to the one present in the human data. These results show that continuous noise manipulations can reproduce the major subtypes of dyslexia defined in the literature. According to the analysis of the underlying deficits (Figure 16.3, right panels), the surface dyslexics in this sample had, on average, strong deficits in phoneme matching (sublexical phonology) and object naming (lexical phonology). In contrast, phonological dyslexics had strong deficits in phoneme matching and also in letter processing.

The ability of the model to simulate subtypes on the basis of deficits in individual subcomponents is rather striking, and is important because previous accounts of dissociated profiles within the context of the dual-route model (Castles & Coltheart, 1993) assumed that surface dyslexia was due to a "lesion" of the orthographic lexical route, whereas phonological dyslexia was due to a lesion of the non-lexical phonological route. The present results tell a different story. In the human data, there was no clear-cut dissociation between impaired lexical versus impaired non-lexical processing associated with surface and phonological dyslexia. Rather, different combinations of lexical and non-lexical deficits were associated with the two profiles. Importantly, the model was able to simulate these dissociated profiles on the basis of multiple underlying deficits without any a priori assumptions about the deficiency of one or the other route.

In particular, in our sample, surface dyslexia was not associated with visual-orthographic deficits but rather with phonological deficits, namely deficits in picture naming and phoneme matching. The severe picture-naming deficit of our surface dyslexics gives an interesting explanation for how irregular-word reading can be impaired in the absence of a strong deficit to the orthographic lexicon. That is, in order to read irregular words via the lexical route, readers need to be able to access not only their orthographic lexicon but also their phonological lexicon. If access to the phonological lexicon were impaired, as suggested in our picture-naming data, a dyslexic reader would show a deficit on irregular-word reading. Indeed, the picture-naming deficit was significantly larger in surface dyslexics compared to phonological dyslexics, which underscores the possibility that irregular-word-reading deficits might be attributable to poor phonological lexical representations and/or poor vocabulary, possibly as a result of a lack of reading or developmental delay (see also Harm & Seidenberg, 1999). It is also possible that in these children the phonological procedure is well remediated while automatic access to whole word representations remains inefficient. One has to keep in mind, however that the present study and simulations concerned French-speaking dyslexics and it is possible that there are important cross-language differences in the nature of subtypes (Sprenger-Charolles et al., 2011). For example, in more transparent languages, nonword reading is often at ceiling, which gives the misleading impression that most dyslexics are "surface" dyslexics.

Interestingly, phonological dyslexia in the present sample was associated with poor letter perception. The present simulations also supported this interpretation by showing that adding noise to the letter level was particularly damaging for nonword reading. The finding that noise at the letter level affected nonword reading is clearly consistent with evidence from spatial attention tasks, which suggests that phonological dyslexics (but not the surface dyslexics) suffer from spatial attention problems which have their most disturbing effect on nonword reading (Facoetti et al., 2006, 2009). This makes perfect sense because precise coding of letter identity and letter position is particularly important for nonword reading (Grainger, Dufau, & Ziegler, 2016;

Grainger & Ziegler, 2011). Note that recent developments of the dual-route model of reading include an attentional window that operates on the input to the non-lexical route (Perry et al., 2007, 2010; Perry, Ziegler, & Zorzi, 2013, 2014a, 2014b). Such a model clearly predicts that deficits in focused visual attention would affect nonword more than irregular-word reading.

The present work on subtypes of dyslexia has important practical implications. First, it shows that it is overly simplistic and potentially dangerous to assume that all developmental surface dyslexics must have deficits in their orthographic systems, whereas all developmental phonological dyslexics must have deficits in their phonological systems. The present data show that surface dyslexia can result from a phonological deficit (i.e., access to the phonological lexicon), at least in languages other than English, whereas nonword reading deficits can result from impaired letter processing. More generally, different underlying deficits or different degrees of severity can give rise to either surface or to phonological dyslexia, and the mere observation of a deficit in irregular-word or nonword reading is not sufficient to infer the underlying causes.

16.4 Toward a Developmental Model of Dyslexia

There is an obvious limitation with the multi-component approach described above. That is, it is entirely possible that there are single developmental causes of dyslexia, such as deficits in low-level auditory processing (Goswami et al., 2002) or deficits in categorical perception of speech (e.g., Serniclaes, 2004, p. 771; Vandermosten et al., 2010, p. 1625), that have cascading effects on the developing reading system. Such cascading effects may affect distinct subcomponents of the reading system in different ways depending on the severity of the initial deficit and individual factors, such as compensatory strategies, training, teaching methods, orthographic transparency of the writing system, oral language skills, or socioeconomic background. For example, one can imagine that a deficit in the categorical perception of speech will not only cause poor phonological development of words (lexical) and phonemes (sublexical) but will also hamper orthographic development, as learning to process letters efficiently depends on the child's ability to map the orthographic code onto a phonological code (Share, 1995). Thus, what looks like a triple deficit at the age of 10 might well have been a single deficit at the age of 5, which demonstrates the need for more longitudinal studies (Goswami, 2015).

16.4.1 Simulating Reading Development via Phonological Decoding and Self-Teaching

To tackle some of these shortcomings, we have recently proposed a connectionist developmental model of learning to read (Ziegler, Perry, & Zorzi, 2014) based on the CDP model described earlier (for a review, see Zorzi, 2010). The developmental model builds upon the idea that children come to the task of learning to read with a phonological lexicon partially in place and rely on phonological decoding skills to acquire the orthographic form of these spoken words (i.e., Share's [1995] phonological decoding and self-teaching theory). That is, during the initial stages of learning to read, children are taught basic phonological decoding skills, that is, a small number of basic letter–sound (grapheme–phoneme) correspondences. Such teaching takes place in an "explicit" and "supervised" way. Phonological decoding allows children to decipher words that they have heard but never seen before, thus giving them access to the thousands of words that are present in their spoken lexicon. In theory, every successfully decoded word provides the child with an opportunity to set up direct connections between a given letter string (orthography) and the spoken word, which results in the development of an orthographic lexicon. Phonological decoding thus provides a powerful self-teaching device because the explicit learning of a small set of spelling–sound correspondences allows the child to decode an increasingly large number of words, which in turn bootstraps orthographic and lexical development. Importantly, only the initial learning of a small set of grapheme–phoneme correspondences requires explicit teaching and feedback (supervised learning). From there on, the child will read more or less autonomously and it is the decoded word itself which provides the teaching signal to improve the decoding network. Thus, phonological decoding can be seen to act as a self-teaching mechanism or "built-in teacher" (non-supervised learning).

We have implemented this learning loop for English in the context of CDP++ (Perry et al., 2010), a recent large-scale version of the CDP model that can handle polysyllabic word reading. A schematic description of the learning process is illustrated in Figure 16.4. The details of the implementation can be found in Ziegler et al. (2014). In a nutshell, initially, the decoding network was pretrained on a small set of grapheme–phoneme correspondences. Next, the network was presented with written words to be learned, actually several thousands of written words. On the basis of the pretraining, the decoding network computed the potential (but possibly incorrect) pronunciation of a novel word, which typically results in the activation of word units in the phonological lexicon. If a word entry was found in the phonological lexicon which was consistent with the letter string, a direct connection was set up between the written word and its phonological counterpart (orthographic development). That is, the word became lexicalized. In turn, the internally activated phonology of the word was then used as a training signal to improve the decoding network by adjusting its connection weights (i.e., an internally generated rather than a supervised teaching signal).

After pretraining, the model was presented with 32,735 words. The first thing the researchers wanted to establish was whether a self-teaching network

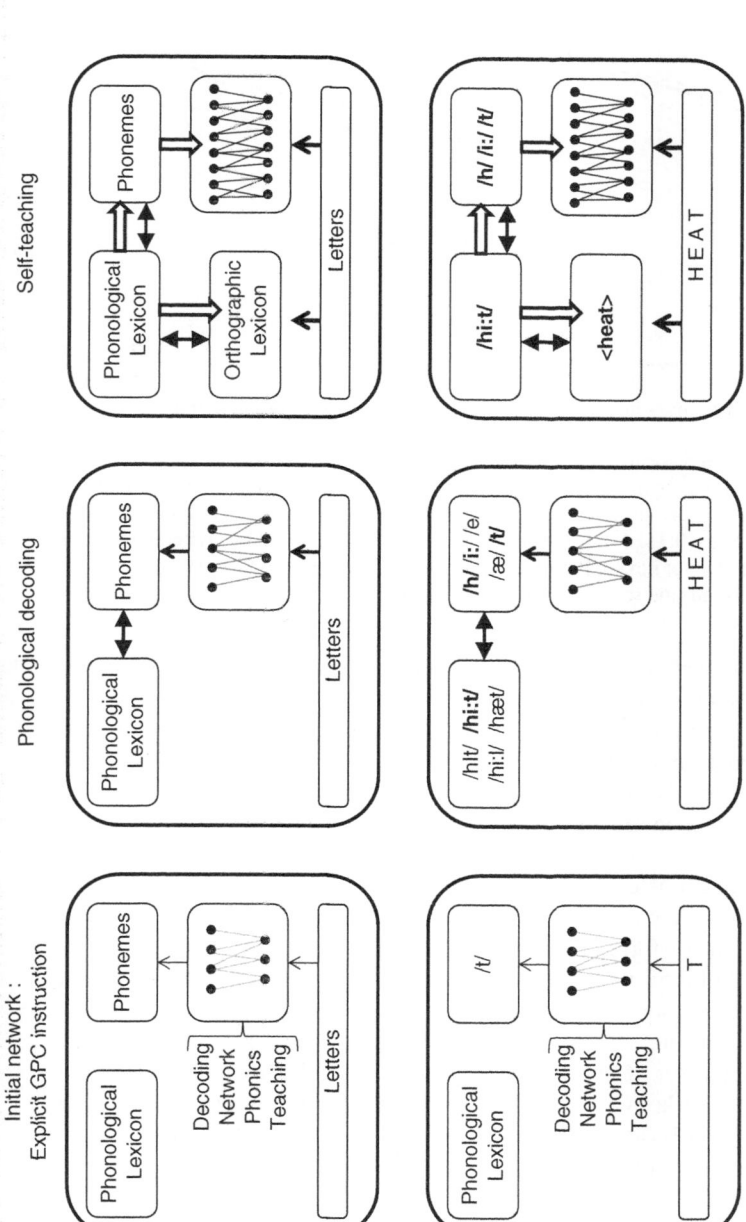

Figure 16.4 Illustration of the phonological decoding and self-teaching mechanisms in the context of the connectionist dual-process model. After initial explicit teaching on a small set of grapheme–phoneme correspondences, such as T->/t/ (left panels), the associative network is able to decode novel words, such as HEAT (middle panels), which has a preexisting representation in the phonological lexicon. If the decoding mechanism activates a word in the phonological lexicon (here the correct word /hi:t/ is more active than its competitors), an orthographic entry is created (<heat>), and the phonology of the "winner" (/hi:t/) is used as an internally generated teaching signal (gray arrows) to improve and strengthen the weights of the decoding network (right panel)

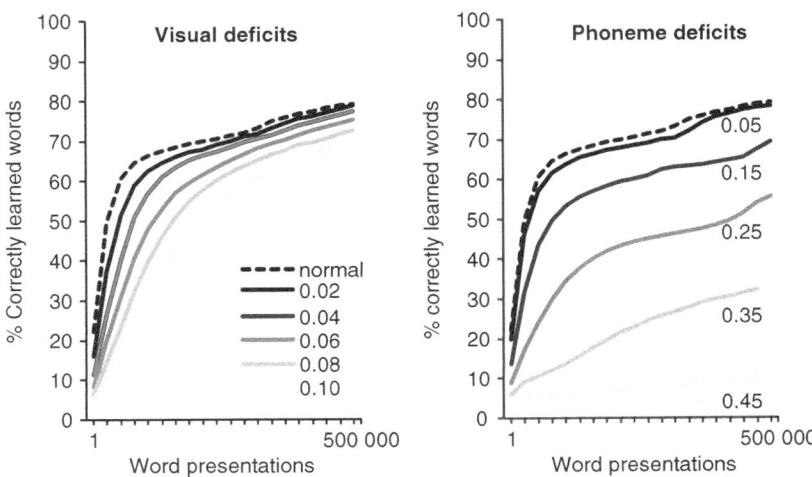

Figure 16.5 Learning to read with phoneme or visual deficits. A: Phoneme deficits were simulated by changing a correctly assembled phoneme with a phonetically similar but incorrect phoneme with a certain probability (0.05, 0.15, 0.25, 0.35, 0.45). B: Visual deficits were simulated by switching a letter with the letter next to it with a certain probability (0.02, 0.04, 0.06, 0.06, 0.10). The dotted line represents the unimpaired network

with minimal supervised learning can actually learn correct orthographic word forms. This is far from trivial, especially for English orthography, which contains many inconsistent letter–sound correspondences (the letter "a" can be pronounced in five different ways even in common English words) and many irregular words (aisle, pint, yacht, etc.). As can be seen in Figure 16.5 (dotted line, non-impaired network), the model learned about 80 percent of the words. The remaining 20 percent of the words were too irregular to be learned through decoding (aisle, yacht, choir . . .). Importantly, very rapidly in the course of learning, the most active item in the phonological lexicon tended to be the correct word form, which is the reason why self-teaching can work so well. In summary, this simulation provides a proof for the claim that phonological decoding and self-teaching combine to form a powerful boot-strapping mechanism, which allows the beginning reader to "start small" (i.e., with a small set of explicitly taught letter–sound correspondences) and then build upon this knowledge to "self-learn" orthographic representations for the majority of words (up to 80 percent) through a simple decoding mechanism that gets more efficient with every successfully decoded word. An effective decoding network is therefore crucial for the development of the model's lexical network.

16.4.2 Simulating Visual and Phoneme Deficits during Processes of Learning to Read

Now that we have a developmentally plausible and functioning learning model, we can ask how different deficits that are present at the outset of learning to read might affect that learning process. The results described above (see Figure 16.1) as well as the literature on developmental dyslexia highlight at least two core deficits, which can be identified prior to reading. The first is related to phonological processing deficits that are most apparent in phonological aware-ness tasks (Bruck, 1992; Swan & Goswami, 1997). This deficit seems to be universal as it is found across transparent and opaque writing systems (Landerl et al., 2013; Ziegler, Bertrand et al., 2010). The second deficit is related to visual and orthographic processing difficulties and can be seen in tasks where children have to process letter strings that are not pronounceable, such as RWTXN (Bosse et al., 2007; Collis, Kohnen, & Kinoshita, 2013; Hawelka, Huber, & Wimmer, 2006; Ziegler, Pech-Georgel et al., 2010). Recent evidence suggests that such letter-in-string processing deficits might result from abnor-mally strong crowding (Zorzi et al., 2012) or impoverished visual-attentional processing (Facoetti et al., 2006), which might be identified even prior to reading (Franceschini et al., 2012). The co-occurrence of phonological proces-sing and visuospatial attention deficits has also been observed in prereading children with familial risk for dyslexia in comparison to their (not-at-risk) peers (Facoetti et al., 2010).

We thus investigated how visual and phoneme deficits that are present prior to learning to read affect the learning-to-read process itself. This allowed us to look at the *causal* link between a specific deficit and the reading outcome across development akin to a longitudinal study. To simulate visual difficulties, each letter in a word was switched with the letter next to it with a certain probability (.02, .04, 06, .06, .10). Thus, for example, instead of presenting CAT to the model, we would present ACT. Such letter-position errors are relatively frequent in children with dyslexia (Collis et al., 2013; Kohnen et al., 2012). To simulate deficits in phonological awareness, each time a correct word was activated in the phonological lexicon, we changed the phonemes in the output of the decoding network, which resulted in an incorrect teaching signal. Again, this was done parametrically by changing each correct phoneme with a certain probability (.05, .15, .25, .35, .45). Changing phonemes was not done ran-domly, but rather we switched a given phoneme with a phonetically similar one (e.g., /b/ was switched to /p/). The results are presented in Figure 16.5.

As can be seen, the effect of the two deficits on performance varied in a non-additive way across the levels of impairments. Basically, the greater the deficit, the more it deteriorated the learning performance of the model. That was especially so for the phonological deficits: subtle phoneme deficits (probability of phoneme swapping of .05) did not affect learning much, as they could be compensated for. However, when phoneme swapping happened on every other trial (probability of phoneme swapping of .45), learning through decoding and self-teaching was no longer possible. The visual deficits also affected the learning process. When comparing the two simulations, it would be tempting to conclude that visual and visual-attentional deficits had a somewhat smaller impact than phoneme deficits, which would be in line with a vast body of research (Ramus et al., 2003; Saksida et al., 2016; White et al., 2006).

16.4.3   Cross-Language Issues

The present modeling approach could be applied to study cross-language differences and similarities in dyslexia (e.g., Paulesu et al., 2001; Ziegler et al., 2003). Indeed, given that CDP++ exists in different languages (Italian: Perry et al., 2014a; French: Perry et al., 2014b), one could investigate whether the same set of deficits produce different reading profiles in different languages (e.g., greater impact on speed than on accuracy in a transparent orthography). This might reveal that the behavioral differences are just different expressions of the same cognitive phenotype and thus might help to settle the longstanding debate about putative differences between dyslexia in transparent versus more opaque (i.e., English) orthographies. Indeed, we believe that the causes of dyslexia are identical but that the same causes express themselves differently in different languages and/or writing systems (e.g., Paulesu et al., 2001; Ziegler, 2006). More research on this topic is needed.

16.5   Discussion and Conclusion

The present chapter has highlighted two interesting facts about developmental dyslexia. On the one hand, there is a considerable amount of heterogeneity, because most dyslexics exhibit a variety of deficits across different domains (letter processing, phoneme processing, phonological lexicon). This finding corroborates the claim that dyslexia is multifactorial in nature (e.g., Pennington, 2006). On the other hand, not all deficits are equal; that is, of similar size and affecting an equal number of children. Indeed, deficits in the phonological domain tend to outweigh deficits in visual-orthographic processing, a finding that has been reported in English (White et al., 2006), French (Saksida et al., 2016), and Italian (Menghini et al., 2010).

   To gain a better understanding of the heterogeneity that is associated with developmental dyslexia, we have outlined a new modeling approach, which consists of simulating individual differences in reading different kinds of words on the basis of underlying deficits in core components of the reading system, as specified by a computational model of reading. The originality of this approach is that individual deficits in reading performance are predicted by individual differences in subcomponents of reading. Practically, this is done by adding noise to those model components for which empirical evidence suggests that they are deficient. The amount of noise added is proportional to the size of the individual deficit. This simulation approach showed a striking match between the human data and the model both for accuracy and latency on a French sample (Ziegler et al., 2008). One of the most striking results was that the individual deficit-based simulations reproduced the patterns of surface and phonological dyslexia found in this sample on the basis of deficits in the subcomponents of reading rather than assumptions about generally impaired routes.

Finally, we have proposed a fully implemented developmentally plausible model of learning to read based on phonological decoding and self-teaching (Ziegler et al., 2014). We have shown that such a model can indeed learn up to 80 percent of words in the fairly opaque English orthography. The upshot of having a fully implemented developmental model is that such a model can be used to investigate how deficits that are present prior to reading or occur during reading development might cause the kind of reading impairments seen in children with dyslexia (e.g., slow reading, poor decoding, and letter-confusion errors).

The present model was used to explain how two of the most established deficits – visual and phoneme deficits – affect orthographic development. In future work, developmental data will be used to estimate the size of the underlying deficit(s) for each individual child and then investigate to what extent impairments during learning would predict inter-individual differences and dyslexia subtypes. If this work were successful, the model could be used to predict developmental trajectories for at-risk children before dyslexia is actually diagnosed (Lyytinen et al., 2001), as well as the outcome of reading interventions that are based on training the critical subcomponents of the reading network. Computer simulations could also be used to develop and assess optimal sequences and materials for reading and intervention programs.

Acknowledgments

This research was supported by grants from the Australian Research Council (DP120100883), the Agence National de la Recherche (ANR-13-APPR-0003), the European Research Council (210922-GENMOD), and the Brain and Language Research Institute (BLRI, ANR-11-LABX-0036), Investments of the Future A*MIDEX (ANR-11-IDEX-0001–02). We would like to thank Ken Pugh, Charles Perfetti, and Ludo Verhoeven for invaluable feedback on a previous version of this chapter.

References

Ahissar, M. (2007). Dyslexia and the anchoring-deficit hypothesis. *Trends in Cognitive Sciences, 11*(11), 458–465.

Ahissar, M., Lubin, Y., Putter-Katz, H., & Banai, K. (2006). Dyslexia and the failure to form a perceptual anchor. *Nature Neuroscience, 9*(12), 1558–1564.

Bosse, M. L., Tainturier, M. J., & Valdois, S. (2007). Developmental dyslexia: The visual attention span deficit hypothesis. *Cognition, 104*(2), 198–230.

Bruck, M. (1992). Persistence of dyslexics' phonological awareness deficits. *Developmental Psychology, 28,* 874–886.

Castles, A., & Coltheart, M. (1993). Varieties of developmental dyslexia. *Cognition, 47* (2), 149–180.

Collis, N. L., Kohnen, S., & Kinoshita, S. (2013). The role of visual spatial attention in adult developmental dyslexia. *Quarterly Journal of Experimental Psychology (Hove), 66*(2), 245–260.

Coltheart, M., Rastle, K., Perry, C., Langdon, R., & Ziegler, J. (2001). DRC: A dual route cascaded model of visual word recognition and reading aloud. *Psychological Review, 108*(1), 204–256.

Di Filippo, G., Zoccolotti, P., & Ziegler, J. C. (2008). Rapid naming deficits in dyslexia: a stumbling block for the perceptual anchor theory of dyslexia. *Developmental Science, 11*(6), F40-F47.

Facoetti, A., Corradi, N., Ruffino, M., Gori, S., & Zorzi, M. (2010). Visual spatial attention and speech segmentation are both impaired in preschoolers at familial risk for developmental dyslexia. *Dyslexia, 16*(3), 226–239.

Facoetti, A., Ruffino, M., Peru, A., Paganoni, P., & Chelazzi, L. (2008). Sluggish engagement and disengagement of non-spatial attention in dyslexic children. *Cortex, 44*(9), 1221–1233.

Facoetti, A., Trussardi, A. N., Ruffino, M. et al. (2009). Multisensory spatial attention deficits are predictive of phonological decoding skills in developmental dyslexia. *J Cogn Neurosci, 22*(5), 1011–1025.

Facoetti, A., Zorzi, M., Cestnick, L. et al. (2006). The relationship between visuospatial attention and nonword reading in developmental dyslexia. *Cognitive Neuropsychology, 23,* 841–855.

Franceschini, S., Gori, S., Ruffino, M., Pedrolli, K., & Facoetti, A. (2012). A causal link between visual spatial attention and reading acquisition. *Current Biology, 22*(9), 814–819.

Goswami, U. (2011). A temporal sampling framework for developmental dyslexia. *Trends in Cognitive Sciences, 15*(1), 3–10.

Goswami, U. (2015). Sensory theories of developmental dyslexia: three challenges for research. *Nature Reviews Neuroscience, 16*(1), 43–54.

Goswami, U., Thomson, J., Richardson, U. et al. (2002). Amplitude envelope onsets and developmental dyslexia: A new hypothesis. *Proceedings of the National Academy of Sciences USA, 99*(16), 10911–10916.

Grainger, J., Dufau, S., & Ziegler, J. C. (2016). A vision of reading. *Trends in Cognitive Sciences, 20*(3), 171–179.

Grainger, J., & Ziegler, J. C. (2011). A dual-route approach to orthographic processing. *Frontiers in Psychology, 2*(45).

Griffiths, Y. M., & Snowling, M. (2002). Predictors of exception word and nonword reading in dyslexic children: The severity hypothesis. *Journal of Educational Psychology*, *94*(1), 34–43.

Harm, M. W., & Seidenberg, M. S. (1999). Phonology, reading acquisition, and dyslexia: Insights from connectionist models. *Psychological Review*, *106*(3), 491–528.

Harm, M. W., & Seidenberg, M. S. (2004). Computing the meanings of words in reading: cooperative division of labor between visual and phonological processes. *Psychological Review*, *111*(3), 662–720.

Hawelka, S., Huber, C., & Wimmer, H. (2006). Impaired visual processing of letter and digit strings in adult dyslexic readers. *Vision Research*, *46*(5), 718–723.

Kohnen, S., Nickels, L., Castles, A., Friedmann, N., & McArthur, G. (2012). When "slime" becomes "smile": Developmental letter position dyslexia in English. *Neuropsychologia*, *50*(14), 3681–3692.

Landerl, K., Ramus, F., Moll, K. et al. (2013). Predictors of developmental dyslexia in European orthographies with varying complexity. *Journal of Child Psychology and Psychiatry*, *54*(6), 686–694.

Lyytinen, H., Ahonen, T., Eklund, K. et al. (2001). Developmental pathways of children with and without familial risk for dyslexia during the first years of life. *Developmental Neuropsychology*, *20*(2), 535–554.

Manis, F. R., Seidenberg, M. S., & Doi, L. M. (1999). See Dick RAN: Rapid naming and the longitudinal prediction of reading subskills in first and second graders. *Scientific Studies of Reading*, *3*(2), 129–157.

McClelland, J. L., & Rumelhart, D. E. (1981). An Interactive activation model of context effects in letter perception: 1. An account of basic findings. *Psychological Review*, *88*(5), 375–407.

Menghini, D., Finzi, A., Benassi, M. et al. (2010). Different underlying neurocognitive deficits in developmental dyslexia: a comparative study. *Neuropsychologia*, *48*(4), 863–872.

Paulesu, E., Demonet, J. F., Fazio, F. et al. (2001). Dyslexia: Cultural diversity and biological unity. *Science*, *291*(5511), 2165–2167.

Pennington, B. F. (2006). From single to multiple deficit models of developmental disorders. *Cognition*, *101*(2), 385–413.

Perry, C., Ziegler, J. C., & Zorzi, M. (2007). Nested incremental modeling in the development of computational theories: The CDP+ model of reading aloud. *Psychological Review*, *114*(2), 273–315.

Perry, C., Ziegler, J. C., & Zorzi, M. (2010). Beyond single syllables: Large-scale modeling of reading aloud with the Connectionist Dual Process (CDP++) model. *Cognitive Psychology*, *61*(2), 106–151.

Perry, C., Ziegler, J. C., & Zorzi, M. (2013). A computational and empirical investigation of graphemes in reading. *Cognitive Science*, 1–29.

Perry, C., Ziegler, J. C., & Zorzi, M. (2014a). CDP++.Italian: Modelling sublexical and supralexical inconsistency in a shallow orthography. *PLoS One*, *9*(4),e94291.

Perry, C., Ziegler, J. C., & Zorzi, M. (2014b). When silent letters say more than a thousand words: An implementation and evaluation of CDP++ in French. *Journal of Memory and Language*, *72*, 98–115.

Perry, C., Zorzi, M., & Ziegler, J. C. (2019). Understanding Dyslexia Through Personalized Large-Scale Computational Models. *Psychological Science*, *30*(3), 386–395.

Plaut, D. C., McClelland, J. L., Seidenberg, M. S., & Patterson, K. (1996). Understanding normal and impaired word reading: Computational principles in quasi-regular domains. *Psychological Review, 103*(1), 56–115.

Ramus, F., & Ahissar, M. (2012). Developmental dyslexia: The difficulties of interpreting poor performance, and the importance of normal performance. *Cognitive Neuropsychology, 29*(1–2), 104–122.

Ramus, F., Rosen, S., & Dakin, S. C. et al. (2003). Theories of developmental dyslexia: insights from a multiple case study of dyslexic adults. *Brain, 126*, 841–865.

Saksida, A., Iannuzzi, S., Bogliotti, C. et al. (2016). Phonological skills, visual attention span, and visual stress in developmental dyslexia. *Developmental Psychology, 52* (10), 1503–1516.

Seidenberg, M. S., & McClelland, J. L. (1989). A distributed, developmental model of word recognition and naming. *Psychological Review, 96*(4), 523–568.

Serniclaes, W., Van Heghe, S., Mousty, P., Carre, R., & Sprenger-Charolles, L. (2004). Allophonic mode of speech perception in dyslexia. *Journal of Experimental Child Psychology, 87*(4), 336–361.

Share, D. L. (1995). Phonological recoding and self-teaching: Sine qua non of reading acquisition. *Cognition, 55*(2), 151–218.

Sperling, A. J., Lu, Z. L., Manis, F. R., & Seidenberg, M. S. (2005). Deficits in perceptual noise exclusion in developmental dyslexia. *Nature Neuroscience, 8*, 862–863.

Sperling, A. J., Lu, Z. L., Manis, F. R., & Seidenberg, M. S. (2006). Motion-perception deficits and reading impairment: It's the noise, not the motion. *Psychological Science, 17*(12), 1047–1053.

Sprenger-Charolles, L., Cole, P., Lacert, P., & Serniclaes, W. (2000). On subtypes of developmental dyslexia: Evidence from processing time and accuracy scores. *Canadian Journal of Experimental Psychology, 54*(2), 87–104.

Sprenger-Charolles, L., Siegel, L. S., Jimenez, J. E., & Ziegler, J. C. (2011). Prevalence and reliability of phonological, surface, and mixed profiles in dyslexia: A review of studies conducted in languages varying in orthographic Depth. *Scientific Studies of Reading, 15*(6), 498–521.

Stein, J. (2014). Dyslexia: The role of vision and visual attention. *Current Developmental Disorders Reports, 1*(4), 267–280.

Stein, J., & Walsh, V. (1997). To see but not to read: The magnocellular theory of dyslexia. *Trends in Neurosciences, 20*(4), 147–152.

Swan, D., & Goswami, U. (1997). Phonological awareness deficits in developmental dyslexia and the phonological representations hypothesis. *Journal of Experimental Child Psychology, 66*(1), 18–41.

Tallal, P., & Piercy, M. (1973). Defects of non-verbal auditory perception in children with developmental aphasia. *Nature, 241*(5390), 468–469.

van Bergen, E., van der Leij, A., & de Jong, P. F. (2014). The intergenerational multiple deficit model and the case of dyslexia. *Frontiers in Human Neuroscience, 8*(346).

Vandermosten, M., Boets, B., & Luts, H. et al. (2010). Adults with dyslexia are impaired in categorizing speech and nonspeech sounds on the basis of temporal cues. *Proceedings of the National Academy of Sciences of the United States of America, 107*(23), 10389–10394.

White, S., Milne, E., Rosen, S. et al. (2006). The role of sensorimotor impairments in dyslexia: A multiple case study of dyslexic children. *Developmental Science, 9*(3), 237–255.

Woollams, A. M. (2014). Connectionist neuropsychology: Uncovering ultimate causes of acquired dyslexia. *Philosophical Transactions of the Royal Society of London B Biological Sciences, 369*(1634), 20120398.

Woollams, A. M., Lambon Ralph, M. A., Plaut, D. C., & Patterson, K. (2007). SD-squared: On the association between semantic dementia and surface dyslexia. *Psychological Review, 114*(2), 316–339.

World Health Organization. (2011). *International statistical classification of diseases and related health problems – 10th revision.* Geneva, Switzerland: World Health Organization.

Ziegler, J. C. (2006). Do differences in brain activation challenge universal theories of dyslexia? *Brain and Language, 98*(3), 341–343.

Ziegler, J. C. (2008). Better to lose the anchor than the whole ship. *Trends in Cognitive Sciences, 12,* 244–245.

Ziegler, J. C., Bertrand, D., Tóth, D. et al. (2010). Orthographic depth and its impact on universal predictors of reading: A cross-language investigation. *Psychological Science, 21*(4), 551–559.

Ziegler, J. C., Castel, C., Pech-Georgel, C. et al. (2008). Developmental dyslexia and the dual route model of reading: Simulating individual differences and subtypes. *Cognition, 107,* 151–178.

Ziegler, J. C., Pech-Georgel, C., Dufau, S., & Grainger, J. (2010). Rapid processing of letters, digits, and symbols: What purely visual-attentional deficit in developmental dyslexia? *Developmental Science, 13,* F8–F14.

Ziegler, J. C., Perry, C., Ma-Wyatt, A., Ladner, D., & Schulte-Korne, G. (2003). Developmental dyslexia in different languages: Language-specific or universal? *Journal of Experimental Child Psychology, 86*(3), 169–193.

Ziegler, J. C., Perry, C., & Zorzi, M. (2014). Modelling reading development through phonological decoding and self-teaching: Implications for dyslexia. *Philosophical Transactions of the Royal Society of London B Biological Sciences, 369*(1634), 20120397.

Zorzi, M. (2010). The connectionist dual process (CDP) approach to modelling reading aloud. *European Journal of Cognitive Psychology, 22,* 836–860.

Zorzi, M., Barbiero, C., Facoetti, A. et al. (2012). Extra-large letter spacing improves reading in dyslexia. *Proceedings of the National Academy of Sciences, 109*(28), 11455–11459.

Zorzi, M., Houghton, G., & Butterworth, B. (1998a). The development of spelling–sound relationships in a model of phonological reading. *Language & Cognitive Processes, 13*(2&3), 337–371.

Zorzi, M., Houghton, G., & Butterworth, B. (1998b). Two routes or one in reading aloud? A connectionist dual-process model. *Journal of Experimental Psychology: Human Perception & Performance, 24*(4), 1131–1161.

17 Modeling Developmental Dyslexia across Languages and Writing Systems

Jason D. Zevin

17.1 Introduction

Computational models of reading have played an important role in theorizing about developmental dyslexia. In particular, simulations of how children learn to read, based on Parallel Distributed Processing (PDP) principles, such as the *triangle model* (Seidenberg & McClelland, 1989) have been influential, because they hold the promise of explaining complex phenomena as emerging from a relatively simple set of assumptions. For example, Harm and Seidenberg (1999) demonstrated how *lower-level* perceptual difficulties that interfere with the formation of phonological categories can give rise to specific deficits observed in phonological dyslexia in English. The theory behind the triangle model is that reading skill emerges as a result of statistically driven learning of the mappings among the written and spoken forms of words and their meanings. At the computational level of analysis, this provides the basis for a universal model of reading across languages (e.g. Frost, 2012). And indeed, by applying the same model architecture and learning rules across different languages and writing systems, we can generate insights into how the reading system might be organized differently (or similarly) across languages, with important consequences for how we think about the diverse ways that reading difficulties manifest across languages (Yang et al., 2009, 2013).

In this chapter, I first lay out the triangle model approach to addressing the notion of *orthographic depth* (Frost, Katz, & Bentin, 1987), and how this has played out in simulations from my own lab of typical and disordered reading acquisition in English and Chinese. I then consider how well these simulations reflect the underlying theory – that the basic architecture of the reading system is the same across languages. In evaluating any model (Quine, 1951; or, really, any hypothesis) it is important to examine the assumptions that connect the theory as stated to the results obtained. In this chapter I focus on the way we have thus far approached cross-language modeling of learning to read, and consider the decisions that have been made to try and bring very different writing systems and languages into register in attempting to compare them fairly. It turns out that language-specific assumptions permeate nearly every decision about how to build a model of reading in a particular language, from what task to train and test the model on, to more obscure – but often crucial – assumptions about details of orthographic and phonological representations. Any attempt to bring multiple different languages together in the same computational model (or modeling framework) will encounter similar difficulties, so the discussion has some general consequences for the question of how languages and writing systems should be compared.

17.2   Orthographic Depth, Reading Disability, and the Triangle Model

The notion of orthographic depth (Frost et al., 1987) provides a descriptive framework that captures important differences among writing systems. Specifically, it suggests that the relative contribution of lexical and sublexical processes for making contact with phonology will depend on the relative "depth" of the writing system. Most work has been done in the English spelling-to-sound system, which has features of both shallow and deep orthographies (Malone, 1925; Venezky, 1999). At its core is an alphabet of letters that correspond roughly to individual speech sounds (Venezky, 1970), as in shallow orthographies like Finnish or Serbian – although in those very shallow orthographies the mapping from letter to phoneme is one to one. At the same time, English has many spellings that encode morphological or etymological information, often with the side effect of creating ambiguities in spelling to sound. For example, words like "buffet" and "biscuit" reflect their French origin, and inflected forms create ambiguity with respect to voicing (consider "bucks" and "bugs").

Chinese, in contrast, is an example of an extremely "deep" orthography (DeFrancis, 1989) in that the pronunciation of a character cannot be computed sound -by sound from its constituent parts.[1] Unlike letters, the basic units of the Chinese writing system – "radicals" – do not contain componential information about pronunciation (Mattingly, 1987). There is no relationship between, e.g., the first radical in a character and the first phoneme in the spoken word it represents. Radicals are often organized into larger units such as phonetic and semantic components. Instead, the majority (85 percent) of characters in Chinese are phonograms (Zhu, 1988), which consist of a phonetic component that provides information about the character's pronunciation, and a semantic component that provides information about the meaning of the character, for

---

[1] Note that throughout, except where noted, I am using "Chinese" to refer to the use of the Chinese writing system for Mandarin, but should acknowledge that this writing system is used by a number of languages and dialects, some of which are not even typologically related to Mandarin.

example that it is likely to be a handheld object, or a four-legged animal (Li & Kang, 1993). Thus, the pronunciation of many characters can be probabilistically determined by their phonetic components. The mapping from print to sound is sometimes entirely arbitrary, however, so that the same character may have completely unrelated pronunciations, and many perfect homophones share no orthographic features at all.

17.3   Learning to Read in Different Orthographies

Differences in the statistical regularities of writing systems also have important consequences for the development of reading skill. One is a marked difference in speed of learning to read across languages: shallower systems are easier to learn than deeper ones (Seymour, Aro, & Erskine, 2003), and there are further differences among deep orthographies; Chinese children can typically read fewer than 1000 characters after first grade (Xing, Shu, & Li, 2004), whereas the average English-reading child can recognize 3000–5000 words at the same age (White, Graves, & Slater, 1990) – and with less intensive training. A second consequence of orthographic depth on reading development concerns the "division of labor" between phonological and semantic codes in reading (Harm & Seidenberg, 2004). In a shallow orthography, pronunciations can easily be computed directly from spelling, resulting in a relatively limited role for semantics in reading aloud (e.g., Kang & Simpson, 2001; Raman & Baluch, 2001). In relatively "deep" languages, such as English, semantic knowledge plays an important role in reading aloud, particularly in the reading of words whose spellings are highly atypical (Strain, Patterson, & Seidenberg, 1995).

Over the course of development, differences in the division of labor mean that distinct preliterate language skills will contribute differentially to reading success across writing systems. Indeed, the relative contributions to reading ability of "phonological awareness" – i.e., the ability to categorize and manipulate individual speech sounds – and "morphological awareness," – the ability to process the meanings of words as componential – depends on orthographic depth. In Chinese, however, morphological awareness is a strong predictor of reading success (Shu et al., 2006), although phonological awareness also appears to play some role (Shu, Peng, & McBride-Chang, 2008).

The differential contributions from more basic cognitive processes to reading may also account for different patterns of reading disorder observed across languages. In English, and to some extent in Chinese, there is evidence for subtypes of developmental dyslexia: phonological dyslexics who have specific difficulty with decoding and surface dyslexics who have difficulty with atypically spelled words, but relatively spared performance on regular words and nonwords (Manis et al., 1996). These subtypes are often explained as resulting from distinct preexisting deficits: in semantic processing for the developmental delay/surface dyslexics and phonological processing for the phonological dyslexics. Developmental dyslexics learning these writing systems tend to present with slow reading, comprehension difficulties and particular difficulty reading nonwords (Lindgren, De Renzi, & Richman, 1985). Recent evidence from Italian that morphological effects are exaggerated in developmental dyslexics (Burani et al., 2008) and case studies of surface dyslexia (Barca et al., 2006; Zoccolotti et al., 1999) suggest that there is more to be understood about the contribution of semantics to reading in transparent orthographies, however.

17.4   Modeling Dyslexia across Languages and Writing Systems

In the triangle model, nonword naming is supported by generalization from experience with words that share structure, e.g., the ability to arrive at a pronunciation for BINK is influenced by BIN, INK, PINK, and many others besides. This ability to generalize depends on having encoded spelling-to-sound regularities, which in turn depends on being able to represent the similarity space over which these regularities emerge. Phonological deficits interfere with this process. In contrast, for an inconsistent item like DOLL, experience with the lexicon provides ambiguous cues because overlapping items like ROLL, POLL, TOLL, and others compete with the many items in which the letter O by itself is pronounced as in DOLL. As in any ambiguity resolution problem, the specific context is important. Knowing the pronunciation of DOLL means, in part, knowing that -OLL has a particular pronunciation in the context of the letter D at the beginning. In this way we can see how semantic information – in the sense of simply knowing that this is the word "doll," – aids in ambiguity resolution, and how deficits in semantic processing can produce a deficit that is more pronounced for words with unusual spellings (Harm & Seidenberg, 2004; Plaut et al., 1996).

Whereas in English, most developmental reading difficulty that is observable at the single-word level is associated with phonological deficits, Chinese character reading exhibits substantial individual variability that is related to measures indexing both phonological and semantic processing (McBride-Chang et al., 2003; Shu et al., 2006). In Chinese, the influence of semantic deficits is much more serious than in English: Poor semantic processing leads to difficulties with all words, even those with more typical spelling-to-sound correspondences, although reading of atypically spelled words does suffer relatively more (Shu et al., 2005). Children with phonological deficits, in contrast, are impaired relative to age-matched controls on reading of all words, but the impairment is greater for words with typical spelling-to-sound correspondences, with the result that phonological dyslexics do not show the typical advantage for regular-consistent over irregular-inconsistent words (Shu et al., 2005). This posed an interesting target for computational modeling: How can the same "core deficit" lead to such different outcomes for reading in the context of a "universal" reading model?

Our initial simulation (Yang et al., 2009) learned orthography-to-phonology mappings for Chinese using the same model architecture and learning rule as Harm and Seidenberg (1999). The model architecture included feed-forward connections via a set of hidden units, as in a basic three-layer perceptron (McClelland, Rumelhart, & PDP Research Group, 1986), and an attractor network to represent the phonological forms of words. Knowledge of print-to-sound correspondences was thus gradually learned as a set of weights that allowed the model to rapidly converge on the correct pronunciation in the phonological layer when presented with the orthographic form of the word on the input. This simulation captured a number of important phenomena in skilled adult reading of Chinese. In extending this model to address developmental dyslexia across languages, Yang et al. (2013) added two layers to the simulation: an English orthographic input, and a semantic layer (also set up as an "input," similar to Plaut et al., 1996). We also modified the phonological output layer so that it could represent both English and Chinese syllables. In this way, we were able to compare reading acquisition across the two writing systems in the same simulation.

In a simulation of typical development, we found differences between the two writing systems that mimicked gross differences observed in studies of learning to read. First, Chinese was learned much more slowly than English in all cases. We then introduced manipulations to simulate phonological and semantic deficits. In English, phonological deficits resulted in a pattern consistent with phonological dyslexia – overall difficulty with reading, with a pronounced impairment on nonword reading – whereas the effect of semantic impairment was relatively small, and limited to a deficit in performance on highly inconsistent items (consistent with surface dyslexia). In Chinese, both phonological and semantic impairments had widespread effects. In addition to simulating gross features of typical and atypical development, we were able to successfully simulate the performance of three cases of developmental dyslexia in Chinese. In each simulation, there was independent motivation to implement the core deficit in a particular subsystem. One child had clear difficulties with morphological processing, but relatively normal phonological awareness. His data were simulated by implementing a deficit in the semantics-to-phonology pathway throughout development and matching the model's overall performance to the patient's. Conversely, two other subjects who showed frank phonological awareness difficulties in the absence of morphological processing deficits were simulated by implementing the same type of deficit on the direct mapping from spelling to sound. In both cases, the pattern of reading disability was correctly predicted by the model when the appropriate core deficit was simulated.

From this we concluded that the differential manifestations of dyslexia in Chinese and English – and its differential association with core processing abilities – are plausibly due to statistical properties of the orthography-to-phonology mappings they represent, and can emerge from the same processing architecture. It seems straightforward that we have, in fact, modeled English and Chinese in the same architecture: After all, it is the same simulation model. The only structural differences between the two languages are the language-specific orthographic inputs, and their connections to the (same) layer of hidden units, and a few phonological features that are used in one language but not the other. Thus far I have asked you to take it on faith that the models I am presenting reflect an "apples-to-apples" comparison between English and Chinese reading. A more explicit examination of the details of these models will help clarify how literally to take this premise.

17.5   Comparison of Reading Models across Writing Systems

17.5.1   Underlying Assumptions

A number of assumptions underlie the assertion that the simulations of Chinese and English described above are truly equivalent. First, we have to consider whether recognizing individual characters in Chinese is legitimately comparable to recognizing words in English. In English text, word boundaries are indicated with spaces, so that there is little ambiguity about what it means to talk about "visual word recognition," although there might be occasional arguments about, e.g., "doghouse" or "dog house" and other compound words. In Chinese, the situation is considerably more complicated, as I will explain in a moment, raising the question of whether a model that learns to recognize individual characters in Chinese is the best analog for a model that learns to recognize whole words in English. If we accept, for the sake of argument, that Chinese character recognition is "equivalent enough" to English word recognition, we must then consider whether the phonological, semantic, and especially orthographic representations used in the models are fairly comparable. I address each of these concerns in turn, with special consideration of the problems they raise for the assertion that the models are actually language-universal.

In English, word boundaries are generally quite clear in text, and monosyllabic words exhibit many of the interesting properties of the spelling-to-sound system. Thus, a substantial literature concerning the reading aloud of single – largely monosyllabic – words in English existed before the first computational models, providing natural target phenomena for Seidenberg and McClelland (1989). The existence of this model (and its direct competitor; Coltheart et al., 2001) prompted many more empirical studies with just such stimuli. One reason for the focus on monosyllabic words is that multisyllabic words raise difficult decisions about how the orthographic and phonological representations should be constructed (however, see Sibley & Kello, 2006, for approaches that are consistent with this framework), but another motivation has been that there is enough to explain about monosyllabic word reading in English that it is possible to model a wide range of phenomena without dealing with the practical issues around syllabification.

In this light, the extension of the triangle framework to simulations of single Chinese character recognition is well motivated. Studies of Chinese character naming are often designed as explicitly analogous to studies of English word reading, and in fact many of the same phenomena can be tested, because it is possible to compute useful descriptive statistics for individual characters, such as frequency and number of strokes, and for phonograms there is consensus about how to characterize phenomena such as consistency and regularity. Further, as will become clear when I discuss representational issues, it is very felicitous that the pronunciations of Chinese characters are all monosyllabic, and can thus be captured in the same feature-and-slot-based representation used for English (albeit extended to include features that are contrastive in Chinese). As far as semantics is concerned, Chinese characters are somewhat defensible as word-like as far as these models are concerned. I say this because the semantic representations we use for words are admittedly oversimplified and capture only the most frequent usage in all cases. Although Chinese characters are generally not the same as words, they have standard dictionary definitions that can be used to describe how they might be arranged in a similarity space.

There are, however, important limits to the analogy between English words and Chinese characters. In English, somewhat arbitrary decisions occasionally need to be made about whether such compounds as "ball field," "ice cream," and "house-made" should be one word, two words, or hyphenated, and different writers may disagree without sacrificing intelligibility. In Chinese this kind of ambiguity is more prevalent because of the rich derivational structure of the language, and also because the writing system permits ambiguity about the location of word boundaries. In connected text, Chinese is written without spaces to indicate word boundaries, so that there is actually some ambiguity about where words begin and end (Inhoff & Wu, 2005). This is in part because Chinese has a rich system of derivational morphology, in which characters play a role as the "basic unit" (Taft & Zhu, 1995). For example, the word for "airport" is composed of the characters for "fly," "machine," and "place." The first two characters combine to form the word for "airplane," so the ambiguity here is about whether "airport" should be one word or two. (Note that the character for "place" occurs in many such arrangements, e.g., words/phrases that can be translated as "supermarket," "ball field," "parking lot," and "horse racing track.") Most words in Chinese comprise two characters, and only a minority of single characters can be used grammatically as words. Thus, the focus on character recognition in simulations of Chinese reading is defensible as a parallel to English given that the richest data on Chinese reading comes from tasks that have treated characters as parallel to English words, and the observed patterns of difficulty in character reading among Chinese dyslexics.

If one were to build a "word-recognition" model for Chinese, it would be critical for the model to deal with multi-character words. In fact, there is no way such a model could explain much of anything without addressing compositionality, so that the model would likely expose important differences between Chinese and English word recognition. A relevant example of this is the "morphological awareness" test that is commonly used as a measure of semantic processing in Chinese (McBride-Chang et al., 2005; Shu et al., 2006). This test essentially asks children to guess the meanings of new words. For example, a child may be asked to identify a fanciful drawing of a "zebra-cow," i.e., a cow with stripes like a zebra's. Children's ability to do this in Chinese is taken as evidence that they have learned the productivity of the morphological system. The word for "zebra," after all, is "stripe" + "horse," so the neologism for a striped cow is easy to figure out. In relating these morphological deficits to single-character reading, we relied on a particular framework for relating morphology to semantics that comes with its own assumptions.

17.5.2   Semantic Representations

Yang et al. (2013) used random-bit semantic representations – literally encoding individual words as random patterns of ones and zeros on a set of unlabeled "semantic" units – similar to those used by Plaut et al. (1996). The motivation in both cases was to examine the role of semantic input as essentially an additional source of constraint in the mapping from orthography to phonology. Further, because we used the same patterns for both languages, we were able to argue that the differences between learning for English and Chinese were due to differences in the mappings from orthography to phonology. The claim that noisy semantics-to-phonology mappings have a different impact on the development of reading skill in Chinese and English in that context can be defended on those grounds, but it would be silly not to admit that those models are leaving out potentially important features that differ between writing systems. For example, in English, many of the irregularities in the spelling-to-sound system are related to both derivational and inflectional morphological processes. Harm and Seidenberg (2004) explored how morphological information could influence single-word reading in their model, which incorporated syntactic features such as "+past tense" and "+plural" within its semantic representation. This reflects a commitment to a view of morphology as emerging from the statistics of mappings among orthography, phonology, and semantics, which has been pursued in related work (Joanisse & Seidenberg, 1998; Seidenberg & Gonnerman, 2000) that has been extended to cross-language work on morphology (Mirković, MacDonald, & Seidenberg, 2005; Mirković, Seidenberg, & MacDonald, 2011), and which is, of course, a sharp departure from the conventional view that morphology is a formal, syntactic process that operates autonomously of semantics.

Interestingly, the arbitrariness of the mapping from orthography to semantics is an important variable that differs between languages. Chinese is particularly unusual in having orthographic structures (semantic radicals) that contribute independently to semantics. For example, the characters for "cat" and "pig" share a semantic radical indicating that they are four-legged animals, which also appears in a character that translates roughly as "crazy." Although behavioral effects of semantic transparency at this level of detail have thus far been elusive, it is an important aspect of the writing system. Indeed, when we consider that each character codes for a single syllable, and Mandarin only has a small number of phonologically legal syllables, the necessarily large number of homophones (Myers, 2010) at the single-character level means that mappings from orthography to semantics are more regular – in the sense of approximating a one-to-one relationship between patterns – than mappings from phonology to semantics. This simply cannot be captured with arbitrary, random-bit semantics that have no fidelity to the similarity space among the meanings of characters that share orthographic structure. Of course, the derivational effects described above would also be outside the scope of a model with random-bit semantics, if it could somehow be expanded to consider multi-character words.

This issue extends beyond comparisons between English and Chinese, of course. In Semitic languages, partial semantics can be computed without phonology: The written form of a word provides deterministic information about its root and word form, but only probabilistic information about its derivational morphology. So, different cases (for example) of the same lemma may be written with the same sequence of characters, but pronounced with different vowels. When reading connected text for comprehension, this is not an issue, because the syntactic and discourse context support disambiguation. But in the same way that researchers generally avoid English words like READ, WIND, or ENTRANCE when testing reading aloud in English, they must avoid large numbers of words when testing Hebrew or Arabic. Thus, it is clear that choices about what to include in the semantic representations of a model, and what format those representations ought to take, are influenced not only by details of the languages under consideration, but also by the tasks and by larger theoretical issues around the relationship between semantics and morphology.

17.5.3   *Phonological Representations*

When reading researchers talk about "phonology," we are mainly talking about the pronunciations of individual words. When phonologists talk about "phonology," they are talking about systematic knowledge of the structures of spoken language, usually with a commitment to a particular format of representations that supports direct comparisons between specific languages. It makes no sense to talk about phenomena like word-final devoicing, or vowel harmony or tone sandhi as being somehow shaped by the same rules, constraints, task models, or what have you, without a way of describing these as somehow the same thing across the languages in which they occur. In computational models of word recognition, representations of "phonology" are quite crude – although they are good enough to capture some phonological phenomena related to inflectional and derivational morphology. Generally, we can get away with this because the role of the phonological representations in these models is simply to give a rough rendering of the relevant similarity space. This is nicely demonstrated by considering the evolution of phonological representations in the "triangle" model for English.

The initial model of Seidenberg and McClelland (1989) used a complex distributed coding scheme involving "Wickelfeatures." The idea was that features would be distributed across phonemes, so that words were represented by clusters of features, none of which corresponded directly to a particular phoneme in the output. This was an interesting idea (and concerns about the psychological reality of phonemes that motivated it have been a persistent topic, e.g. Lotto and Holt, 2000), but it did a relatively poor job of capturing the similarity space of the language as native speakers of the language seem to encode it (Hahn & Bailey, 2005). By shifting to localist representations (each phoneme in each position represented by a single unit), Plaut et al., (1996) dramatically improved pseudoword reading, although this was not the focus of their modeling. Harm and Seidenberg (1999) introduced feature-based representations, and further took pains to represent the features in a way that maintained the similarity space of sounds in the language – rather than simply coding them as binary. Further, they included an attractor network that allowed them to simulate some aspects of speech perception, and which served as the locus for phonological impairments.

We should have no illusions that the slot-based, featural representations used by Harm and Seidenberg (1999) or in the Chinese models that followed their lead (Yang et al., 2009, 2013) advance a serious claim about how the phonological forms of words are represented. What this representation does better than the representations used in earlier work is capture some relevant dimensions of the similarity space of monosyllabic English words and Chinese syllables. This notion of phonological similarity space is also subtle enough that it can be extended to provide a mechanistic explanation of the specific difficulties faced by speakers of dialects that are different from what is used in the classroom (Brown et al., 2015). This is an area where these models are poised to contribute substantially.

Thus far, we have dealt with learning to read as if it were contiguous with learning one's native language. But for many – if not most – beginning readers, the dialect or language spoken in the classroom is different from what is spoken at home. This is certainly true of African American Vernacular English speakers (Washington et al., 2013), but also of many people learning to read throughout South Asia (where reading is often taught primarily or exclusively in a dominant language such as Hindi, Urdu, or English, despite vast language diversity), Africa (where literacy instruction may be focused on colonial, rather than indigenous languages), and China (where Standard Chinese as spoken in Beijing is de facto a minority language, but is the language in which formal literacy instruction is most widely provided). Understanding the mismatch between the language one typically uses for communication and the language one must learn as part of literacy instruction should be a target for more future research.

17.5.4   *Orthographic Representations*

It may seem straightforward to design orthographic representations for English, but in successive models in the "triangle" framework, these have evolved almost as much as the phonological representations. As with phonological representations, the challenge is to appropriately capture the similarity space of the orthography. Because of the way words are input to the model, care must be taken to ensure that overlap that seems "obvious" to anyone familiar with the language is somehow captured by the input to the model. Consider the three words: PIN, PINK, and SPIN. Now imagine you have five sets of "letter detectors" that you can arrange any way you like with respect to these words. If you line the letter detectors up so that the words are left justified, PIN and PINK will overlap, but SPIN will not activate any of the same letter detectors as the other two words. If they are right justified, PINK will activate a completely non-overlapping set of letter detectors. Neither of these seems correct. The solution arrived at by Harm and Seidenberg (1999) was to use a vowel-centered orthographic representation. In our simplified example with five letter detectors (or "slots"), this would produce _PIN_, _PINK, and SPIN_, with the underscores representing a slot that is left blank. As with the phonological representations, this is not a serious proposal for how orthographic representations are organized in the brain, but an attempt to fairly represent the similarity space of written words without too much handcrafting.

In adapting this approach to Chinese models, we took the position that the input coding should (1) capture the visual similarity of characters, and (2) be structured so that the model could discover the left/right structure of "phonograms," which have probabilistic orthographic-to-phonological information. This was accomplished by organizing the radicals (the basic compositional units of Chinese orthography) so that the phonetic components of words overlapped. This involved adapting a coding scheme developed by Xing et al. (2004) representing characters over a set of seven slots, starting from the bottom right (see Yang et al., 2009, for more details). Although the details are difficult to describe concisely without a good deal more discussion of Chinese orthography, an obvious concern with this form of representation is that we may have "built in" information about phonetic components, which convey probabilistic information about the pronunciations of characters. Using multidimensional scaling analyses (MDS), we were able to demonstrate that the similarity space of the orthographic representations was not unduly shaped by the phonetic components: Items that shared a phonetic component were no more similar to one another in the MDS analysis than items that shared the same number of strokes and overall shape.

Thus, devising orthographic representations for these models is a balancing act between making sure that the relevant similarity between written words is *available* to be learned, and prefiguring the results of the simulations by building representations that reflect biases about what there is to learn about orthography. This reflects a broader problem with slot-based representations more generally. We defend this position by saying that what we are interested in is how the mapping between similarity spaces shapes what you learn, and by demonstrating that the inputs are not biased to "create" the phenomena we wish to observe. The computational-level theory in these models is that mappings among written and spoken forms of words and their meanings is learned by a system that encodes statistical regularities – and is thus very sensitive to the similarity of items in their orthography, phonology, and (less critically) semantics. In order for them to be a good model for that theory, it is important to duly represent the similarity spaces under consideration, not to get the orthographic representations exactly right.

This is good news for the models, because slot-based representations are obviously wrong – at least for English – and in fact research has focused recently on how we might organize orthographic representations to address phenomena like insensitivity to letter transpositions. Many of these models are based on the interactive activation framework (McClelland & Rumelhart, 1981), and as such focus on what sort of input representation can make contact with the lexicon in order to simulate adult data (Davis, 2010; Grainger & Van Heuven, 2003), but do not address whether it is possible to learn from such representations (but see Di Bono & Zorzi, 2013; Glotin et al., 2010). An exception is the model of Lerner, Armstrong, and Frost (2014), which learned to map from orthography to semantics using a "noisy" positional code. The researchers represented each letter with nineteen units each of which correspond to a possible position in the word. They encoded overlap by treating position as a Gaussian distribution. So, a letter in the fourth position would maximally activate the third unit, but would also activate the adjacent slots (although somewhat less), and the units adjacent to those, and so on. In this way, position was represented with some uncertainty for both Hebrew and English. The model was trained to map these orthographic representations onto a random-bit semantic space using a random-bit/prototype structure as in the models we have been discussing for spelling-to-sound, with support from semantics. The model showed higher sensitivity to specific letter position in Hebrew than in English, showing that the language specificity of transposed letter effects can emerge from the statistical properties of the languages, and does not require different a priori assumptions about structure of orthographic input.

17.5.5   Cross-Language Issues

It should be clear from the foregoing discussion that approaches to understanding orthographic representations, even among alphabetic languages, potentially involve a number of language-specific assumptions. But if the contribution of orthographic complexity to the development of reading ability and disability is to be properly understood, it would be helpful to find some way of quantifying it. If what we are hoping to produce is a simple metric that predicts something about what difficulties children are likely to have in different writing systems, a good place to start is by simply counting the number of symbols to be learned. Nag (2011) points out that the *akshara* scripts used to represent many Indian languages vary in how extensive the symbol set is, i.e., how many different symbols are used in the writing system. For extensive systems, like Kannada, early reading difficulties are highly correlated with difficulty recognizing individual alpha-syllabic characters (Nag & Snowling, 2012). This is so, even though Kannada is a relatively shallow orthography. It is tempting to pose a simple comparative question along the lines of "are more extensive orthographies harder to learn than more contained ones?" and in fact one does not need any kind of simulation modeling to ask this question; all one needs is a tally of the number of unique characters in each script.

A simple count of the number of characters will likely have some explanatory power, but there may be subtler features that impact learnability of orthographic forms. Chang, Plaut, and Perfetti (2016) have approached this in a way that attempts to make as few language-specific assumptions as possible. They used bitmapped representations of characters from 130 languages and trained an autoencoder on each language. Autoencoders learn to reproduce the input from a relatively small number of hidden units, so that they learn to extract regularities in the input, in order to arrive at a compressed representation. Autoencoder networks are widely used in image compression, for example. But it is not the case that the approach of simply using the same bitmap grid for all orthographies somehow avoids making language-specific assumptions. Consider Korean orthography, which is designed to be completely transparent, and thus contains a small number of letters that correspond precisely (leaving aside dialect and idiolect differences in pronunciation) to the sounds of the language. Letters are organized into square syllables in a roughly clockwise order starting from the top left. Thus the "m" in "mi" is visually identical to the "m" in "jim," but it appears in an entirely different location. As far as the bitmap representation is concerned, they might as well be unrelated. This is, of course, exactly the same problem that arises in slot-based representations. There are models of the visual system that produce position-invariant representations (Serre, Oliva, & Poggio, 2007), and perhaps modeling how these stimuli are encoded in the visual system from the primary visual cortex up to the fusiform gyrus would solve this problem. (It would certainly be interesting.) Finally, it is important to note that even this model involves some language-specific assumptions, particularly with respect to the appropriate level of description within an orthography to use in the training set. For example, in *akshara* scripts, should complex syllables count as one or more graphemes? There is no theory-neutral way to make this decision, but it would have a large impact on the computed orthographic complexity. Nonetheless, this represents an important step in an area that is underrepresented in the modeling literature.

17.6   Discussion and Conclusion

Models require simplifying assumptions, because they are tools for under-standing how a system works (rather than detailed replicas of the system under investigation). The simplifying assumptions modelers make should be consonant with the computational-level description of what it is they are trying to model. Our attempts to compare English and Chinese "in the same model" are limited in important ways; most critically, we have had to focus on tasks for which there are data in both languages, we have had to ignore the difference between Chinese characters and English words, in terms of the roles they play in the languages at large, and we have had to create orthographic representa-tions for each language independently. I have defended these decisions as consistent with the computational-level theory behind these models. The char-acter in Chinese, while it is not the same as the word in English, plays a similar role in the learning of mappings among orthography, phonology, and seman-tics; further, tests of reading both English words and Chinese characters aloud provide insights into how these mappings are represented, and differentiate specific subtypes of reading disability. The orthographic representations were designed to encode the similarity space of written words and characters appro-priately, and to make the overlap that is important in mappings from orthogra-phy to phonology available to the models.

These models produced some interesting insights into how the same impair-ments in phonological or semantic processing could produce very different outcomes in the two languages, within the same simulation. It will be important, however, to broaden the scope of this research to a wider variety of languages, and to adopt methods related to computational modeling that can potentially provide quantitative characterizations of the relative complexity of the written forms of words, and the relative "smoothness" of the relationship between written and spoken forms and meanings of words across languages. For example, we saw that when Chang, Plaut, and Perfetti (2016) developed a metric of orthographic complexity based on autoencoding of bitmaps – as language-general a representation as possible – there were still a number of choices about the input representations that necessarily impacted the relative complexity of different languages.

Nonetheless, the goal of using the tools of computational modeling to develop metrics that can describe basic properties of writing systems is an important one, and one that may be pursued more efficiently than the process of building full-scale models that "learn to read." In this way, we may be able to predict the form that reading difficulties will take in languages where relatively little data is available, but much help is needed in improving literacy outcomes. Although many open questions remain, it is clear that computational modeling has an important role to play in understanding how we can generalize insights about the nature and cause of reading disability across languages.

References

Barca, L., Burani, C., Di Filippo, G., & Zoccolotti, P. (2006). Italian developmental dyslexic and proficient readers: Where are the differences? *Brain and Language, 98*, 347–351. doi: http://dx.doi.org/10.1016/j.bandl.2006.05.001.

Brown, M. C., Sibley, D. E., Washington, J. A. et al. (2015). Impact of dialect use on a basic component of learning to read. *Frontiers in Psychology, 6*, 196. doi: http://dx.doi.org/10.3389/fpsyg.2015.00196

Burani, C., Marcolini, S., De Luca, M., & Zoccolotti, P. (2008). Morpheme-based reading aloud: Evidence from dyslexic and skilled Italian readers. *Cognition, 108*, 243–262. doi: http://dx.doi.org/10.1016/j.cognition.2007.12.010.

Chang, L.-Y., Plaut, D. C., & Perfetti, C. A. (2016). Visual-orthographic complexity in learning to read.: Modeling learning across writing system variations. *Scientific Studies of Reading, 20*(1), 64–85.

Coltheart, M., Rastle, K., Perry, C., Langdon, R., & Ziegler, J. (2001). DRC: A dual route cascaded model of visual word recognition and reading aloud. *Psychological Review, 108*, 204–256. doi: http://dx.doi.org/10.1037/0033-295X.108.1.204.

Davis, C. J. (2010). The spatial coding model of visual word identification. *Psychological Review, 117*(3), 713–758. doi: http://dx.doi.org/10.1037/a0019738.

DeFrancis, J. (1989). *Visible speech: The diverse oneness of writing systems.* Honolulu, HI: University of Hawaii Press.

Di Bono, M. G., & Zorzi, M. (2013). Deep generative learning of location-invariant visual word recognition. *Frontiers in Psychology*, *4*, 635. doi: http://dx.doi.org/10.3389/fpsyg.2013.00635.

Frost, R. (2012). A universal approach to modeling visual word recognition and reading: Not only possible, but also inevitable. *Behavioral and Brain Sciences*, *35*, 310–329. doi: http://dx.doi.org/10.1017/S0140525X12000635.

Frost, R., Katz, L., & Bentin, S. (1987). Strategies for visual word recognition and orthographical depth: A multilingual comparison. *Journal of Experimental Psychology: Human Perception & Performance*, *13*, 104–115. doi: http://dx.doi.org/10.1037/0096-1523.13.1.104.

Glotin, H., Warnier, P., Dandurand, F. et al. (2010). An adaptive resonance theory account of the implicit learning of orthographic word forms. *Journal of Physiology-Paris*, *104*, 19–26. doi: http://dx.doi.org/10.1016/j.jphysparis.2009.11.003.

Grainger, J., & Van Heuven, W. (2003). Modeling letter position coding in printed word perception. In P. Bonin (Ed.), *The mental lexicon* (pp. 1–24). New York, NY: Nova Science.

Hahn, U., & Bailey, T. M. (2005). What makes words sound similar? *Cognition*, *97*, 227–267. doi: http://dx.doi.org/10.1016/j.cognition.2004.09.006.

Harm, M. W., & Seidenberg, M. S. (1999). Phonology, reading, and dyslexia: Insights from connectionist models. *Psychological Review*, *163*, 491–528. doi: http://dx.doi.org/10.1037/0033-295X.106.3.491.

Harm, M. W., & Seidenberg, M. S. (2004). Computing the meanings of words in reading: Cooperative division of labor between visual and phonological processes. *Psychological Review*, *111*, 662–720. doi: http://dx.doi.org/10.1037/0033-295X.111.3.662.

Inhoff, A. W., & Wu, C. (2005). Eye movements and the identification of spatially ambiguous words during Chinese sentence reading. *Memory & Cognition*, *33*, 1345–1356. doi: http://dx.doi.org/10.3758/BF03193367.

Joanisse, M. F., & Seidenberg, M. S. (1998). Dissociations between rule-governed forms and exceptions: A connectionist account. *Poster presented at the 1998 Annual Meeting of the Cognitive Neuroscience Society*, San Francisco, CA.

Kang, H., & Simpson, G. B. (2001). Local strategic control of information in visual word recognition. *Memory & Cognition*, *29*, 648–655. doi: http://dx.doi.org/10.3758/BF03200466.

Lerner, I., Armstrong, B. C., & Frost, R. (2014). What can we learn from learning models about sensitivity to letter-order in visual word recognition? *Journal of Memory and Language*, *77*, 40–58. doi: http://dx.doi.org/10.1016/j.jml.2014.09.002.

Li, Y., & Kang, J. (1993). Analysis of phonetics of the ideophonetic characters in modern Chinese. In Y. Chen (Ed.), *Information analysis of usage of characters in modern Chinese*, 84–98. Shanghai, China: Shanghai Education Press.

Lindgren, S. D., De Renzi, E., & Richman, L. C. (1985). Cross-national comparisons of developmental dyslexia in Italy and the United States. *Child Development*, *56*, 1404–1417. doi: http://dx.doi.org/10.2307/1130460.

Lotto, A. J., & Holt, L. L. (2000). The illusion of the phoneme. In S. J. Billings, J. P. Boyle, & A. M. Griffith (Eds.), *Chicago linguistic society, Volume 35* (pp. 191–204). Chicago, IL: Chicago Linguistic Society.

Malone, K. (1925). Benjamin Franklin on spelling reform. *American Speech, 1*, 96–100. doi: http://dx.doi.org/ 10.2307/452554.

Manis, F. R., Seidenberg, M. S., Doi, L. M., McBride-Chang, C., & Peterson, A. (1996). On the basis of two subtypes of developmental dyslexia. *Cognition, 58*, 157–95. doi: http://dx.doi.org/10.1016/0010–0277(95)00679–6.

Mattingly, I. I. (1987). Morphological structure and segmental awareness. *Cahiers de Psychologie, 7*, 488–493.

McBride-Chang, C., Cho, J.-R., Liu, H. et al. (2005). Changing models across cultures: Associations of phonological awareness and morphological structure awareness with vocabulary and word recognition in second graders from Beijing, Hong Kong, Korea, and the United States. *Journal of Experimental Child Psychology, 92*, 140–160. doi: http://dx.doi.org/10.1016/j.jecp.2005.03.009.

McBride-Chang, C., Shu, H., Zhou, A., Wat, C. P., & Wagner, R. K. (2003). Morphological awareness uniquely predicts young children's Chinese character recognition. *Journal of Educational Psychology, 95*, 743–751. doi: http://dx.doi.org /10.1037/0022–0663.95.4.743.

McClelland, J. L., & Rumelhart, D. E. (1981). An interactive activation model of context effects in letter perception: Part 1. An account of basic findings. *Psychological Review, 88*, 375–407. doi: http://dx.doi.org/10.1037/0033-295X.88.5.375.

McClelland, J. L., Rumelhart, D. E., & PDP Research Group (Eds.). (1986). *Parallel distributed processing: Explorations in the microstructure of cognition. Volume 2: Psychological and biological models.* Cambridge, MA: MIT Press.

Mirković, J., MacDonald, M. C., & Seidenberg, M. S. (2005). Where does gender come from? Evidence from a complex inflectional system. *Language and Cognitive Processes, 20*, 139–167. doi: http://dx.doi.org/10.1080/01690960444000205.

Mirković, J., Seidenberg, M. S., & MacDonald, M. C. (2011). Rules vs. statistics: Insights from a highly inflected language. *Cognitive Psychology, 35*, 638–681. doi: http://dx.doi.org/10.1111/j.1551–6709.2011.01174.x.

Myers, J. (2010). Chinese as a natural experiment. *The Mental Lexicon, 5*, 421–435. doi: http://dx.doi.org/10.1075/ml.5.3.09mye.

Nag, S. (2011). The *akshara* languages: What do they tell us about children's literacy learning? In R. K. Mishra & N. Srinivasan (Eds.), *Language-cognition interface: State of the art* (pp. 291–310). Munich: Lincom Publishers.

Nag, S., & Snowling, M. J. (2012). Reading in an alphasyllabary: Implications for a language universal theory of learning to read. *Scientific Studies of Reading, 16*, 404–423. doi: http://dx.doi.org/10.1080/10888438.2011.576352.

Plaut, D. C., McClelland, J. L., Seidenberg, M. S., & Patterson, K. E. (1996). Understanding normal and impaired word reading: Computational principles in quasi-regular domains. *Psychological Review, 103*, 56–115. doi: http://dx.doi.org/10 .1037/0033-295X.103.1.56.

Quine, W. V. (1951). Main trends in recent philosophy: Two dogmas of empiricism. *The Philosophical Review, 60*, 20–43. doi: http://dx.doi.org/10.2307/2181906.

Raman, I., & Baluch, B. (2001). Semantic effects as a function of reading skill in word naming of a transparent orthography. *Reading and Writing, 14*, 599–614. doi: http:// dx.doi.org/10.1023/A:1012004729180.

Seidenberg, M. S., & Gonnerman, L. M. (2000). Explaining derivational morphology as the convergence of codes. *Trends in Cognitive Sciences, 4*, 353–361. doi: http://dx .doi.org/10.1016/S1364-6613(00)01515–1.

Seidenberg, M. S., & McClelland, J. L. (1989). A distributed, developmental model of word recognition and naming. *Psychological Review, 96*, 523–568. doi: http://dx .doi.org/10.1037/0033-295X.96.4.523.

Serre, T., Oliva, A., & Poggio, T. (2007). A feedforward architecture accounts for rapid categorization. *Proceedings of the National Academy of Sciences, 104*, 6424–6429. doi: http://dx.doi.org/10.1073/pnas.0700622104.

Seymour, P. H. K., Aro, M., & Erskine, J. M. (2003). Foundation literacy acquisition in European orthographies. *British Journal of Psychology, 94*, 143–174. doi: http://dx .doi.org/10.1348/000712603321661859.

Shu, H., McBride-Chang, C., Wu, S., & Liu, H. (2006). Understanding Chinese developmental dyslexia: Morphological awareness as a core cognitive construct. *Journal of Educational Psychology, 98*, 122–133. doi: http://dx.doi.org/10.1037/0022–0663 .98.1.122.

Shu, H., Meng, X., Chen, X., Luan, H., & Cao, F. (2005). The subtypes of developmental dyslexia in Chinese: Evidence from three cases dyslexia. *Dyslexia, 11*, 311–329. doi: http://dx.doi.org/10.1002/dys.310.

Shu, H., Peng, H., & McBride-Chang, C. (2008). Phonological awareness in young Chinese children. *Developmental Science, 11*, 171–181. doi: http://dx.doi.org/10 .1111/j.1467–7687.2007.00654.x.

Sibley, D. E., & Kello, C. T. (2006). Learning representations of orthographic word forms. In *Proceedings of the 27th annual meeting of the Cognitive Science Society.* Vancouver, Canada.

Strain, E., Patterson, K., & Seidenberg, M. S. (1995). Semantic effects in single-word naming. *Journal of Experimental Psychology: Learning, Memory and Cognition, 21*, 1140–1154. doi: http://dx.doi.org/10.1037/0278–7393.21.5.1140.

Taft, M., & Zhu, X. (1995). The representation of bound morphemes in the lexicon: A Chinese study. In L. B. Feldman (Ed.), *Morphological aspects of language processing* (pp. 293–316). Hillsdale, NJ: Erlbaum.

Venezky, R. L. (1970). *The structure of English orthography.* The Hague: Mouton.

Venezky, R. L. (1999). *The American way of spelling: The structure and origins of American English orthography.* New York, NY: Guilford Press.

Washington, J. A., Terry, N. P., Seidenberg, M. S. et al. (2013). Language variation and literacy learning: The case of African American English. In C. A. Stone, E. R. Silliman, B. J. Ehren, & G. P. Wallach (Eds.). *Handbook of language and literacy: Development and disorders* (pp. 204–221). New York, NY: Guilford Press.

White, T. G., Graves, M. S., & Slater, W. H. (1990). Growth of reading vocabulary in diverse elementary schools: Decoding and word meaning. *Journal of Educational Psychology, 82*, 281–290. doi: http://dx.doi.org/10.1037/0022–0663.82.2.281.

Xing, H., Shu, H., & Li, P. (2004). The acquisition of Chinese characters: Corpus analyses and connectionist simulations. *Journal of Cognitive Science, 5*, 1–49.

Yang, J. F., McCandliss, B. D., Shu, H., & Zevin, J. D. (2009). Simulating language-specific and language-general effects in a statistical learning model of Chinese reading. *Journal of Memory & Language, 61*, 238–257. doi: http://dx .doi.org/10.1016/j.jml.2009.05.001.

Yang, J. F., McCandliss, B. D., Shu, H., & Zevin, J. D. (2013). Orthographic influences on division of labor in learning to read Chinese and English: Insights from computational modeling. *Bilingualism Language and Cognition, 16*, 354–366. doi: http://dx .doi.org/10.1017/S1366728912000296.

Zhu, X. (1988). Analysis of cueing function of phonetic components in modern Chinese. In X. Yuan (Ed.), *Proceedings of the symposium on the Chinese language and characters* (pp. 85–99). Beijing: Guang Ming Daily Press (in Chinese).

Zoccolotti, P., De Luca, M., Di Pace, E. et al. (1999). Markers of developmental surface dyslexia in a language (Italian) with high grapheme–phoneme correspondence. *Applied Psycholinguistics, 20*, 191–216. doi: http://dx.doi.org/10.1017/S0142716499002027.

18   Etiology of Developmental Dyslexia

*Richard K. Olson, Janice M. Keenan, Brian Byrne, and
Stefan Samuelsson*

18.1   Introduction

Identical and fraternal twin pairs reared together have been key to understanding
the genetic and environmental etiology of dyslexia and of individual differences
in reading.[1] In this chapter, we begin with a brief overview of the methods of
twin research, and the historical development and application of these methods
to understanding the etiology of individual differences and deficits in reading and
related skills. Then we examine results from predominantly English-language
twin research on dyslexia. The next section on twin studies of individual
differences in reading ability introduces a broader cross-language perspective
that includes comparisons of findings from studies in the United States, the
United Kingdom, Australia, Norway, Sweden, the Netherlands, and China. Then
we expand the reading phenotype beyond word recognition to reading comprehension, the ultimate goal of reading. The final section summarizes the findings
that seem to be similar across all studied languages, notes limitations and
qualifications of twin study results, and concludes with comments on the implications of behavior-genetic research for public policy in education.

18.2   Methods of Twin Studies

18.2.1   Assessing Etiology of Individual Differences

Individual differences in most complex behavioral and physical characteristics
are normally distributed (i.e., the *bell curve*) in the population. This includes

[1] Richard K. Olson, Department of Psychology and Neuroscience, and Institute for Behavioral
Genetics, University of Colorado Boulder, and Department of Behavioral Sciences and
Learning, Linköping University; Janice M. Keenan, Department of Psychology, University of
Denver; Brian Byrne, School of Behavioural, Cognitive and Social Sciences, University of New
England, and Department of Behavioral Sciences and Learning, Linköping University; Stefan
Samuelsson, Department of Behavioral Sciences and Learning, Linköping University.

reading ability (Rodgers, 1983) and many of its related cognitive skills (Christopher et al., 2012). These normal distributions support the comparison of correlations from large samples of identical and fraternal twin pairs reared together to estimate the average influences of genes, shared family environment, and non-shared environment (including measurement error) on individual differences in the sampled population. The estimation of genetic and environmental influences from twins reared together is based on the fact that identical twins are monozygotic (MZ), so they share all their genes and their family environment. Fraternal (dizygotic, DZ) twins also share their family environment, but they share only half their segregating genes on average (Plomin et al., 2013).

The basic method of twin studies can be illustrated through two examples of different correlations for MZ and DZ twin pairs. Under the basic assumptions of twin research, if a trait is completely determined by genes and there is no measurement error, the expected correlations would be a perfect $r = 1$ for MZ twin pairs (because they share all their genes), and $r = 0.5$ for DZ twin pairs (because they share half their segregating genes on average). Note that in the case of 100 percent genetic influence, the difference between the MZ and DZ correlations is 0.5. Therefore, doubling the difference between the MZ and DZ twin correlations in this specific example and the ones presented below yields an approximate estimate of the percentage of additive genetic influence, conventionally labeled as A. In the extreme example of complete genetic influence, A = 1 or 100 percent. For an intermediate example, if the MZ correlation is 0.9 and the DZ correlation is 0.6, twice the difference is 0.6, so A = 0.6 or 60 percent. Shared environment, conventionally labeled C, equals the MZ correlation (0.9) minus A (0.6), so C = 0.3 or 30 percent. Finally, non-shared environment in this example, conventionally labeled E, is simply 1 minus the 0.9 MZ correlation, so E = 0.1 or 10 percent. This computation of E is based on the fact that MZ twins share both their genes (A) and their shared environment (C), so their difference from a perfect correlation of 1 is due to non-shared environment (E). The size of the E estimate often reflects measurement error, but other sources of E include non-shared prenatal development and birth problems, illnesses, accidents that may affect cognitive abilities, differences in peers, and differences between classrooms when twins do not share their classroom. The estimates of A, C, and E from studies reviewed in this chapter are usually based on structural equation modeling of the MZ and DZ twins' variance-covariance matrices in the *OpenMx* program (Boker et al., 2011).

18.2.2   *Assessing Etiology of Dyslexia*

Early evidence for genetic influence on dyslexia came from a handful of small twin studies in English that compared MZ and DZ twin concordance for dyslexia versus no dyslexia. These twin concordance analyses compared the percentages of MZ and DZ pairs with a categorical diagnosis of dyslexia and thus ignored important variance from co-twins who did not quite meet the cutoff for dyslexia. There was also evidence consistent with genetic influence from non-twin family studies that showed that dyslexia tends to be transmitted across generations (DeFries et al., 1978; Vogler, DeFries, & Decker, 1985); however, such familial patterns are not sufficient evidence for genetic influence on dyslexia because families share their environment as well as their genes.

In the late 1970s, the National Institutes of Health (NIH) in the United States became concerned about the genetic and environmental etiology of dyslexia and its possible subtypes. Therefore, NIH solicited a proposal for a twin study of dyslexia from a group of investigators led by John DeFries at the University of Colorado's Institute for Behavioral Genetics. The project developed measures that would be sensitive to potential subtypes of dyslexia, and that would also be suitable for the planned twin study, which began testing Colorado twins in 1982. Testing continues to this day through NIH funding of the Colorado Learning Disabilities Research Center (CLDRC). As of April 2016, the CLDRC sample included 5,370 individuals (936 pairs of MZ twins, 1437 pairs of DZ twins, and 624 non-twin siblings).

The CLDRC sample selection is initially based on soliciting twin pairs through Colorado school districts. Twins who have a loosely defined school history of dyslexia in at least one member of each pair are invited for laboratory testing. A "control" sample of twin pairs with no school history of dyslexia in either twin is also included in the CLDRC study. School history for Attention Deficit Hyperactivity Disorder (ADHD) was added from 1990 onward as a selection criterion, so affected twin pairs can have at least one twin with a school history of dyslexia only, ADHD only, or both. Control twin pairs are also recruited that have no school history for either disorder. The initial school-history diagnoses are confirmed with extensive laboratory testing of word reading, spelling, reading comprehension, ADHD, and related skills, including full scale IQ. Inclusionary criteria include (1) English-speaking home, (2) no evidence of neurological problems such as seizure or history of brain injury, (3) no uncorrected visual or auditory deficits, and (4) no known genetic disorders or syndromes.

The CLDRC has no minimum IQ or IQ-reading discrepancy criterion for inclusion in the study, although no twins fall below a full scale IQ score of 60, and very few are below 75. This lax IQ criterion may seem to violate traditional criteria for the diagnosis of dyslexia that have required a discrepancy between reading and IQ, but it was included because one of the goals of the CLDRC is to test the genetic and environmental etiology of the relation between IQ, its various components, and reading. However, most behavior-genetic analyses of twin data in the CLDRC that do not explore relations between IQ and the etiology of dyslexia require a minimum verbal or performance IQ of 85 or 90.

Because reading ability is continuously and normally distributed in the population (Rodgers, 1983), the early twin concordance analyses based on comparing the percentages of MZ and DZ pairs with a diagnosis of dyslexia ignored important variance in co-twins who did not quite meet the cutoff for dyslexia. To solve this problem, John DeFries and David Fulker developed their "DF" model to more appropriately estimate average genetic and environmental influences on membership in the low tail of the normal reading distribution, the dyslexic group (DeFries & Fulker, 1985). The DF model identifies dyslexic "proband" members of twin pairs by their membership in the low tail of the normal distribution, and then it estimates averages for genetic and environmental influences on membership in this deviant group by examining differences in regression to the population mean for the non-proband MZ and DZ co-twins. For an extreme example, if low group membership were entirely due to genes then: (1) both members of all MZ pairs would be in the low group because they share all their genes, and (2) the DZ co-twins of DZ probands would regress halfway on average to the population mean because they share on average only half their segregating genes with their probands in the low tail. Some MZ co-twins may regress part way to the population mean, and the average co-twin regression of these MZ twins provides an estimate of non-shared-environment influence, including measurement error, on the dyslexic group deficit. Evidence for shared environment influence is present when DZ co-twin regression is less than half the MZ co-twin regression to the population mean. More recently, differential MZ and DZ co-twin regression to the population mean has been modeled in the Mx program to more easily obtain estimates and confidence intervals (Purcell & Sham, 2003).

The reader may have noticed that we have not defined exactly what is meant by the "low tail" of the normal distribution for reading. That is because the definition of dyslexia by degree of severity in a normal distribution of reading ability is arbitrary. Although many authors may state that dyslexia exists in some specific percentage of the population, often 5–10 percent (c.f., Compton et al., 2014), it is because they choose to use a cutoff of 5–10 percent, not because there is a break in the reading-ability distribution at that point. To maintain consistency with these arbitrary criteria in the literature on dyslexia, most behavior-genetic research on the etiology of dyslexia has used approximately the lower 10 percent of readers in the sampled populations to define the proband group with dyslexia.

18.3   Findings on Genetic and Environmental Etiology of Dyslexia

In the present and following sections, we will report only the percentage estimates for genetic (A) and shared environment (C) influences, not E (non-shared environment including measurement error); that is because E simply equals 100 percent – (A percent + C percent). So for example, if A has been estimated at 40 percent and C has been estimated at 50 percent, then it can be assumed that E has been estimated at 10 percent. We use the subscript $_g$ (for group) when the A_g and C_g estimates are for the etiology of low-tail group membership for dyslexia rather than for individual differences.

Friend, DeFries, and Olson (2008) applied the DF model to a composite measure of reading and spelling data from 545 same-sex twin pairs at mean age 11.4 years in which at least one member of each pair scored below the 10th percentile. The average genetic and environmental etiology for dyslexic group membership in this CLDRC sample was A_g = 61 percent for genetic and C_g = 30 percent for shared environment. Harlaar et al. (2005) reported very similar results from their large and representative population sample; this included 3,909 pairs of 7-year-old twins in the United Kingdom who were participating in the Twins Early Development Study (TEDS). The DF modeling estimates for the etiology of word and nonword reading below the tenth percentile in the TEDS sample, averaged across gender, were A_g = 59 percent and C_g = 30 percent. A third study by Kirkpatrick et al. (2011) performed a DF analysis of 266 RD probands selected from 9,430 twins, parents, and adoptees from the Minnesota Twin Family Study and the Sibling Interaction and Behavior Study. The genetic and environmental estimates for the dyslexic proband group deficit in word reading were A_g = 72 percent and C_g = 9 percent.

In summary, the results of these three twin studies of dyslexia are consistent in showing substantial genetic influence. Although the Friend et al. (2008) and the Harlaar et al. (2005) studies also reported significant shared-environment influence of about 30 percent, the average influence of genes on dyslexic group membership was about twice as strong as the shared-environment influence. This significant shared-environment influence raises the question of its etiology among children with dyslexia, a topic we will return to in the section on the etiology of individual differences.

18.3.1 Differences in the Etiology of Dyslexia Related to Socioeconomic Status (SES) and IQ

We would like to know the etiology of an individual child's dyslexia, but behavior-genetic data cannot tell us this; it only provides information about the average etiology of dyslexic group membership. It is therefore possible that for some individual children within the dyslexic group, environmental factors may be the major, or only, influence on their dyslexia, while for others, the major or only influence may be from genes. It is possible, however, to expand the DF regression model to ask if the degree of genetic and environmental influences on dyslexia is significantly related to individual differences on other variables, thus bringing us closer to an understanding of differential genetic and environmental etiology within the group with dyslexia.

Friend et al. (2008) did this using parents' years of education as a proxy for SES to explore the possibility of a "genetic influence by environment" interaction. They found that genetic influence was significantly higher on average for children with dyslexia who had parents with higher education, compared to children with lower parent education. For children with lower parent education level, shared family environment and genes were about equally influential, on average. One interpretation of these results is that children who fail in reading in spite of having highly educated parents (and likely a better environment for learning to read) are more likely to have genetic than environmental constraints on their reading development. A potentially related result is that the twins' IQ scores are significantly associated with the level of genetic influence on their dyslexia. Genetic influence on dyslexia tends to be greater among twins with higher IQ scores (Wadsworth, Olson, & DeFries, 2010). To some extent this may be due to the association between higher IQ and a more supportive educational environment for reading.

It is important that the consistency of these "genetic influence by environment" interactions be tested across different twin samples. To date, we are aware of only one other study that has tested the interaction found by Friend et al. (2008) for dyslexia and parent education. Kirkpatrick et al. (2011) did not replicate the interaction reported by Friend et al., though their proband sample was less than half the size of the Friend et al. sample, and their measure of reading was limited to a single measure of word recognition. Nevertheless, the failure of Kirkpatrick et al. to find an interaction with parent education indicates the need for further research on "genetic influence by environment" interactions in other twin samples.

18.3.2 Subtype Differences in the Etiology of Dyslexia

Early theories of dyslexia subtypes in English distinguished between children who had specific difficulty in their phonological awareness and phonological decoding of words (labeled "dysphonetic"), while other children had specific difficulty in visually establishing whole-word representations (labeled "dyseidetic") (Boder, 1973). A related distinction among normal readers of English was proposed by Baron (1977). He distinguished "Phoenician" normal readers, who seemed to read primarily through phonological coding, from "Chinese" normal readers, who relied more on visual whole-word processing. More recent times have seen research on related "dual-route" models of word reading that can also be viewed as a basis for subtypes in dyslexia (Castles & Coltheart, 1993; Castles et al., 1999).

To explore related subtypes for dyslexia in the CLDRC twins, Olson et al. (1985) developed computer-based forced-choice tasks to assess the twins' phonological and orthographic coding skills. The phonological choice task required subjects to silently select which of two pronounceable printed non-words (e.g., caik daik) is the one that would sound like a common word. Phonological coding was also assessed traditionally through subjects' oral reading of nonwords. Orthographic coding was assessed with two tasks. One asked subjects to listen to a sentence such as "Which is a fruit?" and then rapidly select the correct word from two homophones (pair pear). The other orthographic coding task asked subjects to quickly choose the word in word–pseudohomophone pairs (e.g., rane rain). Thus, the correct answer in the orthographic coding tasks could not be derived from phonological decoding alone (Olson et al., 1989, 1994).

The first behavior-genetic analysis of phonological and orthographic coding deficits derived from using these tasks concluded that while phonological coding deficits were significantly influenced by genes, orthographic coding deficits were not (Olson et al., 1989). This result was widely cited because many theorists believed that dyslexia was caused by a biologically based phonological processing deficit, and deficits in orthographic coding were more likely due to a lack of print exposure in the environment (Stanovich & West, 1989). However, subsequent analyses by Gayán and Olson (2001) of phonological and orthographic coding deficits in a much larger twin sample clarified that both were significantly influenced by genes; $A_g = 62$ percent, $C_g = 23$ percent, and $A_g = 63$ percent, $C_g = 16$ percent, respectively. In addition, both skills had a very high genetic correlation with dyslexia defined by the group deficit in word recognition: $r = 0.88$ with orthographic coding and $r = 0.98$ with phonological coding, a nonsignificant difference. A very similar pattern of results was reported by Gayán and Olson (2003) for the genetic and environmental etiology of individual differences in orthographic coding, phonological coding, and word recognition. In summary, the amount of genetic influence and the genetic correlation with dyslexia were similarly high for orthographic and phonological coding. Therefore, the behavior-genetic evidence does not support distinct etiological subtypes in dyslexia based on differential deficits in orthographic and phonological coding.

The prominence of orthographic and phonological subtype theory in the dyslexia literature may reflect the fact that English includes relatively large numbers of homophones and distinctly irregular words that seem to suggest the need for a specialized orthographic mechanism for word-specific representations. Similarly, research on bilinguals showing that they can be dyslexic in their alphabetic language but not in their non-alphabetic language, or vice versa, is similarly suggestive (McBride-Chang et al., 2013). Our results do not deny the existence of such a mechanism. Indeed, recent research suggests that word-specific neural representations, regardless of their orthographic regularity, are rapidly learned in the so-called visual word form areas of the brain (Glezer et al., 2015), and this process is important for the development of reading fluency in any writing system (Perfetti, Cao, & Booth, 2013).

While the behavior-genetic results of Gayán and Olson (2001, 2003) seemed to argue against etiologically distinct orthographic and phonological subtypes of RD, the results of Peterson, Pennington, & Olson (2013; Peterson et al., 2014) support at least a dimension of phonological deficit relative to subjects' level of both word recognition and orthographic coding skills. Also, the degree of phonological deficit, but not the orthographic deficit, remains relatively stable from mean age 10 to mean age 16. However, subtype diagnosis did not inform prognosis for growth in word recognition from age 10 to 16, after controlling for word recognition at age 10 (Hulslander et al., 2010; Peterson et al., 2014). This latter result questions the clinical utility of this particular subtype diagnosis after age 10 for readers of English.

18.3.3   Comorbidity between Dyslexia and ADHD

Before turning to behavior-genetic studies of individual differences across different countries and languages, we will comment briefly on a subtype distinction in dyslexia related to its significant phenotypic and genetic comorbidity with ADHD. Several studies in English have noted this comorbidity for some children with dyslexia, particularly with the Attention Deficit (AD) component of ADHD (Willcutt et al., 2010), and this comorbidity has been significantly associated with the same quantitative trait locus for dyslexia on chromosome 6p (Gayán et al., 2005). Consistent with this molecular genetic result, bivariate DF behavior-genetic analyses of dyslexia and AD have shown that there is a significant genetic correlation between these two disorders, and their genetic correlation is significantly mediated by deficits in processing speed (Willcutt et al., 2007, 2010). Although most children with dyslexia do not have ADHD, those who do share dyslexia and ADHD tend to have more severe deficits in dyslexia, and their dyslexia tends to be more highly heritable.

18.4   Genetic and Environmental Influences on Individual Differences in Reading

We now turn to results from behavior-genetic studies of individual differences in reading across the full distribution of reading skill, as opposed to behavioral-genetic studies of dyslexia, i.e. membership in the low tail of the reading-ability distribution. As we mentioned earlier the etiology of dyslexia is not necessarily the same as the etiology of individual differences across the full range of reading ability. However, Kovas and Plomin (2007) have argued that if the estimates of A, C, and E are fairly similar for dyslexia and for individual differences in reading ability then this would imply that the same genes are involved. If this is true, results from twin studies on individual differences in reading ability in different languages can also speak to the etiology of dyslexia in different languages.

18.4.1   The International Longitudinal Twin Study

The International Longitudinal Twin Study (ILTS) (Byrne et al., 2002; Samuelsson et al., 2005) is the only study that has used extensive parallel measures to assess the genetic and environmental etiology of reading and related skills in orthographically irregular English in the United States (Colorado) and Australia, and two very similar and relatively orthographically regular Scandinavian languages, Norwegian and Swedish. Since Norwegian and Swedish languages and orthographies are quite similar, and both began formal reading instruction in the first grade at the time of the study, the Norwegian and Swedish samples are combined as the "Scandinavian" sample to increase statistical power. The Australian and Colorado samples are not combined for language-group comparisons because formal reading instruction begins earlier in Australia.

The ILTS initially tested twins on prereading skills in their homes or pre-schools during the year prior to kindergarten entry. They were subsequently tested on reading and related skills at the end of kindergarten, first grade, and second grade in all three samples (Byrne et al., 2009; Christopher et al., 2013a; Samuelsson et al., 2008), and also at the end of fourth grade in the Colorado sample (Christopher et al., 2013b, 2015; Olson et al., 2011).

Regardless of language, at preschool most individual differences on print knowledge (mainly letter-name and sound knowledge) were due to differences in shared family environment (A = 20 percent – 26 percent; C = 62 percent – 74 percent) (Samuelsson et al., 2007). The vast majority of preschool children could not read, so we could not estimate genetic and environmental influences on their reading ability. By the end of kindergarten, most children could read enough words and nonwords on the TOWRE test of word and nonword reading efficiency (Torgesen, Wagner, & Rashotte, 1999) that we could estimate genetic and environmental influences on their individual differences (Samuelsson et al., 2008). Those individual differences were mostly due to genes in Australia (A = 84 percent; C = 9 percent) and Colorado (A = 68 percent; C = 25 percent). In contrast, individual differences for the Scandinavian twins' reading at the end of kindergarten were mostly due to shared environment (A = 33 percent; C = 52 percent). However, this contrast was probably not related to the difference in orthographic regularity between English and

Scandinavian. Samuelsson et al. noted that reading is not formally taught in Scandinavia until the first grade, so the Scandinavian twins' reading scores at the end of kindergarten were significantly lower than for the Australian and Colorado twins. Thus, it was variation in the Scandinavian twins' shared home, preschool, and kindergarten environment that was the major influence on individual differences at the end of kindergarten.

After children in the ILTS samples had all received at least a year of formal reading instruction, normally by the end of first grade, genetic influence was about as strong in Scandinavia (A = 79 percent; C = 7 percent) as it was in Australia (A = 80 percent; C = 2 percent) and Colorado (A = 83 percent; C = 7 percent) (Samuelsson et al., 2008). Similarly high genetic and low shared-environment estimates have been found for spelling and reading comprehension at the end of first grade, and the genetic correlations between word recognition, spelling, and reading comprehension were all above $r_a = .9$ (Byrne et al., 2007). The pattern of high genetic and low shared-environment estimates continued to the end of second grade in all three samples (Byrne et al., 2009; Christopher et al., 2013a), and to the end of fourth grade in Colorado for word and nonword reading, reading comprehension, and spelling (Christopher et al., 2013b, 2015; Olson et al., 2011). In summary, after a year of formal reading instruction, individual differences in word reading, spelling, and reading comprehension are highly influenced by genes for the alphabetic languages in this study, regardless of country and orthographic regularity.

Behavior-genetic estimates of genetic and environmental influences may depend on the environmental range in the sampled twin population. Therefore, it is important to compare results across samples where the environmental range may differ. Other studies in English have sometimes yielded slightly higher estimates than ours of shared environment and slightly lower estimates of genetic influence (Harlaar et al., 2005; Hart et al., 2013; Logan et al., 2013), and one study reports lower shared-environment influences Kirkpatrick et al., 2011). Some of these differences can be attributed to such things as within-wave differences in months of education (see Olson et al., 2014, for an explanation). But in general, the results present a consistent picture: When it comes to explaining variation across performance levels, the variation in shared home and classroom environments has less influence on individual differences in reading than genetic influences, once children have completed a year of formal reading instruction.

Of course environmental influences also have a big effect – they affect the performance level of reading in the population because we learn to read in classrooms and homes. When compared to the strong shared-environment influences on preschool print knowledge, it seems that what formal reading instruction in schools does is to considerably reduce the environmental variance for reading development. This is a very good result. It would be unfortunate if strong family-based environmental influences persisted beyond the early stages of school. Indeed, this is partly what schools are about, overcoming factors that produce big differences among children before they go to school, particularly when those environmental influences are negative.

18.4.2   Twin Studies in Other Languages

To date there have been relatively few twin studies of individual differences in reading in languages other than English. We have already discussed the ILTS results from Scandinavia that were very similar to those in English after the first year of formal reading instruction. A twin study in the Netherlands also reported similar estimates for word-reading accuracy and fluency on the One Minute Reading Test from 112 pairs of 9-year-old twins recruited from the Netherlands Twin Registry (van Leeuwen et al., 2009). In this study, A = 83 percent and C = 0 percent, but the authors acknowledged that their sample size was quite small and they had little power to detect C.

Of particular interest are two twin studies of Chinese readers in Hong Kong. Chow et al. (2011) recruited 339 Chinese twin pairs aged 3 to 11 years who used Cantonese as their mother tongue. The twins were assessed on a wide range of reading-related skills, but for comparison to other studies of word recognition in alphabetic orthographies we focus on their results for the twins' reading ability for printed Chinese characters. The A = 73 percent and C = 18 percent estimates for individual differences in Chinese character reading were remarkably similar to those from the twin studies we have reviewed for word reading in alphabetic orthographies.

The second study by the same researchers, Ho et al. (2012) reported similar estimates for Chinese character reading (A = 75 percent, C = 16 percent) in a sample of 270 pairs aged 5 to 11 years that overlapped with the sample in Chow et al. (2011). But the focus of this study was on the genetic and environmental relations between language comprehension (oral vocabulary), word reading, and reading comprehension. They found that word recognition and vocabulary had significant independent genetic influences, and together they accounted for most of the genetic influence on a measure of reading comprehension in Chinese. As such, the Ho et al. study provides a perfect segue to our next section on the genetic and environmental etiology of individual differences in English reading comprehension.

18.5   Studies of Individual Differences in Reading Comprehension

Across the last two decades there has been increasing attention to children's difficulties in reading comprehension and oral language comprehension where these may be partly independent from their difficulties in printed-word recognition. There is some dispute about the idea that dyslexia should be defined only by deficits in printed-word recognition and related phonological skills, and that specific deficits in reading comprehension should be separately diagnosed as a language disorder. Regardless of the dyslexia definition issue, we believe that it is important for research and practice to better understand the phenotypic relations between these skills, their developmental course, and their genetic and environmental etiology. In this section we expand our review to include reading comprehension, oral language comprehension, and word recognition. There is independence between decoding and comprehension skills because there are children who have problems in reading comprehension, despite having adequate word-reading skill (Cain & Oakhill, 2007). To date, there have been no DF analyses of comprehension deficits, so here we focus on the results from behavior-genetic analyses of individual differences in the population.

Keenan et al. (2006) explored the genetic and environmental etiology of Hoover and Gough's (1990) simple view of reading comprehension, wherein individual differences in reading comprehension can be entirely accounted for by individual differences in word recognition or decoding and listening comprehension. Keenan et al. found that for children between 8 and 18 years of age (mean 11 years) in the CLDRC sample, the genetic correlation between individual differences in word reading and listening comprehension was modest, $r = 0.37$; so, most of the genetic influence on comprehension was independent of the genetic influences on word recognition and was highly significant. Taken together, genetic influences on word reading and listening comprehension accounted for all of the genetic influence on reading comprehension. In contrast, the shared-environment correlations between these skills were all quite high, suggesting that what is a good environment for word reading is also a good environment for comprehension. Thus, it was the largely independent genetic influences on listening comprehension and word recognition that accounted for their unique contributions to individual differences in reading comprehension. This basic result has been confirmed by Harlaar et al. (2010) in an independent twin sample from Ohio, and by Betjemann et al. (2011) in an expanded sample from the CLDRC.

Betjemann et al. (2011) also found that the choice of tests for assessing reading comprehension had a significant influence on the degree of phenotypic and genetic covariance between word decoding, listening comprehension, and reading comprehension. Latent traits for reading comprehension tests most closely associated with word decoding (RC-D) and tests most closely associated with listening comprehension (RC-LC) were similar in their levels of genetic and environmental influence (respectively, A = 60 percent, C = 32 percent and A = 66 percent, C = 23 percent). Both types of test shared significant genetic influence with decoding and listening comprehension, but RC-D tests shared most genetic variance with decoding and RC-LC tests shared most genetic variance with listening comprehension. The authors noted that different tests used to measure the same general construct of reading comprehension may manifest very different patterns of genetic covariation, consistent with their differential dependence on decoding and oral comprehension (Keenan, Betjemann, & Olson, 2008).

We conclude this section on the etiology of individual differences in reading comprehension with an exploration of their genetic and environmental relations to prereading skills. Christopher et al. (2015) examined the genetic and environmental etiology of the phenotypic correlations between prereading and subsequent word reading, spelling, and reading comprehension at the end of the first and fourth grades. At the end of first grade, relations between prereading skills and word reading, spelling, and reading comprehension were largely due to genetic influences. This was true even when individual differences in pre-school print knowledge and vocabulary were primarily due to shared family environment. However, for fourth-grade reading comprehension, the phenotypic correlations with preschool print knowledge ($r = 0.50$), phonological awareness ($r = 0.61$), and vocabulary ($r = 0.57$) were primarily mediated by the twins' shared environment.

Why are shared family environment influences on three of the preschool skills more closely associated with fourth-grade reading comprehension than with word recognition or spelling, and why is their shared-environment influence more strongly related to reading comprehension at the end of Grade 4 than at the end of the first grade? The answer may be that individual differences in reading comprehension are more influenced by individual differences in word-decoding skills at first grade when many children are still learning to read (Elwér et al., 2013). When children are primarily reading to learn, at the end of Grade 4, most have sufficient word-decoding skills to accurately read the text. Therefore, individual differences in reading comprehension become relatively more dependent on vocabulary and world knowledge. Of course this begs the question of why word recognition and spelling are less related to these shared environmental influences. We suggest that individual differences in word decoding and spelling are more closely tied to basic genetically influenced differences in learning rates for accurate and fluent print-to-sound (decoding) and sound-to-print (spelling) relations (Byrne, Wadsworth et al., 2013).

It will be interesting to see if the greater shared-environment influences linking prereading skills to reading comprehension at the end of Grade 4 are maintained when our twins complete their follow-up assessments at the end of Grade 9. Preliminary results from a nearly complete Grade 9 follow-up sample in Colorado suggests that they are (Christopher, personal communication, April 2016).

We should add that in univariate behavior-genetic analyses of reading comprehension, the level of genetic influences on individual differences in reading comprehension tend to be quite high and nearly comparable to those for word recognition in the ILTS and Ohio unselected population samples (Soden et al., 2015). It remains to be seen if DF analyses of reading comprehension deficits will yield A_g and C_g estimates similar to those reported for word recognition. Our view is that deficits in reading comprehension deserve as much as or more attention than deficits in printed-word recognition, and the shared environmental links from preschool skills to later reading comprehension signal important avenues for early intervention (Christopher et al., 2015).

18.6   Discussion and Conclusion

Dyslexia, defined by a group deficit in printed-word recognition below approximately the 10th percentile, has been shown in three independent English samples to have significant genetic etiology. Genetic influence is, on average, at least twice that of shared family environment. Note, however, that the balance of genetic and environmental influences on individuals within the dyslexia group may differ as a function of family SES, and of the twins' IQ and ADHD status. It is also important to understand that behavior-genetic studies are not able to specify the balance of genetic and environmental influences for any individual with RD. They only provide estimates for the average influence from genes and environment in the sampled population, and for the average influence of moderating variables such as SES on the balance of genetic and environmental influences across the dyslexic sample. This important qualification also holds not just for twin studies of dyslexia but also for twin studies of individual differences across the full range.

Most behavior-genetic twin studies on reading and related skills have focused on individual differences across the full normal distribution in their sampled populations. These studies have included alphabetic orthographies with varying orthographic regularity, and the non-alphabetic character script of Cantonese in Hong Kong. The results of these studies are remarkably consistent. As we found for dyslexia in the three English samples, genetic influence on individual differences is significantly stronger than shared environmental influence, and it accounts for the majority of individual differences in the sampled populations. Based on these consistent results across languages, we hypothesize that when the etiology of group deficits in word-reading accuracy and fluency (dyslexia) are studied in languages other than English, the results will be similar to those from English studies.

There are several important qualifications concerning behavior-genetic estimates of genetic and environmental influences on dyslexia and on individual differences in reading. First, the estimates always depend on the reading-related environmental range in the sampled populations. All studies we have reviewed in this chapter tested twin samples with universal state-supported education in reading, and all children in the studies were attending school. The environmental range in countries without universal literacy instruction will be much greater, resulting in lower genetic and higher shared-environment influence.

A related concern is that even within samples with universal education, the most environmentally disadvantaged families may be less likely to participate in twin research, thus restricting the environmental range of the sample. For example, the Colorado component of the ILTS used a birth twin registry to contact the 90 percent of twin families who did not explicitly reject future participation in twin studies at the time of birth. Sixty percent of these families were able to be contacted by letter or phone to enlist their participation in the study when their twins were approximately 4 years of age, and 88 percent of the contacted families agreed to participate. It is certainly possible that there were proportionally more environmentally disadvantaged families among those who could not be contacted, and among those who were contacted but refused participation. Furthermore, the Colorado sample excluded children whose first language in their home was not English. These factors likely combined to reduce the effective environmental range below its actual representation in the Colorado sampling area.

A different limitation or source of uncertainty about the results of behavior-genetic research with twins emerges from the possibility that there may be violations of basic assumptions of twin models. First, there may be some genetic non-additivity (dominance and/or epistasis). Under the common additive genetic model of the reviewed twin studies, violation of the additivity assumption would overestimate genetic and underestimate shared-environment influence (Keller & Coventry, 2005; Keller, Medland, & Duncan, 2010). Some researchers have argued there is little direct evidence that non-additive genetic variance has a major influence on complex cognitive traits (e.g., Hill, Goodard, & Visscher, 2008). Others have noted that adoption studies of reading generally find very low correlations between reading scores of adopted siblings, and shared-environment estimates are similar to those from twin studies (e.g., Petrill et al., 2006; Wadsworth et al., 2006). We are open to the possibility of some non-additivity bias in the reviewed twin studies, particularly when estimates of shared-environment influence are at or close to 0, as they were in the ILTS samples from Australia, Colorado, and Scandinavia, and a Florida sample for word-reading efficiency at the end of first grade. However, we concur with Hill et al. (2008) that a non-additivity bias is not likely to be very strong for a complex cognitive trait like reading, and all this does not question the predominant role of genetic factors in dyslexia and individual differences in the reviewed studies.

Finally, there is an important qualification of genetic and environmental estimates for dyslexia and for individual differences in reading due to an active gene–environment correlation. It is known that there is a positive correlation between reading ability and amount of reading practice (Mol & Bus, 2011; Stanovich & West, 1989), and that genetic influences on differences in reading ability in early elementary school come partly from correlated genetic influences on differences in reading practice (Harlaar et al., 2011, 2014). It seems that if a child has genes that make learning to read difficult, they are less likely to enjoy and engage in reading practice, a gene–environment correlation that contributes importantly to slower reading growth in children with dyslexia.

This gene–environment correlation poses a problem for intervention. Many children with genetically compromised learning rates for reading may need much more practice than their normal reading peers to reach or more closely approach the grade-level criterion prescribed, as for example in the United States by the No Child Left Behind education act (107th Congress, 2002). The educational challenge is to motivate the necessary additional reading practice for children with dyslexia, the amount of which is likely to be correlated with the severity of their dyslexia. As we have argued elsewhere, some children with severe dyslexia in word reading and/or reading comprehension may fail to reach grade level regardless of much greater reading practice in their schools and homes, with the attendant loss of other valued home and school activities (Olson et al., 2014). We believe that a major implication of behavior-genetic research on dyslexia for public policy in education is that it is unreasonable to expect grade-level performance in reading for all children. We believe that a better understanding of and acknowledgment of the powerful influence of genes on many children's dyslexia will lead to more reasonable student expectations and a better appreciation of the extraordinary effort required for those children to reach or more closely approach functional levels of literacy.

Acknowledgments

Funding was provided by the National Institutes of Health, grant numbers P50 HD027802 for the Colorado Learning Disabilities Research Center, and R01 HD038526 for the Colorado component of the International Longitudinal Twin Study (ILTS). The Australian component of the ILTS was supported by the Australian Research Council, A79906201, DP0663498, DP0770805. The Scandinavian component of the ILTS was supported by the Research Council of Norway 154715/330, the Swedish Research Council grants 345–2002-3701, PDOKJ028/2006:1, and 2011–1905, and the Swedish Council for Working Life and Social Research (2011–0177). We thank the twins and their families who participated in our research. The Australian

Twin Registry is supported by an enabling grant from the National Health and Medical Research Council. Correspondence concerning this chapter should be addressed to Richard Olson, Department of Psychology and Neuroscience, University of Colorado Boulder, Boulder, CO 80309. Email: Richard.Olson@Colorado.edu.

References

107th Congress. (2002). The No Child Left Behind Act of 2001. Pub. L. No. 107–110, Stat. 1425. Washington, DC: United States Congress.

Betjemann, R. S., Keenan, J. M., Olson, R. K., & DeFries, J. C. (2011). Choice of reading comprehension test influences the outcomes of genetic analyses. *Scientific Studies of Reading, 15*(4), 363–382. doi: http://dx.doi.org/10.1080/10888438.2010.493965.

Baron, J. (1977). Mechanisms for pronouncing printed words: use and acquisition. In D. LaBerge & S. J. Samuels (Eds.), *Basic processes in reading: perception and comprehension* (pp. 175–216). Hillsdale, NJ: Earlbaum.

Boder, E. (1973). Developmental dyslexia: A diagnostic approach based on three atypical reading-spelling patterns. *Developmental Medicine and Child Neurology, 15*, 663–687.

Boker, S. M., Neale, M. C., Maes, H. H. et al. (2011). OpenMx: An open source extended structural equation modeling framework. *Psychometrika*.

Byrne, B., Christopher, M., Coventry, W. et al. (2013). Subsample standardization in twin studies of academic achievement. *Paper presented at the meeting of the Behavior Genetics Association*, Marseilles, France, June 29, 2013.

Byrne, B., Coventry, W. L., Olson, R. K. et al. (2009). Genetic and environmental influences on aspects of literacy and language in early childhood: Continuity and change from preschool to grade 2. *Journal of Neurolinguistics, 22*, 219–236.

Byrne, B., Delaland, C., Fielding-Barnsley, R. et al. (2002). Longitudinal twin study of early reading development in three countries: Preliminary results. *Annals of Dyslexia, 52*, 49–74.

Byrne, B., Samuelsson, S., Wadsworth, S. et al. (2007). Longitudinal twin study of early literacy development: Preschool through Grade 1. *Reading and Writing: An Interdisciplinary Journal, 20*, 77–102.

Byrne, B., Wadsworth, S., Boehme, K. et al. (2013). Multivariate genetic analysis of learning and early reading development. *Scientific Studies of Reading, 17*(3), 224–242. doi: http://dx.doi.org/10.1080/10888438.2011.654298.

Cain, K. & Oakhill, J. (2007). Reading comprehension difficulties: Correlates, causes, and consequences. In K. Cain & J. Oakhill (Eds.), *Children's comprehension problems in oral and written text: A cognitive perspective*. New York: Guilford Press, pp. 41–75.

Castles, A. E., & Coltheart, M. C. (1993). Varieties of developmental dyslexia. *Cognition, 47*, 149–180.

Castles, A., Datta, H., Gayán, J., & Olson, R.K. (1999). Varieties of developmental reading disorder: Genetic and environmental influences. *Journal of Experimental Child Psychology, 72*, 73–94. PMID: 9927524.

Chow, B. W. Y., Ho, C. S. H., Wong, S. W. L., Waye, M., & Bishop, D. V. M. (2011). Genetic and environmental influences on Chinese language and reading abilities. *PLoS One, 6*(2): e16640. doi: http://dx.doi.org/10.1371/journal.pone.0016640.

Christopher, M. E., Hulslander, J., Byrne, B. et al. (2013a). The genetic and environmental etiologies of individual differences in early reading growth in Australia, the United States, and Scandinavia. *Journal of Experimental Child Psychology*, *115*, 453–467. doi: http://dx.doi.org/10.1016/j.jecp.2013.03.008.

Christopher, M. E., Hulslander, J., Byrne, B. et al. (2013b). Modeling the etiology of individual differences in early reading development: Evidence for strong genetic influences. *Scientific Studies of Reading*, *17*, 350–368. doi: http://dx.doi.org/10.1080/10888438.2012.729119.

Christopher, M. E., Hulslander, J., Byrne, B. et al. (2015). Genetic and environmental etiologies of the longitudinal relations between pre-reading skills and reading. *Child Development*, *86*, 342–361. doi: http://dx.doi.org/10.1111/cdev.12295.

Christopher, M. E., Miyake, A., Keenan, J. M. et al. (2012). Predicting word reading and comprehension with executive function and speed measures: A latent variable analysis. *Journal of Experimental Psychology: General*, *141*, 470–488. doi: http://dx.doi.org/10.1037/a0027375.

Compton, D. L., Miller, A. C., Elleman, A. M., & Steacy, L. M. (2014). Have we forsaken reading theory in the name of "quick fix" interventions for children with reading disability? *Scientific Studies of Reading*, *18*, 55–73. doi: http://dx.doi.org/10.1080/10888438.2013.836200.

DeFries, J. C., & Fulker, D. W. (1985). Multiple regression analysis of twin data. *Behavior Genetics*, *15*, 467–478. doi: http://dx.doi.org/10.1007/BF01066239.

DeFries, J. C., Singer, S. M., Foch, T. T., & Lewitter, F. I. (1978). Familial nature of reading disability. *British Journal of Psychiatry*, *132*, 361–367.

Ehri, L. C. (2014). Orthographic mapping in the acquisition of sight word reading, spelling memory, and vocabulary learning. *Scientific Studies of Reading*, *18*, 5–21. doi: http://dx.doi.org/10.1080/10888438.2013.819356.

Elwér, Å., Keenan, J. M., Olson, R. K., Byrne, B., & Samuelsson, S. (2013). Longitudinal stability and predictors of poor oral comprehenders and poor decoders. *Journal of Experimental Child Psychology*, *115*, 497–516. doi: http://dx.doi.org/10.1016/j.jecp.2012.12.001.

Friend, A., DeFries, J. C., & Olson, R. K. (2008). Parental education moderates genetic influences on reading disability. *Psychological Science*, *19*, 1124–1130. doi: http://dx.doi.org/10.1111/j.1467-9280.2008.02213.x.

Gayán, J., & Olson, R. K. (2001). Genetic and environmental influences on orthographic and phonological skills in children with reading disabilities. *Developmental Neuropsychology*, *20*, 483–507. doi: http://dx.doi.org/10.1207/S15326942DN2002_3.

Gayán, J., & Olson, R. K. (2003). Genetic and environmental influences on individual differences in printed word recognition. *Journal of Experimental Child Psychology*, *84*, 97–123. doi: http://dx.doi.org/10.1016/S0022-0965(02)00181-9.

Gayán, J., Willcutt, E. G., Fisher, S. E. et al. (2005). Bivariate linkage scan for reading disability and attention-deficit/hyperactivity disorder localizes pleiotropic loci. *Journal of Child Psychology and Psychiatry*, *46*, 1045–1056. doi: http://dx.doi.org/10.1111/j.1469-7610.2005.01447.x.

Glezer, L. S., Kim, J., Rule, J., Jiang, X., & Riesenhuber, M. (2015). Adding words to the brain's visual dictionary: Novel word learning selectively sharpens orthographic representations in the VWFA. *The Journal of Neuroscience*, *35*, 4965–4972. doi: http://dx.doi.org/10.1523/JNEUROSCI,4031-14.2015.

Harlaar, N., Cutting, L., Deater-Deckard, K. et al. (2010). Predicting individual differences in reading comprehension: a twin study. *Annals of Dyslexia, 60*, 265–288. doi: http://dx.doi.org/10.1007/s11881-010-0044-7.

Harlaar, N., Deater-Deckard, K., Thompson, L. A., DeThorne, L. S., & Petrill, S. A. (2011). Associations between reading achievement and independent reading in early elementary school: A genetically informative cross-lagged study. *Child Development, 82*, 2123–2137. doi: http://dx.doi.org/10.1111/j.1467-8624.2011.01658.x.

Harlaar, N., Spinath, F. M., Dale, P. S., & Plomin, R. (2005). Genetic influences on early word recognition abilities and disabilities: A study of 7-year-old twins. *Journal of Child Psychology and Psychiatry, 46*, 373–384. doi: http://dx.doi.org/10.1111/j.1469-7610.2004.00358.x.

Harlaar, N., Trzaskowski, M., Dale, P. S., & Plomin, R. (2014). Word reading fluency: Role of genome-wide single-nucleotide polymorphisms in developmental stability and correlations with print exposure. *Child Development, 85*, 1190–1205. doi: http://dx.doi.org/10.1111/cdev.12207.

Hart, S. A., Logan, J. A. R., Soden-Hensler, B. et al. (2013). Exploring how nature and nurture affect the development of reading: An analysis of the Florida Twin Project on reading. *Developmental Psychology, 49*, 1971–1981. doi: http://dx.doi.org/10.1037/a0031348.

Hill, W. G., Goddard, M. E., & Visscher, P. M. (2008). Data and theory point to mainly additive genetic variance for complex traits. *PLoS Genetics, 4*(2), e1000008. doi: http://dx.doi.org/10.1371/journal.pgen.1000008.

Ho, C. S.-H., Chow, B. W.-Y., Wong, S. W.-L. et al. (2012). The genetic and environmental foundation of the simple view of reading in Chinese. *PLoS One, 7* (10), e47872. doi: http://dx.doi.org/10.1371/journal.pone.0047872.

Hoover, W. A. & Gough, P. B. (1990). The simple view of reading. *Reading and Writing, 2*, 127–160. doi: http://dx.doi.org/10.1007/BF00401799.

Hulslander, J., Olson, R. K., Willcutt, E. G., & Wadsworth, S. J. (2010). Longitudinal stability of reading-related skills and their prediction of reading development. *Scientific Studies of Reading, 14*, 111–136. doi: http://dx.doi.org/10.1080/10888431003604058.

Keenan, J. M., Betjemann, R. S., & Olson, R. K. (2008). Reading comprehension tests vary in the skills they assess: Differential dependence on decoding and oral comprehension. *Scientific Studies of Reading, 12*, 281–300. doi: http://dx.doi.org/10.1080/10888430802132279.

Keenan, J. M., Betjemann, R. S., Wadsworth, S. J., DeFries, J. C., & Olson, R. K. (2006). Genetic and environmental influences on reading and listening comprehension. *Journal of Research in Reading, 29*, 75–91. doi: http://dx.doi.org/10.1111/j.1467-9817.2006.00293.x.

Keller M. C., & Coventry, W. L. (2005). Quantifying and addressing parameter indeterminacy in the classical twin design. *Twin Research and Human Genetics, 8*, 201–213.

Keller, M. C., Medland, S. E., & Duncan, L. E. (2010). Are extended twin family designs worth the trouble? A comparison of the bias, precision, and accuracy of parameters estimated in four twin family models. *Behavior Genetics, 40*, 377–393. doi: http://dx.doi.org/10.1007/s10519-009-9320-x.

Kirkpatrick, R. M., Legrand, L. N., Iacono, W. G., & McGue, M. (2011). A twin and adoption study of reading achievement: Exploration of shared environmental and gene-environment-interaction effects. *Learning and Individual Differences, 21,* 368–375. doi: http://dx.doi.org/10.1016/j.lindif. 2011.04.008.

Kovas, Y., & Plomin, R. (2007). Learning abilities and disabilities: Generalist genes, specialist environments. *Current Directions in Psychological Science, 16,* 284–288. doi: http://dx.doi.org/10.1111/j.1467-8721.2007.00521.x.

Logan, J. A. R., Hart, S. A., Cutting, L. et al. (2013). Reading development in children ages 6 to 12: Genetic and environmental influences. *Child Development, 84,* 2131–2144. doi: http://dx.doi.org/10.1111/cdev.12104.

McBride-Chang, C., Shu, H., Chan, W. et al. (2013). Poor readers of Chinese and English: Overlap, stability, and longitudinal correlates. *Scientific Studies of Reading, 17*(1), 57–70. doi:10.1080/10888438.2012.689787

Mol, S. E., & Bus, A. G. (2011). To read or not to read: A meta-analysis of print exposure from infancy to early adulthood. *Psychological Bulletin, 137,* 267–296. doi: http://dx.doi.org/10.1037/a0021890.

Olson, R., Forsberg, H., Wise, B., & Rack, J. (1994). Measurement of word recognition, orthographic, and phonological skills. In G. R. Lyon (Ed.), *Frames of reference for the assessment of learning disabilities: New views on measurement issues* (pp. 243–277). Baltimore, MD: Paul H. Brookes Publishing.

Olson, R. K., Keenan, J. M., Byrne, B., & Samuelsson, S. (2014). Why do children differ in their reading and related skills. *Scientific Studies of Reading, 18,* 38–54. doi: http://dx.doi.org/10.1080/10888438.2013.800521.

Olson, R. K., Keenan, J. M., Byrne, B. et al. (2011). Genetic and environmental influences on vocabulary and reading development. *Scientific Studies of Reading, 15,* 26–46. doi: http://dx.doi.org/10.1080/10888438.2011.536128.

Olson, R. K., Kliegl, R., Davidson, B. J., & Foltz, G. (1985). Individual and developmental differences in reading disability. In G. E. MacKinnon & T. G. Waller (Eds.), *Reading research: Advances in theory and practice, Vol. 4* (pp. 1–64). New York, NY: Academic Press.

Olson, R. K., Wise, B., Conners, F., Rack, J., & Fulker, D. (1989). Specific deficits in component reading and language skills: Genetic and environmental influences. *Journal of Learning Disabilities, 22,* 339–348. doi: http://dx.doi.org/10.1177 /002221948902200604.

Perfetti, C., Cao, F. & Booth, J. (2013). Specialization and universals in the development of reading skill: How Chinese research informs a universal science of reading. *Scientific Studies of Reading, 17*(1), 5–21, doi: http://dx.doi.org/10.1080/10888438 .2012.689786.

Peterson, R. L., Pennington, B. F., & Olson, R. K. (2013). Subtypes of developmental dyslexia: Testing the predictions of the dual-route and connectionist frameworks. *Cognition, 126,* 20–38. doi: http://dx.doi.org/10.1016/j.cognition.2012.08.007.

Peterson, R. L., Pennington, B. F., Olson, R. K., & Wadsworth, S. (2014). Longitudinal stability of phonological and surface subtypes of developmental dyslexia. *Scientific Studies of Reading, 18,* 347–362. doi: http://dx.doi.org/10.1080/10888438 .2014.904870.

Petrill, S. A., Deater-Deckard, K., Thompson, L. A., DeThorne, L. S., & Schatschneider, C. (2006). Reading skills in early readers: Genetic and shared environmental influences. *Journal of Learning Disabilities, 39,* 48–55. doi: http://dx .doi.org/10.1177/00222194060390010501.

Plomin, R., DeFries, J. C., Knopik, V. S., & Neiderhiser, J. M. (2013). *Behavioral genetics* (6th ed.). New York, NY: Worth Publishers.

Powers, N. R., Eicher, J. D., Butter, F. et al. (2013). Alleles of a polymorphic ETV6 binding site in DCDC2 confer risk of reading and language impairment. *American Journal of Human Genetics, 93*, 19–28. doi: http://dx.doi.org/10.1016/j.ajhg.2013.05.008.

Purcell, S., & Sham, P. C. (2003). A model-fitting implementation of the DeFries-Fulker model for selected twin data. *Behavior Genetics, 33*, 271–278. doi: http://dx.doi.org /10.1023/A:1023494408079.

Rodgers, B. (1983). The identification and prevalence of specific reading retardation. *British Journal of Educational Psychology, 53*, 369–373. doi: http://dx.doi.org/10 .1111/j.2044-8279.1983.tb02570.x.

Rutter, M., & Yule, W. (1975). The concept of specific reading retardation. *Journal of Child Psychology and Psychiatry, 16*, 181–197. doi: http://dx.doi.org/10.1111/j.1469-76http:// dx.doi.org/10.1975.tb01269.x

Samuelsson, S., Byrne, B., Olson, R. K. et al. (2008). Response to early literacy instruction in the United States, Australia, and Scandinavia: A behavior-genetic analysis. *Learning and Individual Differences, 18*, 289–295. doi: http://dx.doi.org/10 .1016/j.lindif.2008.03.004.

Samuelsson, S., Byrne, B., Quain, P. et al. (2005). Environmental and genetic influences on prereading skills in Australia, Scandinavia, and the United States. *Journal of Educational Psychology, 97*, 705–722.

Samuelsson, S., Olson, R. K., Wadsworth, S. et al. (2007). Genetic and environmental influences on prereading skills and early reading and spelling development in the United States, Australia, and Scandinavia. *Reading and Writing, 20*, 51–75. doi: htt p://dx.doi.org/10.1007/s11145-006-9018-x.

Soden, B., Christopher, M. E., Hulslander, J. et al. (2015). Longitudinal stability in reading comprehension is largely heritable from grades 1 to 6. *PLoS One, 10*(1), e0113807. doi: http://dx.doi.org/10.1371/journal.pone.0113807.

Stanovich, K. E., & West, R. F. (1989). Exposure to print and orthographic processing. *Reading Research Quarterly, 24*, 402–433. doi: http://dx.doi.org/10.2307/747605.

Torgesen, J. K., Wagner, R. K., & Rashotte, C. A. (1999). *Test of Word Reading Efficiency (TOWRE)*. Austin, TX: Pro-Ed.

van Leeuwen, M., van den Berg, S. M., Peper, J. S., Hulshoff Pol, H. E., & Boomsma, D. I. (2009). Genetic covariance structure of reading, intelligence, and memory in children. *Behavior Genetics, 39*, 245–254. doi: http://dx.doi.org/10.1007 /s10519-009-9264-1.

Vogler, G. P., DeFries, J. C., & Decker, S. N. (1985). Family history as an indicator of risk for reading disability. *Journal of Learning Disabilities, 18*, 419–421. doi: http:// dx.doi.org/10.1177/002221948501800711.

Wadsworth, S. J., Corley, R. P., Plomin, R., Hewitt, J. K., & DeFries, J. C. (2006). Genetic and environmental influences on continuity and change in reading achievement in the Colorado Adoption Project. In A. C. Huston & M. N. Ripke (Eds.), *Developmental contexts of middle childhood: Bridges to adolescence and adulthood* (pp. 87–106). New York, NY: Cambridge University Press.

Wadsworth, S. J., Olson, R. K., & DeFries, J. C. (2010). Differential genetic etiology of reading difficulties as a function of IQ: An update. *Behavior Genetics, 40*, 751–758. doi: http://dx.doi.org/10.1007/s10519-010-9349-x.

Willcutt, E. G., Betjemann, R. S., McGrath, L. et al. (2010). Etiology and neuropsychology of comorbidity between RD and ADHD: The case for multiple-deficit models. *Cortex, 46*, 1345–1361. doi: http://dx.doi.org/10.1016/j.cortex.2010.06.009.

Willcutt, E. G., Pennington, B. F., Olson, R. K., & DeFries, J. C. (2007). Understanding comorbidity: A twin study of reading disability and attention-deficit/hyperactivity disorder. *American Journal of Medical Genetics Part B: Neuropsychiatric Genetics, 144B*, 709–714. doi: http://dx.doi.org/10.1002/ajmg.b.30310.

19   Intergenerational Transmission in Developmental Dyslexia

Fumiko Hoeft and Cheng Wang

19.1   Introduction

Developmental dyslexia is a neurologically based learning disorder that often runs in families (Fisher & DeFries, 2002). This chapter focuses on its intergenerational transmission, which refers to the transfer of traits and behaviors from parents to offspring, including genetic factors and nongenetic factors such as epigenetics and environment. Traditionally, transmission of genomic information (i.e., inheritance of DNA sequence) has been considered to be the key pathway by which behavior, cognitive abilities, character traits, and susceptibility to a disorder are inherited. However, growing evidence suggests that nongenetic factors play important roles in influencing gene function and modifying heritability. Combined, the effects of these factors likely result in the various phenotypes of dyslexia. Delineating the intergenerational transmission patterns of dyslexia provides means to further understand its etiology and may provide insight into early identification and preventive intervention. Thus, the goal of the current chapter is to highlight studies that advance our understanding of potential mechanisms of intergenerational transmission in this brain-based disorder. Relevance to cross-literacy research in dyslexia, which is the topic of this book, will be included as we see fit.

Throughout the chapter, we explore a number of key questions such as

1. What are the neurobiological factors that are implicated in dyslexia?
2. Is there evidence to support that the behavioral and neural patterns of dyslexia and literacy transmit across generations? If so, what do we know about the contribution from genetic risks, environmental factors, epigenetic processes, and the complex interaction among them?
3. What are some models that give the most comprehensive interpretation of observations to date?
4. What causes sex differences in dyslexia manifestation and how it might impact transmission of dyslexia?

5. What new insights can intergenerational designs bring to us? What implications does it provide for clinical assessment and intervention?

As part of this process, we further propose a new paradigm, intergenerational neuroimaging, to help provide a neurobiological link between various factors that are associated with dyslexia. Here, we define intergenerational neuroimaging as an approach that examines transmission of brain-behavioral relationships between parents and offspring (Ho et al., 2016). This new paradigm may expand our understanding of the etiologies and factors that influence manifestation of dyslexia.

19.2   Dyslexia as a Neurobiological Disorder

Developmental dyslexia is a learning disability characterized by reading and spelling impairment that cannot be explained by intelligence or education (Lyon, Shaywitz, & Shaywitz, 2003; Schulte-Körne, 2010). Many theories have been proposed in regard to its etiology, and substantial evidence has been accumulated that favors a dysfunction of the neurobiological systems that are known to participate in reading development and other related cognitive processes.

The earliest neuroscience findings were obtained from postmortem case studies of brains from individuals with severe reading difficulties. Galaburda and colleagues (Galaburda & Kemper, 1979; Galaburda et al., 1985; Humphreys, Kaufmann, & Galaburda, 1990) contributed significantly to the neurology of dyslexia by revealing specific cortical anomalies of dyslexic brains, including neuronal ectopias and dysplasia primarily in perisylvian regions, based on their detailed examination of postmortem brains from dyslexic and non-dyslexic individuals. Ectopias refer to small congregations of neurons in an abnormally superficial layer of the cortex, while dysplasia refers to a loss of characteristic architectural organization of the cortical neurons, and these malformations at the microscopic level suggest abnormal cortical development (Habib, 2000). Since neuronal migration is thought to occur as early as the second trimester, the mechanism leading to these cortical anomalies presumably happens during or before this period of fetal brain development. However, the impact of testosterone on brain development may also occur later, during the perinatal period. While postmortem studies allow detailed examination of brain anatomy and continue to provide crucial information that is not possible with modern noninvasive neuroimaging, they are often small in sample size and do not allow examination of brain functions that are of interest in real time and in a controlled way. Since then researchers have started to resort to studying the living brain *in vivo* with neuroimaging methods.

Neuroimaging studies in general show some subtle neurobiological anomalies in dyslexic readers in gray-matter structure and functional activation, as well as structural and functional connectivity among brain regions involved in reading and writing, across different cultures. Since the topic has been covered extensively in other chapters of this volume, only a brief summary of the neuroimaging findings of dyslexia across languages and cultures is presented here as a grounding for later discussion of intergenerational transmission in dyslexia.

The most consistent findings in neuroimaging research of dyslexia have been the reduced activation and corresponding structural abnormalities in a left temporo-parietal area primarily important for phonological processes, a left occipito-temporal region primarily important for orthographic processes, and their connectivity with related cortical regions (Linkersdörfer et al., 2012; Richlan, Kronbichler, & Wimmer, 2009, 2011, 2013; Vandermosten et al., 2012). The more ventral region of the left temporo-parietal area (e.g., posterior superior temporal gyrus [pSTG]) is likely involved in phonological storage and retrieval (Chang et al., 2010; Pasley et al., 2012); the more dorsal region (e.g., supramarginal gyrus [SMG]) is likely important for grapheme–phoneme conversion (Booth et al., 2004); and the most dorsal region, near the intraparietal sulcus, possibly plays an important role in attention (Ravizza et al., 2004). Moreover, the left temporo-parietal region in dyslexics has been shown to be functionally and structurally anomalous not only when compared to age-matched controls, but also when compared to reading-matched controls, indicating that these regions are persistently anomalous rather than simply a maturational delay or related to reading performance (Hoeft et al., 2006, 2007; Xia et al., 2016). The left occipito-temporal region primarily includes the fusiform gyrus (FG) and the inferior temporal gyrus (ITG). While activation in the left FG becomes more selective for higher-order visual stimuli moving along its posterior-to-anterior axis (Vinckier et al., 2007), such hierarchical organization in the left FG is altered in dyslexia (van der Mark et al., 2009). Adjacent to the left FG, the left ITG plays an important role in integrating multimodal information, and its impairment has also been reported in dyslexia at both functional and structural levels (Paulesu et al., 2001; Silani et al., 2005). It is also notable that dyslexic individuals show more activation in the bilateral ventral frontal and striatal region as well as right-hemisphere regions that are homologous to the anomalous left posterior regions. Many of these are often considered as compensatory processes, some of which may be important for articulatory processes (Hancock, Richlan, & Hoeft, 2017), whose involvement increases with development.

Although earlier work on dyslexia has focused primarily on the English language, typical and atypical reading in other languages and writing systems are increasingly being investigated, showing the universal neural systems involved in reading and dyslexia (reviewed in Peterson & Pennington, 2012). For example, activation of lexical processing in auditory and visual domains in typical readers shows similar coupling in English, Spanish, Chinese, and

Hebrew, especially in the dorsal pathway, including the left temporo-parietal region (Rueckl et al., 2015). Poor readers across English, French, and Italian, languages that use the Roman alphabet with varying orthographic depth, show a similar pattern of reduced functional activation in the left temporal and occipital regions (Paulesu et al., 2001). Cross-linguistic similarities also extend to the Chinese morphosyllabic writing system, which is opaque and has weak character-to-sound mapping, presumably leading to a greater reliance on ortho-semantic processes; despite the language-specific neural activity, impaired readers in English and Chinese show very similar reduced activation in the posterior and anterior left hemisphere regions (Hu et al., 2010). Structurally, Chinese dyslexic children also show anomalous left temporo-parietal structure even when compared to reading-matched controls, similar to those with dyslexia in many other writing systems (Xia et al., 2016). In general, cross-cultural studies show more universality than would be expected based on different properties of languages and writing systems. (Editors' note: See Xu et al., Chapter 10 in this volume for evidence on differences across writing systems.)

19.2.1   Role of Genetics

Dyslexia is highly heritable (Fisher & DeFries, 2002). The role of genetics in this intergenerational transmission has been investigated with molecular genetic studies of risk genes for dyslexia, behavioral genetic studies in twins and families, and the more recent imaging genetic studies.

Twin studies have long been employed to estimate the environmental and genetic contribution to the etiology of dyslexia (Olson et al., 1989). A typical twin study recruits a large set of monozygotic twins (who share approximately 100 percent of their genes) and same-sex dizygotic twins (who share approximately 50 percent of their genes). By comparing the concordance rate of dyslexia between the two groups of twins, researchers are able to estimate the sources that lead to individual differences in reading development. A higher concordance rate of dyslexia in monozygotic twins compared to dizygotic twins would suggest a genetic influence on dyslexia; this has been reported consistently across many studies (e.g., Byrne et al., 2009; Harlaar et al., 2005; Light & DeFries, 1995; Petrill et al., 2007; Stevenson et al., 1987; Swagerman et al., 2015).

Even though the genetic basis is complex and identifying genetic risk factors is a formidable challenge, a number of susceptibility genes have been reported to be associated with dyslexia risk through quantitative genetic research across languages and writing systems, providing evidence of the universal effects of those susceptibility genes in dyslexia. For instance, *DYX1C1*, one of the most replicated loci on chromosome 15, was supported by evidence from English, German, and Chinese populations (Kere, 2011; Lim et al., 2011). The genetic studies converged on the conclusion that many genes of small effects confer risk for dyslexia, as it is the case for many other complex traits. This characteristic is termed *polygenic*, which means the trait is governed by simultaneous action of many gene loci. Typically, a trait that depends on the interaction and additive action of a number of small-effect causes will follow a bell-shaped normal distribution in the population, and reading skill is no exception.

Although a lot of work on functions of those genes has been done with animal models and may not necessarily translate to humans, it is clear that the most replicated susceptibility genes (*DYX1C1, DCDC2, KIAA0319, ROBO1*, etc.) share a putative role in brain development, or more specifically, in neuronal migration (*DCDC2*: Burbridge et al., 2008; Meng et al., 2005; *DYX1C1*: Wang et al., 2006; *KIAA0319*: Paracchini et al., 2006; *ROBO1*: Hannula-Jouppi et al., 2005; see review Scerri & Schulte-Körne, 2010). This complements the cortical malformations observed in dyslexic brains (e.g., ectopias), which are likely formed as the result of disrupted neuronal migration at an early developmental stage. Several susceptibility genes may also play important roles in other neural phenotypes such as axon guidance and dendrite morphology (e.g., Hannula-Jouppi et al., 2005; Peschansky et al., 2010). Evidence also supports that some putative susceptibility genes may increase neural noise through enhanced glutamatergic signaling and disrupted neural migration, disturbing the excitation–inhibition balance in cortical networks that are important to sensory processing and multisensory integration (Hancock, Pugh, & Hoeft, 2017). These findings are consistent with existing findings on the neurobiological basis of dyslexia and imply that those susceptibility genes might impact behavioral phenotypes – reading outcome in our case – through coding neural structure and function, and offer important directions for future research.

One thing worth noting is that for the majority of behaviorally defined complex disorders including dyslexia, the pathway from genotype to phenotype is long and complicated and needs to take into account the interactions between genes. For example, the *DYX1C1* gene was found to affect the expression of other genes involved in neuronal migration and development of the nervous system (Tammimies et al., 2013). Given the complexity, it is not surprising, then, that only a few susceptibility genes have been identified so far with varying replication rate across those genes, that together they make only a small contribution to the increased risk of dyslexia and leave a large amount of phenotypic variation unaccounted for. The discrepancy between the amount of risk that individual genes can explain and the heritability estimate from twin and family studies is notorious among researchers and is referred to as *missing heritability*, whereby the known risk genes/loci explain very little of the heritability reported from twin studies (each prominent gene explained less than 0.5 percent in the case of dyslexia; Meaburn et al., 2008), while the overall heritability estimates for dyslexia are between 41 percent and 74 percent (Grigorenko, 2004).

Recent studies have begun combining genetics and imaging to understand the impacts of dyslexia-susceptibility genes on reading-related brain morphology and function. This approach to assessing the impact of genetic variation on the brain is termed *imaging genetics*. Imaging genetics can complement behavioral genetics by identifying the biological effects of genetic risk factors at the level of integrated neural systems (Hariri, Drabant, & Weinberger, 2006). Since dyslexia is a brain-based disorder, naturally, neural measures could be intermediate phenotypes that lie between genotypes and behavioral phenotypes and presumably are closer to the underlying biology. In fact, using smaller sample sizes than similar behavioral genetic studies, imaging genetics studies on dyslexia have confirmed the association of susceptibility genes with a number of prominent neural markers, including structural and functional activation anomalies implicated in dyslexia (Cope et al., 2012; Darki et al., 2012; Kirsten et al., 2012; Landi et al., 2013; Meda et al., 2008; Pinel et al., 2012; Scerri et al., 2012; Szalkowski et al., 2013). Imaging genetics should therefore expedite the search for and discovery of genetic variants that increase the risk of dyslexia. For a review of imaging genetics in dyslexia, see Eicher and Gruen (2013), but a caveat to keep in mind is that this approach of searching for intermediating neural measures is conceptually not different from searching for behavioral phenotypes, and it is therefore of crucial importance that neural mechanisms underlying disease processes are captured (Flint, Timpson, & Munafò, 2014). If the neural markers are chosen appropriately, their association with genotypes will be less influenced by measurement error, environmental influences, or multiple pathway effects, making the search more efficient (Flint et al., 2014).

The studies reviewed in this section show that genetics plays an indisputable role in the transmission of dyslexia. Molecular, behavioral, and imaging genetic studies complement each other to inform the genetic etiology of dyslexia at different levels. Further research into functions and interactions of the susceptibility genes could lead to a systematic understanding of the etiology of dyslexia as well as its mechanism of transmission.

19.2.2   *Role of Gene–Environment Interaction*

Aside from the genetic etiology of dyslexia previously discussed, there is a wide range of environmental factors that are found to impact the risk of developing neurodevelopmental disorders. These environmental factors include, but are not limited to: exposure to hormones during prenatal stage; nutrition, exposure to toxins; infections; traumatic injury; parental care; home setting; peer relationships; school experience; and culture. There are a number of studies that examined the effect of environment, predominantly socioeconomic status (SES), on brain functional and structural patterns, with mixed findings. Some findings to date suggest that reading-related brain activation and structure generally co-vary positively with SES (Jednoróg et al., 2012; Raizada et al., 2008). In line with this, a twin study showed that orthographic processing is not strongly heritable at a neurofunctional level, although it may be anatomically constrained by heritable factors (Polk et al., 2007). These results are in contrast to findings from Pinel et al. (2015); they reported that functional activation in the visual word form area was more similar in monozygotic twins who share 100 percent of their genes than in dizygotic twins who share only 50 percent of their genes, indicating strong heritability. Supporting the finding of strong heritability, individuals with dyslexia also show similar dysfunctional activation patterns regardless of SES background (Monzalvo et al., 2012).

The interaction of genes and environment has been an important theme widely explored in various developmental disorders (Caspi & Moffitt, 2006). Gene-by-environment (G×E) interaction refers to a phenomenon in which sensitivity to environmental risk factors depends on one's genotype. A number of psychological and genetic models attempt to explain individual variability in complex traits as a combination of predispositional vulnerability (genetic liability) and stressors (environmental liability). Theoretically, two seemingly contradictory patterns are possible in regard to how environment modulates genetic effects: (1) genetic influence is greater in a less optimal environment, as poorer environment may increase vulnerability to the detrimental effects of dyslexia-susceptibility genes, akin to the diathesis-stress model (Rende & Plomin, 1992), with *diathesis* referring to biological or genetic predisposition to a disorder and *stress* referring to environmental stressors; or (2) genetic influence is greater in more supportive/enriched environments, as minimizing contributions of nongenetic factors will increase relative contributions of genetic factors to the total phenotypic variation in a population. The distinction between these two patterns, which we describe below, may partly be due to the different fields each stems from, with the former deriving from the development of psychopathology and the latter from behavioral genetics.

One of the earliest molecular genetic studies examining G×E interactions in children with dyslexia and their siblings found results consistent with the diathesis-stress model (Mascheretti et al., 2013). Their findings showed that the effects of the *DYX1C1* gene on reading and phonological memory were dependent on environmental risk factors such as birth weight, SES, and maternal smoking during pregnancy. Specifically, the dyslexia-related genetic markers investigated in their study can exert a detrimental effect upon reading phenotypes in the context of disadvantageous environments. These environmental factors have been associated with learning disabilities in previous studies (Bowen, Gibson, & Hand, 2002; Byrne et al., 2006; Gilger, Pennington, & DeFries, 1992). Twin studies, often employed in behavioral genetic studies, generally report that environmental factors could change the extent of genetic influence on reading outcome. Most of these studies show that genetic influence is greater in supportive than in less optimal environments. For example, genetic influence was higher and environmental influence was lower in children whose parents had a higher level of education, as compared to children whose parents' level of education was lower (Friend, DeFries, & Olson, 2008).

To summarize, gene-by-environment interaction is a common and important source of variability in complex behavioral traits including dyslexia. Despite inconsistency in empirical findings and seemingly contradictory theoretical models, taking G×E interaction into consideration has important implications for dyslexia assessment, intervention, and the impact of different cultures and writing systems. It allows us to recognize the effectiveness of remedial intervention programs in helping individuals reach their potential, and also to acknowledge the existence of genetic and biological constraints. More importantly, the interplay between nature and nurture contributes to the variability in the dyslexia phenotypes; therefore, it should also be noted that culture and writing systems shape children's environment, and in this regard, these factors may impact the presentation of reading difficulty.

19.2.3   Role of Epigenetics

Other than genetic and environmental factors and their complex interplay, the influence of epigenetic factors on dyslexia has also been brought to light (Smith, 2011). An *epigenetic* trait is a "stably heritable phenotype resulting from changes in a chromosome without alterations in the DNA sequence" (Berger et al., 2009, p. 781). The missing heritability problem discussed earlier gives rise to growing interest in possible epigenetic processes in complex traits. Epigenetic effects occur throughout the life span and are influenced by age, lifestyle, and disease state (van Vliet, Oates, & Whitelaw, 2007). Many different mechanisms can produce epigenetic changes, including but not limited to DNA methylation,[1] histone modification, and the process of cell differentiation. It has been shown that the contribution made by environmental factors as described in the prior section may also be mediated through epigenetics.

To our knowledge, there has only been one epigenetic study of dyslexia and reading to date. In this study, the expression of the dyslexia-susceptibility *DYX1C1* gene was regulated by estrogen receptors, which are activated by the primary female sex hormone (Tammimies et al., 2012). This study also

---

[1] DNA methylation is a biochemical process whereby a methyl group is added to the cytosine or adenine DNA nucleotides, and is one of the major epigenetic mechanisms that alter how genes are expressed without altering the underlying DNA sequence.

demonstrated that a single nucleotide polymorphism in the *DYX1C1* is crucial for epigenetic regulation of this gene in that it affects a possible methylation site. Epigenetic effects may also vary according to the sex of the offspring and whether the inherited gene is received from the mother or from the father, and this is referred to as *parent-of-origin* effect (Lawson, Cheverud, & Wolf, 2013). It has been recently suggested that many complex traits, including disease states, may show some form of parent-of-origin effect (Mott et al., 2014). Sex-specific transmission pattern has also been documented in psychiatric disorders such as depression (e.g., Davies & Windle, 1997; Yamagata et al., 2016). In the case of dyslexia, although it has not been widely explored, examination of behavioral and neural transmission of dyslexia in different parent–child dyads (e.g., father to son) might shed light on the etiology and sex differences in dyslexia.

Alterations in epigenetic processes such as DNA methylation and histone modification are likely to play important roles in the causes of complex disorders, including dyslexia. Future work along this line is needed in order to understand the complex epigenetic mechanisms by which dyslexia could be inherited, including factors that impact the selective expression of dyslexia-related susceptibility genes. Epigenetic research holds great potential to explain much of the influence of environment on genotypes and to elucidate the missing heritability problem in dyslexia. Animal work has also shown that genetic defects in histone modification could be reversed using therapeutic interventions (reviewed in Smith, 2011), making it a worthwhile direction to pursue.

19.2.4 Role of Sex Differences

Sex difference in the prevalence rate of dyslexia is now well established and is considered to be attributable to biological differences and not a result of ascertainment bias, although the ratio is not as extreme as in some other disorders, such as autism spectrum disorders (ASD). For instance, Hawke et al. (2009) found that the male-to-female ratio in dyslexia ranges from 1.27:1 to 4.33:1, with a higher gender ratio in more severely impaired samples, as compared to 4–5:1 in ASD (e.g. Yeargin-Allsopp et al., 2003). These sex differences may provide us with clues in theorizing pathways involved in intergenerational transmission patterns.

In addition to sex difference in the prevalence rate, a number of human neuroimaging studies have revealed that individuals with dyslexia have different neuro-functional and structural patterns based on sex, although here there has been much less consensus. A pioneering imaging study on reading and language revealed that phonological processing engaged left-lateralized neural activation in males, mostly in the left inferior frontal gyrus (IFG), but recruited more diffuse neural systems of both left and right IFG in females (Shaywitz et al., 1995). Their work provided direct evidence of sex difference in the functional brain organization engaged in reading-related processes. The right-hemisphere language regions in general have been considered key pathways that individuals with dyslexia employ to compensate for their weaker left hemisphere function (Hoeft et al., 2011; Maisog et al., 2008; Richlan et al., 2009). Perhaps this diffuse and bilateral involvement in females buffers (i.e., acts as a brain reserve in) them from developing symptoms of dyslexia, hence leading to a sex difference in the prevalence rate. Consistent with this idea, cortical thickness reduction in the left ventral occipito-temporal regions that are responsive to words was found only in dyslexic girls, not in dyslexic boys (Altarelli et al., 2013). This suggests that given similar severity of behavioral manifestation of dyslexia, the biological underpinnings in females may be more pronounced than in males. In other words, females with the same biological (e.g. genetic, neural) risk load might be buffered from developing symptoms of dyslexia at the same level of severity as compared to males.

On the other hand, using structural MRI, the same research group found altered patterns of asymmetry of the planum temporale, one of the earliest neural markers related to dyslexia, in dyslexic boys but not in dyslexic girls (Altarelli et al., 2014). This is in accord with the earlier postmortem studies (Galaburda et al., 1985; Humphreys et al., 1990), but does not fit with the aforementioned buffering hypothesis in females with dyslexia. Another study found an interaction between development (i.e., children vs. adults) and sex in dyslexia, further complicating the picture (Evans et al., 2014). While incon-sistency among these studies could partially be attributed to regional differ-ences, roles of these brain regions and networks, or effects of maturation and environment, future large-scale research on the molecular, neural, and neuro-cognitive mechanisms underlying sex differences, and sex-specific interge-nerational transmission patterns, are needed to advance our understanding of the biological mechanisms underlying dyslexia.

According to the now more than thirty-year-old Geschwind-Galaburda Hypothesis, the male dominance of dyslexia manifestation may partly be attrib-uted to higher levels of testosterone synthesized by developing male fetuses, which is considered to retard the growth rate of parts of the left hemisphere and influence lateralization (Geschwind & Galaburda, 1985). Since the original Geschwind-Galaburda Hypothesis, prenatal testosterone has also been shown to influence sexually dimorphic anatomy and function of the human brain, such as local gray-matter volume of specific brain regions, corpus callosum size and asymmetry, and the myelination process (e.g., Chura et al., 2010; Lombardo et al., 2012). On the other hand, Boets et al. (2007) found that compared to typically developing children, dyslexic children showed no significant difference in the second/fourth digit ratio, which is considered to reflect prenatal testoster-one exposure at the molecular level (Lutchmaya et al., 2004). Another line of work has shown a positive link between dyslexia and estrogen signaling pathway by examining functional interactions between the dyslexia candidate protein DYX1C1 and estrogen receptors, suggesting involvement of hormonal pathways in dyslexia (Massinen et al., 2009).

Sex differences have also been observed in the genetic transmission of dyslexia. For example, Pennington and colleagues (1991) reported that the penetrance estimate of AA and Aa genotypes, where A is the abnormal allele associated with dyslexia, was always equal for males but not for females. This study complements the previously discussed sex differences in dyslexia and suggests that females might have more protective factors against dyslexia and therefore need more genetic risk load to show the same level of impairment when compared with males (buffering hypothesis). Dahdouh and colleagues (2009) were the first to apply sex-separated analyses in a molecular genetics study and found a significant association between a three-marker haplotype in the *DYX1C1* gene, which was associated with dyslexia across samples from the United Kingdom and the United States, and dyslexia diagnosis in female probands but not in males. This might explain some of the inconsistency in *DYX1C1* dyslexia association reported so far, since female-to-male ratio varied largely across different studies.

Despite the progress achieved to date, more research and consensus is needed on whether there is a sex-specific transmission pattern in reading and dyslexia, and if so, what the mechanism is. The prenatal environment has been proposed as a particularly promising pathway to exploring sex-specific transmission. Such research could provide critical and novel information about the neurobiological mechanism underlying literacy and dyslexia.

19.3   Multifactorial Deficit and Intergenerational Transmission

19.3.1   Single- versus Multiple-Deficit Hypotheses

Historically, different theories have dominated dyslexia research at different time points and many of them have assumed that differences between dyslexic and typical readers could in principle be derived from a single underlying cause (e.g., deficit in low-level auditory processing). The most recent dominant single-deficit hypothesis of dyslexia is the phonological deficit hypothesis (Rack, Snowling, & Olson, 1992). It assumes that reading disability has its root in the deficits of phonological processing, which is the process of segmenting and manipulating the minimal unit of spoken speech (i.e., phoneme; e.g., Bruck, 1992). It is still an open debate as to what cognitive deficits contribute to the risk for developmental dyslexia, and various possibilities have been proposed in addition to the phonological deficit, including impaired temporal processing, visuospatial attention, and cerebellar/motor development (see Ramus, 2003 for a review).

With the substantial advances made to date, however, it is becoming evident that a single-deficit model cannot in itself provide comprehensive explanations for the heterogeneity observed in dyslexia. In parallel to its polygenic character on the genetic level, dyslexia is unlikely to be caused by a single isolated neurocognitive deficit. Instead, dyslexia is likely a heterogeneous disorder with different phenotypes, causes, and underlying biological risk factors. As is the case for most developmental disorders and complex traits, single-deficit models are giving way to models that consider multiple factors underlying liability (Pennington, 2006; van Bergen, van der Leij, & de Jong, 2014). In Pennington's multiple-deficit model (MDM), multiple etiological factors produce the behavioral symptoms of developmental disorders by influencing the relevant neural systems and cognitive processes. It therefore offers a useful framework with which to incorporate genetic and environmental endowment from parents in order to understand the transmission process. We have recently called this the cumulative risk and protection model based on the notion that protective factors should also be considered.

19.3.2   Integration of Parental Information

Reading disability is considered a product of the effects of many genes in interaction with their environment, therefore it follows that the liability or risk of reading failure is a gradient rather than an "all-or-none" dichotomy. Dyslexia is therefore a multifactorial trait that can be explained by a liability threshold model. Taken together, the extant findings from behavioral, genetics, and neuroimaging studies may be best understood within the framework of the MDM, where genetic and environmental factors as well as interaction among them are considered as risk and protective factors that explain complex traits such as reading ability (Pennington, 2006). MDM can be considered as an extension of the polygenic theory of developmental disorders. Intergenerational designs, especially in families with children at familial risk of developing dyslexia, can contribute to formulating and testing hypotheses of the model. Van Bergen et al. (2014) further proposed an intergenerational multiple-deficit model (iMDM; see Figure 19.1), which is based on the idea that both parents share liability through the interplay of genetic and environmental influences.

Findings from recent family-risk studies give direct support to the iMDM. For instance, in a prospective longitudinal study, Dutch children with differing family risk for dyslexia were followed from kindergarten through fifth grade, when dyslexia status was determined (van Bergen et al., 2011). It was found in this study that the parents of at-risk non-dyslexic children had a higher educational level and better reading fluency when compared to the parents of at-risk dyslexic children, suggesting a gradient in the family risk. Torppa et al. (2011) examined whether

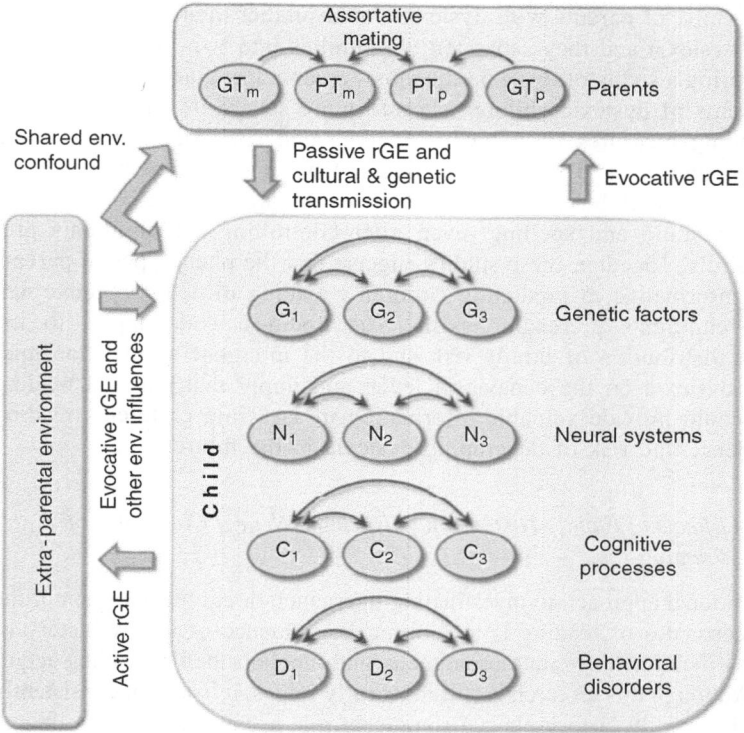

Figure 19.1 The intergenerational multiple-deficit model. Double-headed arrows indicate interactions. Causal connections between levels of analysis are omitted. GTm = maternal genotype, PTm = maternal phenotype, GTp = paternal genotype, PTp = paternal phenotype, G = genetic risk or protective factor, N = neural system, C = cognitive process, D = complex behavioral disorder, env. = environmental, rGE = gene–environment correlation. Terminology: A phenotype is any measurable characteristic of an individual (e.g., reading ability or parenting style); a genotype is an individual's genetic makeup. There is shared environmental confound if an environmental factor influences both the parental and child phenotype. Genetic transmission refers to the genotypic factors passed down from parent to offspring that influence the phenotypes in both generations. Cultural transmission is the genuine environmental influence of parental characteristics on child outcome, so controlled for environmental and genetic confounds. Assortative mating is nonrandom mating. Gene–environment correlation (rGE) refers to the situation in which exposure to environments is not independent but correlated to the child's genotype (see the text for explanation about the three forms of rGE). The figure depicts the situation for one individual child and his/her (biological) parents. At the group level (i.e., multiple children), a second form of gene–environment interplay emerges: gene–environment interaction. That is, heredity depends on the environment, or sensitivity to the environment depends on genotype. Reproduced with permission from van Bergen, van der Leij, & de Jong (2014), p. 346.

literacy skills of parents with dyslexia could predict their children's liability for dyslexia and they separated the families into two groups based on the offspring's status of dyslexia diagnosis assessed in grade 3. They found that parents of dyslexic children showed more severe impairment in several reading measures (pseudoword reading and spelling accuracy, rapid word recognition, and text-reading fluency) when compared with parents of non-dyslexic children. Furthermore, parental skills predicted children's grade 3 reading and spelling, even after controlling for children's preschool skills. Together, these studies suggest that the phenotypes of parents can be informative in predicting children's reading difficulties above and beyond children's prereading skills. The findings lend support to the gradient distribution of family risk and to the intergenerational transmission of dyslexia on the behavioral level, and imply that parental reading profile could provide valuable information in assessing children's reading performance and risk of developing dyslexia in the future.

19.3.3   *Effects of Family History on Offsprings' Neural Correlates of Reading*

The traditional approach to investigating intergenerational transmission of the neural correlates of reading is to look at the influence of family history of dyslexia on children's brain morphometry and functions before reading acquisition. Although this research is still in its early stages, it has been consistently shown that family history plays a significant role in the preliterate to literate brain and behavior of children, especially in the bilateral occipito-temporal and left temporo-parietal regions, corresponding to the previous findings of hypoactivation in the left posterior regions of dyslexic brains (reviewed qualitatively and quantitatively using meta-analysis in Vandermosten, Hoeft, & Norton, 2016).

Most of these imaging studies have thus far focused simply on presence or absence of familial risk. For example, beginning readers with a family history of reading difficulty showed altered topological properties of structural correlation network based on cortical surface areas compared to beginning readers without family history (Hosseini et al., 2013). Another study also identified structural brain alteration as predating reading onset in a small sample of children at risk of dyslexia, suggesting that the neural alteration in dyslexia may be present at birth or develop in early childhood prior to reading onset (Raschle, Chang, & Gaab, 2011). Reduced functional activation has also been reported in prereading children with a family history of dyslexia (Raschle, Zuk, & Gaab, 2012). In addition to showing evidence of intergenerational transmission, the results also suggest that those neural differences identified in prior studies are not the results of reading failure, but are present before reading acquisition starts. A longitudinal study looking at the reading network followed Norwegian children from the preliterate stage until dyslexia was diagnosed and found that the primary neural abnormalities that precede dyslexia are in the lower-level brain regions responsible for auditory and visual processing and core executive functions, and that abnormalities in the reading network were only observed at age 11, after children had learned how to read (Clark et al., 2014). Their study, while very small in sample size and hence controversial (Ramus, 2001), further supports the presence of neural abnormality before formal literacy training, but also shows that the alterations of the emergent higher-order reading network may not show until a later stage.

There has only been one study to date that examined sex-specific transmission patterns in how maternal and paternal risk is related to the offspring's reading brain. In this study, we showed greater maternal history of reading difficulty being associated with reduced gray matter in language-related regions in beginning readers (Black et al., 2012). Further analyses revealed a significant negative correlation between cortical surface area, but not cortical thickness, and greater severity of maternal history of reading disability, especially in the left inferior parietal lobule. Since the cortical surface area is considered to be more prone to prenatal influences (Kapellou et al., 2006), the results suggest that the effect of maternal reading history on children's reading-related brain structure is more likely due to prenatal influence during pregnancy. Future work on sex-specific transmission patterns will be helpful in understanding the mechanism underlying intergenerational transmission.

19.4   Clinical Implications of Intergenerational Research

At the practical level, as scientific discoveries emerge, researchers will need to make clear how such findings help inform educational and clinical practice. We have the obligation to help children with dyslexia, their parents, teachers, and policymakers so they will not draw the wrong conclusions regarding the etiology and modifying factors, risk and protective factors, and biological and environmental factors associated with dyslexia. Using this information in a constructive way would help maximize the potential of children with dyslexia.

Currently, dyslexia is still considered the most prevalent learning disability and poor readers report more emotional and behavioral symptoms when compared to typical readers (e.g., Arnold et al., 2005). Most children with dyslexia do not receive assessment and intervention until they have already experienced repeated failures after several years of formal literacy training. In the past several decades, researchers have drawn attention to the importance of early identification of and intervention in dyslexia, and as a result, there is more awareness of the need to maximize the efficiency of prevention efforts. As supported by a number of studies, timely intervention is crucial in overcoming the challenges brought by dyslexia, and early identification is a key step in this process. By taking account of the factors impacting intergenerational transmission, it would be feasible to identify the risk of developing dyslexia even before reading instruction starts, which would make timely intervention more feasible. Therefore, the ideal program must utilize the scientific advances gained from intergenerational study in order to inform assessment and intervention.

The intergenerational research in dyslexia shows that children whose parents have a history of reading difficulty are at higher risk of developing dyslexia. Furthermore, as discussed in Section 19.3.2, many studies on gene–environment interactions in dyslexia show that genetic influence is greater in more supportive environments. This implies that positive environmental factors such as higher parental level of education, SES, or instruction quality do not negate the effect of genetic risk inherited from parents. While recognizing the importance of remedial intervention, it is important to acknowledge these genetic and biological constraints so as to honor the extraordinary effort that these children, their parents, and their teachers may have expended on improving reading skills, even if they do not reach the ideal level (Friend et al., 2008). On the other hand, although large-scale and longitudinal studies are needed to understand the underlying mechanisms, it is evident that parental history of reading difficulty is one of the most important predictors of children's risk; it is thus of critical importance for those families to start assessment early on, even before formal reading instruction starts.

19.5   Discussion and Conclusion

This chapter reviewed a number of studies, including twin and family studies, in an effort to understand the factors contributing to the intergenerational transmission of dyslexia. The results have suggested that dyslexia is etiologically heterogeneous and many factors, including the genetic, epigenetic, and environmental, are involved in its transmission, and that there is also a complex interplay among these. The prior studies reveal a common cognitive deficit, altered neural correlates, and genetic risk markers in impaired readers across languages and writing systems. We proposed that factors including genetic, environmental, and epigenetic influences contribute to the intergenerational inheritance of dyslexia across different languages. We also highlighted findings of sex differences in manifestation and inheritance of dyslexia in order to reach a deeper understanding of its etiology and offer directions for future research. To conclude, the employment of intergenerational designs is a fruitful direction to achieve a more comprehensive framework of the universal etiology of dyslexia. We further discussed how family information could be incorporated in the MDM to improve accuracy in predicting children's risk for developing dyslexia. It is also important to understand how transmission of developmental disorders differs and is similar across languages and writing systems. Due to a lack of research taking this perspective, we cannot make an evidence-based claim, but we speculate that the factors governing intergenerational transmission of dyslexia share more similarities than differences across languages.

While the scientific inquiry of intergenerational transmission patterns in dyslexia has a long history, many questions remain to be addressed, including how the neural measures mediate the influences of family risk on reading outcome. Marrying neuroimaging techniques to the traditional intergenerational design allows us to investigate parent–offspring resemblance and the transmission of neural patterns. Such studies will likely extend current research effort in identifying the etiology of dyslexia and its transmission mechanism. Specifically, they enable us to examine the transmission of reading-related neural markers (such as morphometry characteristic of a specific reading responsive region, or properties of a constructed reading network) and how they are shaped via intertwined genetic and environmental pathways at different developmental stages. Additionally, neuroimaging may reveal sensitive neural phenotypes that link genes and behavior, and expand our knowledge of the underlying biological pathways.

There is no preexisting research on intergenerational neuroimaging to investigate the neural resemblance of reading processes between parents and their offspring. One likely reason for the lack of research in this area is that the neural activity is dynamic both on a developmental and on a millisecond scale and dependent on the children's reading abilities. It could be susceptible to many transient factors such as children's developmental stage (Richlan et al., 2011), experience, or attentional state (Yoncheva et al., 2010), which makes it difficult to compare inter-subject neural networks. Another limitation of familial risk research is that it is difficult to disentangle different contributors to the variability in children's reading ability, since parents provide both genetic and environmental endowments. Children at familial risk might inherit genetic risk as well as experience a less rich literacy environment. Adoption designs and studies of families with children born through *in vitro* fertilization (IVF) might be promising in this regard (Ho et al., 2016). This is an important direction we can advance, especially given that different neural patterns might underlie different subtypes of dyslexia. Another fruitful avenue would be to incorporate both molecular genetic and neuroimaging approaches in the intergenerational design. It would then be feasible to directly address the effects of and interaction among genetic and environment factors at the level of neural network and molecular/cellular mechanisms, in addition to the cognitive level. This research direction shows promise in its potential to verify old theories and generate new hypotheses.

Additionally, when additional factors are identified in transmission of reading behavior (including genetic risk factors, and parental and postnatal environmental factors that are dissociable through intergenerational neuroimaging designs in IVF families), it will be feasible to utilize multivariate pattern analysis to make more precise predictions of children's liability to develop dyslexia in the future on the basis of parental neurobiological and cognitive profiles, as well as various environmental factors, including home and school literacy environment.

Acknowledgments

Both authors contributed equally to this chapter. FH was funded by the National Institute Health (NIH) grants K23HD054720, R01HD078351, R01HD086168, R01HD094834, R01HD096261, R01HD067254/R01HD044073 (PI: L. Cutting, Vanderbilt U), R01HD065794 (PI: K. Pugh, Haskins Labs), P01HD001994 (PI: J. Rueckl, Haskins Labs); National Science Foundation (NSF) grant 1540854 (PI: A. Gazzaley, UCSF); University of California Office of the President (UCOP) grant MRP-17–454925; The Oak Foundation grant ORIO-16–012; University of California, San Francisco (UCSF) grants Academic Senate Pilot Grant for Junior Investigators, Catalyst Award (PI: R. Hancock, UCSF), and Digital Health Research Grant (PI: R. Hancock, UCSF); UCSF – Center for Creativity (CCC) Neuroscience Fellowship, UCSF Dyslexia Center; Dyslexia Training Institute; The Potter Family; Holy Names University and Raskob School; and Currey Ingram Academy. CW was funded by the NARSAD Young Investigator Award.

References

Altarelli, I., Leroy, F., Monzalvo, K. et al. (2014). Planum temporale asymmetry in developmental dyslexia: Revisiting an old question. *Human Brain Mapping, 35*, 5717–5735. doi: http://dx.doi.org/10.1002/hbm.22579.

Altarelli, I., Monzalvo, K., Iannuzzi, S. et al. (2013). A functionally guided approach to the morphometry of occipitotemporal regions in developmental dyslexia: Evidence for differential effects in boys and girls. *The Journal of Neuroscience, 33*, 11296–11301. doi: http://dx.doi.org/10.1523/JNEUROSCI.5854-12.2013.

Arnold, E. M., Goldston, D. B., Walsh, A. K. et al. (2005). Severity of emotional and behavioral problems among poor and typical readers. *Journal of Abnormal Child Psychology, 33*, 205–217. doi: http://dx.doi.org/10.1007/s10802-005-1828-9.

Berger, S. L., Kouzarides, T., Shiekhattar, R., & Shilatifard, A. (2009). An operational definition of epigenetics. *Genes & Development, 23*, 781–783. doi: http://dx.doi.org/10.1101/gad.1787609.

Black, J. M., Tanaka, H., Stanley, L. et al. (2012). Maternal history of reading difficulty is associated with reduced language-related gray matter in beginning readers. *NeuroImage, 59*, 3021–3032. doi: http://dx.doi.org/10.1016/j.neuroimage.2011.10.024.

Boets, B., De Smedt, B., Wouters, J., Lemay, K., & Ghesquie, P. (2007). No relation between 2D: 4D fetal testosterone marker and dyslexia. *NeuroReport, 18*, 1487–1491. doi: http://dx.doi.org/ 10.1097/WNR.0b013e3282e9a754.

Booth, J. R., Burman, D. D., Meyer, J. R. et al. (2004). Development of brain mechanisms for processing orthographic and phonologic representations. *Journal of Cognitive Neuroscience, 16*, 1234–1249. doi: http://dx.doi.org/10.1162/0898929041920496.

Bowen, J. R., Gibson, F. L., & Hand, P. J. (2002). Educational outcome at 8 years for children who were born extremely prematurely: A controlled study. *Journal of Paediatrics and Child Health, 38*, 438–444. doi: http://dx.doi.org/10.1046/j.1440-1754.2002.00039.x.

Bruck, M. (1992). Persistence of dyslexics' phonological awareness deficits. *Developmental Psychology, 28*, 874–886. doi: http://dx.doi.org/10.1037/0012-1649.28.5.874.

Burbridge, T. J., Wang, Y., Volz, A. J. et al. (2008). Postnatal analysis of the effect of embryonic knockdown and overexpression of candidate dyslexia susceptibility gene homolog Dcdc2 in the rat. *Neuroscience, 152*, 723–733. doi: http://dx.doi.org/10.1016/j.neuroscience.2008.01.020.

Byrne, B., Coventry, W. L., Olson, R. K. et al. (2009). Genetic and environmental influences on aspects of literacy and language in early childhood: Continuity and change from preschool to Grade 2. *Journal of Neurolinguistics, 22*, 219–236. doi: http://dx.doi.org/10.1016/j.jneuroling.2008.09.003.

Byrne, B., Olson, R. K., Samuelsson, S. et al. (2006). Genetic and environmental influences on early literacy. *Journal of Research in Reading, 29*, 33–49. doi: http://dx.doi.org/ 10.1111/j.1467-9817.2006.00291.x.

Caspi, A., & Moffitt, T. E. (2006). Gene-environment interactions in psychiatry: Joining forces with neuroscience. *Nature Reviews Neuroscience, 7*, 583–590. doi: http://dx.doi.org/10.1038/nrn1925.

Chang, E. F., Rieger, J. W., Johnson, K. et al. (2010). Categorical speech representation in human superior temporal gyrus. *Nature Neuroscience, 13*, 1428–1432. doi: http://dx.doi.org/10.1038/nn.2641.

Chura, L. R., Lombardo, M. V., Ashwin, E. et al. (2010). Organizational effects of fetal testosterone on human corpus callosum size and asymmetry. *Psychoneuroendocrinology, 35*, 122–132. doi: http://dx.doi.org/10.1016/j.psyneuen.2009.09.009.

Clark, K. A., Helland, T., Specht, K. et al. (2014). Neuroanatomical precursors of dyslexia identified from pre-reading through to age 11. *Brain, 137*, 3136–3141. doi: http://dx.doi.org/10.1093/brain/awu229.

Cope, N., Eicher, J. D., Meng, H. et al. (2012). Variants in the DYX2 locus are associated with altered brain activation in reading-related brain regions in subjects with reading disability. *NeuroImage, 63*, 148–156. doi: http://dx.doi.org/10.1016/j.neuroimage.2012.06.037.

Dahdouh, F., Anthoni, H., Tapia-Páez, I. et al. (2009). Further evidence for DYX1C1 as a susceptibility factor for dyslexia. *Psychiatric Genetics, 19*, 59–63. doi: http://dx.doi.org/10.1097/YPG.0b013e32832080e1.

Darki, F., Peyrard-Janvid, M., Matsson, H., Kere, J., & Klingberg, T. (2012). Three dyslexia susceptibility genes, DYX1C1, DCDC2, and KIAA0319, affect temporo-parietal white matter structure. *Biological Psychiatry, 72*, 671–676. doi: http://dx.doi.org/10.1016/j.biopsych.2012.05.008.

Davies, P. T., & Windle, M. (1997). Gender-specific pathways between maternal depressive symptoms, family discord, and adolescent adjustment. *Developmental Psychology, 33*, 657–668. doi: http://dx.doi.org/10.1037/0012-1649.33.4.657.

Eicher, J. D., & Gruen, J. R. (2013). Imaging-genetics in dyslexia: Connecting risk genetic variants to brain neuroimaging and ultimately to reading impairments. *Molecular Genetics and Metabolism, 110,* 201–212. doi: http://dx.doi.org/10.1016/j .ymgme.2013.07.001.

Evans, T. M., Flowers, D. L., Napoliello, E. M., & Eden, G. F. (2014). Sex-specific gray matter volume differences in females with developmental dyslexia. *Brain Structure & Function, 219,* 1041–1054. doi: http://dx.doi.org/10.1007/s00429-013-0552-4.

Fisher, S. E., & DeFries, J. C. (2002). Developmental dyslexia: Genetic dissection of a complex cognitive trait. *Nature Reviews. Neuroscience, 3,* 767–780. doi: http://dx .doi.org/10.1038/nrn936.

Flint, J., Timpson, N., & Munafò, M. (2014). Assessing the utility of intermediate phenotypes for genetic mapping of psychiatric disease. *Trends in Neurosciences, 37,* 733–741. doi: http://dx.doi.org/10.1016/j.tins.2014.08.007.

Friend, A., DeFries, J. C., & Olson, R. K. (2008). Parental education moderates on reading genetic influences disability parental. *Psychological Science, 19,* 1124–1130. doi: http://dx.doi.org/ 10.1111/j.1467-9280.2008.02213.x.

Galaburda, A. M., & Kemper, T. L. (1979). Cytoarchitectonic abnormalities in developmental dyslexia: A case study. *Annals of Neurology, 6,* 94–100. doi: http://dx .doi.org/10.1002/ana.410060203.

Galaburda, A. M., Sherman, G. F., Rosen, G. D., Aboitiz, F., & Geschwind, N. (1985). Developmental dyslexia: Four consecutive patients with cortical anomalies. *Annals of Neurology, 18,* 222–233. doi: http://dx.doi.org/10.1002/ana.410180210.

Geschwind, N., & Galaburda, A. M. (1985). Cerebral lateralization. Biological mechanisms, associations, and pathology: I. A hypothesis and a program for research. *Archives of Neurology, 42,* 428–459. doi: http://dx.doi.org/10.1001/archneur .1985.04060070024012.

Gilger, J. W., Pennington, B. F., & DeFries, J. C. (1992). A twin study of the etiology of comorbidity: Attention-deficit hyperactivity disorder and dyslexia. *Journal of the American Academy of Child & Adolescent Psychiatry, 31,* 343–348. doi: http://dx .doi.org/ 10.1097/00004583-199203000-00024.

Grigorenko, E. L. (2004). Genetic bases of developmental dyslexia: A capsule review of heritability estimates. *Enfance, 56,* 273–288. doi: http://dx.doi.org/10.3917/enf .563.0273.

Habib, M. (2000). The neurological basis of developmental dyslexia: An overview and working hypothesis. *Brain, 123,* 2373–2399. doi: http://dx.doi.org/10.1093/brain/123 .12.2373

Hancock, R., Pugh, K. R., & Hoeft, F. (2017). Neural noise hypothesis of developmental dyslexia. *Trends in Cognitive Science, 6,* 434–48. doi: http://dx.doi.org/10.1016/j .tics.2017.03.008.

Hancock, R., Richlan, F., & Hoeft, F. (2017). Possible roles for fronto-striatal circuits in reading disorder. *Neuroscience & Biobehavioral Reviews, 72,* 243–260. doi: http://dx .doi.org/10.1016/j.neubiorev.2016.10.025.

Hannula-Jouppi, K., Kaminen-Ahola, N., Taipale, M. et al. (2005). The axon guidance receptor gene ROBO1 is a candidate gene for developmental dyslexia. *PLoS Genetics, 1*(4), e50. doi: http://dx.doi.org/10.1371/journal.pgen.0010050.

Hariri, A. R., Drabant, E. M., & Weinberger, D. R. (2006). Imaging genetics: Perspectives from studies of genetically driven variation in serotonin function and

corticolimbic affective processing. *Biological Psychiatry, 59*, 888–897. doi: http://dx
.doi.org/10.1016/j.biopsych.2005.11.005.

Harlaar, N., Spinath, F. M., Dale, P. S., & Plomin, R. (2005). Genetic influences on early
word recognition abilities and disabilities: A study of 7-year-old twins. *Journal of
Child Psychology and Psychiatry and Allied Disciplines, 46*, 373–384. doi: http://dx
.doi.org/10.1111/j.1469-7610.2004.00358.x.

Hawke, J. L., Olson, R. K., Willcut, E. G., Wadsworth, S. J., & Defries, J. C. (2009).
Gender ratios for reading difficulties. *Dyslexia, 15*, 239–242. doi: http://dx.doi.org/10
.1002/dys.389.

Ho, T. C., Sanders, S. J., Gotlib, I. H., & Hoeft, F. (2016). Intergenerational neuroimaging of human brain circuitry. *Trends in Neurosciences, 39*, 644–648. doi: http://dx
.doi.org/10.1016/j.tins.2016.08.003.

Hoeft, F., Hernandez, A., McMillon, G. et al. (2006). Neural basis of dyslexia:
A comparison between dyslexic children and non-dyslexic children equated for
reading ability. *Journal of Neuroscience, 26*, 10700–10708. doi: http://dx.doi.org/10
.1523/JNEUROSCI.4931-05.2006.

Hoeft, F., McCandliss, B. D., Black, J. M. et al. (2011). Neural systems predicting long-
term outcome in dyslexia. *Proceedings of the National Academy of Sciences of the
United States of America, 108*, 361–366. doi: http://dx.doi.org/10.1073/pnas
.1008950108.

Hoeft, F., Meyler, A., Hernandez, A. et al. (2007). Functional and morphometric brain
dissociation between dyslexia and reading ability. *Proceedings of the National
Academy of Sciences of the United States of America, 104*, 4234–4239. doi: http://dx
.doi.org/10.1073/pnas.0609399104.

Hosseini, S. M. H., Black, J. M., Soriano, T. et al. (2013). Topological properties of
large-scale structural brain networks in children with familial risk for reading
difficulties. *NeuroImage, 71*, 260–274. doi: http://dx.doi.org/10.1016/j
.neuroimage.2013.01.013.

Hu, W., Lee, H. L., Zhang, Q. et al. (2010). Developmental dyslexia in Chinese and
English populations: Dissociating the effect of dyslexia from language differences.
Brain, 133, 1694–1706. doi: http://dx.doi.org/10.1093/brain/awq106.

Humphreys, P., Kaufmann, W. E., & Galaburda, A. M. (1990). Developmental dyslexia
in women: Neuropathological findings in three patients. *Annals of Neurology, 28*,
727–738. doi: http://dx.doi.org/10.1002/ana.410280602.

Jednoróg, K., Altarelli, I., Monzalvo, K. et al. (2012). The influence of socioeconomic
status on children's brain structure. *PLoS One, 7*(8), e42486. doi: http://dx.doi.org/10
.1371/journal.pone.0042486.

Kapellou, O., Counsell, S. J., Kennea, N. et al. (2006). Abnormal cortical development after premature birth shown by altered allometric scaling of brain
growth. *PLoS Medicine, 3*(8), e265. doi: http://dx.doi.org/10.1371/journal
.pmed.0030265.

Kere, J. (2011). Molecular genetics and molecular biology of dyslexia. *Wiley
Interdisciplinary Reviews: Cognitive Science, 2*, 441–448. doi: http://dx.doi.org/10
.1002/wcs.138

Kirsten, H., Wilcke, A., Ligges, C., Boltze, J., & Ahnert, P. (2012). Association study of
a functional genetic variant in KIAA0319 in German dyslexics. *Psychiatric Genetics,
22*, 216–217. doi: http://dx.doi.org/10.1097/YPG.0b013e32834c0c97.

Landi, N., Frost, S. J., Mencl, W. E. et al. (2013). The COMT Val/Met polymorphism is associated with reading-related skills and consistent patterns of functional neural activation. *Developmental Science, 16*(1), 13–23. doi: http://dx.doi.org/10.1111/j.1467-7687.2012.01180.x.

Lawson, H. A., Cheverud, J. M., & Wolf, J. B. (2013). Genomic imprinting and parent-of-origin effects on complex traits. *Nature Reviews Genetics, 14*, 609–617. doi: http://dx.doi.org/10.1038/nrg3543.

Light, J. G., & DeFries, J. C. (1995). Comorbidity of reading and mathematics disabilities: Genetic and environmental etiologies. *Journal of Learning Disabilities, 28*, 96–106. doi: http://dx.doi.org/10.1177/002221949502800204.

Lim, C. K. P., Ho, C. S. H., Chou, C. H. N., & Waye, M. M. Y. (2011). Association of the rs3743205 variant of DYX1C1 with dyslexia in Chinese children. *Behavioral and Brain Functions, 7*(1), 16. doi: http://dx.doi.org/10.1186/1744-9081-7-16.

Linkersdörfer, J., Lonnemann, J., Lindberg, S., Hasselhorn, M., & Fiebach, C. J. (2012). Grey matter alterations co-localize with functional abnormalities in developmental dyslexia: An ALE meta-analysis. *PLoS One, 7*(8), e43122. doi: http://dx.doi.org/10.1371/journal.pone.0043122.

Lombardo, M. V., Ashwin, E., Auyeung, B. et al. (2012). Fetal testosterone influences sexually dimorphic gray matter in the human brain. *The Journal of Neuroscience, 32*, 674–680. doi: http://dx.doi.org/10.1523/JNEUROSCI.4389-11.2012.

Lutchmaya, S., Baron-Cohen, S., Raggatt, P., Knickmeyer, R., & Manning, J. T. (2004). 2nd to 4th Digit ratios, fetal testosterone and estradiol. *Early Human Development, 77*, 23–28. doi: http://dx.doi.org/10.1016/j.earlhumdev.2003.12.002.

Lyon, G. R., Shaywitz, S. E., & Shaywitz, B. A. (2003). A definition of dyslexia. *Annals of Dyslexia, 53*, 1–14. doi: http://dx.doi.org/10.1007/s11881-003-0001-9.

Maisog, J. M., Einbinder, E. R., Flowers, D. L., Turkeltaub, P. E., & Eden, G. F. (2008). A meta-analysis of functional neuroimaging studies of dyslexia. *Annals of the New York Academy of Sciences, 1145*, 237–259. doi: http://dx.doi.org/10.1196/annals.1416.024.

Mascheretti, S., Bureau, A., Battaglia, M. et al. (2013). An assessment of gene-by-environment interactions in developmental dyslexia-related phenotypes. *Genes, Brain, and Behavior, 12*, 47–55. doi: http://dx.doi.org/10.1111/gbb.12000.

Massinen, S., Tammimies, K., Tapia-Páez, I. et al. (2009). Functional interaction of DYX1C1 with estrogen receptors suggests involvement of hormonal pathways in dyslexia. *Human Molecular Genetics, 18*, 2802–2812. doi: http://dx.doi.org/10.1093/hmg/ddp215.

Meaburn, E. L., Harlaar, N., Craig, I. W., Schalkwyk, L. C., & Plomin, R. (2008). Quantitative trait locus association scan of early reading disability and ability using pooled DNA and 100 K SNP microarrays in a sample of 5760 children. *Molecular Psychiatry, 13*, 729–740. doi: http://dx.doi.org/10.1038/sj.mp.4002063.

Meda, S. A., Gelernter, J., Gruen, J. R. et al. (2008). Polymorphism of DCDC2 reveals differences in cortical morphology of healthy individuals – A preliminary voxel based morphometry study. *Brain Imaging and Behavior, 2*, 21–26. doi: http://dx.doi.org/10.1007/s11682-007-9012-1.

Meng, H., Smith, S. D., Hager, K. et al. (2005). DCDC2 is associated with reading disability and modulates neuronal development in the brain. *Proceedings of the National Academy of Sciences of the United States of America, 102*, 17053–17058. doi: http://dx.doi.org/10.1073/pnas.0508591102.

Monzalvo, K., Fluss, J., Billard, C., Dehaene, S., & Dehaene-Lambertz, G. (2012). Cortical networks for vision and language in dyslexic and normal children of variable socio-economic status. *NeuroImage*, *61*(1), 258–274. doi: http://dx.doi.org/10.1016/j.neuroimage.2012.02.035.

Mott, R., Yuan, W., Kaisaki, P. et al. (2014). The architecture of parent-of-origin effects in mice. *Cell*, *156*, 332–242. doi: http://dx.doi.org/10.1016/j.cell.2013.11.043.

Olson, R., Wise, B., Conners, F., Rack, J., & Fulker, D. (1989). Specific deficits in component reading and language skills: Genetic and environmental influences. *Journal of Learning Disabilities*, *22*(6), 339–348. doi: http://dx.doi.org/10.1177/002221948902200604.

Paracchini, S., Thomas, A., Castro, S. et al. (2006). The chromosome 6p22 haplotype associated with dyslexia reduces the expression of KIAA0319, a novel gene involved in neuronal migration. *Human Molecular Genetics*, *15*, 1659–1666. doi: http://dx.doi.org/10.1093/hmg/ddl089.

Pasley, B. N., David, S. V., Mesgarani, N. et al. (2012). Reconstructing speech from human auditory cortex. *PLoS Biology*, *10*(1), e1001251. doi: http://dx.doi.org/10.1371/journal.pbio.1001251.

Paulesu, E., Démonet, J. F., Fazio, F. et al. (2001). Dyslexia: Cultural diversity and biological unity. *Science*, *291*(5511), 2165–2167. doi: http://dx.doi.org/10.1126/science.1057179.

Pennington, B. F. (2006). From single to multiple deficit models of developmental disorders. *Cognition*, *101*, 385–413. doi: http://dx.doi.org/10.1016/j.cognition.2006.04.008.

Pennington, B. F., Gilger, J. W., Pauls, D. et al. (1991). Evidence for major gene transmission of developmental dyslexia. *The Journal of the American Medical Association*, *266*, 1527–1534. doi: http://dx.doi.org/10.1001/jama.1991.03470110073036.

Peschansky, V. J., Burbridge, T. J., Volz, A. J. et al. (2010). The effect of variation in expression of the candidate dyslexia susceptibility gene homolog Kiaa0319 on neuronal migration and dendritic morphology in the rat. *Cerebral Cortex*, *20*, 884–897. doi: http://dx.doi.org/10.1093/cercor/bhp154.

Peterson, R. L., & Pennington, B. F. (2012). Developmental dyslexia. *The Lancet*, *379*(9830), 1997–2007. doi: http://dx.doi.org/10.1016/S0140-6736(12)60198-6.

Petrill, S. A., Deater-Deckard, K., Thompson, L. A. et al. (2007). Longitudinal genetic analysis of early reading: The Western reserve reading project. *Reading and Writing*, *20*, 127–146. doi: http://dx.doi.org/10.1007/s11145-006-9021-2.

Pinel, P., Fauchereau, F., Moreno, A. et al. (2012). Genetic variants of FOXP2 and KIAA0319/TTRAP/THEM2 locus are associated with altered brain activation in distinct language-related regions. *The Journal of Neuroscience*, *32*, 817–825. doi: http://dx.doi.org/10.1523/JNEUROSCI.5996-10.2012.

Pinel, P., Lalanne, C., Bourgeron, T. et al. (2015). Genetic and environmental influences on the visual word form and fusiform face areas. *Cerebral Cortex*, *25*, 2478–2493. doi: http://dx.doi.org/10.1093/cercor/bhu048.

Polk, T. A, Park, J., Smith, M. R., & Park, D. C. (2007). Nature versus nurture in ventral visual cortex: A functional magnetic resonance imaging study of twins. *The Journal of Neuroscience*, *27*, 13921–13925. doi: http://dx.doi.org/10.1523/JNEUROSCI.4001-07.2007.

Rack, J. P., Snowling, M. J., & Olson, R. K. (1992). The nonword reading deficit in developmental dyslexia: A review. *Reading Research Quarterly*, *27*, 29–53. doi: http://dx.doi.org/10.2307/747832.

Raizada, R. D. S., Richards, T. L., Meltzoff, A., & Kuhl, P. K. (2008). Socioeconomic status predicts hemispheric specialisation of the left inferior frontal gyrus in young children. *NeuroImage*, *40*, 1392–1401. doi: http://dx.doi.org/10.1016/j .neuroimage.2008.01.021.

Ramus, F. (2001). Dyslexia: Talk of two theories. *Nature*, *412*, 393–395. doi: http://dx .doi.org/10.1038/35086683.

Ramus, F. (2003). Developmental dyslexia: Specific phonological deficit or general sensorimotor dysfunction? *Current Opinion in Neurobiology*, *13*, 212–218. doi: http://dx.doi.org/10.1016/S0959-4388(03)00035-7.

Raschle, N. M., Chang, M., & Gaab, N. (2011). Structural brain alterations associated with dyslexia predate reading onset. *NeuroImage*, *57*, 742–749. doi: http://dx.doi.org /10.1016/j.neuroimage.2010.09.055.

Raschle, N. M., Zuk, J., & Gaab, N. (2012). Functional characteristics of developmental dyslexia in left-hemispheric posterior brain regions predate reading onset. *Proceedings of the National Academy of Sciences of the United States of America*, *109*, 2156–2161. doi: http://dx.doi.org/10.1073/pnas.1107721109.

Ravizza, S. M., Delgado, M. R., Chein, J. M., Becker, J. T., & Fiez, J. A. (2004). Functional dissociations within the inferior parietal cortex in verbal working memory. *NeuroImage*, *22*, 562–573. doi: http://dx.doi.org/10.1016/j.neuroimage.2004.01.039.

Rende, R., & Plomin, R. (1992). Diathesis-stress models of psychopathology: A quantitative genetic perspective. *Applied and Preventive Psychology*, *1*, 177–182. doi: http://dx.doi.org/10.1016/S0962-1849(05)80123-4.

Richlan, F., Kronbichler, M., & Wimmer, H. (2009). Functional abnormalities in the dyslexic brain: A quantitative meta-analysis of neuroimaging studies. *Human Brain Mapping*, *30*, 3299–3308. doi: http://dx.doi.org/10.1002/hbm.20752.

Richlan, F., Kronbichler, M., & Wimmer, H. (2011). Meta-analyzing brain dysfunctions in dyslexic children and adults. *NeuroImage*, *56*, 1735–1742. doi: http://dx.doi.org/10 .1016/j.neuroimage.2011.02.040.

Richlan, F., Kronbichler, M., & Wimmer, H. (2013). Structural abnormalities in the dyslexic brain: A meta-analysis of voxel-based morphometry studies. *Human Brain Mapping*, *34*, 3055–3065. doi: http://dx.doi.org/10.1002/hbm.22127.

Rueckl, J. G., Paz-Alonso, P. M., Molfese, P. J. et al. (2015). Universal brain signature of proficient reading: Evidence from four contrasting languages. *Proceedings of the National Academy of Sciences*, *112*(50), 15510–15515. doi: http://dx.doi.org/10.1073 /pnas.1509321112.

Scerri, T. S., Darki, F., Newbury, D. F. et al. (2012). The dyslexia candidate locus on 2p12 is associated with general cognitive ability and white matter structure. *PLoS One*, *7*(11), e50321. doi: http://dx.doi.org/10.1371/journal.pone.0050321.

Scerri, T. S., & Schulte-Körne, G. (2010). Genetics of developmental dyslexia. *European Child & Adolescent Psychiatry*, *19*, 179–197. doi: http://dx.doi.org/10 .1007/s00787-009-0081-0.

Schulte-Körne, G. (2010). The prevention, diagnosis, and treatment of dyslexia. *Deutsches Ärzteblatt International*, *107*, 718–726. doi: http://dx.doi.org/10.3238/arz tebl.2010.0718.

Shaywitz, B. A., Shaywitz, S. E., Pugh, K. R. et al. (1995). Sex differences in the functional organization of the brain for language. *Nature, 373*, 607–609. doi: http://dx .doi.org/10.1038/373607a0.

Silani, G., Frith, U., Demonet, J.-F. et al. (2005). Brain abnormalities underlying altered activation in dyslexia: A voxel based morphometry study. *Brain, 128*, 2453–2461. doi: http://dx.doi.org/10.1093/brain/awh579.

Smith, S. D. (2011). Approach to epigenetic analysis in language disorders. *Journal of Neurodevelopmental Disorders, 3*(4), 356–364. doi: http://dx.doi.org/10.1007/s116 89-011-9099-y.

Stevenson, J., Graham, P., Fredman, G., & McLoughli, V. (1987). A twin study of genetic influences on reading and spelling ability and disability. *Journal of Child Psychology and Psychiatry, 28*(2), 229–247. doi: http://dx.doi.org/10.1111/j.1469-7 610.1987.tb00207.x.

Swagerman, S. C., van Bergen, E., Dolan, C. et al. (2015). Genetic transmission of reading ability. *Brain and Language, 172*, 3–8. doi: http://dx.doi.org/10.1016/j .bandl.2015.07.008.

Szalkowski, C. E., Fiondella, C. F., Truong, D. T. et al. (2013). The effects of Kiaa0319 knockdown on cortical and subcortical anatomy in male rats. *International Journal of Developmental Neuroscience, 31*(2), 116–122. doi: http://dx.doi.org/10.1016/j .ijdevneu.2012.11.008.

Tammimies, K., Tapia-Páez, I., Rüegg, J. et al. (2012). The rs3743205 SNP is important for the regulation of the dyslexia candidate gene DYX1C1 by estrogen receptor β and DNA methylation. *Molecular Endocrinology, 26*, 619–629. doi: http://dx.doi.org/10 .1210/me.2011-1376.

Tammimies, K., Vitezic, M., Matsson, H. et al. (2013). Molecular networks of DYX1C1 gene show connection to neuronal migration genes and cytoskeletal proteins. *Biological Psychiatry, 73*, 583–590. doi: http://dx.doi.org/10.1016/j.biopsych.2012.08.012.

Torppa, M., Eklund, K., van Bergen, E., & Lyytinen, H. (2011). Parental literacy predicts children's literacy: A longitudinal family-risk study. *Dyslexia, 17*, 339–355. doi: http://dx.doi.org/10.1002/dys.437.

van Bergen, E., de Jong, P. F., Regtvoort, A. et al. (2011). Dutch children at family risk of dyslexia: Precursors, reading development, and parental effects. *Dyslexia, 17*, 2–18. doi: http://dx.doi.org/10.1002/dys.423.

van Bergen, E., van der Leij, A., & de Jong, P. F. (2014). The intergenerational multiple deficit model and the case of dyslexia. *Frontiers in Human Neuroscience, 8*(346). doi: http://dx.doi.org/10.3389/fnhum.2014.00346.

van der Mark, S., Bucher, K., Maurer, U. et al. (2009). Children with dyslexia lack multiple specializations along the visual word-form (VWF) system. *NeuroImage, 47*, 1940–1949. doi: http://dx.doi.org/10.1016/j.neuroimage.2009.05.021.

van Vliet, J., Oates, N. A., & Whitelaw, E. (2007). Epigenetic mechanisms in the context of complex diseases. *Cellular and Molecular Life Sciences, 64*, 1531–1538. doi: http:// dx.doi.org/10.1007/s00018-007-6526-z.

Vandermosten, M., Boets, B., Wouters, J., & Ghesquière, P. (2012). A qualitative and quantitative review of diffusion tensor imaging studies in reading and dyslexia. *Neuroscience and Biobehavioral Reviews, 36*, 1532–1552. doi: http://dx.doi.org/10 .1016/j.neubiorev.2012.04.002.

Vandermosten, M., Hoeft, F., & Norton, E. S. (2016). Integrating MRI brain imaging studies of pre-reading children with current theories of developmental dyslexia: A review and quantitative meta-analysis. *Current Opinion in Behavioral Science*, *10*, 155–161. doi: http://dx.doi.org/10.1016/j.cobeha.2016.06.007.

Vinckier, F., Dehaene, S., Jobert, A. et al. (2007). Hierarchical coding of letter strings in the ventral stream: Dissecting the inner organization of the visual word-form system. *Neuron*, *55*, 143–156. doi: http://dx.doi.org/10.1016/j.neuron.2007.05.031.

Wang, Y., Paramasivam, M., Thomas, A. et al. (2006). DYX1C1 functions in neuronal migration in developing neocortex. *Neuroscience*, *143*, 515–22. doi: http://dx.doi.org /10.1016/j.neuroscience.2006.08.022.

Xia, Z., Hoeft, F., Zhang, L., & Shu, H. (2016). Neuroanatomical anomalies of dyslexia: Disambiguating the effects of disorder, performance, and maturation. *Neuropsychologia*, *81*, 68–78. doi: http://dx.doi.org/10.1016/j.neuropsychologia.2015.12.003.

Yamagata, B., Murayama, K., Black, J. M. et al. (2016). Female-specific intergenerational transmission patterns of the human corticolimbic circuitry. *Journal of Neuroscience*, *36*, 1254–1260. doi: http://dx.doi.org/10.1523/JNEUROSCI.4974-14 .2016.

Yeargin-Allsopp, M., Rice, C., Karapurkar, T., Boyle, C., & Murphy, C. (2003). Prevalence of autism in a US metropolitan area. *The Journal of the American Medical Association*, *289*, 49–55.

Yoncheva, Y. N., Zevin, J. D., Maurer, U., & McCandliss, B. D. (2010). Auditory selective attention to speech modulates activity in the visual word form area. *Cerebral Cortex*, *20*, 622–632. doi: http://dx.doi.org/10.1093/cercor/bhp129.

Epilogue

20 Developmental Dyslexia across Languages and Writing Systems: The Big Picture

Charles Perfetti, Kenneth Pugh, and Ludo Verhoeven

In this final chapter, we provide our view on some of the main conclusions that can be drawn from the research on developmental dyslexia across languages. The overarching questions concern how our understanding of reading disability benefits from considering a broad array of languages. If there is a universal biological basis of developmental dyslexia, there should be shared observations on reading disability across languages and writing systems. Or, so one might expect. It is possible, however, that observations of differences in the manifestations of dyslexia – whether subtyping within a language (e.g., phonological vs surface dyslexia) or comparisons across languages (e.g., alphabetic vs morphosyllabic) – reflect some unitary cause or combinations of multiple causes.

20.1 Dyslexia across Nine Languages and Four Writing Systems

In our recent volume on learning to read across languages and writing systems (Verhoeven & Perfetti, 2017), seventeen authors, each an expert on reading in a given language, collectively examined seventeen different languages representing all major writing systems. We searched across these languages and writing systems for evidence on both universal aspects of learning to read and differences associated with specific languages and writing systems. In reviewing the research across these languages, we presented a table comparing the seventeen languages, their orthographies, and the relevant research on each, focusing on precursors to reading and reading development. We concluded that there were eleven generalizations across languages, five concerning awareness of language units and six concerning learning to read. These generalizations are summarized in Table 20.1, along with our assessment of their relevance for dyslexia.

Because the nine languages examined in the present volume, which represent four major writing systems, are a subset of these seventeen languages, we can be sure that the generalizations about learning to read apply to them. The question is how the factors that are important in learning to read across

Table 20.1 *Cross-language generalizations about learning to read and their relation to dyslexia*

Language awareness	Word identification
1. *Linguistic awareness at multiple levels supports learning to read.* Linguistic awareness at multiple levels can be low in dyslexia.	1. *Orthographic knowledge is foundational for reading.* Both orthographic pathways can be affected: sublexical phonology and lexical-semantic connections can be impaired. But whether the role of orthography is independent of its connection to phonology and meaning is less clear.
2. *Syllable awareness universally emerges earlier than phonemic awareness and is predictive of early reading.* Lack of syllable-level awareness is not a factor in alphabetic writing, but may be in syllable- and morpheme-level writing.	2. *For alphabetic literacy, spelling develops more slowly than reading and relies heavily on morphological knowledge.* Spelling and reading difficulties are generally connected as twin deficits in dyslexia. Spelling and reading are connected through bidirectional but asymmetric mapping functions that allow some disassociations to occur.
3. *Phonemic awareness in alphabetic reading is uniformly important, not dependent on orthographic transparency. It is not a uniformly important factor in reading syllabaries and morphosyllabaries.* A preschool failure in phonemic awareness does not predict dyslexia; however, a lack of awareness with or after reading instruction is an indicator. Phoneme awareness emerges later for children reading Chinese and Japanese, but its absence is not a marker for dyslexia.	3. *The development of word identification benefits from phonological transparency.* Transparency supports ease of learning to read. However, dyslexia occurs for children reading in any orthography. Transparency may affect whether phonological awareness or processing fluency is observed as the marker of dyslexia.
4. *Phonemic awareness and learning to read alphabetically develop reciprocally.* Dyslexics' difficulty in learning to read impedes the development of awareness, as well as vice versa.	4. *The role of morphology in word identification depends on the morphology of the language and the phonological transparency of the orthography.* The use of morphology in word reading may be impaired in dyslexia generally. In morpheme-based writing systems, impaired use of morphology can indicate dyslexia. In alphabetic reading, the use of morphology may compensate for a phonological deficit.
5. *Morphological knowledge is variably associated with reading across languages and writing systems.* A lack of morphological knowledge may be associated with dyslexia in some languages; its status as a primary factor is not yet clear.	5. *Word identification shifts from computation to memory-based retrieval for words as they become familiar.* Dyslexia is generally marked by low fluency: fluency is here defined as a memory-based retrieval of word pronunciation and meaning.

languages and writing systems are relevant for characterizing developmental dyslexia across languages.

There is a simple connection between learning to read and dyslexia, perhaps deceptively simple. At its core, learning to read requires a child to learn how his or her writing system connects to his or her language. For this, the child must connect written symbols to units of the language – mapping graphs to the words, morphemes, or phonemes of that language. Although this is only the start, the longer-term development of reading skill depends critically on a foundation built on these connections, even as reading experience strengthens and extends the mappings. This longer-term development, fueled by reading experience, gradually shifts reading from a process of computing language units from written units to one of memory retrieval, as words come to be represented as high-quality lexical units with tightly bonded orthographic, phonological, and semantic constituents. Graphic strings then come to more or less automatically retrieve word meanings and pronunciations from memory, producing fluent word reading.

These developments are universal, holding across writing systems that map onto language in different ways – through morphemes, syllables, and phonemes. As Table 20.1 summarizes, research across languages and writing systems shows generalizations on the role of language awareness and the development of word identification. However, these generalizations require accommodations that are imposed by writing systems and languages. Thus, whereas phonological awareness is an important predictor of reading, *phoneme* awareness is less important than *syllable* awareness for syllabic and morphosyllabic writing systems. Although both language and writing need to be taken into account, writing systems are not arbitrary choices for languages; rather they accommodate, to some extent, the properties of the language (Frost, 2012; Seidenberg, 2011; Perfetti & Harris, 2013). Thus, we can focus on the writing system with the understanding that at least some properties of the language are reflected in the choice of writing system.

A basic conclusion that can be drawn is that the factors relevant for learning to read are also relevant for reading disabilities. Failures to develop language awareness prior to or at least concurrently with reading are risk factors for dyslexia; but the necessary level of language awareness depends on the writing system. Lack of phoneme awareness during the development of early reading signals a risk for alphabetic reading, but not necessarily for Chinese reading, in which syllable awareness is both more relevant and easier to attain. Similarly, failures to demonstrate phonological processes in reading suggest a reading problem, but the relevant level of phonology depends on the writing system. Phonemic processing problems indicate dyslexia in alphabetic reading but not necessarily for reading syllabic or morphosyllabic writing.

In what follows we consider the behavioral indicators of dyslexia, its "phenotypes" as shown by cognitive and language skills that are associated with it. Of course, the main phenotype behaviors are difficulties in reading and spelling words. Providing the foundations for reading and spelling are the linguistic subsystems (phonology, morphology) and cognitive processes (perception, attention, memory retrieval) that reading requires.

20.1.1   Is a Phonological Deficit a Universal Cause of Dyslexia?

The conclusion that phonological problems are at the core of reading disability seems to have achieved the status of a universal consensus. The reviews of the nine languages in Part I of this volume concluded, for each language, that phonological difficulties were associated with dyslexia. However, this generalization may deserve some qualification. First, the phonological grain size that is relevant for reading depends on the writing system. In alphabets, abjads, and alphasyllabaries, single graphic units map onto phonemes (abjads and alphasyllabaries map additional units as well). Syllabaries (Japanese Kana, Cree) and morphosyllabaries (Chinese, Japanese Kanji) map graphs to syllables. Both the logic of mappings and the research on reading suggest that, for these writing systems, phoneme awareness is less essential. Further, although syllable awareness is important in reading syllable-based writing systems, syllable awareness is universally attained by most children, suggesting that lack of phonological awareness at the syllable level is not a major contributor to dyslexia in syllabary reading. In fact, neither Japanese nor Chinese produces clear evidence on a central role for phonological awareness. As pointed out by Xu et al. (Chapter 10 in this volume), research by McBride-Chang et al. (2004) and Siok and Fletcher (2001) concludes that phonological awareness at the onset-rime and syllable levels are more important in Chinese, in contrast to the role of phoneme awareness in alphabetic reading. This does not mean that phoneme-level awareness is irrelevant in Chinese and Japanese. If phonological difficulties are universal in reading, tests that are more sensitive to these difficulties (e.g., phoneme-level tests) will be more diagnostic than tests that are less sensitive (syllable-level tests).

20.1.2   Is Orthographic Transparency Relevant for a Phonological Deficit?

It is not just Japanese and Chinese that are less affected by phonological awareness. Within the family of alphabetic writing systems, the impact of phonological problems seems to vary somewhat with the transparency of the orthography – the consistency of graphs-to-phoneme mappings. Among the alphabetic languages reviewed here, Finnish provides the most consistent mappings of individual graphs (letters) to phonemes. Children readily learn the mappings and come to identify printed words accurately (Lyytinen et al., Chapter 6 in this volume). Nevertheless, children who show reading problems appear to benefit from phonological interventions. This suggests that, for a transparent orthography, reading difficulties reflect more complex phonological (e.g., multisyllabic coding) problems. A comparison of English, French, German, Dutch, Hungarian, and Finnish dyslexics by a European research network (Landerl et al., 2013) suggests a way to conceptualize the complex relation between the transparency of an alphabetic orthography and the importance of phonological processing. Phoneme awareness (measured by phoneme deletion) proved a significant associate of dyslexia in all six languages, demonstrating that phoneme awareness is important even in transparent systems as a marker of dyslexia. However, phoneme awareness was more strongly associated with dyslexia in the most complex orthographies (English, French) than both the medium complex (German, Dutch) and the least complex (Hungarian, Finnish) orthographies. (See Landerl, Chapter 11 in this volume.) It is tempting to conclude that children with low phonemic awareness are more likely to fail to learn to read in a complex orthography because its greater mapping demands put more pressure on phonological processes. However, because these results are based on concurrent correlations, they do not establish causality. Awareness of phonemes, especially as measured in a phoneme-deletion task, develops with reading experience, complicating the inference that can be made. Nevertheless, the stronger association of phoneme knowledge and reading success or failure in the less transparent orthographies of English and French compared with the more transparent Finnish and Hungarian is interesting on any interpretation of the causal chain.

The answer to the question of this section is a "yes," but with a qualification. The phonological basis for reading disability is not an artifact of orthographic transparency, even if it does seem that English was doomed to be the language of choice for dyslexia. Phonological problems display a role across languages, but the writing system seems to affect the extent to which these problems are expressed in dyslexia. Orthographies vary in the pressure they place on phonological processes and the level of phonology that receives this pressure.

20.1.3   Is Failure of Automatization of Retrieval a Universal Indicator of Dyslexia?

Rapid Automatized Naming (RAN) is the second major indicator of reading problems at the behavioral-cognitive level. The inability to rapidly name stimuli of various kinds (digits and color names as well as orthographic stimuli) may be the major marker for dyslexia as a fluency problem. Like phonological awareness, RAN-marked disabilities are general across writing systems: "Phonological awareness and RAN are cognitive predictors of reading acquisition and dyslexia in all orthographic systems that have been investigated up to date" (Landerl, Chapter 11 in this volume). This includes Chinese, in which RAN seems more indicative of reading problems than phonological awareness. It is possible that the two indicators are linked to both shared (decoding) and nonshared (fluency) components of reading. They may share a phonological component that is prominent in phonological tasks and backgrounded in RAN, which prominently measures a speed-of-memory-retrieval process that involves output phonology. RAN differs from phonological awareness, or phonological processing more generally, in not having a clear theoretical basis. Phonological awareness gains its theoretical status because phonological representations are needed for the mapping from orthography. Although rapid naming has a less clear status within a causal chain that results in dyslexia, rapid memory retrieval is a recurring event that is part of both simple perceptual and more complex perceptual-cognitive processes.

20.1.4   *Is There Also a Morphology Deficit in Dyslexia?*

As we suggest in Table 20.1, a significant role for morphology is not yet clear. This uncertainty partly reflects the enduring research focus on a phonological deficit as the main factor in dyslexia. However, research on the role of morphology, both as language awareness and as a component of lexical knowledge that functions in reading, has grown. With this increasing research comes a tentative conclusion that morphology must have a role across all languages and writing systems, because morphology is a fundamental building block of language, linking grammatical forms to meanings. Like phonology, its importance in dyslexia and learning to read depends on the writing system and the language it encodes.

This dependence is complex, however. Reading Finnish requires morphological knowledge, because it has a complex agglutinative morphology. The result is long words that, while simple in their mappings to phonology, are complex morphologically, nearly always containing several morphemes. This should place considerable pressure on a child's morphological knowledge, but, somewhat surprisingly, morphological awareness is largely unstudied in Finnish (Lyytinen et al., Chapter 6 in this volume). In high contrast is reading Chinese, which is claimed to be dependent on morphological knowledge (McBride-Chang et al., 2003) and a factor in dyslexia (Shu et al., 2006). (See Xu et al., Chapter 10 in this volume.) Unlike Finnish, however, Chinese does not have a complex, agglutinative morphology that creates strings of grammatical morphemes. Rather it has derivational compounding: the combination of morphemes that often can stand alone into larger multi-morpheme units. And the morphological processes at issue are the ability to recognize or produce these compounds, usually as written characters, sometimes as spoken syllables.

Although compositional processes are involved in both, Chinese and Finnish clearly put different pressures on reading. For a third case, consider the abjads of Hebrew and Arabic, in which consonant letters, rather than being adjacent, are distributed across a word. Reading these words requires the extraction of a root morpheme, which combines with other information (the "pattern" in the word) to yield a grammatically inflected complex morpheme. Deficits in this morphological knowledge are a factor in dyslexia in Hebrew. (See Share et al., Chapter 8 in this volume.) The study of morphology as a factor in reading disability needs to move beyond attention to a generic morphological factor to a more specific and nuanced analysis of the morphological demands imposed by the language and its writing system.

Finally, there is the question of how a deficit in morphological knowledge connects with a phonological deficit as a factor in dyslexia. The two are intrinsically connected through the fundamental nature of language, which relates forms to each other across levels (phonological to grammatical) and to meanings. Deacon et al. (Chapter 15 in this volume) note that recent studies suggest that phonological sources may be fundamental in dyslexia even when there is an association of morphological awareness with dyslexia. Further, they raise the possibility that the use of morphology, which was observed in their dyslexic sample, may be an adaptation – a compensatory mechanism – to the participants' disability.

It is clear that knowledge and use of morphology is an important component of literacy. There is not yet evidence that it is a causal factor in dyslexia across writing systems. Morphology may be the factor that is most dependent on language and writing system, both in its particular manifestation and in its significance for dyslexia.

20.2   The Search for Deeper Causes of Developmental Dyslexia

20.2.1   Behavioral Indicators of Dyslexia

The behavioral indicators of dyslexia provide a level of explanation that is readily tractable and can be linked to the cognitive and linguistic systems involved in reading. But they also stimulate a search for causes that are a step closer to biology. This search is compelling, given that from its earliest discoveries, dyslexia has been understood as a disorder rooted in neural disturbances. Between behavior and brain, however, is an intermediate level of description, based on behavioral measurement but linked by inference to sensory and perceptual brain mechanisms.

These descriptions include basic visual processes, in particular a weakened magnocellular-dorsal stream that is said to lead to an attentional dysfunction (Facoetti et al., Chapter 14 in this volume). Other approaches have sought deeper explanations of the phonological cause of dyslexia – for example, oversensitivity to non-systematic variation in speech leads to unstable phoneme categories (Serniclaes et al., 2004); poor perception of amplitude modulation interferes with the development of phonological representations (Goswami, 2011); and a disorder in sensitivity to frequency changes across short temporal durations produces difficulties in processing stop consonants (Tallal, 2004), among others. As pointed out by Perfetti and Harris (Chapter 2 in this volume), the research generated by these ideas shifts explanatory levels from cognitive-behavioral concepts to finer-grained sensory-perceptual concepts. Additional shifts have followed, to neuroanatomical and then to genetic and biochemical concepts, leaving a potentially bewildering array of causes. It helps to realize that these explanations are not strictly competitive but rather coexist at different conceptual levels.

20.2.2   *Neural Indicators of Speech Perception Deficits*

These shifts downward to biological causes seem, at first pass, to be helpful for the cause of universals. The "classic" behavioral indicators are obtained while children are interacting with printed or spoken language; if the sensory-perceptual indicators are obtained with at least partly non-linguistic tasks, processing problems that are free of language and writing system influences can be exposed. Although research has pursued these various deeper causes, there is not enough cross-language research to provide a clear conclusion about the generality of sensory-perceptual factors. One such factor, however, has received considerable attention in more than one language: the ability to show auditory discrimination in passive listening, as detected through the oddball paradigm and an event-related potential (ERP) component – the mismatch negativity (MMN) – that the oddball elicits. Auditory discrimination is relevant for speech processing, including the formation of stable phoneme boundaries. Problems in auditory processing, at least those reflected in the auditory MMN, may be part of the causal chain that leads to the phonological cause of dyslexia. (See the chapters by Lyytinen et al. [Chapter 6], Verhoeven [Chapter 4], and Norton et al. [Chapter 12], in this volume.) When other paradigms sensitive to speech perception are considered, however, the results are mixed. (See Sprenger-Charolles, Chapter 3 in this volume.)

20.2.3   *Precursors and Early Predictors of Dyslexia*

A continuing quest in treating dyslexia effectively is to identify early markers or risk factors. The current status of this quest is not optimistic. As Norton et al. (Chapter 12 in this volume) put it, "Predicting which children will develop dyslexia before they have learned to read is still a challenge in all languages."

Nevertheless, the results of some longitudinal studies are very interesting. The Jyväskylä Longitudinal Study of Dyslexia (Lyytinen et al., 2015; see Chapter 6 in this volume), which has followed children who are at familial risk for dyslexia from birth to puberty, has found predictive signs of dyslexia as early as 3 to 5 days after birth. Event-related potentials (ERPs), recorded while newborns were exposed to auditory stimuli, both syllables and sinusoidal sounds, produced stimulus-related voltage shifts that turned out to correlate with reading acquisition years later. ERP indicators for both speech and nonspeech stimuli – essentially indicators of sound discrimination – were predictive of later reading problems. Another factor turned out to be predictive. At 6 months, babies were tested on their ability to discriminate phonemes on the basis of length. Children with familial risk showed low discrimination, and thus poor phoneme categorical perception. This is important because Finnish phonemes include length contrasts for both vowels and consonants, which are marked in the transparent Finnish orthography by one vs. two letters. Although the causal chain here is not clear, it appears that the ability to form stable phoneme categories is at risk for children who fail to show relevant auditory discriminations from a very early age.

It is important to keep in mind that these early ERP indicators have been found for children who are at familial risk for dyslexia. This fact not only points to a genetic predisposition among these children, but also means that we cannot generalize the value of these early indicators to children without familial risk. Thus, universal screening by either ERPs or fMRIs is not only impractical, but is also not warranted on the basis of the present evidence. Norton et al. (Chapter 12 in this volume) make the same point. Testing at a young age only for children who have family risk factors, not all children, may prove useful. It will also be important to identify the universal etiology of dyslexia separately, if indeed it is separable from its dependence on language and writing system.

20.3   The Neurobiology of Developmental Dyslexia

The assumption of a biological basis for a developmental reading disability has endured at least since Orton's (1929) description of word blindness in children. By now, there are detailed descriptions of the neuroanatomy of reading and reading disability and the genetics of dyslexia that combine to provide a neurobiological description that links to the central behavioral features of the disability, especially the phonological deficit.

20.3.1   The Functional Neuroanatomy of Dyslexia

Imaging research with typical readers, both children and adults, has identified neural networks that are largely shared across languages and writing systems. The writing system appears to influence the functionality of this reading network through the demands it places on the cognitive functions that are associated with the various components of the network.

This network and related elaborated networks were developed in PET and fMRI studies of alphabetic reading, first in English, then in other alphabetic orthographies. As imaging studies extended to non-alphabetic writing, both divergence from the alphabetic network and convergence with it were reported. For alphabetic reading, the basic network consists of at least three nodes in the left hemisphere, with the first node – the processing of graphic strings – being the most posterior part of the temporal lobe adjacent to visual cortex, the posterior fusiform gyrus. From this occipital-temporal (OT) "visual word form" area there is a ventral pathway and a dorsal pathway. The ventral pathway moves forward through the temporal lobe to the middle/inferior temporal gyrus (MTG/ITG). The dorsal pathway moves upward to the temporal-parietal (TP) cortex, including the posterior superior temporal gyrus (pSTG) and the inferior parietal lobule and its angular and supramarginal gyri (AG and SMG). (See Shuai et al., Chapter 13 in this volume.) The anterior component of the reading network is the left inferior frontal gyrus (IFG) (Broca's region), which is involved in, among other things, phonological processes in reading. The general picture included the idea that the dorsal pathway is more engaged by more complex phonological analysis, whereas the ventral pathway is engaged when reading is simpler or more automatized. Studies found that, within this network, reading disability is associated with reduced activation and functional connectivity in the dorsal (TP) areas and also in the left fusiform gyrus.

However, this general picture needs to be modified, according to a meta-analysis and reviews by Richlan, Kronbichler, and Wimmer (2009) and Richlan (2012). Instead, reading disability may be associated with underactivation in three left-hemisphere areas – the left fusiform gyrus, consistent with the earlier research, and the left inferior parietal lobule (IPL) and the left IFG. These results go along with refinement of the three-node network into five components that include differentiation of the dorsal node and of the left anterior node (including the IFG; Richlan, 2012). One important caveat on generalizations, however, is that the meta-analysis (Richlan et al., 2009) reporting dyslexia comparisons with typically developing readers is restricted to European alphabetic orthographies. More cross-language research is needed to determine the extent to which specific brain areas are universally implicated in dyslexia.

Whether or not the reading network is characterized as universal, i.e. applying to non-alphabetic reading (e.g., Chinese or Japanese) seems to be a matter of emphasis. There are clearly shared brain regions across languages and writing systems. This is a compelling consequence of the basic dependence of reading on language: Written language encodes spoken language in conveying meaning; thus, reading engages the reader's spoken language as part of reading for meaning. To accommodate this, the reading network must connect the posterior areas of the brain to the language areas, regardless of the writing system. Evidence that these connections occur across languages comes from the study across English, Spanish, Hebrew, and Chinese by Rueckl et al. (2015), which showed common areas of convergence between brain areas activated by print and by speech across languages. These results are an impressive affirmation of the universal connection of reading with spoken language.

This does not mean, however, that languages and writing systems do not matter for the reading network. Chinese provides the clearest contrast with alphabetic writing. Abjads and alphasyllabaries encode individual phonemes; pure syllabaries (Japanese kana and Cree) encode syllable-level phonology. Only the written morphosyllabary of Chinese seems to encode meaning and phonology on the same level (the syllable). It is actually a complex story to determine what it means when we say that a character encodes meaning. The usual assumption is that a character directly encodes meaning. An alternative is that the character encodes a syllable and also selects which syllable among many similar ones is the morpheme associated with the character. Importantly, the results of imaging studies of Chinese readers show areas of brain activation that partly overlap with alphabetic reading, while also showing some differences, as reviewed in early meta-analyses by Bolger et al. (2005) and Tan et al. (2005). Shared areas include the left fusiform gyrus, a fact that highlights its function of coding graphic input to connect it with left-hemisphere language areas, regardless of the forms of the writing-system graphs or their mapping levels. The most noted difference reported between Chinese and alphabetic reading is the greater involvement of the left middle frontal gyrus (LMFG) in Chinese.

For studies comparing dyslexic with typically developing readers in Chinese, imaging studies have found areas that are shared in alphabetic dyslexia (especially Hu et al., 2010) and brain regions that are more distinctive for Chinese dyslexics. One shared area across Chinese and alphabetic dyslexia is the under-activation of the left OT (visual word form) area. Prominent among differences is the LMFG, which is underactivated in Chinese dyslexics. (See Xu et al., Chapter 10 in this volume.) The role of the LMFG in typically developing readers of Chinese has received various interpretations that center on integration processes across the orthographic, phonological, and semantic components of Chinese characters, including the possibility of pre-motor functions related to character writing (Cao & Perfetti, 2017). Across writing systems, the importance of the left IPL has emerged, both in alphabetic reading (Richlan et al., 2009) and in Chinese reading (Cao et al., 2006). The development of reading skill in both Chinese and English seems to lead to the increased functionality of the left IPL, which may function as part of an integrating network for orthography, phonology, and meaning (Perfetti, Cao, & Booth, 2013).

20.3.2   Genetic Factors

Dyslexia has a genetic component, observable in families and transmitted across generations by genetic, epigenetic, and environmental factors (Hoeft & Wang, Chapter 19 in this volume). Behavioral genetics studies, using the classic approach of comparing monozygotic twins with dizygotic twins and ordinary siblings, have consistently found substantial genetic variance in reading measures. The combined results of three English twin studies reviewed by Olson et al. (Chapter 18 in this volume) are that sharing genes accounts for at least twice as much variance in reading measures as does sharing environment. It is important to emphasize, as Olson et al. do, that environmental variance, especially family socioeconomic status (SES), influences the balance found statistically between genetic and environmental influences. When children are sampled from a narrow range of SES, then genetic factors are allowed to have larger influences than when a broader range of SES is sampled. Further, the genetic influence may be partly mediated by the relevant behaviors in interaction with the environment, producing gene–environment interactions. When genes make reading difficult, a child is not likely to seek the reading experiences that are so important for acquiring high levels of skill. Nor are the same opportunities likely to be present in the home environment. Olson et al. make the important point that the general heritability of dyslexia, based on the statistical methods of behavioral genetics, cannot be applied to an individual child. It is possible that for a given child nearly all the influence on reading is environmental; for another, it could be nearly all genetic.

Associating the heritability factors of behavioral genetic studies with the components of word reading has proved inconclusive overall. Although one might expect a phonological deficit to emerge as one clear component, studies have produced differing conclusions on the question of whether a phonological factor can be separated from an orthographic factor. This may be because the behavioral tasks involved responses to printed words and nonwords, with the logic that phonology is relevant for deciding the pronunciation of a nonword, whereas orthography is relevant for deciding the correct spelling of a real word. The problem with this is that once a child has learned something about reading, the orthographic and phonological components of reading become intertwined. Probing a phonological deficit with a strictly phonological task is a better way to determine whether genetic influences target phonology independent of orthography.

A strong genetic influence in reading may suggest that twin studies in different languages should produce comparable variance estimates for a genetic component. Indeed, this was the case for a comparison of English (in Australia and the United States) with Norwegian and Swedish (collectively, "Scandinavian") in the International Longitudinal Twin Study (Byrne et al.,

2002; Samuelsson et al., 2005). Comparable levels of high genetic influence were observed across these alphabetic orthographies. It remains to be seen how results for non-alphabetic writing compare, but data for Hong Kong Cantonese children show a genetic influence on character reading (Chow et al., 2011) that is similar to that observed in the International Longitudinal Study.

20.4   Intervention

Interventions for children with reading disabilities are in place around the world. Although there is considerable variation, most programmatic interventions appear to be consistent with the factors causing dyslexia that have been identified through research. For the United States, as noted in Perfetti and Harris (Chapter 2 in this volume), the United States Institute for Education Sciences maintains a periodically updated clearing house, *What Works* [*ies.ed.gov*], which, in 2016, listed seventy literacy interventions, including twelve for children with reading disabilities. Many interventions reviewed in the present volume's chapters on specific languages include strong phonological components. (See the chapters on Czech and Slovak, Dutch, English, French, Finnish, Hebrew, and Finnish). In China, where efforts to identify dyslexia are relatively recent, interventions have targeted visual-perceptual (Meng et al., 2014) and visual-motor (Qian & Bi, 2015) factors, consistent with the observations that reading Chinese puts pressure on visual-orthographic processing. A comprehensive intervention program in Hong Kong, which also includes a phonological component, has shown success, with the authors conjecturing that orthographic and morphological components of the intervention are especially important (Ho et al., 2014). (See Xu et al., Chapter 10 in this volume.)

The value of early interventions is increasingly coming to be recognized internationally. Russia has long emphasized universal early screening and interventions, available from age 2, with speech screening at kindergarten. (See Zhukova and Grigorenko, Chapter 7 in this volume.) The value of early interventions appears to be highlighted by the discovery that auditory risk factors are detectable shortly after birth for children with family risk factors (Lyytinen et al., Chapter 6 in this volume). As we noted, in the absence of family risk, identifying individual children who will struggle in reading after instruction is underway is probably not reliable enough to be recommended at this point.

We note the increasing use and clear value – at least where early prereading intervention is not done – of the Response-to-Intervention (RTI) framework. (See Perfetti & Harris, Chapter 2 in this volume.) The RTI idea is to offer support to a child as soon as signs of struggling to read emerge despite adequate instruction – which, in the case of alphabetic reading, must follow sound, evidence-based principles that include decoding. A child who shows inadequate learning under these circumstances then receives specifically tailored instruction.

A major issue for all interventions is the long-term results. In Dutch, for example, research-informed interventions emphasize that phonological and orthographic support are effective for at-risk children in kindergarten. However, as Verhoeven (Chapter 4 in this volume) observed, transferring the immediate gains to reading in the first grade has proved difficult. The transfer of training gains may be a matter of the shifting challenges of reading across age and literacy tasks. (Horizontal transfer – attaining skill at reading words that were not part of training – is often obtained.) Training in phoneme awareness prior to reading may lead to gains in phoneme awareness without providing enough support for the child when reading words is required a year later. Indeed, longer-term transfer does occur when the content of training is congruent with the tasks of reading. Verhoeven (Chapter 4 in this volume) reports positive effects for fifth-grade children who had undergone a fifty-week training program.

Interventions based on the sensory-perceptual theories have also been developed – auditory temporal training, visual-spatial and visual-attention training, and even brain stimulation in the dorsal visual cortex (functional in the magnocellular pathway) have been applied; e.g., a multi-component program that includes phonology (Fast ForWord) based on the temporal-processing-disorder hypothesis (Tallal, 2004). (See Share et al., Chapter 8 in this volume, for other examples.) Specifically targeted programs may be effective where a single cause or interrelated causes have been identified. However, more comprehensive programs that have a chance to boost multiple components of reading may be more useful on average. For example, the research strongly points to two factors that are manifest in children with dyslexia: a central phonological deficit and a secondary deficit in rapid naming. An English-language intervention that targets both deficits (Morris et al., 2010) shows effectiveness. A slightly different strategy is embodied in the reading acceleration program (RAP, Breznitz, 2006; see Share et al., Chapter 8 in this volume), which indirectly affects several components of reading, including phonological decoding and rapid naming, but also task attention and working memory, while (theoretically) increasing synchronization of the brain's reading network. Across many studies, the RAP has shown gains in both decoding accuracy and reading rate, extending even to reading comprehension.

There is thus good news on the intervention front. Effective programs have been developed and tested. Continued research is needed on how to sustain gains over longer periods.

20.5   Universality and Simplicity in Developmental Dyslexia Reconsidered

A central question throughout this discussion is the prospect of a parsimonious, universal description (or better, an explanatory etiology) of developmental dyslexia. There are two closely related aspects to this question: (1) is there a single cause of dyslexia? and (2) is this cause the same regardless of language and writing system? We can assume that these two questions do not get a simple answer, but it is worth considering the possibilities.

One possibility for the first question is to conclude that, although a child with dyslexia may show various weaknesses related to language, visual attention, cross-modal integration, etc., there is a single sufficient cause of these: a deficit in phonological functioning. By using the term "phonological functioning," we evade distinctions that are usually made between phonological knowledge, phonological awareness, phonological representations, phonological memory, phonological encoding, and other designations. We also leave open the relevant phonological units. Equally important, deeper levels of explanation remain open as well. For example, the claim that a phonological deficit is the cause of dyslexia allows an elaboration of the causal chain to go downward to auditory processing as well as upward to mappings of orthography to phonology. Note that the logic of the single cause can apply to any favored "basic cause." We refer to a phonological deficit here, because that appears to be what the evidence currently suggests. Perseverance in pursuit of evidence for a different basic cause can change things.

A second possibility for the first question is to conclude that there are multiple causes of dyslexia, not merely multiple levels of description. In a study of Italian children with dyslexia, Menghini et al. (2010) report that although 85 percent showed a deficit in phonological awareness (and 75 percent in nonword repetition), most of these showed deficits in other areas, including tasks tapping sustained attention, visual-spatial attention, and executive function – in addition to the 15 percent who showed weakness in one or the other of these tasks without phonological awareness or nonword repletion problems. Ziegler et al. (Chapter 16 in this volume) report that studies of French children with dyslexia also found that most children showed phonological deficits, although these were measured with a range of different tasks (object naming, phoneme matching); but most of these children also showed weaknesses in other tasks, especially a non-phonological letter-detection task. Other studies reviewed by Facoetti et al. (Chapter 14 in this volume) add findings across methods and languages that link dyslexia with deficits in visual attention and the magnocellular-dorsal pathway.

Finding multiple weaknesses across tasks does not imply the existence of multiple causes. Although identifying unique and shared variances across tasks can help support the plausibility of any given inference about causal structures, the possibility exists that a single cause, including an unmeasured or unrecognized factor, underlies multiple differences across tasks. This is especially true when children are already showing signs of dyslexia, because a single cause can influence behaviors that affect performance on multiple tasks.

Nevertheless, finding multiple weaknesses gives no support to a single-cause theory. Faced with these limitations on inferences, we can reach for an empirically plausible universalist conclusion: that a deficit in phonological function is the most important cause of reading disability, that it is nearly always present when a child shows a reading disability, and that other factors may contribute. This means other causes (e.g., visual-spatial or attention problems) are involved in the small number of cases where there is no phonological deficit.

The second question, whether a cause is universal, is closely related to the first. To the extent that dyslexia is biological and that writing systems map graphs to language, then any cause rooted in biology should be expressed universally. The complexity of inferring evidence for this is roughly the same as for the first question. If there is a single cause, say a phonological deficit, then manifestations of dyslexia will vary with the extent that the writing system makes demands on phonology. If all writing systems map phonology at some level, this means that the language variations in dyslexia depend on the level of phonological mapping – the grain size (phoneme or syllable; see Wydell, Chapter 9 in this volume) – and on the extent to which meaning encoded in the ortho-morphology can assist the reader in compensation for a phonological deficit. Because written Chinese provides meaning cues in its ortho-morphology, it may reduce further the demands of phonology beyond the fact that it maps phonology at the syllable level. Other systems, such as the abjads of Hebrew and Arabic, seem to make additional demands on morphological processing without, in any obvious way, reducing the demands of phonology.

Thus, the Chinese–alphabetic comparison is the clearest test case for a universal dyslexia, one in which a single cause is responsible for all reading disabilities. At first pass, the analysis of Chinese supports the multiple-cause model, with non-phonological causes being more prominent in that language – which would still produce cases of phonological dyslexia, just relatively fewer of them compared with alphabetic reading, and with even fewer cases in which phonology was the only factor. Given the demands of learning around 3000 characters over six years of schooling, we should expect an important role for visual processes (attention and visual-spatial processes), and there is some evidence that visual-attention tasks predict reading ability in Hong Kong children (Liu, Chen, & Chung, 2015). The overall picture for the causes of reading problems in Chinese remains complex, with phonological, morphological, and visual-orthographic processes identified in behavioral research and inferred from brain-imaging research.

Where complexity is in abundance, simplicity can sometimes come from modeling. Theoretical conceptual models and computational models both strive for causal simplification, a central goal of scientific inquiry. In the case of reading, computational models have proved their value, both as classic theoretical models that predict experimental results (e.g., Coltheart et al., 2001) and, especially, as PDP learning models that simulate learning outcomes. These learning models allow co-occurrence patterns to emerge over iterations of input, thus creating implicit orthography-to-phonology mappings. Ziegler et al. (Chapter 16 in this volume) describe an innovative learning-to-read model with an initial decoding (sublexical) component and an acquired orthographic (whole-word) component. Exemplifying its simplification value, the model can simulate both the phonological and visual impairments that produce word-reading disability.

Models also can provide some simplification to cross-language comparisons. PDP models, with the addition of a semantic layer in the network, are able to reflect the division of labor between meaning and orthographic influences on reading words. These models, by capturing the effects of statistical regularities that occur in mapping orthography to phonology, can account for the differences in learning to read words aloud between shallow and deep orthographies. As reviewed by Zevin (Chapter 17 in this volume), the models have been extended to simulate learning Chinese (Yang et al., 2009) and to provide comparison of learning English and Chinese in a single model, one with a semantic layer and both English and Chinese orthographic inputs and phonological outputs (Yang et al., 2013). Simulating phonological deficits and semantic deficits within the model produced a comparison of English and Chinese simulated reading problems. The result for English was that a phonological deficit produced diminished ability in word reading and, especially, in nonword reading; simulating a semantic deficit led to a more restricted problem regarding words with highly inconsistent mappings of spelling to pronunciation. Chinese, in contrast, showed wide-spread effects in reading characters following either phonological or semantic deficits. The interesting implication of this modeling outcome is its congruence with empirical and theoretical approaches to dyslexia in English and Chinese. The English results mimic the subtyping into the more prominent phonological dyslexia and a less prominent surface dyslexia. The Chinese results reflect the logic of the language's writing system – character forms that have both phonological values (but not ordered phoneme strings) and semantic values – and the results of studies suggesting orthographic, morphological, and phonological factors in reading difficulties.

Any given simulation, which depends on multiple assumptions about model architectures, input and output units, and, in this case, on comparable units across languages, cannot be an arbiter of the complex questions surrounding the etiology of dyslexia. Nevertheless, the models provide simplifying theoretical perspectives that can accommodate the variety of empirical observations that have emerged in the study of dyslexia.

20.6   Final Conclusion

We conclude that there has been much progress made in how to understand the sources of reading disability and how to address them. The research, far from its early days when its focus was on dyslexia in English, now has a broader foundation across languages and writing systems. The key components of language – phonology and morphology – are involved in reading because the written word encodes both. Although morphology is differentially represented in writing – a morphology that is especially rich in Finnish (derivational and inflectional), more restricted in Chinese (mainly compounding), and intermediate in English – phonology is encoded in all writing systems. What varies is only the mapping level – syllables or phonemes. We thus observe a phonological component for dyslexia across languages with variation in the level of phonology that is encoded in the writing. When that level is at the syllable, a reduced pressure on fine-grained phonology allows other factors to become more important.

The early understanding of developmental dyslexia as a biologically influenced disorder has been verified in more specific ways. Behavioral genetic studies have convincingly demonstrated the high heritability of dyslexia. Neuroimaging studies have identified neural structures that function during successful reading and shown functional anomalies in children with reading disabilities. Although the exact components of the brain's reading network may turn out to be somewhat different from the earliest conclusions drawn fifteen to twenty years ago, the overall picture seems clear. Visual input is processed through multiple layers of bilateral visual cortex, resulting in graphic forms that are used in writing systems being processed in the left temporal-occipital cortex, to be connected with the left-hemisphere language areas. In a previous section, we reviewed the different follow-ups to this simple story that have arisen as the research base has grown. Here, we emphasize that the details are important, but also that there is considerable agreement on them. The bulk of the research suggests that language and writing-system variations make somewhat different demands on the neural substrates of reading, especially for the high-contrast comparison of alphabetic and morphosyllabic (Chinese) reading. This variation reflects differential demands on orthographic, phonological, and semantic information in identifying printed words and morphemes. An important point is that, counter to differences in brain areas observed during reading, reading and spoken language show overlapping areas in languages encoded in different writing systems. Details aside, reading depends on language. Dyslexia disrupts the necessary connections.

We can expect that in the future the biological picture will be further enriched, not just through imaging, but at the genetic and neural developmental levels. Gene studies at the molecular level, which have increased in number in recent years, may eventually acquire large enough samples to verify specific gene-transmission mechanisms of dyslexia risk. Hypotheses involving neuronal development (e.g., neuronal migration) and neurochemical processes (e.g., glutamate and choline concentrations) may gain traction.

Meanwhile, we note that the progress across languages and across multiple research methods have converged on a rich view of dyslexia as a multifactor disability, with phonology central in most cases. Further progress may come through simplification that brings explanatory coherence to this richness. Sound interventions are not awaiting further progress. In fact, effective interventions based on what is known have already been developed and applied around the world.

References

Bolger, D. J., Perfetti, C. A., & Schneider, W. (2005). A cross-cultural effect on the brain revisited: Universal structures plus writing system variation. *Journal of Human Brain Mapping, 25*(1), 92–104.

Breznitz, Z. (2006). *Fluency in reading: Synchronization of processes.* Mahwah, NJ: Lawrence Erlbaum.

Byrne, B., Delaland, C., Fielding-Barnsley, R., Quain, P. et al. (2002). Longitudinal twin study of early reading development in three countries: Preliminary results. *Annals of Dyslexia, 52,* 49–74.

Cao, F., Bitan, T., Chou, T. L., Burman, D. D., & Booth, J. R. (2006). Deficient orthographic and phonological representations in children with dyslexia revealed by brain activation patterns. *Journal of Child Psychology and Psychiatry, 47,* 1041–1050.

Cao, F., & Perfetti, C. A. (2017). Neural signatures of the reading-writing connection: Greater involvement of writing in Chinese reading. *PLoS One, 11*(12), e0168414. https://doi.org/10.1371/journal.pone.0168414.

Chow, B. W.-Y., Ho, C. S.-H., Wong, S. W.-L., Waye, M. M., & Bishop, D. V. (2011). Genetic and environmental influences on Chinese language and reading abilities. *PLoS One, 6*(2), e16640.

Coltheart, M., Rastle, K., Perry, C., Langdon, R., & Ziegler, J. (2001). DRC: A dual route cascaded model of visual word recognition and reading aloud. *Psychological Review, 108,* 204–256.

Frost, R. (2012). Towards a universal model of reading. *Behavioral and Brain Sciences, 35,* 263–279.

Goswami, U. (2011). A temporal sampling framework for developmental dyslexia. *Trends in Cognitive Sciences, 15,* 3–10.

Ho, C. S.-H., Wong, Y.-K., Lo, C.-M. et al. (2014). Helping children with reading disability in Chinese: The response to intervention approach with effective evidence-based curriculum. In X. Chen, Q. Wang, & C. Yang (Eds.) *Reading development and difficulties in monolingual and bilingual Chinese children* (pp. 103–124). New York: Springer.

Hu, W., Lee, H. L., Zhang, Q. et al. (2010). Developmental dyslexia in Chinese and English populations: dissociating the effect of dyslexia from language differences. *Brain, 133*(6), 1694–1706.

Landerl, K., Ramus, F., Moll, K. et al. (2013). Predictors of developmental dyslexia in European orthographies with varying complexity. *Journal of Child Psychology and Psychiatry, 54,* 686–694.

Liu, D., Chen, X., & Chung, K. K. H. (2015). Performance in a visual search task uniquely predicts reading abilities in third-grade Hong Kong Chinese children. *Scientific Studies of Reading*, *19*, 307–324.

Lyytinen, H., Erskine, J., Hämäläinen, J., Torppa, M., & Ronimus, M. (2015). Dyslexia – early identification and prevention: Highlights from the Jyväskylä longitudinal study of dyslexia. *Current Developmental Disorders Reports*, *2*, 330–338.

McBride-Chang, C., Bialystok, E., Chong, K. K., & Li, Y. (2004). Levels of phonological awareness in three cultures. *Journal of Experimental Child Psychology*, *89*, 93–111.

McBride-Chang, C., Shu, H., Zhou, A., Wat, C. P., & Wagner, R. K. (2003). Morphological awareness uniquely predicts young children's Chinese character reading. *Journal of Experimental Psychology*, *95*, 743–751.

Meng, X., Lin, O., Wang, F., Jiang, Y., & Song, Y. (2014). Reading performance is enhanced by visual texture discrimination training in Chinese-speaking children with developmental dyslexia. *PLoS One*, *9*(9), e108274.

Menghini, D., Finzi, A., Benassi, M. et al. (2010). Different underlying neurocognitive deficits in developmental dyslexia: a comparative study. *Neuropsychologia*, *48*(4), 863–872.

Morris, R. D., Lovett, M. W., Wolf, M. et al. (2010). Multiple-component remediation for developmental reading disabilities: IQ, socioeconomic status, and race as factors in remedial outcomes. *Journal of Learning Disabilities*, *45*(2), 99–127.

Orton, S. T. (1929). The three levels of cortical elaboration to certain psychiatric symptoms. *American Journal of Psychiatry*, *8*, 647–659.

Perfetti, C. A., Cao, F., & Booth, J. (2013). Specialization and universals in the development of reading skill: How Chinese research informs a universal science of reading. *Scientific Studies of Reading*, *17*(1), 5–21.

Perfetti, C. A., & Harris, L. N. (2013). Universal reading processes are modulated by language and writing system. *Language Learning and Development*, *9*(4), 296–316.

Qian, Y., & Bi, H.-Y. (2015). The effect of magnocellular-based visual-motor intervention on Chinese children with developmental dyslexia. *Frontiers in Psychology*, 6 (1529). doi: http://dx.doi.org/10.3389/fpsyg.2015.01529.

Richlan, F. (2012). Developmental dyslexia: Dysfunction of a left hemisphere reading network. *Frontiers in Human Neuroscience*, *6*, 120. doi: http://dx.doi.org/10.3389/f nhum.2012.00120.

Richlan, F., Kronbichler, M., & Wimmer, H. (2009). Functional abnormalities in the dyslexic brain: A quantitative meta-analysis of neuroimaging studies. *Human Brain Mapping*, *30*(10): 3299–3308.

Rueckl J. G., Paz-Alonso P. M., Molfese, P. J. et al. (2015). Universal brain signature of proficient reading: Evidence from four contrasting languages. *Proceedings National Academy of Sciences*, *112*, 15510–15515.

Samuelsson, S., Byrne, B., Quain, P. et al. (2005). Environmental and genetic influences on prereading skills in Australia, Scandinavia, and the United States. *Journal of Educational Psychology*, *97*, 705–722.

Seidenberg, M. S. (2011). Reading in different writing systems: One architecture, multiple solutions. In P. McCardle, J. Ren, O. Tzeng, & B. Miller (Eds.), *Dyslexia across languages: Orthography and the brain-gene-behavior link* (pp. 146–168). Baltimore, MD: Brookes.

Serniclaes, W., van Heghe, S., Mousty, P., Carre, R., & Sprenger-Charroles, L. (2004). Allophonic mode of speech perception in dyslexia. *Journal of Experimental Child Psychology*, *87*, 336–361.

Shu, H., McBride-Chang, C., Wu, S., & Liu, H. (2006). Understanding Chinese developmental dyslexia: Morphological awareness as a core cognitive construct. *Journal of Educational Psychology*, *98*, 122–133.

Siok, W. T., & Fletcher, P. (2001). The role of phonological awareness and visual-orthographic skills in Chinese reading acquisition. *Developmental Psychology*, *37*, 886–899.

Tallal, P. (2004). Improving language and literacy is a matter of time. *Nature Reviews Neuroscience*, *5*, 721–728.

Tan, L. H., Laird, A. R., Li, K., & Fox, P. T. (2005). Neuroanatomical correlates of phonological processing of Chinese characters and alphabetic words: A meta-analysis. *Human Brain Mapping*, *25*(1), 83–91.

Verhoeven, L., & Perfetti, C. (2017). *Learning to read across languages and writing systems*. Cambridge, UK: Cambridge University Press.

Yang, J. F., McCandliss, B. D., Shu, H., & Zevin, J. D. (2009). Simulating language-specific and language-general effects in a statistical learning model of Chinese reading. *Journal of Memory & Language*, *61*, 238–257.

Yang, J. F., McCandliss, B. D., Shu, H., & Zevin, J. D. (2013). Orthographic influences on division of labor in learning to read Chinese and English: Insights from computational modeling. *Bilingualism Language and Cognition*, *16*, 354–366.

Index